# DESIGNING FOODS

*Animal Product Options in the Marketplace*

Committee on Technological Options
to Improve the Nutritional Attributes
of Animal Products

Board on Agriculture

National Research Council

NATIONAL ACADEMY PRESS
Washington, D.C.   1988

**NATIONAL ACADEMY PRESS**     **2101 Constitution Avenue, NW**     **Washington, DC 20418**

NOTICE: The project that is the subject of this report was approved by the Governing Board of the National Research Council, whose members are drawn from the councils of the National Academy of Sciences, the National Academy of Engineering, and the Institute of Medicine. The members of the committee responsible for the report were chosen for their special competences and with regard for appropriate balance.

This report has been reviewed by a group other than the authors according to procedures approved by a Report Review Committee consisting of members of the National Academy of Sciences, the National Academy of Engineering, and the Institute of Medicine.

The National Academy of Sciences is a private, nonprofit, self-perpetuating society of distinguished scholars engaged in scientific and engineering research, dedicated to the furtherance of science and technology and to their use of the general welfare. Upon the authority of the charter granted to it by the Congress in 1863, the Academy has a mandate that requires it to advise the federal government of scientific and technical matters. Dr. Frank Press is president of the National Academy of Sciences.

The National Academy of Engineering was established in 1964, under the charter of National Academy of Sciences, as a parallel organization of outstanding engineers. It is autonomous in its administration and in the selection of its members, sharing with the National Academy of Sciences the responsibility for advising the federal government. The National Academy of Engineering also sponsors engineering programs aimed at meeting national needs, encourages education and research, and recognizes the superior achievements of engineers. Dr. Robert M. White is president of the National Academy of Engineering.

The Institute of Medicine was established in 1970 by the National Academy of Sciences to secure the services of eminent members of appropriate professions in the examination of policy matters pertaining to the health of the public. The Institute acts under the responsibility given to the National Academy of Sciences by its congressional charter to be an adviser to the federal government and, upon its own initiative, to identify issues of medical care, research, and education. Dr. Samuel O. Thier is president of the Institute of Medicine.

The National Research Council was organized by the National Academy of Sciences in 1916 to associate the broad community of science and technology with the Academy's purposes of furthering knowledge and advising the federal government. Functioning in accordance with general policies determined by the Academy, the Council has become the principal operating agency of both the National Academy of Sciences and the National Academy of Engineering in providing services to the government, the public, and the scientific and engineering communities. The Council is administered jointly by both Academies and the Institute of Medicine. Dr. Frank Press and Dr. Robert M. White are chairman and vice chairman, respectively, of the National Research Council.

This project was supported by the U.S. Department of Agriculture and the U.S. Department of Health and Human Services, under agreement 59-3159-5-25.

Preparation of the publication was supported by funds from the W. K. Kellogg Foundation; the American Meat Institute; the American Sheep Producers Council, Inc.; EXCEL Corporation; IBP, Inc.; Monfort of Colorado, Inc.; the National Cattlemen's Association; the National Live Stock & Meat Board; the National Pork Producers Council; Swift Independent, Corp.; and Val-Agri, Inc.

**Library of Congress Cataloging-in-Publication Data**

National Research Council (U.S.). Committee on Technological Options
  to Improve the Nutritional Attributes of Animal Products.
   Designing foods: animal product options in the marketplace /
  Committee on Technological Options to Improve the Nutritional
  Attributes of Animal Products, Board on Agriculture, National
  Research Council.
     p.      cm.
  Includes index.
  ISBN 0-309-03798-0.     ISBN 0-309-03795-6 (pbk.)
  1. Animal products—United States.   2. Nutrition.    I. Title
TS1955.N38 1988
641.3'06—dc19
                                   88-2065
                                    CIP

# Committee on Technological Options to Improve the Nutritional Attributes of Animal Products

DAVID L. CALL, *Chairman*, Cornell University
C. EUGENE ALLEN, University of Minnesota
HENRY A. FITZHUGH, Winrock International
RICHARD H. FORSYTHE, Campbell Institute for Research and Technology
RICHARD D. GOODRICH, University of Minnesota
SCOTT M. GRUNDY, University of Texas Health Science Center
TIMOTHY HAMMONDS, Food Marketing Institute
R. GAURTH HANSEN, Utah State University
NORGE W. JEROME, University of Kansas Medical Center
JOHN KINSELLA, Cornell University
KRISTEN W. MCNUTT, Consumer Choices Unlimited, Inc.
GARY C. SMITH, Texas A&M University
VAUGHN C. SPEER, Iowa State University
JOHN H. VENABLE, Colorado State University
WILLARD J. VISEK, University of Illinois
THOMAS E. WAGNER, Ohio University

**Staff**

BARBARA LUKE, *Project Director*
PATRICIA LOCACCIATO, *Staff Assistant**
ALICE JONES, *Senior Secretary*

---

* Through December 1986

# Board on Agriculture

# Preface

Animal products have always been a mainstay of the American diet, and thanks to new production technologies, a wider range of products are available today than ever before. About 36 percent of the food energy and between 36 and 100 percent of each of the major nutrients in the food supply come from animal products. But they also contribute more than half the total fat, nearly three-fourths of the saturated fatty acids, and all the cholesterol—dietary components that may increase the risk of heart disease and cancer for some individuals.

The link between diet, the maintenance of health, and the development of chronic disease has become increasingly evident in recent years. The advice from national health organizations has become more focused, identifying dietary excesses of calories, fat, saturated fatty acids, and cholesterol and deficiencies of iron and calcium as adversely affecting the health of the people in the United States. Although federal surveys show that healthful trends in diet are improving, many individuals still must make substantial changes to meet current recommendations.

New technologies and production methods appear to hold promise for improving the nutritional attributes of animal products. Recent research has shown that the use of growth hormone in beef and pork may result in increased feed efficiency in the live animal and an improved lean to fat ratio in the carcass. Producers may soon be using the latest biotechnology methods to enhance growth and improve carcass quality, and processors are already applying new techniques such as restructuring, ultrafiltration, enzymatic modification, and supercritical fluid or solvent extraction to the manufacture of new animal products.

In January 1985, the U.S. Department of Agriculture asked the National Research Council's Board on Agriculture to evaluate the effectiveness of new technologies, their possible current and future applications, their effect on regulatory policies, and their potential benefits to the consumer. Specifically, the board's charge was to —

* Identify the targets for preferred nutritional characteristics of animal products, based on dietary recommendations of national health organizations;

• Quantify current consumption patterns of animal products using federal dietary surveys and food supply data;

• Assess current options available to consumers and existing technologies to alter the characteristics of animal products;

• Develop a strategy for constructive change consistent with contemporary dietary recommendations; and

• Develop a strategy to foster widespread adoption of economical and practical innovations, taking into account existing and possible future economic incentives and disincentives for adherence.

To accomplish these objectives, the board convened the Committee on Technological Options to Improve the Nutritional Attributes of Animal Products. The committee held nine meetings between December 1985 and February 1987 to gather information and hear testimony from experts. One meeting was held as a public session to solicit input from organizations, special interest and consumer groups, and individuals. In addition, scientific papers presented at two workshops provided the committee with new information and research results on improved production practices and technologies to alter growth.

This report contains the committee's analyses of food supply and dietary data on consumption patterns; identification of targets for change in the nutritional composition of animal products; and recommendations on marketing and policy issues and research imperatives. The reader should note that throughout the report, the committee defines the term *animal products* as all foods derived from animals.

Chapters 1, 2, and 3 define the role of animal products in the diet, review dietary recommendations from the major health organizations, and identify specific levels, or targets, of nutrients for a healthful diet. Chapter 4 presents data from national surveys on changing consumer attitudes toward nutrition and food practices. It also describes traditional and nutritionally modified versions of dairy products, meats, poultry, and fish and applies these options in example diets to meet the target levels of nutrients defined in Chapter 1. Chapter 5 identifies policies and programs that either impede further progress or that should be refocused to maximize the benefits of dietary choice. Chapter 6 defines promising technologies in production and manufacturing for creating animal products that would better match the targeted levels of nutrients.

The committee's recommendations will require the efforts and cooperation of many groups, whether the issues relate to providing consumers with better nutrition information, consolidating data bases, or developing advertising and promotional guidelines. Current cooperative efforts are to be commended; however, the committee believes that federal agencies, private industry, and academia can work together more effectively by seizing new opportunities to jointly address many of the issues discussed in this report.

The American marketplace is a dynamic forum in which producers have historically responded to consumer demand by providing an ever-growing array of products. It is clear that consumers are willing to try new kinds of foods, including highly processed or newly fabricated products that differ from traditional versions. As scientific evidence mounts implicating specific dietary components in the development of major diseases, the food industry must respond by providing new products that match current scientific knowledge. The committee hopes this report will aid both private and federal sources in meeting this challenge.

DAVID L. CALL
Chairman

# Acknowledgments

A report of this magnitude represents the combined efforts of many individuals and organizations. The committee thanks all those individuals who gave of their time and talents to contribute to this report, especially those who wrote papers included in the Appendix, testified, gave presentations, or wrote supporting documents for the study.

The committee acknowledges Karen Bunch and her associates at the Economic Research Service, U.S. Department of Agriculture, for contributing to the analysis of food supply data and trends; Catherine Wotecki and her staff at the National Center for Health Statistics, U.S. Department of Health and Human Services, for providing nutritional status and health data; and Katsuto Ono, Anthony Kotula, and Brad Berry of the Meat Science Research Laboratory, Agricultural Research Service, U.S. Department of Agriculture, for verifying meat composition data.

Many individuals in private industry and academia contributed to the development of this report. Scientists in the animal science department at Texas A&M University deserve special thanks for their contributions, and the Food Marketing Institute and the National Live Stock & Meat Board are acknowledged for providing valuable data for the committee's analysis. The committee also thanks the Center for Science in the Public Interest for providing Michael Jacobson's Nutrition Wizard™ computer software program.

The committee especially thanks Betty B. Peterkin, former associate administrator of the Human Nutrition Information Service (HNIS), U.S. Department of Agriculture, and her staff members for their exceptional assistance in gathering and verifying data from the dietary and food supply surveys, and for providing additional analysis of Continuing Survey of Food Intake by Individuals data, cited as HNIS unpublished data, 1987, in the tables.

# Contents

## ASSESSING BODY COMPOSITION

## PRODUCTION AND PROCESSING OPTIONS TO ALTER COMPOSITION

## POLICY

# Tables and Figures

## FIGURES

# DESIGNING FOODS

# Executive Summary

This century has witnessed tremendous advances in all fields of human endeavor, particularly the sciences. Our daily lives have been enriched, our standard of living improved, and the average life span prolonged. This report examines the changing interface between agriculture and human health—two fields that have been progressing geometrically during this century—and the role of animal products in the diet. Animal products contribute more than a third of the calories and between a third and all of the other major nutrients in the food supply. They also contribute more than half of the total fat, three-fourths of the saturated fatty acids, and all the cholesterol, food components that may adversely affect an individual's health.

The food industry in the United States began during the late nineteenth and early twentieth centuries, when the population began to shift from rural communities to urban centers. Early food companies applied the scientific knowledge of the day to produce products that would meet the needs of the consumer's changing life-style. During those early years, the major innovations in the industry included canning, refriger-ation, and freezing—techniques that are taken for granted today.

The major public health problems at the turn of the century were very different from those seen today. Nutritional deficiencies and infectious diseases were responsible for most of the disability and death. With the implementation of public health measures and the development and widespread use of antibiotics and vaccines, most of the infectious diseases prevalent decades ago have been all but eradicated today. Improvements in economic status along with the enrichment and fortification of a variety of foods and improvements in product quality and distribution have reduced the occurrence of nutritional deficiencies in the United States to a fraction of what was commonplace 90 years ago.

The nutrition-related health problems experienced by a large segment of the U.S. population today arise from the overconsumption of fat, saturated fatty acids, and cholesterol. For another group the main dietary problems center around underconsumption of iron, calcium, and calories. The incidence of nutrition-related health problems is significant, affecting either directly or indirectly nearly every American family. For example, it has been estimated that 34 million adults in the United States are overweight; nearly 1 million adults die each year of cardiovascular disease;* 15 million to 20 million adults are afflicted by osteoporosis; 8 million adults and 12 million children go hungry due to inadequate diets (Physician Task Force on Hunger in America, 1987); and iron deficiency has been cited as the most common form of childhood anemia.

The following specific target levels for caloric intake and nutrients in the diet were chosen by the Committee on Technological Options to Improve the Nutritional Attributes of Animal Products on the basis of the dietary recommendations of major national health organizations and the health findings of federal surveys. These targets are used as the foundation of this report and the committee's analysis and recommendations.

• Caloric intake matched to individual needs and appropriate to achieve and maintain desirable body weight (American Cancer Society, 1984; American Heart Association, 1986; National Institutes of Health, 1984; National Research Council, 1980, 1982; Office of the Assistant Secretary for Health and the Surgeon General, 1979; U.S. Department of Agriculture/U.S. Department of Health and Human Services, 1985; U.S. Senate Select Committee on Nutrition and Human Needs, 1977);
• 30 percent or less of calories from fat for adults (American Cancer Society, 1984; American Heart Association, 1986; National Institutes of Health, 1984; National Research Council, 1982);
• 10 percent or less of calories from

saturated fatty acids; 10 percent or less of calories from polyunsaturated fatty acids; and 15 percent or less of calories from monounsaturated fatty acids for adults (American Heart Association, 1986);
• 300 mg or less of cholesterol per day for adults (American Heart Association, 1986);
• Calcium intake of the Recommended Dietary Allowances (RDA) for age and sex (National Research Council, 1980); and
• Iron intake of the RDA for age and sex (National Research Council, 1980).

These targets are chosen by the committee as constituting the consensus of dietary and nutrition recommendations made by the government and nongovernment agencies cited. It is not the intention of the committee to establish new dietary guidelines. The Food and Nutrition Board of the National Research Council is currently undertaking a major study of diet and health issues, and a new National Research Council report may eventually be published that makes specific recommendations.

In evaluating how well the current U.S. food supply and marketplace options match these target levels, the committee relied upon several sources of data. Food supply data (also known as per capita disappearance data) from 1965 to 1985 provided information on trends for individual commodities. Federal dietary survey data from 1977 to 1978 and 1985 were used to study dietary habits for selected segments of the population. (The Nationwide Food Consumption Survey is conducted every 10 years. The data from the 1977 to 1978 are used in this report, as well as data from the linking survey in 1985.) Data on supermarket food sales for 1984 and 1985 provided insight on the latest trends in the marketplace. In addition, the nutritional compositions of individual animal products, both traditional and modified versions, were evaluated.

Food supply trends varied markedly from product to product during the 20–year period from 1965 to 1985. There was a rise in

---

* In 1985, 948,145 people in the United States died of cardiovascular disease, including 771,169 from diseases of the heart, 153,050 from cerebrovascular diseases, and 23,926 from atherosclerosis; 461,563 individuals died from cancer (National Center for Health Statistics, 1987).

the consumption of some reduced or naturally low-fat animal products, such as low-fat milk and fish, but there was increased use of high-fat foods, such as hard processed cheese and baking and frying fats of both vegetable and animal origin. One of the fastest growing food items, according to dietary survey data and supermarket sales, was meat mixtures—entrees containing one or more types of meat, poultry, or fish as a major ingredient. The intake of processed foods in general also increased; consumers were eating more frequent, smaller meals but buying foods that required less preparation time.

These trends indicate a shift in the consumption of fats, with a decrease in the intake of visible, separable fats and an increase in the intake of fats in processed foods such as mixtures, baked goods, carryout food items, and partially prepared foods that require little additional preparation at home.

The committee concluded that, overall, Americans consume too much fat. Fat in foods, whether present in the food's original state, as with well-marbled beef, or added during preparation, such as with deep frying in fat, adds calories, saturated fatty acids, and cholesterol. Conversely, the removal of fat from a food lowers its caloric, cholesterol, and fatty acid contents, and favorably alters its nutritional composition by increasing its other nutrients in relation to its caloric value.

There is a movement among food producers, processors, and manufacturers in the United States toward lowering the fat content of animal products. But at present, this mostly consists of the physical removal of fat at one point in the food production process (for example, closely trimmed retail cuts of beef) with the reintroduction of the trimmed fat at another point (for example, french fries fried in beef tallow). The committee believes that economic, marketing, and research policies should be redefined to encourage the production of leaner animals and the processing and manufacturing of lower fat animal products by economically discouraging the production of fat in live animals and their carcasses and the use of fat in food products. From a research standpoint, this involves the further development and practical application of growth promoters and repartitioning agents in live animals to shift the utilization of nutrients from fat deposition to protein accretion while enhancing growth rate. In production, changes in such policies as standards of identity are necessary to facilitate the manufacture and marketing of lower fat animal products. Standards of identity are an established range of mandatory ingredients for certain foods such as catsup, mayonnaise, frankfurters, and bologna that do not have to appear on the product label.

The U.S. food industry has responded to the consumer's demands for variety, convenience, and taste by providing an ever-expanding array of options in the marketplace. Supermarket sales indicate that consumers are willing to try new products, including new versions of traditional foods, even when priced at a premium. However, consumers may not be aware of the quality of nutrition they are trading for convenience and at what price. Survey data indicate that consumers are confused about grades of beef, product labeling, and the content of food products and are demanding more detailed and clearer information about the products they buy and the foods they eat. The trends signify that the marketplace is responding, despite current limitations.

The present grading system for retail meats is not only costly and inefficient but it encourages the overfattening of beef and lamb (but not pork). Consumer demand for leaner animal products must reach the producer so that excessive amounts of fat are not added to any point in the food chain. Trimming of fat at slaughter or at purchase is only a partial, short-term response. The real solution lies in the production of leaner animals.

## CHANGES IN POLICY

The committee makes 18 policy recommendations covering the areas of production, grading, labeling, standards of identity, point-of-purchase information, sources of data, advertising and promotion, the government's role in nutrition education, and integrated research and education programs. A principal finding is that public policy influences consumer choice. New policies are now needed to sustain the positive trends evident among consumers and throughout the animal product industries, trends like nutrition education programs in supermarkets, closer retail trim of meats, and the growing array of lower fat animal product options. The committee's goals are to provide consumers the opportunity to exercise personal choice in the marketplace, to encourage the development of a range of products consistent with those choices, and to ensure sufficient consumer education and information to make those choices informed decisions.

The starting point is for producers and their industry associations to recognize the need to understand marketplace trends and the role of foods in a healthy diet and to implement appropriate animal feeding, breeding, and selection programs. They should also support public policy reforms that will facilitate progress toward the shared goals of offering consumers a consistently high-quality product at the lowest possible price.

### The Grading System

The committee makes several recommendations regarding the current grading system. First, it supports the recent change in the name of the Good grade to Select, to provide the beef industry with an opportunity for improved marketing of beef with less marbling than is found in Prime or Choice. The objectives in adopting grading system changes should be to provide con-

sumers with clearer, more accurate information about the meat products they purchase and to send to producers and packers distinct economic signals on the types of products consumers prefer. The current system fails on both counts.

Second, the committee recommends that the U.S. Department of Agriculture (USDA) carefully study the potential benefits of changes in regulations to allow hot-fat trimming at slaughter— removal of the subcutaneous fat from the carcass immediately after slaughter (thus, the term *hot fat* referring to the temperature of the carcass). Such a change from current regulations would mean that price would be determined from the pounds of carcass remaining after trimming, in effect penalizing the producer for additional fat.

A change in official USDA grade standards would be needed to uncouple the simultaneous determination of yield and quality grades of a single carcass. Yield grades are based on estimates of relative cutability, that is, the yield of trimmed cuts from the carcass. Yield grade 1 signifies the highest comparative cutability (yield of trimmed wholesale or retail cuts as a percentage of carcass weight), whereas yield grade 4 for pork carcasses and 5 for beef and lamb carcasses denotes the lowest relative cutability. Quality grades such as Prime, Choice, and Good/Select are based on estimates of relative palatability (flavor, juiciness, and tenderness) of the meat when cooked. The uncoupling of yield and quality grades would allow packers wishing to hot-fat trim on the slaughter or dressing floor to still have carcasses quality graded while giving other packers the freedom to continue the current practice of assigning both quality and yield grades.

Before uncoupling is effected, the committee recommends that the USDA investigate methods such as ultrasound for reliably determining carcass yield grade so that yield grades of 4 and 5 (carcasses with a higher amount of fat between cuts of meat) can be detected and treated differently (for example, muscle-boned to remove seam fat) from yield grade 3, 2, and 1 carcasses, which have less fat. The lean to fat ratio in the meat as it would be prepared for retail display is important to both retailer and consumer. A rapid and economical method for determining yield grade or the proportion of lean to fat tissue in carcasses would make removal of fat at slaughter feasible without the yield grade uncertainty and the risk of excessive seam fat in wholesale or retail cuts.

## Labeling and Standards of Identity

Three of the committee's policy recommendations involve labeling and standards of identity. First, the committee agrees with the Food and Drug Administration (FDA) that regulations should not restrict truthful information at the point of purchase or on food product packaging.

Second, the committee recommends that use of the term *Natural* for meat products be standardized in a manner similar to the current FDA effort to standardize use of terms in cholesterol labeling. In standardizing the term, care must be taken that use of the term Natural not connote that meat from animals otherwise designated is somehow unnatural and thus unhealthy.

Finally, the committee recommends that the USDA restrict use of the terms *Light*, *Lite*, or *Lean* to products in the form that would be presented to the retail consumer. Certification of the relative leanness of carcasses should not simply be carried over to retail cuts as is now often done. Rather, use of descriptive terminology on retail cuts should require some objective standard for the cut itself.

## Information and Consumer Education

The creation of a wide range of marketplace options allows consumers maximum flexibility in matching products to their own dietary and life-style needs. However, for the system to work effectively, shoppers must have the information needed for informed choice. The information available on labels is an important first step, but additional information available at the point of purchase should also be promoted. The committee recommends that the FDA encourage the development of point-of-purchase information programs (additional nutrition education information beyond that mandated by law) in light of the continued growth in popularity of these programs and the demonstrated willingness of retailers and processors to supply information beyond that given on the label. This could be done by issuing specific guidelines for providing factual nutrition data without judgment or comment. The committee also recommends that restaurants be encouraged to provide point-of-purchase information to their customers. Point-of-purchase information programs should be subjected to the same standards and scrutiny as advertising programs monitored by the Federal Trade Commission.

The committee recommends that all government food data banks be periodically reviewed by an oversight group and consolidated when appropriate. This process of review and management of data bases should not be done in a vacuum. Rather, food retailers and processors should be encouraged to share their expertise and information and to ensure that the information compiled will meet the needs of a wide range of users. Currently, there are no standards for serving sizes; consistency would facilitate comparisons among products, labels, point-of-purchase information, and federal and private data bases. The committee further recommends the establishment of standards governing serving sizes. This is important in terms of nutrition education and research and for a wide range of data base users.

Probably no policy issue has received more attention from regulators, consumer advocacy groups, and food manufacturers than claims of health promotion and disease prevention. Aside from the fact that such claims may initiate mandatory nutrition labeling, the most recurrent problem is the inability of manufacturers to document them. The committee recommends that the private sector seriously consider developing advertising and promotional guidelines that would restrict or eliminate the use of misleading claims or claims that specific foods are cures for, or preventers of, diseases.

Government has a dual role in nutrition education: communication of clear and accurate nutrition information to consumers and communication of up-to-date scientific information and marketplace trends to producers. Unfortunately, misinformation often passes for scientific fact, particularly in the mass media. Because of the many conflicting claims and counterclaims made in the field of nutrition, government agencies play a vital role in separating fact from fallacy for both consumers and producers. Organizations such as the Food and Nutrition Board of the National Research Council and the American Heart Association translate research into practical information for use by nutrition educators. The Food and Nutrition Board's RDAs, which are widely used around the world, are an example of this process. USDA's Extension Service provides a nationwide nutrition education system that connects nutrition and agricultural concerns. Through its vast network to nutrition professionals, educators, scientists, and consumer groups, it can effectively communicate nutrition information to targeted audiences. The committee recommends that federal agencies strive to reach consensus positions that would enable them to speak with one voice on nutrition and health issues. The committee further recommends a coordinated effort by the government to dispel false notions among consumers and encourages federal agencies and private industry to work together to deliver consumer information.

One piece of information that is essential to making dietary recommendations is the level of fat consumed by the typical American. In the past, government data sources may have inaccurately estimated the amount of fat consumed, particularly fat of animal origin. Attempts are currently under way within the USDA to improve dietary survey methodologies to more accurately reflect actual intake. The committee commends this and recommends that the food disappearance data also be modified to better reflect actual use. In addition, the federal government should take steps to more accurately distinguish and monitor the fatty acid composition of fats consumed in the diet. The committee also recommends that the USDA obtain data on the fat content of partially trimmed meats and, if possible, on the percentage of consumers who trim their meats completely, partially, or not at all.

## Research and Development

The committee recommends that all research pertaining to animal agriculture take a systems approach whenever possible. This extends to the expenditure of funds raised by producer groups through check-off programs. Check-off programs include a per-head fee assessed when animals are slaughtered. The organizations charged with collecting check-off funds use the money for special programs such as research or education. Producer groups that have already supported research projects along with their promotion programs are to be commended. Such activity should be encouraged. The committee recommends that producer check-off programs include regular funding for total systems research as it pertains to the producer's products.

Government policies that may inhibit the implementation of new technologies should also be evaluated. It is imperative that the United States maintain both the high quality and stringent safety standards associated with its foods and food products. However, inhibition of research and development initiatives in both public and private sectors is occurring because of overly strict regulations and an unwillingness to accept research data from other countries. Currently, food technology research conducted in another country is not accepted in the United States without being duplicated, which significantly increases the cost of producing new foods and food ingredients. The committee encourages a responsive regulatory policy that does not inhibit creativity or innovation.

### RESEARCH RECOMMENDATIONS

The committee makes 18 research recommendations (see Chapter 6) covering such areas as preharvest technology transfer, preharvest research related to the reduction or alteration of animal fat, and postharvest technology. The committee concluded that current pre- and postharvest technologies provide ample opportunity for reducing the fat content of animal products. Even though some options are now being applied, others have not yet been adopted because of high costs, lack of demand, product labeling standards, or, in some cases, the stability of the product's quality (such as shelf life) in the marketplace. Clearly, these problems must be addressed through basic and applied research.

The more that is known about the basic biology of factors controlling the partitioning of nutrients into protein or fat in animals, the higher the probability of changing these processes through genetic or metabolic control. Just as animal biology is advancing, so is our understanding of food science and postharvest research needs. These research advances are the basis for improved and new foods composed of or containing animal products.

### Preharvest Technology

Several of the committee's recommendations center on technologies that could be applied before slaughter to alter the composition of the animal during growth. These recommendations include identifying the cellular and molecular mechanisms that control partitioning of feed nutrients into fat or lean tissues and altering the fatty acid composition and the lean to fat ratio of meat, milk, and eggs through breeding, nutrition, and management. In addition, the committee recommends implementing available technologies for determining the fat and protein contents of live animals and carcasses.

Research is also recommended to determine the extent of genetic variation in the cholesterol content of animals, the reduction of oxidative rancidity of animal products through feeding or management, and the development of more cost-effective methods of efficiently producing low-fat animal products by integrated production management systems.

### Postharvest Technology

Postharvest technologies to reduce fat in animal products can be used satisfactorily in many situations. However, these technologies are not without costs and are usually associated with some change in product characteristics such as texture, flavor, and shelf life. In addition (and depending on the product and the changes) a variety of regulatory and labeling issues must be addressed.

One of the main research recommendations echoes a previously discussed policy change: the adoption of standards of identity that would reflect today's technology and consumer needs. Less prescriptive standards could permit beneficial applications of new technologies to reduce the fat content of animal products in new ways. The committee also recommends the use of technologies to remove fat at the earliest possible stage in processing and to improve methods to evaluate and monitor the resulting fat content of the product after processing. The use of non-fat or low-fat ingredients are recommended to simulate the textural and quality characteristics and properties of fat and to alter the fatty acid composition of processed animal products.

Several of the committee's recommendations center around altering the cholesterol content of animal products during processing. These include the use of molecular genetics and other biotechnologies to generate new microorganisms to reduce the cholesterol content of products through fermentation and the use of selective extraction to reduce both the cholesterol and fat contents of processed animal products.

Sodium chloride plays a critical role in delaying microbial growth, providing flavor, and contributing to the functional characteristics of many processed products, but it is also cited as being excessive in the American diet. The committee recommends that methods be developed to safely and organoleptically (taste and texture appeal) reduce or replace sodium in manufactured animal products.

Animal products have always been part of the fundamental fabric of the American diet, offering a rich array of choices, tastes, and nutrients, and providing the very basis of the traditional diet in this country. This report presents a wide variety of information and data through which to view the current American diet and suggests directions for its course in the future. Some of the changes are relatively simple to implement; others involve a coordinated effort between industry and government. In all cases, the need to improve the composition of the foods in our diets is evident, and the necessary technology is within our grasp.

## REFERENCES

American Cancer Society. 1984. Nutrition and cancer, cause and prevention. An American Cancer Society special report. Ca—A Cancer Journal for Clinicians 34(2):121–126.

American Heart Association. 1986. Dietary guidelines for healthy adult Americans. Circulation 74:1465A.

National Center for Health Statistics. 1987. Advance Report of Final Mortality Statistics, 1985, 36(5), August 28. Hyattsville, Md.: Public Health Service.

National Institutes of Health. 1984. NIH Consensus Development Statement on Lowering Blood Cholesterol to Prevent Heart Disease, Vol. 5, No. 7. Washington, D.C.: National Institutes of Health.

National Research Council. 1980. Recommended Dietary Allowances, 9th ed. Washington, D.C.: National Academy Press.

National Research Council. 1982. Diet, Nutrition, and Cancer. Washington, D.C.: National Academy Press.

Office of the Assistant Secretary for Health and the Surgeon General. 1979. Healthy People, the Surgeon General's Report on Health Promotion and Disease Prevention. DHEW (PHS) Publication No. 79–55071. Washington, D.C.: U.S. Public Health Service.

Physician Task Force on Hunger in America. 1987. Hunger Reaches Blue Collar America: An Unbalanced Recovery in a Service Economy. Boston: Harvard School of Public Health.

U.S. Department of Agriculture/Health and Human Services. 1985. Nutrition and Your Health: Dietary Guidelines for Americans, 2nd ed. Home and Garden Bulletin No. 232. Washington, D.C.: U.S. Government Printing Office.

U.S. Senate Select Committee on Nutrition and Human Needs. 1977. Dietary Goals for the United States, 2nd ed. No. 052-070-04376-8. Washington, D.C.: U.S. Government Printing Office.

# 1

# Data Sources, Key Nutrients, and Selection of Targets for Change

The current issues surrounding the adequacy of the American diet no longer center primarily on nutrient deficiency. Overconsumption of calories, fat, saturated fatty acids, cholesterol, and sodium has become a serious problem for many consumers, and animal products have been implicated as major sources of these food components. At the same time, it is recognized that meats, fish, dairy products, and eggs are important sources of many essential nutrients, including protein, B vitamins, iron, zinc, and calcium.

In this report, the committee recommends various options for improving the nutritional value of animal products. First, however, it is important to understand clearly the contemporary role of animal products in the American diet. The following questions were essential to the committee's charge:

- What are the uses and limitations of the data available to study consumption and nutrient contribution of animal products?
- What have been the trends in consumption of animal products in the United States?
- What contribution do animal products

make to the nutrients available in the food supply?
- What is the role of animal products in the diets of different age and sex groups of the population?

## SOURCES OF DATA AND THEIR LIMITATIONS

The U.S. Department of Agriculture (USDA) provides data on food and nutrient consumption at three levels: the U.S. food supply, food use by households, and food intake by individuals. In addition, data on nutritional status from federal surveys are used throughout the report.

### Food Supply Data (1965–1985)

The food supply data (per capita disappearance) measure the amount of food available for consumption in the United States, based on annual estimates of production of food products adjusted for imports, exports, and stock exchanges. The data are collected at the wholesale or retail level of distribution. The result is an estimate of the total amount of food that is produced and mar-

9

keted for national consumption. Dividing this total by the U.S. population results in an estimate of consumption per capita. This series is often referred to as disappearance data to indicate that it is based on the disappearance of food through marketing channels and is not a direct estimate of consumption. In 1986, the USDA began referring to this series as "apparent consumption" to distinguish it from more direct estimates of consumption. A companion series, the Nutrient Content of the Food Supply, is derived by calculating the nutritive value of the total amount of foods available for national consumption (Marston and Raper, 1987). In using these data bases, the committee found the term *apparent consumption* confusing and elected to use per capita disappearance or food supply data instead throughout the report.

### Federal Surveys

#### Nationwide Food Consumption Survey (1977–1978)

More direct estimates of food consumption are provided by the USDA's Nationwide Food Consumption Survey (NFCS), last conducted in 1977–1978. The NFCS, which is conducted every 10 years, is the most comprehensive source of data available on the food and nutrient intake of the U.S. population. In total, 36,142 individuals were surveyed over four consecutive seasons beginning in the spring of 1977. A detailed description of the survey methodology is provided in Peterkin (1981) and will not be presented in this report. Even though the NFCS is now 10 years old, it is still useful for several reasons. For one, it is the most recent information available on food and nutrient intake for the household population and is useful for comparing dietary intakes among age and sex groups, especially when analyzing the data at an aggregated level such as food groups.

Furthermore, the survey measured dietary intake by individuals. In this phase of the survey, members of the participating households provided information on foods they ate on 3 consecutive days. Each was asked by an interviewer to recall the foods eaten the day before the interview and to keep records of foods eaten on the interview day and the day following. Nutrient intakes of the individuals were derived from food composition data for approximately 4,500 foods and food combinations in the USDA's Nutrient Data Bank, a file of food composition maintained and updated by USDA's Human Nutrition Information Service.

#### Continuing Survey of Food Intake by Individuals (1985)

The most recent source of data available on the dietary intake of individuals is the USDA's Continuing Survey of Food Intake by Individuals (CSFII). This survey was designed to complement the decennial NFCS by providing continuous data on dietary status of selected subgroups, especially those that may be at nutritional risk (Welsh, 1986). It is the first nationwide dietary intake survey designed to be conducted annually. Dietary recall data for 1 day by 1,503 women 19 to 50 years of age and by 548 children 1 to 5 years of age were collected by personal interview from April through June 1985, and for 5 days at 2-month intervals by telephone interview (U.S. Department of Agriculture, 1985). This core respondent group was selected because previous surveys had shown that women of childbearing age and young children were more likely than other age and sex groups to have diets low in certain nutrients. The 1985 survey was augmented by a 1-day intake record for 1,134 men (U.S. Department of Agriculture, 1986). Whenever possible, the committee compared data from the 1977–1978 NFCS and the 1985 CSFII.

#### National Health and Nutrition Examination Survey

Another nationwide survey that includes data on dietary intake is the National Health and Nutrition Examination Survey (NHANES), performed by the U.S. Department of Health and Human Services (DHHS). NHANES I took place between 1971 and 1974 and had a sample size of 28,043 individuals from its target population of 1– to 74–year-olds. NHANES II was conducted from 1976 to 1980 on a target population of individuals ages 6 months to 74 years. The sample size was 27,801, with oversampling of children ages 6 months to 5 years, adults ages 60 to 74 years, and those individuals living in poverty areas. NHANES is primarily a health survey designed to gather information on the total prevalence of disease conditions and physical status as well as clinical data on the interrelationships of health and nutrition variables. Individuals who participated in the survey were interviewed for diet and health information and underwent clinical examinations by health professionals.

The dietary component of NHANES consisted of a recall of dietary intake for the previous day and an additional recall of usual food consumption for the previous month. NHANES is the only nationwide survey available to measure the relationship between food and nutrient intake and biochemical nutritional status (McDowell et al., 1981). It is used as an important source of information on the health and nutritional status of the U.S. population.

### Pediatric Nutrition Surveillance System of the Centers for Disease Control

Since 1973, the Centers for Disease Control have coordinated the Pediatric Nutrition Surveillance System (PNSS) to continuously monitor the nutritional status of high-risk pediatric populations (Centers for Disease Control, 1985). The PNSS uses nutrition-related data collected by local health departments during delivery of routine child health services. The data include demographic information, height, weight, birth weight, and hemoglobin or hematocrit determinations, or both. The anthropometric

data on height, weight, and age are converted to percentiles of height for age and weight for height using the National Center for Health Statistics reference population. During 1984, data were submitted for 610,439 children ages birth to 9 years (Centers for Disease Control, 1985). Although this source does not contain direct estimates of dietary intake, it does provide valuable data on the nutritional status of children.

### Other Data Sources

The National Live Stock & Meat Board study (Breidenstein and Williams, 1987) and the Stanton (1987) study for the American Meat Institute both concentrate on the role of red meat in the diet, particularly their contribution to the overall fat content of the diet. The Household Refuse Analysis Project, headed by University of Arizona archeologist William Rathje (1984), focuses on trends in consumption of meats and discard patterns of separable fat through the analysis of residential garbage. Each of these sources has its limitations and advantages but is valuable for its unique analytical approach.

### Limitations of the Data Bases

The per capita disappearance data, NFCS, CSFII, and private studies are important sources of information, but none provide exact measures of food or nutrient intakes. In addition, each measures a different aspect of food intake, and each has advantages and limitations for assessing particular issues. It is preferable, therefore, to use as many suitable sources as possible to more closely assess the consumption of animal products and their contribution to the diet.

The per capita disappearance data are primarily designed to measure gross trends in food nutrient availability. They are valuable for determining the contribution of specific animal products to total nutrients in the food supply because they measure distinct commodities. Because the data are measured at the wholesale or retail level of the food system, they measure nutrients inherent in primary commodities before processing, such as fresh meats, milk, and cheese. In addition, the data have not been adjusted for waste that may occur beyond the retail level of distribution, such as plate waste or trimming during meal preparation. Moreover, no estimate of the discard of food due to spoilage and other reasons that would preclude human consumption is made.

In contrast, the NFCS data measure food intake in the form consumed, such as cheeseburgers and beef stew. Such dietary survey data customarily group food mixtures by the nutrient contribution of the mixture's main ingredient. Such groups cannot correctly account for all nutrients derived from animal products like milk and cheese, meat, poultry, and fish. Nutrients from the cheese and meat in pizza, for example, will be credited to the grain products group because grain is the main ingredient. On the other hand, categories referred to as poultry or meat may include nutrients from other categories, such as the fat used in frying chicken or the vegetables used in beef stew. Thus, assessing fat intake and the contribution of various foods to total fat or any nutrient is not a straightforward exercise and requires numerous assumptions and interpretation of the various sources of data.

The food supply data provide information on the total amount of fat available. There is specific information on the exact type of fat and oil available (such as soybean oil and lard, as well as fat occurring in foods), but the data overstate the amount actually ingested because they are not adjusted for waste, spoilage, trimming, or cooking losses. In contrast, NFCS data attempt to include only the fat ingested, but information regarding type of fat or the food from which it is derived is imprecise, mainly because considerable amounts of fat consumed are in processed or mixed foods. However, survey data more accurately reflect food and nutrient intake than do per capita disappearance data because they are based on individual records of foods eaten and therefore do not need to be adjusted for waste.

All sources of food consumption data are imprecise. Food supply data are derived from gross estimates. The accuracy of the survey food intake data is limited by the extent to which individuals can recall and describe the types and amounts of foods they ate. It is likely that the NFCS data generally underestimate food intake because it is so difficult for an individual to recall accurately everything eaten (Weir, 1976). In some cases, when precise descriptions of foods eaten are not known or not specified by the individual surveyed, they are entered by the USDA. This could result in errors in the quantities of nutrients consumed. For example, if the respondent does not know if the fat on his or her baked potato is margarine or butter, the USDA assumes it is margarine—the most often used fat. If roast beef is reported, without information about whether the fat was eaten, USDA assumes that the lean and fat parts are both eaten. In the 1985 CSFII, additional questions were asked to minimize this problem.

Despite these limitations, each data source is valuable because it offers a different perspective on possible avenues for improvement in the diet. The food supply data estimate the nutrients inherent in the animal products before processing, which may suggest changes achievable through genetic manipulation, production, or processing practices. The NFCS and CSFII survey data point to population subgroups that may be in need of modifying their dietary patterns or the amount or proportion of individual nutrients within the diet. The private studies, based largely on the federal dietary surveys, evaluate trends in the dietary intake of animal fat and red meat.

## IDENTIFICATION OF KEY FOOD COMPONENTS

In July 1986, the Joint Nutrition Monitoring Evaluation Committee (JNMEC), a federal advisory committee jointly sponsored by USDA and DHHS, issued a progress report entitled *Nutrition Monitoring in the United States* (U.S. Department of Agriculture/U.S. Department of Health and Human Services, 1986). Because this report represents the most current data on the nutritional status of the U.S. population, the committee chose to rely heavily on its content. The JNMEC concluded that the principal nutrition-related health problems in the United States arise from the overconsumption of fat, saturated fatty acids, cholesterol, and sodium, the same nutrients emphasized by all the national health organizations issuing dietary recommendations. It stated that more than one-fourth of the adults in the United States are overweight; for many of these individuals, obesity probably resulted from consuming more food energy than needed for their level of physical activity. It also concluded that certain subgroups of the U.S. population have special nutrition-related health problems, specifically, low intakes of iron and vitamin C among young children and females of childbearing age, especially if they are black, poor, or both. The JNMEC also expressed concern over the low intake of calcium among women.

The JNMEC emphasized that inadequacies or excesses of food components in the diet and the effects on nutritional status were indeed cause for concern. It singled out the following 10 food components for highest-priority monitoring on the basis of the relationship of the component to nutritional status:

| *High Dietary Consumption* | *Low Dietary Consumption* |
|---|---|
| Food energy* | Vitamin C |
| Total fat* | Calcium* |
| Saturated fatty acids* | Iron* |
| Cholesterol* | Fluoride |
| Sodium* | |
| Alcohol | |

The seven food components marked with an asterisk are of particular importance to the committee because they are found in animal products.

Other national organizations have also recognized these nutrients as exerting the greatest influence on health and have offered a variety of specific recommendations for altering their level in the diet. In 1984 a National Institutes of Health consensus development panel on lowering blood cholesterol to prevent heart disease suggested that the food industry be encouraged to intensify efforts to develop and market products that would facilitate adherence to the dietary guidelines for fat and cholesterol. The panel recommended that school food services and restaurants serve meals consistent with those recommendations (National Institutes of Health, 1984). The panel also recommended that food labeling include the specific source or sources of fat; the amounts of total fat, saturated and polyunsaturated fatty acids, and cholesterol; and other nutrition information. It further recommended that the public be educated on how to best use this information to achieve dietary goals. In the most recent American Heart Association dietary guidelines, food manufacturers were urged to "gradually reduce the sodium and fat content of the food supply as well as to modify the type of fat in food products" (American Heart Association, 1986).

## TARGET LEVELS FOR CALORIC INTAKE AND SELECTED NUTRIENTS

Dietary recommendations issued by the major national health organizations in the United States, as summarized in Table 1–1, acknowledge the importance of eating a varied diet; achieving and maintaining ideal body weight; and limiting intake of total fat, saturated fatty acids, polyunsaturated fatty acids, and cholesterol as positive health measures for optimal nutritional status. The advice given is similar for all these organi-

TABLE 1-1 Summary of National Dietary Guidelines

| Component | Current Level in U.S. Diet | Target Levels for This Report | American Heart Association | American Cancer Society | National Research Council RDAs | NIH Consensus Development Panel | U.S. Senate Select Committee on Nutrition | Surgeon General's Report | USDA/Dept. of Health and Human Services |
|---|---|---|---|---|---|---|---|---|---|
| Calories | | Achieve and maintain desirable weight | Maintain ideal weight | Avoid obesity | Adequate to meet needs | Maintain ideal weight | Avoid being overweight | Maintain desirable weight | Maintain ideal weight |
| Fats (% kcal) | 36–37 | ≤30 | <30 | ≤30 | ≤35 | ≤30 | 27–33 | | Avoid too much |
| Fatty Acids | | | | | | | | | |
| Saturated | 13 | ≤10 | <10 | | Consume less | ≤10 | 8–12 | Consume less | Avoid too much |
| Monounsaturated | 14 | ≤15 | | | | ≥10 | 10 | | |
| Polyunsaturated | 7 | ≤10 | <10 | | 8–10 | 10 | 8–12 | | |
| Cholesterol | 300–450 mg[a] | ≤300 mg/day | <300 mg/day total <100 mg/ 1,000 kcal | | | <250–300 mg/day | 250–350 mg/day | Consume less | Avoid too much |
| Calcium | | 800 mg[b] 1,200 mg[c] | | | 800 mg[b] 1,200 mg[c] | | | | |
| Iron | | 10 mg[d] 15 mg[e] 18 mg[f] | | | 10 mg[d] 15 mg[e] 18 mg[f] | | | | |

[a]The lower value is for women ages 19 to 50; the higher value, for men ages 19 to 50.
[b]This value is for children ages 1 to 10 and adults ages 19 and up.
[c]This value is for males and females ages 11 to 18.
[d]This value is for children ages 4 to 10, males ages 19 to 51+, and females ages 51+.
[e]This value is for children ages six months to three years.
[f]This value is for males and females ages 11 to 18 years and females ages 19 to 50 years.

SOURCES:  U.S. Senate Select Committee on Nutrition and Human Needs. 1977. Dietary Goals for the United States, 2nd ed. No. 052-070-04376-8. Washington, D.C.: U.S. Government Printing Office.

Office of the Assistant Secretary for Health and the Surgeon General. 1979. Healthy People, the Surgeon General's Report on Health Promotion and Disease Prevention. DHEW (PHS) Publication 79-500.71. Washington, D.C.: U.S. Department of Health, Education, and Welfare.

National Research Council. 1980. Recommended Dietary Allowances, 9th ed. Washington, D.C.: National Academy Press.

National Research Council. 1982. Diet, Nutrition, and Cancer. Washington, D.C.: National Academy Press.

American Cancer Society. 1984. Nutrition and cancer, cause and prevention. An American Cancer Society special report. Ca—A Cancer Journal for Clinicians 34(2):121–126.

National Institutes of Health Consensus Development Panel. 1985. Lowering blood cholesterol to prevent heart disease. J. Am. Med. Assoc. 253:2080–2086.

U.S. Departments of Agriculture/Health and Human Services. 1985. Nutrition and Your Health: Dietary Guidelines for Americans, 2nd ed. Home and Garden Bulletin 232. Washington, D.C.: U.S. Government Printing Office.

American Heart Association. 1986. Dietary guidelines for healthy adult Americans. Circulation 74:1465A.

Human Nutrition Information Service, U.S. Department of Agriculture, unpublished data, 1987. (The HNIS, USDA supplied data for the current level in the U.S. diet.)

zations, although some groups are more specific than others. In light of these recommendations and the charge to the committee to identify options to improve the nutritional attributes of animal products, the committee has chosen the following specific target levels for caloric intake and nutrients in the diet:

- *Caloric intake matched to individual needs and appropriate to achieve and maintain desirable body weight* (American Cancer Society, 1984; American Heart Association, 1986; National Institutes of Health, 1984; National Research Council, 1980, 1982; Office of the Assistant Secretary for Health and the Surgeon General, 1979; U.S. Department of Agriculture/U.S. Department of Health and Human Services, 1985; U.S. Senate Select Committee on Nutrition and Human Needs, 1977). Data from the 1976–1980 NHANES indicate that approximately 34 million U.S. adults are obese, of which 12.4 million are severely obese. The incidence of obesity varies widely according to age and sex, with black adults having the highest incidence (61.2 percent for females and 41.4 percent for males). Childhood obesity is more difficult to estimate, but may range from 4 to 14 percent among low-income populations.

- *Thirty percent or less of calories from fat for adults* (American Cancer Society, 1984; American Heart Association, 1986; National Institutes of Health, 1984; National Research Council, 1982). Data from the 1977–1978 NFCS indicated that 6 percent of the population overall had diets from which 30 percent or less of the calories came from fat; data from the 1985 CSFII showed that about 15 percent of children and 12 percent of adult women had diets that met the target.

- *Ten percent or less of calories from saturated fatty acids for adults* (American Heart Association, 1986; National Institutes of Health, 1984). Data from the 1985 CSFII indicated that about 10 percent of women

ages 19 to 50 years and 4 percent of children ages 1 to 5 years had diets that met the target level for percentage of calories from saturated fatty acids.

- *Ten percent or less of calories from polyunsaturated fatty acids for adults* (American Heart Association, 1986; National Institutes of Health, 1984; National Research Council, 1980). Data from the 1985 CSFII indicated that 86 percent of women ages 19 to 50 years and 98 percent of children ages 1 to 5 years had diets that met the target for polyunsaturated fatty acids.

- *Fifteen percent or less of calories (remainder of calories from the fatty acids) from monounsaturated fatty acids for adults* (National Institutes of Health, 1984). Data from the 1985 CSFII indicated that about 65 percent of women ages 19 to 50 years and 78 percent of children ages 1 to 5 years had diets that met the target level for monounsaturated fatty acids.

- *Three hundred milligrams or less of cholesterol per day for adults* (American Heart Association, 1986; National Institutes of Health, 1984). Data from the 1985 CSFII indicated that cholesterol levels averaged 254 mg/day for children ages 1 to 5 years, 304 mg/day for women ages 19 to 50 years, and 435 mg/day for men ages 19 to 50 years. Between 72 and 80 percent of children ages 1 to 5 years and 62 percent of women ages 19 to 50 years had diets that met the target level for cholesterol; comparable data for men were not available, but the trends are thought to be similar.

- *Calcium intake of the Recommended Dietary Allowances (RDAs) for age and sex* (National Research Council, 1980). Data from the 1977–1978 NFCS indicated that 32 percent of individuals had diets that met the target level for calcium (100 percent of the RDA), including 48 percent of children ages 1 to 8 years, 42 percent of males ages 9 to 18 years, and 23 percent of females ages 9 to 18 years. Data from the 1985 CSFII indicated that both total calcium intake (mg/day) and mg/1,000 kcal have increased in the diets of all population groups since the 1977–1978 survey, but women's mean intakes still fell short of meeting the target level. About three-fourths of the women did not meet 100 percent of the RDA; of this group, half did not achieve 70 percent of the RDA.

• *Iron intake of the RDA for age and sex* (National Research Council, 1980). Data from the 1977–1978 NFCS indicated that 44 percent of individuals had diets that met the target level for iron (100 percent of the RDA), including 38 percent of children ages 1 to 8 years, 36 percent of males ages 9 to 18 years, and 18 percent of females ages 9 to 18 years. Data from the 1985 CSFII indicated that mean intakes (mg/day) increased for women and children but not for men, and that mg/1,000 kcal increased for children but not for women or men since the 1977–1978 survey. About 95 percent of the women did not meet 100 percent of the RDA; of this group, three-fourths did not achieve 70 percent of the RDA.

These targeted levels are chosen by the committee as constituting the consensus of dietary and nutrition recommendations made by the various government and nongovernment agencies cited. It is not the intention of the committee to establish new dietary guidelines for the American public. The Food and Nutrition Board of the National Research Council is currently conducting a major study of diet and health issues, and a new National Research Council report may eventually be issued dealing with specific recommendations for these guidelines. For the purpose of assessing target levels of various food components in the diet, the committee has followed the basic recommendations that have been made by other organizations.

The target levels do not include all important characteristics of diets thought to promote health and prevent disease. For example, protein is not targeted because it is plentiful in the diets of most people in the United States. Of the many essential vitamins and minerals, only calcium and iron are targeted because their levels in many diets are below that recommended and animal products are rich sources of them.

## REFERENCES

American Cancer Society. 1984. Nutrition and cancer, cause and prevention. An American Cancer Society special report. Ca—A Cancer Journal for Clinicians 34(2):121–126.

American Heart Association. 1986. Dietary guidelines for healthy adult Americans. Circulation 74:1465A.

Breidenstein, B. C., and J. C. Williams. 1987. Contribution of Red Meat to the U.S. Diet. Chicago, Ill.: National Live Stock & Meat Board.

Centers for Disease Control. 1985. Nutrition Surveillance 1983. U.S. Department of Health and Human Services, Public Health Service, DHHS Publication No. (CDC) 85–8295. Atlanta, Ga.: Centers for Disease Control.

Marston, R., and N. Raper. 1987. Nutrient content of the U.S. food supply. Pp. 18–23 in National Food Review, NFR-36, Economic Research Service. Washington, D.C.: U.S. Department of Agriculture.

McDowell, A., A. Engel, J. T. Massey, and K. Maurer. 1981. Plan and Operation of the Second National Health and Nutrition Examination Survey, 1976–80. Series 1, No. 15. DHHS Publication No. (PHS) 81–1317. Vital and Health Statistics. Washington, D.C.: U.S. Public Health Service.

National Institutes of Health. 1984. NIH Consensus Development Statement on Lowering Blood Cholesterol to Prevent Heart Disease. Vol. 5, No. 7. Washington, D.C.: National Institutes of Health.

National Research Council. 1980. Recommended Dietary Allowances, 9th ed. Washington, D.C.: National Academy Press.

National Research Council. 1982. Diet, Nutrition, and Cancer. Washington, D.C.: National Academy Press.

Office of the Assistant Secretary for Health and the Surgeon General. 1979. Healthy People, the Surgeon General's Report on Health Promotion and Disease Prevention. DHEW (PHS) Publication No. 79–55071. Washington, D.C.: U.S. Public Health Service.

Peterkin, B. B. 1981. Nationwide Food Consumption Survey, 1977–1978. Pp. 59–69 in Nutrition in the 1980s: Constraints on Our Knowledge. New York: Alan R. Liss.

Rathje, W. L. 1984. Where's the beef? Red meat and reactivity. Am. Behav. Sci. 28:71–91.

Stanton, J. L. 1987. An Investigation of Fat Intake. Paper presented to the American Meat Institute, Washington, D.C., January 1987.

U.S. Department of Agriculture. 1985. P. 48 in Women 19–50 Years and Their Children 1–5 Years, 1 Day, 1985. Nationwide Food Consumption Survey, Continuing Survey of Food Intakes by Individuals, Report 85–1, Human Nutrition Information Service. Hyattsville, Md.: U.S. Department of Agriculture.

U.S. Department of Agriculture. 1986. P. 46 in Men 19–50 Years, 1 Day, 1985. Nationwide Food Consumption Survey, Continuing Survey of Food Intakes by Individuals, Report 85–3, Human Nutrition Information Service. Hyattsville, Md.: U.S. Department of Agriculture.

U.S. Department of Agriculture/U.S. Department of Health and Human Services. 1985. Nutrition and Your Health: Dietary Guidelines for Americans, 2nd ed. Home and Garden Bulletin No. 232. Washington, D.C.: U.S. Government Printing Office.

U.S. Department of Agriculture/U.S. Department of Health and Human Services. 1986. Nutrition Monitoring in the United States: A Progress Report from the Joint Nutrition Monitoring Evaluation Committee. DHHS Publication No. (PHS) 86–1255. Washington, D.C.: U.S. Government Printing Office.

U.S. Senate Select Committee on Nutrition and Human Needs. 1977. Dietary Goals for the United States, 2nd ed. No. 052–070–04376–8. Washington, D.C.: U.S. Government Printing Office.

Weir, C. E. 1976. Overview of the role of animal products in human nutrition. Pp. 5–23 in Fat Content and Composition of Animal Products. Washington, D.C.: National Academy Press.

Welsh, S. 1986. The joint nutrition monitoring committee. Pp. 7–20 in What is America Eating? Washington, D.C.: National Academy Press.

# 2

# Current Trends in Consumption
# of Animal Products

## NUTRIENTS IN ANIMAL PRODUCTS AND THEIR BIOAVAILABILITY

Data on the nutrient content of the food supply provide information about the contribution of various food groups to nutrients available for consumption. This series is computed and reported by the U.S. Department of Agriculture (USDA). It is designed to study trends in the levels of nutrients since the early part of the century and changes in food sources of these nutrients. The data have the same limitations as the food supply data in that they are not adjusted for spoilage, trimming, waste, or cooking loss. They measure the nutrients available for consumption by the population rather than nutrient intake. Except for a few processed fruits and vegetables, nutrient values are based on raw food values.

The nutrients consumed represent only a fraction of those present in the food supply. Numerous factors, including metabolic, physiological, and nutritional parameters, all influence the absorption, digestion, and ultimate utilization of nutrients within a food. The bioavailability of a nutrient may not be equivalent in all food sources due to

the nutrient's altered chemical state or to associated factors within the food or within the meal that cause the nutrient to be in a more available or less available form. For instance, in dairy products, calcium is present with lactose, a carbohydrate that enhances calcium's absorption. Some vegetable sources such as spinach also contain considerable amounts of calcium, but the presence of oxalates, which bind calcium as insoluble salts, prevents much of its absorption.

Animal products contribute significantly to the total nutrients in the food supply (Table 2–1 and Figure 2–1). They are a primary source of vitamins $B_{12}$ and $B_6$, riboflavin, niacin, zinc, phosphorus, and calcium and account for 68 percent of the protein available in the food supply.

### Calories

Overall, animal products provide about 36 percent of the caloric content of the food supply while contributing more than a third of the iron, vitamin A, thiamine, and magnesium content; about half of the niacin, riboflavin, and vitamin $B_6$ content; more

TABLE 2-1  Selected Nutrients Provided by Animal Products, 1985 (in percent)

| Nutrient | Animal Product | | | | | | | |
|---|---|---|---|---|---|---|---|---|
| | Milk and Milk Products | Eggs | Red Meat[a] | Poultry | Fish and Shellfish | Animal Fats | Total for All Animal Products (%) | Total from All Foods (per capita/day) |
| Calories | 10.0 | 1.6 | 15.5 | 3.5 | 0.9 | 4.2 | 35.6 | 3,560.0[b] |
| Protein | 20.9 | 4.2 | 27.6 | 11.2 | 4.6 | 0.0 | 68.5 | 102.0 g |
| Total fat | 11.4 | 2.3 | 27.7 | 4.9 | 0.7 | 9.6 | 56.6 | 172.0 g |
| Saturated fatty acids | 20.5 | 2.0 | 32.8 | 4.0 | 0.5 | 14.3 | 74.2 | 59.0 g |
| Cholesterol | 14.0 | 40.4 | 25.8 | 11.1 | 3.4 | 5.3 | 100.0 | 480.0 mg |
| Vitamins | | | | | | | | |
| Niacin | 1.6 | 0.1 | 27.3 | 14.3 | 5.3 | 0.0 | 48.6 | 26.0 mg |
| Riboflavin | 34.6 | 4.5 | 16.3 | 4.9 | 1.1 | 0.1 | 61.4 | 2.4 mg |
| Thiamine | 8.8 | 1.4 | 23.5 | 1.8 | 0.6 | 0.0 | 36.1 | 2.2 mg |
| Vitamin A | 9.6 | 1.9 | 12.5 | 4.3 | 0.3 | 1.9 | 30.5 | 9,900 IU |
| Vitamin $B_6$ | 11.0 | 2.0 | 25.6 | 10.3 | 3.7 | 0.0 | 52.8 | 2.1 mg |
| Vitamin $B_{12}$ | 20.0 | 6.3 | 51.5 | 8.4 | 12.1 | 0.0 | 98.3 | 8.8 µg |
| Minerals | | | | | | | | |
| Calcium | 76.2 | 2.2 | 2.2 | 0.8 | 1.2 | 0.2 | 82.8 | 920.0 mg |
| Iron | 2.4 | 4.0 | 23.1 | 4.7 | 1.5 | 0.0 | 35.7 | 18.3 mg |
| Magnesium | 20.0 | 1.3 | 9.0 | 3.8 | 2.1 | 0.0 | 36.3 | 320.0 mg |
| Zinc | 19.8 | 4.1 | 36.2 | 8.1 | 3.3 | 0.1 | 71.5 | 12.3 mg |

NOTE:  Values are based on disappearance of retail weight without correction for waste or other loss such as nutrient losses during cooking.

[a]Red meat is beef, veal, pork, and lamb.
[b]This figure may differ slightly from other published sources because of rounding.

SOURCE:  Human Nutrition Information Service, U.S. Department of Agriculture, unpublished data, 1987. The nutrient composition values for meats is not updated. A revision of procedures and data for estimating the nutrient contribution of meat is in progress.

than 70 percent of the zinc content; more than 80 percent of the calcium content; and nearly 100 percent of the vitamin $B_{12}$ content.

Red meats account for the largest proportion of the calories (about 15 percent), followed by dairy products (10 percent), animal fats (4 percent), poultry (3.5 percent), eggs (1.6 percent), and fish and shellfish (0.9 percent). From 1977 to 1985, the total calories available per capita in the food supply have increased by 7 percent, from 3,330 to 3,560. This parallels an increase in caloric intake indicated by dietary survey data from 1977 to 1985 for children ages 1 to 5 years of 8.3 percent, women ages 19 to 50 years of 5.6 percent, and men ages 19 to 50 years of 15 percent.

In the 1977–1978 Nationwide Food Consumption Survey (NFCS), animal products contributed an average of about 45 percent of total calories to the diets of all individuals, with dairy products accounting for about 14 percent; meat, poultry, and fish about 28 percent; and eggs 2.4 percent (Table 2-2).  The meat, poultry, and fish group was the primary source of calories for adults, contributing 24 to 34 percent of total intake. Children of ages 3 to 14 years derived slightly fewer calories from this category (20 to 25 percent) and more from the dairy and grain products groups than did adults.

It is possible that the fat, and therefore the calories, derived from meats, poultry, and fish is overstated in the NFCS analysis. In analyzing the dietary survey responses, if an individual did not specify whether he or she ate the separable fat on meat or the

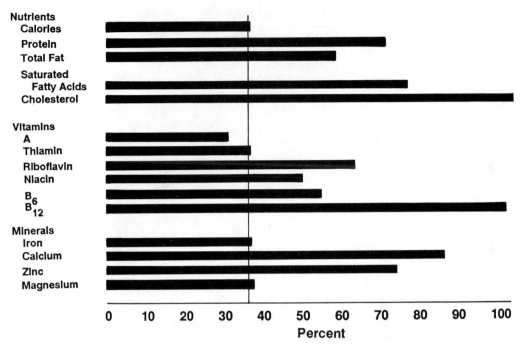

**FIGURE 2–1**　Selected nutrients provided by animal products (in percent). See also Table 2–1. Source: Human Nutrition Information Service, U.S. Department of Agriculture, unpublished data, 1987. (The nutrient composition values for meats are not updated. A revision of procedures and data for estimating the nutrient contribution of meat is in progress.)

poultry skin, the methodology stipulated that it be assumed that all these components were eaten. The American Meat Institute study (Stanton, 1987) addresses this issue.

### Protein

The protein from animal products differs in several respects from that from vegetable sources. First, animal products are richer than vegetable sources of the eight essential amino acids, those components of proteins that cannot be synthesized by the body and must be supplied in food. Animal products provide almost three-fourths of the eight essential amino acids in the food supply and contribute about 67 percent of the total protein, reflecting the greater concentration of these vital nutrients (Table 2–3) (Linkswiler, 1982).

Few proteins from either animal or vegetable sources are consumed without some further processing, usually cooking. How this affects the bioavailability of the proteins for utilization by the body is important, particularly when estimating the amount of protein available in the food supply. Proper cooking facilitates digestion and utilization by partially breaking down the protein structure. Excessive or prolonged heating, however, may actually produce new chemical bonds, decreasing the digestibility of the protein. An example is the decreased physiological availability of lysine, tryptophan, and other amino acids in toasted cereal products (Love, 1982). Lysine, for example, under high heat, links with carbohydrate to form a bond resistant to cleavage. Severe heating of animal proteins has also been shown to destroy cystine and result in reduced digestibility and availability of amino acids (Cheftel, 1977).

TABLE 2-2  Contribution of Animal Products to Total Calories in the Diet Based on 3-Day Intake (in percent)

| Group and Age | Number of Survey Participants | Animal Product | | | |
| | | Milk and Milk Products | Eggs | Red Meat, Poultry, and Fish[a] | Total[b] |
|---|---|---|---|---|---|
| Children | | | | | |
| <1 | 421 | 57.2 | 1.0 | 6.7 | 64.9 |
| 1–2 | 1,035 | 24.9 | 2.9 | 20.3 | 48.1 |
| 3–5 | 1,719 | 20.1 | 2.3 | 21.4 | 43.8 |
| 6–8 | 1,841 | 20.3 | 1.6 | 22.1 | 44.0 |
| Females | | | | | |
| 9–11 | 1,011 | 19.4 | 1.6 | 22.7 | 43.7 |
| 12–14 | 1,148 | 17.9 | 1.6 | 24.8 | 44.3 |
| 15–18 | 1,473 | 15.7 | 1.7 | 27.5 | 44.9 |
| 19–22 | 1,317 | 13.0 | 2.4 | 29.4 | 44.8 |
| 23–34 | 3,879 | 11.9 | 2.4 | 30.3 | 44.6 |
| 35–50 | 3,759 | 10.2 | 2.9 | 32.2 | 45.3 |
| 51–64 | 2,936 | 10.9 | 2.7 | 31.0 | 44.6 |
| 65–74 | 1,376 | 12.3 | 2.7 | 28.4 | 43.4 |
| 75+ | 751 | 14.1 | 2.7 | 25.2 | 42.0 |
| Males | | | | | |
| 9–11 | 939 | 18.9 | 1.7 | 23.9 | 44.5 |
| 12–14 | 1,150 | 18.4 | 1.7 | 24.6 | 44.7 |
| 15–18 | 1,394 | 16.7 | 2.1 | 27.6 | 46.4 |
| 19–22 | 1,030 | 12.6 | 2.3 | 32.0 | 46.9 |
| 23–34 | 2,716 | 11.0 | 2.5 | 31.8 | 45.3 |
| 35–50 | 2,571 | 9.6 | 2.9 | 33.5 | 46.0 |
| 51–64 | 2,161 | 10.6 | 3.0 | 32.5 | 46.1 |
| 65–74 | 1,049 | 11.7 | 3.2 | 29.3 | 44.2 |
| 75+ | 465 | 12.1 | 3.9 | 28.0 | 44.0 |
| Total | 36,142 | 14.3 | 2.4 | 28.4 | 45.1 |

NOTE:  Food groups include mixtures with main ingredient from the group; therefore, calories from some vegetable sources in such mixtures are included. Calories from small amounts of animal sources in mainly vegetable mixtures are excluded.

[a]Red meat is beef, veal, pork, and lamb.
[b]The total is for the three groups of animal products shown.

SOURCE:  U.S. Department of Agriculture. 1984. P. 64 in Nutrient Intakes: Individuals in 48 States, Year 1977–78. Nationwide Food Consumption Survey 1977–78. Report I-2, Human Nutrition Information Service. Hyattsville, Md.: U.S. Department of Agriculture.

From the food supply data, about 102 grams of protein are available per capita, with 68.5 percent derived from animal products. Of this amount, red meat contributes the largest percent (27.6), followed by dairy products (20.9) and poultry (11.2), with the fish/shellfish and egg groups contributing about 4.6 and 4.2 percent, respectively. The trend in the percentage of calories from protein, fat, and carbohydrate in the food supply from 1957 to 1984 is evident in Table 2–4.

In line with the per capita disappearance data, animal products contributed about 70 percent of the protein in the 1977–1978 NFCS (Table 2–5). The red meat, poultry, and fish group was the largest source of protein, contributing 40 to 56 percent of

TABLE 2-3   Percentage of Contribution of Essential Amino Acids from Animal Products to Total Essential Amino Acids in the U.S. Food Supply

| Amino Acid | Amino Acids from Animal Protein (% total) |
| --- | --- |
| Isoleucine | 74.2 |
| Leucine | 72.8 |
| Lysine | 83.6 |
| Phenylalanine | 66.7 |
| Threonine | 75.4 |
| Total sulfur-containing | 74.9 |
| Tryptophan | 71.5 |
| Valine | 73.7 |

SOURCE:   Adapted from H. M. Linkswiler. 1982. Importance of animal protein in human nutrition. P. 270 in Animal Products in Human Nutrition, D. C. Beitz, and R. G. Hansen, eds. New York: Academic Press.

TABLE 2-4   Sources of Food Energy in the U.S. Food Supply for Selected Years (in percent)

| Source | 1957–1959 | 1967–1969 | 1984 |
| --- | --- | --- | --- |
| Protein | 12 | 12 | 12 |
| Fat | 41 | 43 | 43 |
| Carbohydrate | 47 | 45 | 46 |

SOURCE:   Adapted from N. R. Raper and R. M. Marston. 1986. Levels and sources of fat in the U.S. food supply. P. 131 in Dietary Fat and Cancer, C. Ip, D. F. Birt, A. E. Rogers, and C. Mettlin, eds. New York: Alan R. Liss, Inc.

the protein in the diets of adults and 35 to 39 percent of the protein in children's diets. Eggs accounted for roughly 3 to 5 percent of the total protein in the diets of most age and sex groups, except for elderly males, who derived 6 percent of their daily protein from eggs. Table 2–6 compares NFCS and Continuing Survey of Food Intake by Individuals (CSFII) data in terms of the percentage of calories from protein and fat.

### Fat, Saturated Fatty Acids, and Cholesterol

Although animal products are important sources of many nutrients, they are also a significant source of fat. On a raw basis, animal products account for 57 percent of the fat available for consumption (Table 2–1). However, the data based on nutrients in raw food may overstate the fat eaten as part of meat products because meats lose substantial amounts of fat during cooking. This is not true for foods like milk and milk products or grains. Waste is also an important consideration when trying to determine food sources of fat. For example, all the separable fat on meat may not be consumed.

Data from the food supply indicate that the contribution of fat from animal sources has been decreasing, while that from vegetable sources has been increasing (Figure 2–2). Changes in the level and sources of fat in the food supply have also affected the fatty acid content. Table 2–7 presents trend data on the percentage of saturated fatty acids and two unsaturated fatty acids (oleic and linoleic) in the food supply.

Knowledge of the fatty acid composition of dietary fats (visible/invisible) is important because different fatty acids, both saturated and unsaturated, exert different metabolic or physiological effects. Also, in some instances the effects of certain component fatty acids are not known.

Except for milk fat (butterfat), most animal fats contain palmitic and stearic acids as the major saturated fatty acids. In addition, milk fat contains significant amounts of short-chain ($C_4$, $C_6$) and medium-chain ($C_8$, $C_{10}$, $C_{12}$) fatty acids (Table 2–8). (The nomenclature used to describe a fatty acid includes carbon chain length and numbers of double bonds, if present. For example, an 18-carbon fatty acid with one double bond would be written as $C_{18:1}$; an 18-carbon fatty acid without double bonds, that is, completely saturated, would be written as $C_{18:0}$.) Current evidence indicates that different dietary saturated fatty acids may have different physiological effects. For example, stearic acid ($C_{18:0}$) has negligible effects on serum cholesterol levels as compared to

TABLE 2-5   Contribution of Animal Products to Protein in the Diet Based on 3-Day Intake (in percent)

| Group and Age | Number of Survey Participants | Animal Product | | | |
| | | Milk and Milk Products | Eggs | Red Meat, Poultry, and Fish[a] | Total[b] |
|---|---|---|---|---|---|
| Children | | | | | |
| <1 | 421 | 62.9 | 1.6 | 13.0 | 77.5 |
| 1–2 | 1,035 | 32.7 | 4.5 | 34.9 | 72.1 |
| 3–5 | 1,719 | 26.9 | 3.7 | 38.0 | 68.6 |
| 6–8 | 1,841 | 26.7 | 2.6 | 39.4 | 68.7 |
| Females | | | | | |
| 9–11 | 1,011 | 25.0 | 2.6 | 40.2 | 67.8 |
| 12–14 | 1,148 | 22.4 | 2.5 | 43.9 | 68.8 |
| 15–18 | 1,473 | 19.9 | 2.8 | 48.2 | 70.9 |
| 19–22 | 1,317 | 16.4 | 3.7 | 50.7 | 70.8 |
| 23–34 | 3,879 | 15.4 | 3.7 | 52.0 | 71.1 |
| 35–50 | 3,759 | 12.9 | 4.3 | 54.1 | 71.3 |
| 51–64 | 2,936 | 13.9 | 4.2 | 52.6 | 70.7 |
| 65–74 | 1,376 | 15.8 | 4.3 | 48.9 | 69.0 |
| 75+ | 751 | 18.2 | 4.4 | 45.0 | 67.6 |
| Males | | | | | |
| 9–11 | 939 | 24.0 | 2.7 | 42.0 | 68.7 |
| 12–14 | 1,150 | 23.2 | 2.7 | 42.8 | 68.7 |
| 15–18 | 1,394 | 20.9 | 3.2 | 46.6 | 70.7 |
| 19–22 | 1,030 | 15.7 | 3.6 | 52.9 | 72.2 |
| 23–34 | 2,716 | 13.8 | 3.9 | 53.7 | 71.4 |
| 35–50 | 2,571 | 11.5 | 4.4 | 55.7 | 71.6 |
| 51–64 | 2,161 | 12.8 | 4.6 | 54.6 | 72.0 |
| 65–74 | 1,049 | 14.8 | 5.2 | 50.1 | 70.1 |
| 75+ | 465 | 15.2 | 6.3 | 47.6 | 69.1 |
| Total | 36,142 | 18.1 | 3.8 | 48.7 | 70.6 |

NOTE:   Food groups include mixtures with main ingredient from the group; therefore, protein from some vegetable sources in such mixtures is included. Protein from small amounts of animal sources in mainly vegetable mixtures is excluded.

[a]Red meat is beef, veal, pork, and lamb.
[b]The total is for the three groups of animal products shown.

SOURCE:   U.S. Department of Agriculture. 1984. P. 70 in Nutrient Intakes: Individuals in 48 States, Year 1977–78. Nationwide Food Consumption Survey 1977–78. Report I-2, Human Nutrition Information Service. Hyattsville, Md.: U.S. Department of Agriculture.

palmitic acid ($C_{16:0}$) (Hegsted et al., 1965; Keys et al., 1965). Furthermore, the metabolic effects of the short- and medium-chain fatty acids of milk fat have not been determined, and it is questionable whether they should be grouped (for nutritional considerations) with the saturated fatty acids with known hyperlipidemic effects, such as palmitic acid.

Oleic acid ($C_{18:1}$), a major fatty acid component of animal fats, has hypocholesterolemic (cholesterol-lowering) effects (Grundy, 1986), and therefore in moderate amounts is not considered to be an undesirable dietary fatty acid. All animal fats contain polyunsaturated fatty acids, usually in relatively small amounts (Table 2–8). The common tendency to broadly categorize all an-

TABLE 2-6  Calories from Protein and Fat (in percent)

| Group and Age | Protein 1977 | Protein 1985 | Fat 1977 | Fat 1985 |
|---|---|---|---|---|
| Children (1–5) | 15.7 | 15.7 | 37.6 | 34.3 |
| Females (19–50) | 17.1 | 16.1 | 40.8 | 36.6 |
| Males (19–50) | 16.5 | 15.9 | 41.3 | 36.4 |

SOURCES: Adapted from U.S. Department of Agriculture 1985. P. 48 in Women 19–50 Years and Their Children 1–5 Years, 1 Day, 1985. Nationwide Food Consumption Survey, Continuing Survey of Food Intakes by Individuals, Report 85-1, Human Nutrition Information Service. Hyattsville, Md.: U.S. Department of Agriculture. U.S. Department of Agriculture. 1986. P. 46 in Men 19–50 Years, 1 Day, 1985. Nationwide Food Consumption Survey, Continuing Survey of Food Intakes by Individuals. Report 85-3, Human Nutrition Information Service. Hyattsville, Md.: U.S. Department of Agriculture. See these reports for information on changes in methods and data bases that may affect differences in results between 1977 and 1985.

imal fats as high in saturated fatty acids is inaccurate; animal fats are made up of a mixture of saturated and unsaturated fatty acids, as shown in Table 2–8. The potential physiological effects of animal fats containing significant amounts of stearic ($C_{18:0}$), oleic ($C_{18:1}$), short-chain fatty acids, or all three need to be evaluated.

Contrary to popular opinion, vegetable oils rank as one of the primary sources of saturated fatty acids in the food supply. As shown in Table 2–8, vegetable oils such as coconut, palm, and palm kernel oils are as much or more saturated than most animal fats, and considerable amounts are used in commercial baking and as frying fats. Other vegetable oils contain a smaller percentage of saturated fatty acids, but contribute substantially to the total because of the volume in which they are consumed.

Data on the contribution of animal products to total dietary fat from the 1977–1978 NFCS are presented in Table 2–9. Dietary levels of fat averaged 41 percent of total calories for the survey population. More than 63 percent of the total fat was derived from three groups of animal products: 42 percent from red meats, poultry, and fish; 17 percent from milk and milk products; and 4 percent from eggs.

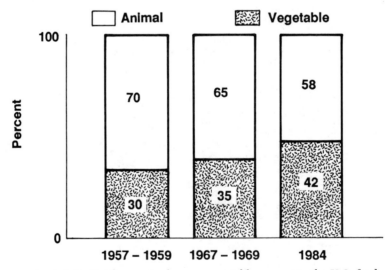

FIGURE 2–2  Fat from animal versus vegetable sources in the U.S. food supply for selected years (in percent). Source: Data from N. R. Raper, and R. M. Marston. 1986. Levels and sources of fat in the U.S. food supply. Pp. 127–152 in Dietary Fat and Cancer, C. Ip, D. F. Birt, A. E. Rogers, and C. Mettlin, eds. New York: Alan R. Liss, Inc.

TABLE 2-7   Selected Fatty Acids in the U.S. Food Supply (in percent)

| Fatty Acid | Year | | | | | | | | |
|---|---|---|---|---|---|---|---|---|---|
| | 1909–1913 | 1925–1929 | 1935–1939 | 1947–1949 | 1957–1959 | 1967–1969 | 1975 | 1980 | 1984 |
| Saturated | 42 | 42 | 42 | 40 | 40 | 37 | 35 | 34 | 35 |
| Oleic | 37 | 38 | 37 | 38 | 38 | 38 | 39 | 38 | 38 |
| Linoleic | 7 | 8 | 9 | 10 | 11 | 13 | 15 | 16 | 15 |

SOURCE:   Adapted from N. R. Raper and R. M. Marston. 1986. Levels and sources of fat in the U.S. food supply. P. 142 in Dietary Fat and Cancer, C. Ip, D. F. Birt, A. E. Rogers, and C. Mettlin, eds. New York: Alan R. Liss, Inc.

TABLE 2-8   Fatty Acid Composition of Selected Fats and Oils, Expressed as Percentage of Total Fatty Acids

| Fat or Oil | Fatty Acid | | | | | | |
|---|---|---|---|---|---|---|---|
| | Saturated | | | Monounsaturated | Polyunsaturated | Other |
| | $\leq C_{10:0}$ | $C_{12:0}$, $C_{14:0}$, $C_{16:0}$ | $C_{18:0}$ | $C_{16:1}$, $C_{18:1}$ | $C_{18:2}$, $C_{18:3}$ | |
| Coconut oil | 14.0 | 74.5 | 2.5 | 6.5 | 1.5 | 0.1 |
| Palm kernel oil | 8.2 | 73.6 | 2.4 | 13.7 | 2.0 | 0.1 |
| Butter oil | 9.2 | 47.0 | 12.5 | 30.1 | 3.4 | — |
| Palm oil | — | 46.5 | 4.7 | 38.9 | 9.4 | 0.5 |
| Beef fat | 0.1 | 28.9 | 21.6 | 42.1 | 2.8 | 4.6 |
| Lard (pork) | 0.1 | 26.4 | 12.3 | 48.2 | 0.0 | 3.0 |
| Chicken fat | — | 24.7 | 6.4 | 48.1 | 0.2 | 0.6 |
| Duck fat | — | 23.4 | 5.5 | 47.0 | 5.5 | — |
| Mutton fat | 0.2 | 29.1 | 24.5 | 35.8 | 5.3 | 5.1 |
| Cocoa butter | — | 25.9 | 34.5 | 35.6 | 2.9 | 1.1 |
| Corn oil | — | 12.2 | 2.2 | 27.6 | 3.7 | — |
| Olive oil | — | 13.7 | 2.5 | 72.3 | 1.5 | — |
| Rapeseed oil | — | 3.9 | 1.9 | 64.3 | 9.9 | — |
| Sunflower seed oil | — | 7.5 | 4.7 | 18.7 | 9.1 | — |
| Soybean oil | — | 11.1 | 4.0 | 23.5 | 1.4 | — |
| Egg yolk | — | 26.1 | 9.9 | 49.9 | 4.7 | — |
| Salmon oil | — | 15.1 | 3.8 | 42.5 | 8.6 | — |
| Cod liver oil | — | 3.2 | 3.7 | 34.6 | 7.3 | 1.2 |
| Herring oil | — | 8.0 | 1.4 | 35.2 | 2.4 | 3.0 |

NOTE:   Fats and oils are listed from most to least saturated. The numbers in the column headings indicate the length of the carbon chain of individual fatty acids and the number of double bonds. For example, a 10-carbon-chain fatty acid without double bonds is expressed as $C_{10:0}$.

SOURCES:   Adapted from Durkee's Typical Compositions and Chemical Constants of Common Edible Fats and Oils. 1970. Cleveland, Ohio: SCM Corp. C. Lenter, ed. 1981. P. 264 in Geigy Scientific Tables, 8th rev. ed., Vol. 1. Basel, Switzerland: CIBA-GEIGY Corp.

In the 1977–1978 NFCS, red meats provided the major source of fat (32 to 49 percent) in the diets of all age groups other than infants. The contribution of red meat, poultry, and fish to total fat was highest for men and women ages 35 to 50. However, males ages 15 to 18 derived a smaller proportion of fat from the red meat group and a greater proportion from milk and milk products than did adult males. These young males had the highest fat intake of any group. Grains, milk, and milk products contributed roughly comparable amounts of fat to the diets of adults (11 to 15 percent). These food groups were greater sources of fat for children and teenagers than for adults.

TABLE 2-9    Contribution of Animal Products to Fat in the Diet Based on 3-Day Intake (in percent)

| Group and Age | Number of Survey Participants | Animal Product | | | |
| | | Milk and Milk Products | Eggs | Red Meat, Poultry, and Fish[a] | Total[b] |
|---|---|---|---|---|---|
| **Children** | | | | | |
| <1 | 421 | 69.5 | 2.0 | 10.3 | 81.8 |
| 1–2 | 1,035 | 30.1 | 5.1 | 32.2 | 67.4 |
| 3–5 | 1,719 | 24.4 | 4.0 | 34.3 | 62.7 |
| 6–8 | 1,841 | 24.2 | 2.8 | 34.8 | 61.8 |
| **Females** | | | | | |
| 9–11 | 1,011 | 23.0 | 2.8 | 35.6 | 61.4 |
| 12–14 | 1,148 | 21.0 | 2.7 | 38.0 | 61.7 |
| 15–18 | 1,473 | 18.3 | 3.0 | 41.1 | 62.4 |
| 19–22 | 1,317 | 15.3 | 4.0 | 43.5 | 62.8 |
| 23–34 | 3,879 | 14.1 | 4.0 | 44.1 | 62.2 |
| 35–50 | 3,759 | 11.8 | 4.6 | 46.7 | 63.1 |
| 51–64 | 2,936 | 12.8 | 4.5 | 45.3 | 62.6 |
| 65–74 | 1,376 | 14.7 | 4.6 | 43.1 | 62.4 |
| 75+ | 751 | 17.4 | 4.7 | 38.9 | 61.0 |
| **Males** | | | | | |
| 9–11 | 939 | 22.2 | 2.9 | 36.8 | 61.9 |
| 12–14 | 1,150 | 21.4 | 2.9 | 37.6 | 61.9 |
| 15–18 | 1,394 | 19.1 | 3.4 | 41.3 | 63.8 |
| 19–22 | 1,030 | 14.9 | 3.8 | 47.0 | 65.7 |
| 23–34 | 2,716 | 13.1 | 4.0 | 46.7 | 63.8 |
| 35–50 | 2,571 | 11.1 | 4.6 | 48.8 | 64.5 |
| 51–64 | 2,161 | 12.4 | 4.7 | 47.3 | 64.4 |
| 65–74 | 1,049 | 14.0 | 5.3 | 44.1 | 63.4 |
| 75+ | 465 | 15.0 | 6.2 | 42.7 | 63.9 |
| Total | 36,142 | 16.9 | 4.0 | 42.4 | 63.3 |

NOTE:   Food groups include mixtures with main ingredient from the group; therefore, fat from some vegetable sources in such mixtures is included. Fat from small amounts of animal sources in mainly vegetable mixtures is excluded.

[a]Red meat is beef, veal, pork, and lamb.
[b]The total is for the three groups of animal products shown.

SOURCE:   U.S. Department of Agriculture. 1984. P. 76 in Nutrient Intakes: Individuals in 48 States, Year 1977–78. Nationwide Food Consumption Survey 1977–78. Report I-2, Human Nutrition Information Service. Hyattsville, Md.: U.S. Department of Agriculture.

Within the meats group, beef was the primary source of fat for most age and sex groups, particularly adult males (Table 2–10). Males ages 19 to 50 derived 17 percent of their dietary fat from beef, compared with 15.2 percent for females of the same age. Poultry was a slightly more important source of fat for women than for men. Pork contributed proportionately more to fat in-

take for children ages 1 to 5 than for other ages. This age group consumed a greater proportion of its meat in the form of processed pork, in particular, frankfurters and bologna (Pao et al., 1982).

Table 2–11 summarizes 1985 CSFII data on the fat and cholesterol in women's diets. The red meat, poultry, and fish group (including mixtures) was the primary source of fat, fatty acids, and cholesterol in women's diets, with red meat providing about half of these components. Red meat was the most significant source of cholesterol, although the contribution of poultry was only slightly less than that of beef or other red meats. Shell eggs accounted for only 29 percent of total cholesterol intake because most eggs are consumed as ingredients in other foods, so that the cholesterol originating from eggs is distributed among other food groups such as grain products.

The USDA is developing an automated system for classifying ingredients of mixtures reported in its surveys into appropriate groups. For example, the beef and vegetables in beef stew now classified as a mixture will be moved to the beef and vegetable groups. This classification system will be used to supplement the system now used, not replace it. The partly completed system was used to determine the proportion of fat and cholesterol in the 4-day diets of women surveyed in 1985. Commercially prepared bakery products such as bread, doughnuts, and snacks have not yet been separated into ingredients and some ingredients are in raw form.

TABLE 2-10  Contribution of Animal Products to Mean Intake of Fat and Percentage of Fat Based on 1-Day Intake

| Group and Age | Total Fat Intake (g/day) | Animal Product | | | | | | |
| | | Milk and Milk Products | Eggs | Total Red Meat, Poultry, Fish, and Mixtures[a] | Beef | Pork | Lamb, Veal, and Game | Poultry |
|---|---|---|---|---|---|---|---|---|
| Children | | | | | | | | |
| <1 | 30.4 | 67.9 | 2.4 | 12.9 | 3.0 | 1.6 | 0.7 | 1.5 |
| 1–2 | 48.9 | 30.3 | 5.5 | 29.9 | 8.5 | 10.5 | 0.1 | 4.7 |
| 3–5 | 61.0 | 24.5 | 5.1 | 32.9 | 9.7 | 10.3 | 0.04 | 4.7 |
| 6–8 | 72.4 | 24.3 | 3.2 | 34.7 | 11.3 | 11.2 | 0.2 | 4.4 |
| Females | | | | | | | | |
| 9–11 | 79.1 | 21.8 | 2.6 | 35.4 | 11.8 | 10.8 | 0.1 | 5.1 |
| 12–14 | 85.3 | 21.3 | 3.3 | 36.6 | 12.6 | 10.7 | 0.2 | 4.4 |
| 15–18 | 80.5 | 18.5 | 3.1 | 38.1 | 13.0 | 9.7 | 0.8 | 5.4 |
| 19–22 | 75.9 | 17.1 | 4.8 | 42.2 | 14.3 | 13.0 | 0.3 | 5.2 |
| 23–34 | 73.7 | 15.1 | 4.8 | 42.3 | 14.3 | 11.7 | 0.3 | 5.3 |
| 35–50 | 70.8 | 12.2 | 4.3 | 45.4 | 16.5 | 11.9 | 0.6 | 5.4 |
| 51–64 | 71.2 | 12.3 | 4.7 | 43.9 | 16.3 | 11.4 | 0.7 | 5.6 |
| 65–74 | 65.8 | 15.6 | 4.2 | 39.8 | 11.9 | 13.1 | 0.9 | 6.2 |
| 75+ | 59.0 | 19.8 | 4.4 | 36.6 | 12.5 | 11.4 | 0.8 | 4.7 |
| Males | | | | | | | | |
| 9–11 | 87.6 | 21.9 | 4.0 | 36.4 | 12.3 | 10.6 | 0.7 | 4.3 |
| 12–14 | 105.5 | 19.9 | 4.1 | 37.6 | 12.5 | 11.1 | 0.02 | 3.6 |
| 15–18 | 123.3 | 18.2 | 3.7 | 41.7 | 16.4 | 11.1 | 0.1 | 4.2 |
| 19–22 | 118.4 | 16.0 | 3.7 | 44.4 | 17.8 | 11.2 | 0.2 | 5.8 |
| 23–34 | 114.8 | 13.1 | 4.1 | 44.7 | 16.8 | 12.6 | 0.2 | 4.1 |
| 35–50 | 109.3 | 12.2 | 5.2 | 46.8 | 16.8 | 12.8 | 0.2 | 4.5 |
| 51–64 | 101.6 | 12.0 | 4.8 | 46.3 | 16.0 | 14.6 | 0.5 | 4.7 |
| 65–74 | 92.8 | 13.9 | 5.5 | 42.2 | 15.0 | 13.6 | 0.4 | 4.8 |
| 75+ | 86.2 | 15.2 | 6.2 | 42.7 | 13.0 | 18.3 | 1.1 | 5.7 |

[a]Red meat is beef, veal, pork, and lamb.

SOURCE:  Adapted from R. L. Rizek and E. M. Jackson. 1982. Current food consumption practices and nutrient sources in the American diet. Pp. 150–151 in Animal Products in Human Nutrition, D. C. Beitz and R. G. Hansen, eds. New York: Academic Press.

TABLE 2-11  Percentage of Fat, Fatty Acids, and Cholesterol in Diets of Women, Ages 19–50 Years Based on 1-Day Intake

| Food Source[a] | Total Fat | Saturated Fatty Acids | Cholesterol |
|---|---|---|---|
| Milk and milk products | 14.4 | 24.8 | 11.8 |
| Eggs (as shell eggs) | 3.8 | 3.0 | 29.2 |
| Meat, poultry, and fish | 32.2 | 31.3 | 37.7 |
| Total red meat[b] | 16.6 | 17.6 | 15.7 |
| Beef | 7.6 | 8.6 | 8.0 |
| Poultry | 3.6 | 2.7 | 6.1 |
| Fish | 1.7 | 1.2 | 3.7 |
| Mixtures | 10.3 | 9.7 | 12.3 |
| Total animal[c] | 50.4 | 59.1 | 78.7 |
| Fats and oils[d] | 12.8 | 9.4 | 2.4 |
| Fruits and vegetables | 9.3 | 7.6 | 2.5 |
| Grain products | 22.2 | 19.6 | 16.0 |
| Legumes, nuts, and seeds | 3.4 | 1.8 | 0.3 |
| Miscellaneous | 2.0 | 2.6 | 0.2 |

[a]Food groups include mixtures with main ingredient from the group; therefore, lipids from some vegetable sources in such mixtures are included. Lipids from small amounts of animal sources in mainly vegetable mixtures are excluded.

[b]Red meat is beef, veal, pork, and lamb. In this case, the category also includes organ meats and processed meats.

[c]The total is for the three groups shown.

[d]Includes butter and other animal fats and oils in table fats and salad dressings.

SOURCES:  U.S. Department of Agriculture. 1985. Women 19–50 Years and Their Children 1–5 Years, 1 Day, 1985. Nationwide Food Consumption Survey, Continuing Survey of Food Intakes by Individuals. Report 85-1, Human Nutrition Information Service. Hyattsville, Md.: U.S. Department of Agriculture. Human Nutrition Information Service, U.S. Department of Agriculture, unpublished data, 1987.

Preliminary results suggest that the red meat, poultry, and fish category provided about one-fourth of the fat and more than one-third of the cholesterol. Fresh, unprocessed red meat provided almost one-fifth of the total fat and cholesterol. Eggs provided more than 40 percent of the cholesterol. Fats and oils provided about one-tenth of the fat, one-tenth of saturated fatty acids, and only 5 percent of the cholesterol, all of which was from animal sources. This information is summarized in Table 2–12.

### Vitamins

Animal products contribute between 33 and 100 percent of available quantities of specific vitamins in the food supply. They are good sources of most of the B vitamins,

particularly riboflavin, niacin, vitamin $B_6$, and vitamin $B_{12}$.

In the 1977–1978 NFCS, milk and milk products contributed 14 percent of calories but larger proportions of several nutrients. They were the primary source of riboflavin and vitamin $B_{12}$ in the diet, contributing an average of nearly 30 percent. Milk and milk products also contributed over 16 percent of vitamin A and smaller percentages of other vitamins. Eggs contributed over 4 percent of vitamin A and riboflavin.

Table 2–13 summarizes the contribution of animal products to the vitamin content of the diet, using data from the 1977–1978 NFCS. The category of red meat, poultry, and fish is the major source of the preformed niacin (44.3 percent), vitamin $B_6$ (39.9 percent), riboflavin (24.2 percent), thiamine

(23.6 percent), and vitamin A (12 percent) in the diet.

## Minerals

Animal products also contribute substantially to the mineral content of the food supply, as indicated in Table 2–1, providing 42 percent of the iron, more than a third of all magnesium, and over 60 percent of the calcium and phosphorus.

### Iron

Prior to 1979, the red meat, poultry, and fish group was the primary source of iron in the food supply. Increased fortification of foods with iron (for example, in flour) and the decline in red meat consumption, however, have made grain products (composed entirely of nonhemoglobin iron) the primary iron source in the diet. Animal products contribute about 28 percent of the total iron to the food supply; cereals and grains account for 39.3 percent; fruits and vegetables, 19.2 percent; and dry beans, peas, nuts, and all others, 13.7 percent.

Data from the 1977–1978 NFCS indicate that animal products contribute about 42 percent of the total iron to the diet (Table 2–14). Of this amount, the red meat, poultry, and fish category provides the highest percentage, 34.5, with milk and milk prod-

ucts and eggs each contributing about 4 percent.

### Calcium

Animal products contribute more than 80 percent of the total calcium available in the food supply (Table 2–1). Milk and milk products provide 76.2 percent; fruits and vegetables, 8.8 percent; red meat, poultry, and fish, 4.2 percent; cereals and grains, 3.6 percent; beans, peas, and nuts, 3.1 percent; and other foods, 2.4 percent. The level of calcium in the food supply and the contribution from dairy products has remained fairly constant during the last 20 years. Despite significant declines in the consumption of fluid milk, milk is still the primary source of calcium, contributing 28 percent to the total calcium derived from dairy products; cheese is a close second at 27 percent. If current consumption trends continue, both cheese and low-fat milk should surpass whole milk as the main source of calcium in the food supply within the next year.

A number of factors influence the absorption and utilization of dietary calcium. Vitamin D facilitates the movement of calcium into the duodenal mucosal cells and increases absorption. High-protein diets also increase calcium absorption because of the action of specific amino acids, especially

TABLE 2-12   Estimated Percentage of Contribution of Fat, Saturated Fatty Acids, and Cholesterol by Animal Products in Diets of Women, Ages 19–50 Years

| Food Source | Total Fat | Saturated Fatty Acids | Cholesterol |
|---|---|---|---|
| Milk and milk products | 15 | 30 | 15 |
| Eggs | 5 | 5 | 40 |
| Red meat, poultry, and fish[a] | 25 | 25 | 35 |
| Fats, animal origin | 10 | 10 | 5 |

NOTE:   Estimates are from a partly completed system to classify ingredients in mixtures by the appropriate food group. Ingredients in some commercially prepared foods such as breads, cereals, and snack foods have not yet been classified. Percentages are shown to the nearest 5.0 percent.

[a]Red meat is beef, veal, pork, and lamb.

SOURCE:   Human Nutrition Information Service, U.S. Department of Agriculture, unpublished data, 1987.

TABLE 2-13  Contribution of Animal Products to Selected Vitamins and Minerals in the Diet Based on 3-Day Intake (in percent)

| Nutrient | Animal Product | | | |
| | Milk and Milk Products | Eggs | Red Meat, Poultry, and Fish[a] | Total[b] |
| --- | --- | --- | --- | --- |
| Food energy | 14.3 | 2.4 | 28.4 | 45.1 |
| Vitamins | | | | |
|   Preformed niacin | 2.4 | 0.2 | 44.3 | 46.9 |
|   Riboflavin | 29.7 | 4.4 | 24.2 | 58.3 |
|   Thiamine | 11.0 | 1.6 | 23.6 | 36.2 |
|   Vitamin A | 16.4 | 4.1 | 12.0 | 32.5 |
|   Vitamin $B_6$ | 10.9 | 2.1 | 39.9 | 52.9 |
|   Vitamin $B_{12}$ | 30.4 | 7.9 | 51.1 | 89.4 |
|   Vitamin C | 5.8 | —[c] | 5.2 | 11.0 |
| Minerals | | | | |
|   Calcium | 50.4 | 2.8 | 7.5 | 60.7 |
|   Iron | 3.7 | 3.8 | 34.5 | 42.0 |
|   Magnesium | 18.0 | 1.4 | 17.4 | 36.8 |
|   Phosphorus | 28.9 | 3.9 | 29.0 | 61.8 |

NOTE:  Food groups include mixtures with main ingredient from the group; therefore, vitamins and minerals from some vegetable sources in such mixtures are included. Vitamins and minerals from small amounts of animal sources in mainly vegetable mixtures are excluded.

[a]Red meat is beef, veal, pork, and lamb.
[b]The total is for the three groups of animal products shown.
[c]Value is less than 0.05 but more than 0.0.

SOURCE:  U.S. Department of Agriculture. 1984. Pp. 88–149 in Nutrient Intakes: Individuals in 48 States, Year 1977–78. Nationwide Food Consumption Survey 1977–78. Report I-2, Human Nutrition Information Service. Hyattsville, Md.: U.S. Department of Agriculture.

serine, arginine, and lysine. The presence of lactose (the carbohydrate found exclusively in animal products) and/or acidophilic flora (such as lactobacilli in cultured dairy products) also increases calcium absorption.

Substances that form insoluble complexes with calcium hinder its normal absorption; these include phytates (found in the outer layers of cereal grains), oxalates (present in spinach, Swiss chard, beet tops, cocoa, and rhubarb), and free fatty acids. Foods high in saturated fatty acids are likely to produce free fatty acids that will then combine with calcium to form insoluble complexes.

Data from the 1977–1978 NFCS indicate that animal products contribute about 60.7 percent of the total calcium in the diet (Table 2–15). Of this amount, the milk and milk products category provides 50.4 per-

cent and the meats and eggs categories contribute 7.5 and 2.8 percent, respectively. Grain products provide 22 percent, some of which is provided by ingredients from animal sources such as milk and eggs.

## TRENDS IN INDIVIDUAL COMMODITIES

### Red Meat, Poultry, and Fish

*Food Supply Data (1965–1985)*

In 1985 the total food supply of red meat, poultry, and fish was at an all-time high of 185 pounds per capita, edible weight (Table 2–16)—a 15 percent increase over 1965 and an 8 percent increase over 1975. This edible weight series is new from the USDA as of 1985. Data on fish, which is reported by the U.S. Department of Commerce, have always been reported on an edible weight basis, but a comparable series was not available for red meat and poultry. The purpose of reporting the data on an edible weight basis is to facilitate quantity comparisons between types of meat. The edible weight measure excludes all bones but does include the 0.25 to 0.5 inch of separable fat

normally sold on retail cuts of red meat. The trends for individual commodities, though, have differed greatly, with changes in different directions and of different magnitudes.

The largest increase in per capita disappearance has been for poultry; between 1965 and 1985, chicken increased 72 percent and turkey increased 62 percent. From 1980 to

TABLE 2-14  Contribution of Animal Products to Iron in the Diet Based on 3-Day Intake (in percent)

| Group and Age | Number of Survey Participants | Animal Product | | | |
| | | Milk and Milk Products | Eggs | Red Meat, Poultry, and Fish[a] | Total[b] |
|---|---|---|---|---|---|
| Children | | | | | |
| <1 | 421 | 32.6 | 1.4 | 6.2 | 40.2 |
| 1–2 | 1,035 | 6.5 | 5.0 | 25.3 | 36.8 |
| 3–5 | 1,719 | 5.0 | 3.8 | 26.6 | 35.4 |
| 6–8 | 1,841 | 5.0 | 2.7 | 28.1 | 35.8 |
| Females | | | | | |
| 9–11 | 1,011 | 4.9 | 2.6 | 29.1 | 36.6 |
| 12–14 | 1,148 | 4.7 | 2.6 | 32.1 | 39.4 |
| 15–18 | 1,473 | 4.1 | 2.9 | 35.4 | 42.4 |
| 19–22 | 1,317 | 3.4 | 3.8 | 36.6 | 43.8 |
| 23–34 | 3,879 | 2.9 | 3.8 | 37.1 | 43.8 |
| 35–50 | 3,759 | 2.4 | 4.2 | 37.6 | 44.2 |
| 51–64 | 2,936 | 2.3 | 4.1 | 35.4 | 41.8 |
| 65–74 | 1,376 | 2.4 | 4.1 | 31.9 | 38.4 |
| 75+ | 751 | 2.9 | 4.3 | 28.9 | 36.1 |
| Males | | | | | |
| 9–11 | 939 | 4.7 | 2.8 | 30.2 | 37.7 |
| 12–14 | 1,150 | 4.7 | 2.7 | 31.0 | 38.4 |
| 15–18 | 1,394 | 4.3 | 3.4 | 35.4 | 43.1 |
| 19–22 | 1,030 | 3.2 | 3.8 | 40.5 | 47.5 |
| 23–34 | 2,716 | 2.7 | 4.0 | 40.3 | 47.0 |
| 35–50 | 2,571 | 2.2 | 4.4 | 40.3 | 46.9 |
| 51–64 | 2,161 | 2.2 | 4.6 | 38.3 | 45.1 |
| 65–74 | 1,049 | 2.3 | 5.1 | 33.4 | 40.8 |
| 75+ | 465 | 2.6 | 6.0 | 31.2 | 39.8 |
| Total | 36,142 | 3.7 | 3.8 | 34.5 | 42.0 |

NOTE: Food groups include mixtures with main ingredient from the group; therefore, iron from some vegetable sources in such mixtures is included. Iron from small amounts of animal sources in mainly vegetable mixtures is excluded.

[a]Red meat is beef, veal, pork, and lamb.
[b]The total is for the three groups of animal products shown.

SOURCE: U.S. Department of Agriculture. 1984. P. 94 in Nutrient Intakes: Individuals in 48 States, Year 1977–78. Nationwide Food Consumption Survey 1977–78. Report I-2, Human Nutrition Information Service. Hyattsville, Md.: U.S. Department of Agriculture.

TABLE 2-15   Contribution of Animal Products to Calcium in the Diet Based on 3-Day Intake (in percent)

| | | Animal Product | | | |
| Group and Age | Number of Survey Participants | Milk and Milk Products | Eggs | Red Meat, Poultry, and Fish[a] | Total[b] |
|---|---|---|---|---|---|
| Children | | | | | |
| <1 | 421 | 74.4 | 0.6 | 1.7 | 76.7 |
| 1–2 | 1,035 | 71.0 | 2.4 | 3.3 | 76.7 |
| 3–5 | 1,719 | 66.3 | 2.1 | 3.7 | 72.1 |
| 6–8 | 1,841 | 66.9 | 1.4 | 4.0 | 72.3 |
| Females | | | | | |
| 9–11 | 1,011 | 65.0 | 1.4 | 4.3 | 70.7 |
| 12–14 | 1,148 | 60.5 | 1.6 | 5.5 | 67.6 |
| 15–18 | 1,473 | 56.0 | 2.0 | 7.3 | 65.3 |
| 19–22 | 1,317 | 48.5 | 2.9 | 8.9 | 60.3 |
| 23–34 | 3,879 | 45.7 | 2.9 | 8.9 | 57.5 |
| 35–50 | 3,759 | 40.3 | 3.6 | 9.2 | 53.1 |
| 51–64 | 2,936 | 42.1 | 3.3 | 8.5 | 53.9 |
| 65–74 | 1,376 | 44.9 | 3.0 | 7.1 | 55.0 |
| 75+ | 751 | 48.8 | 3.0 | 5.7 | 57.5 |
| Males | | | | | |
| 9–11 | 939 | 64.3 | 1.6 | 4.7 | 70.6 |
| 12–14 | 1,150 | 62.6 | 1.5 | 5.1 | 69.2 |
| 15–18 | 1,394 | 58.9 | 2.2 | 6.6 | 67.7 |
| 19–22 | 1,030 | 49.4 | 2.8 | 9.4 | 61.6 |
| 23–34 | 2,716 | 44.7 | 3.2 | 9.7 | 57.6 |
| 35–50 | 2,571 | 39.3 | 3.9 | 10.1 | 53.3 |
| 51–64 | 2,161 | 42.4 | 3.8 | 9.2 | 55.4 |
| 65–74 | 1,049 | 44.8 | 4.0 | 8.0 | 56.8 |
| 75+ | 465 | 45.0 | 4.5 | 6.6 | 56.1 |
| Total | 36,142 | 50.4 | 2.8 | 7.5 | 60.7 |

NOTE:   Food groups include mixtures with main ingredient from the group; therefore, calcium from some vegetable sources in such mixtures is included. Calcium from small amounts of animal sources in mainly vegetable mixtures is excluded.

[a]Red meat is beef, veal, pork, and lamb.
[b]The total is for the three groups of animal products shown.

SOURCE:   U.S. Department of Agriculture. 1984. P. 88 in Nutrient Intakes: Individuals in 48 States, Year 1977–78. Nationwide Food Consumption Survey 1977–78. Report I-2, Human Nutrition Information Service. Hyattsville, Md.: U.S. Department of Agriculture.

1985, total poultry increased more than 13 percent; from 1975 to 1985, it rose more than 40 percent.

In 1985 per capita disappearance of red meat was about .7 percent higher than it was in 1965, but it has dropped about 2.5 percent since 1975 and about 2 percent since 1980. Per capita disappearance of red meat has decreased more than 10 percent from its highest level of 135.3 pounds in 1971 to its 1985 level of 121.4 pounds.

Beef accounts for more than 60 percent of the four items (beef, veal, lamb, and pork) in the red meat category. In 1985 per capita disappearance was up about 7 percent compared to 20 years ago (74.4 pounds in 1985 versus 69.5 pounds in 1965). Per capita disappearance of beef peaked in 1976, at

89.0 pounds. Both veal and lamb, which together make up a little over 2 percent of total red meat, have remained stable over the past 10 years at about 1.5 pounds per capita, although they are both at less than half their 1965 levels.

Per capita disappearance of pork has fluctuated considerably during the past 15 years, from a high of 52.7 pounds in 1971 to a low of 37.1 pounds in 1975. In 1985, it was 44.2 pounds. At present, pork accounts for more than a third of the total red meat in the food supply.

Fish in the food supply was at a record high of 14.5 pounds per capita in 1985, up nearly 19 percent since 1975 and 34 percent since 1965.

A number of theories attempt to explain these trends. Short-term reactions to situations such as shifts in consumer price relationships owing to increased supplies of one commodity relative to another may account for some changes. Other, longer term factors, such as diet and health concerns, might also play an important role (Stucker and Parham, 1984).

Although the food supply data do not directly measure food intake, they have been used to estimate the amount of food potentially available on a cooked, edible

TABLE 2-16   Per Capita Disappearance of Red Meat, Poultry, and Fish by Edible Weight (in pounds)

| Year | Red Meat | | | | | Poultry | | | Fish | Total |
|------|------|------|------|------|-------|---------|--------|-------|------|-------|
|      | Beef | Veal | Pork | Lamb | Total | Chicken | Turkey | Total |      |       |
| 1965 | 69.5 | 3.6 | 45.0 | 2.4 | 120.5 | 23.1 | 5.8 | 28.9 | 10.8 | 160.2 |
| 1966 | 72.7 | 3.2 | 44.0 | 2.6 | 122.5 | 24.7 | 6.2 | 30.9 | 10.9 | 164.3 |
| 1967 | 74.3 | 2.6 | 48.2 | 2.6 | 127.7 | 25.4 | 6.7 | 32.1 | 10.6 | 170.4 |
| 1968 | 76.6 | 2.5 | 49.2 | 2.4 | 130.7 | 25.4 | 6.2 | 31.6 | 11.0 | 173.3 |
| 1969 | 77.3 | 2.3 | 47.8 | 2.3 | 129.7 | 26.6 | 6.6 | 33.2 | 11.2 | 174.1 |
| 1970 | 79.3 | 2.0 | 48.6 | 2.1 | 131.9 | 28.0 | 6.3 | 34.3 | 11.8 | 178.0 |
| 1971 | 78.7 | 1.8 | 52.7 | 2.1 | 135.3 | 28.0 | 6.6 | 34.6 | 11.5 | 181.4 |
| 1972 | 80.6 | 1.5 | 47.5 | 2.2 | 131.8 | 29.0 | 7.0 | 36.0 | 12.5 | 180.3 |
| 1973 | 75.9 | 1.2 | 42.5 | 1.7 | 121.3 | 28.1 | 6.7 | 34.8 | 12.8 | 168.9 |
| 1974 | 80.8 | 1.6 | 45.9 | 1.5 | 129.8 | 28.3 | 7.0 | 35.3 | 12.1 | 177.2 |
| 1975 | 82.9 | 2.8 | 37.1 | 1.3 | 124.1 | 27.8 | 6.7 | 34.5 | 12.2 | 170.8 |
| 1976 | 89.0 | 2.7 | 39.3 | 1.2 | 132.2 | 29.5 | 7.2 | 36.7 | 12.9 | 181.8 |
| 1977 | 86.6 | 2.6 | 40.5 | 1.1 | 130.8 | 30.6 | 7.2 | 37.8 | 12.7 | 181.3 |
| 1978 | 82.3 | 2.0 | 40.4 | 1.0 | 125.8 | 32.3 | 7.3 | 39.6 | 13.4 | 178.8 |
| 1979 | 73.6 | 1.4 | 46.1 | 1.0 | 122.1 | 35.0 | 7.8 | 42.8 | 13.0 | 177.9 |
| 1980 | 72.2 | 1.2 | 49.2 | 1.0 | 123.6 | 34.7 | 8.3 | 43.0 | 12.8 | 179.4 |
| 1981 | 72.7 | 1.3 | 46.8 | 1.1 | 121.9 | 35.8 | 8.5 | 44.3 | 12.9 | 179.1 |
| 1982 | 72.8 | 1.4 | 41.9 | 1.1 | 117.2 | 36.8 | 8.5 | 45.3 | 12.3 | 174.8 |
| 1983 | 74.1 | 1.4 | 44.4 | 1.1 | 120.9 | 37.3 | 8.9 | 46.2 | 13.1 | 180.2 |
| 1984 | 74.0 | 1.4 | 44.0 | 1.1 | 120.5 | 38.6 | 9.0 | 47.6 | 13.7 | 181.8 |
| 1985 | 74.6 | 1.5 | 44.2 | 1.1 | 121.4 | 39.7 | 9.4 | 49.1 | 14.5 | 185.0 |

NOTE: The edible weight measure excludes all bones but includes the 0.25 to 0.50 inch of separable fat normally sold on retail cuts of red meat. Conversion factors from carcass to edible weight are beef, 0.698; pork, 0.67; veal, 0.685; lamb, 0.658; broilers, 0.69; other chicken, 0.73; and turkey, 0.79.

SOURCE: K. L. Bunch. 1987. P. 15 in Food Consumption, Prices, and Expenditures, 1985. Statistical Bulletin 749, Economic Research Service, U.S. Department of Agriculture. Washington, D.C.: U.S. Government Printing Office.

basis. The 185 pounds of red meat, poultry, and fish available per capita in 1985 translates to roughly 8.1 ounces per day, raw weight. The USDA estimates that cooking losses for meat, poultry, and fish range from 15 to 30 percent, depending on the type of commodity and the method of preparation (U.S. Department of Agriculture, 1975). Using this adjustment for the conversion of the data indicates that roughly 5.7 to 7.0 ounces of cooked, edible red meat, poultry, and fish were available from the food supply per person per day in 1985. Spoilage, plate waste, and trimming during preparation further reduced the amount actually ingested. Also, this estimate does not take into account differences in intake by age and sex groups or variations that occur in daily intake.

### Dietary Survey Data

In general, the dietary survey data reflect the decline in red meat consumption indicated by the food supply data (Table 2–17). Comparison of data from the 1977–1978 NFCS and the 1985 CSFII indicates that the average daily intake of beef by women ages 19 to 50 declined by 45 percent compared with 22 percent for pork and 19 percent for processed meats. In contrast to the food supply data, the survey of women's diets indicated a 14 percent decline in chicken intake. Comparison of data from the 1977–1978 NFCS and 1985 CSFII indicate that the intake of fish increased 18 percent.

Despite significant declines in the intake of red meat by women between 1977 and 1985, intake of the total red meat, poultry, and fish category declined only slightly. Mixtures accounted for half of the total intake of the red meat, poultry, and fish category in 1985, compared with one-third in 1977. The shift to mixtures signifies that meats are being used more as an ingredient in meals and less as a separate menu item.

The 1985 CSFII data indicate that changes in men's intake of meat were similar to those for women. Mixtures that may have included foods other than meats (such as grains) accounted for two-thirds of the total intake of red meat, poultry, and fish.

### National Live Stock & Meat Board Study

The National Live Stock & Meat Board study, "Contribution of Red Meat to the U.S. Diet" (Breidenstein and Williams, 1987), estimated meat intake using per capita disappearance data and private survey data (Yankelovich, Skelly and White, Inc., 1985). The private survey segmented the population into different user levels (light, moderate, or heavy) on the basis of telephone interviews of 1,211 individuals identified as the primary food shopper for the household. This analysis differs from recall data from dietary surveys in that estimates for "ingested" and "available" red meats are reconciled numerically. The surveyors estimated that daily per capita cooked red meat intake for light users was 41.4 grams (1.45 ounces); for moderate users, 117 grams (4.14 ounces); and for heavy users, 216.31 grams (7.66 ounces). The estimated breakdown by different types of meat is given in Table 2–18. The nutrient contribution of red meat by use level is summarized in Table 2–19. The committee believes that the data provide a useful analysis of red meat consumption in the United States.

## Milk, Milk Products, and Eggs

### Food Supply Data (1965–1985)

Historically, milk and milk products have been an important part of the U.S. diet. But as for red meats, trends for individual milk and milk products differ greatly (Table 2–20): low-fat milk, yogurt, and hard cheese have increased the most of all products in this category from 1965 to 1985, whereas

TABLE 2-17   Meat, Poultry, and Fish: Trends in Consumption and Mean Intake

| Group and Food | Number of Survey Participants | | Mean Intake (g/day) | | Percent Consuming | |
|---|---|---|---|---|---|---|
| | 1977 | 1985 | 1977 | 1985 | 1977 | 1985 |
| Children, 1–5 | 690 | 548 | | | | |
| Beef | | | 21 | 14 | 29.1 | 17.5 |
| Pork | | | 7 | 7 | 20.5 | 16.2 |
| Lamb, veal, and game | | | —[b] | 1 | 0.3 | 1.4 |
| Organ meats | | | —[b] | —[b] | 0.7 | 0.3 |
| Frankfurters, sausages, and luncheon meats | | | 15 | 12 | 33.1 | 28.2 |
| Chicken | | | 17 | 16 | 17.0 | 19.6 |
| Fish and shellfish | | | 5 | 5 | 7.0 | 8.1 |
| Mixtures[a] | | | 45 | 45 | 34.7 | 32.0 |
| Females, 19–50 | 2,228 | 1,503 | | | | |
| Beef | | | 49 | 27 | 34.9 | 23.1 |
| Pork | | | 18 | 14 | 24.0 | 20.5 |
| Lamb, veal, and game | | | 1 | 1 | 1.3 | 1.0 |
| Organ meats | | | 1 | 1 | 0.9 | 1.0 |
| Frankfurters, sausages, and luncheon meats | | | 16 | 13 | 25.1 | 24.6 |
| Chicken | | | 22 | 19 | 16.1 | 16.8 |
| Fish and shellfish | | | 11 | 13 | 9.8 | 11.5 |
| Mixtures[a] | | | 65 | 88 | 33.2 | 37.1 |
| Males, 19–50 | 1,778 | 1,134 | | | | |
| Beef | | | 80 | 52 | 42.0 | 28.3 |
| Pork | | | 28 | 26 | 28.2 | 25.3 |
| Lamb, veal, and game | | | 3 | 1 | 1.9 | 0.5 |
| Organ meats | | | 2 | 1 | 1.4 | 0.4 |
| Frankfurters, sausages, and luncheon meats | | | 32 | 27 | 35.7 | 31.4 |
| Chicken | | | 28 | 23 | 14.0 | 13.3 |
| Fish and shellfish | | | 14 | 21 | 8.5 | 11.4 |
| Mixtures[a] | | | 105 | 110 | 39.0 | 39.7 |

[a]Mixtures are mainly meat, poultry, or fish.
[b]Values are less than 0.5 but more than 0.0.

SOURCES:   Adapted from U.S. Department of Agriculture. 1985. Pp. 10 and 12 in Women 19–50 Years and Their Children 1–5 Years, 1 Day, 1985. Nationwide Food Consumption Survey, Continuing Survey of Food Intakes by Individuals. Report 85-1, Human Nutrition Information Service. Hyattsville, Md.: U.S. Department of Agriculture. U.S. Department of Agriculture. 1986. Pp. 8–9 in Men 19–50 Years, 1 Day, 1985. Nationwide Food Consumption Survey, Continuing Survey of Food Intakes by Individuals. Report 85-3, Human Nutrition Information Service. Hyattsville, Md.: U.S. Department of Agriculture. See these reports for information on changes in methods and data bases that may affect differences in results between 1977 and 1985.

whole and processed milk (condensed and evaporated) have shown the largest decrease during the same period.

Whole, low-fat, skim and flavored milks and buttermilk currently constitute nearly three-fourths of the milk and milk products group on a product weight basis. In 1985 per capita sales of fluid whole milk was at about half the level it was in 1965 (116.5 pounds versus 236.5 pounds). In contrast, per capita sales of low-fat milk increased more than 680 percent during this same period, from 10.9 pounds in 1965 to 85.0 pounds in 1985. This dramatic shift from

TABLE 2-18  Estimated Average Daily Consumption of Cooked Red Meats in the U.S. Diet, 1984

| Red Meat | Light Grams | Light Ounces | Moderate Grams | Moderate Ounces | Heavy Grams | Heavy Ounces |
|---|---|---|---|---|---|---|
| Beef | 16.31 | 0.57 | 42.16 | 1.49 | 67.44 | 2.38 |
| Ground beef | 7.89 | 0.28 | 17.50 | 0.62 | 30.14 | 1.06 |
| Pork | 2.80 | 0.10 | 11.17 | 0.39 | 21.99 | 0.78 |
| Lamb | 0.32 | 0.01 | 0.62 | 0.02 | 1.23 | 0.04 |
| Veal | 0.63 | 0.02 | 1.22 | 0.04 | 2.41 | 0.09 |
| Processed meat | 13.18 | 0.47 | 44.33 | 1.56 | 93.11 | 2.38 |
| Total red meat ingested | 41.14 | 1.45 | 117.00 | 4.14 | 216.31 | 7.66 |

NOTE:  The values are reconciled from data on total amounts of red meat available for consumption in the United States. (The values are corrected for cooking losses and for amounts of trimmable fat discarded by consumers, assuming that no meat spoiled.)

SOURCE:  Adapted from B. C. Breidenstein and J. C. Williams. 1987. Contribution of Red Meat to the U.S. Diet. Chicago, Ill.: National Live Stock & Meat Board.

TABLE 2-19  Nutrient Contribution of Total Cooked Red Meat Ingestion by Consumption Level in the U.S. Diet, 1984

| Nutrient | Consumption Level Light | Consumption Level Moderate | Consumption Level Heavy | Total Ingested by Average User | RDA (%)[a] |
|---|---|---|---|---|---|
| Total red meat,[b] g | 41.14 | 117.00 | 216.31 | 118.89 | |
| Total red meat, oz | 1.45 | 4.13 | 7.63 | 4.19 | |
| Calories, kcal | 117.5 | 334.9 | 618.1 | 340.1 | 17.0 |
| Cholesterol, mg | 33.4 | 92.2 | 167.8 | 93.2 | — |
| Lipids, g | 8.48 | 24.46 | 45.55 | 24.95 | — |
| Protein, g | 9.47 | 26.33 | 47.57 | 26.44 | 47.2 |
| Vitamins | | | | | |
|   Niacin, mg | 1.751 | 4.911 | 9.062 | 4.998 | 27.8 |
|   Riboflavin, mg | 0.063 | 0.189 | 0.372 | 0.198 | 12.4 |
|   Thiamine, mg | 0.091 | 0.302 | 0.605 | 0.317 | 22.7 |
|   Vitamin $B_{12}$, µg | 0.830 | 2.207 | 3.899 | 2.200 | 73.3 |
| Minerals | | | | | |
|   Iron, mg | 0.91 | 2.49 | 4.44 | 2.50 | 25.0 |
|   Sodium, mg | 160.9 | 526.4 | 1,086.4 | 568.4 | 17.2–51.7 |
|   Zinc, mg | 1.77 | 4.75 | 8.27 | 4.71 | 31.4 |

NOTE:  The values are reconciled from data on total amounts of red meat available for consumption in the United States. (The values are corrected for cooking losses and for amounts of trimmable fat discarded by consumers, assuming that no meat spoiled.)

[a]This column represents the percentage of recommended dietary allowances (RDAs) for males ages 23–50 except for lipids, cholesterol, calories, and sodium entries. There are no RDAs for lipids and cholesterol. The calorie percentage is based on 2,000 kcal mean energy needs of a 154-lb sedentary U.S. adult male or active female. The sodium percentage is based on a 1,100- to 3,300-mg range of estimated safe and adequate daily intake for adults (National Research Council. 1980. Recommended Dietary Allowances. Washington, D.C.: National Academy Press).

[b]Red meat is beef, veal, pork, and lamb. In this case, the category also includes processed meats.

SOURCE:  Adapted from B. C. Breidenstein and J. C. Williams. 1987. Contribution of Red Meat to the U.S. Diet. Chicago, Ill.: National Live Stock & Meat Board.

TABLE 2-20  Per Capita Trends for Selected Milk, Milk Products, and Eggs

| | Milk (lb) | | | | Milk Products (lb) | | | | | | | |
| | Whole[a] | Low-fat[a] | Skim[a] | Flavored and Buttermilk[a] | Butter[b] | Cheese (Whole and Part-Whole Milk)[b] | Condensed and Evaporated (Processed) Milk[b] | Cottage Cheese[b] | Cream Products[a] | Frozen Dairy Products (Desserts)[b] | Yogurt[a] | Eggs (number)[c] |
| Year | | | | | | | | | | | | |
|---|---|---|---|---|---|---|---|---|---|---|---|---|
| 1965 | 236.5 | 10.9 | 12.6 | 14.9 | 6.4 | 9.6 | 22.8 | 4.7 | 6.7 | 28.1 | 0.3 | 313.2 |
| 1966 | 234.1 | 14.5 | 11.0 | 15.0 | 5.7 | 9.8 | 22.6 | 4.6 | 6.3 | 28.1 | 0.4 | 312.3 |
| 1967 | 223.7 | 18.4 | 10.7 | 14.5 | 5.5 | 10.1 | 21.4 | 4.5 | 5.9 | 27.8 | 0.5 | 320.5 |
| 1968 | 218.6 | 22.7 | 11.3 | 14.8 | 5.7 | 10.6 | 21.5 | 4.6 | 5.6 | 28.8 | 0.6 | 315.7 |
| 1969 | 212.1 | 27.3 | 11.7 | 14.6 | 5.4 | 10.9 | 20.6 | 4.8 | 5.2 | 28.8 | 0.9 | 310.2 |
| 1970 | 206.9 | 30.7 | 11.9 | 14.5 | 5.3 | 11.5 | 19.4 | 5.2 | 5.0 | 28.4 | 0.8 | 309.1 |
| 1971 | 199.3 | 35.8 | 11.5 | 14.8 | 5.1 | 12.1 | 19.4 | 5.4 | 4.9 | 28.1 | 1.2 | 310.6 |
| 1972 | 195.0 | 40.1 | 12.6 | 15.3 | 4.9 | 13.5 | 17.8 | 5.5 | 4.9 | 28.0 | 1.4 | 302.9 |
| 1973 | 186.2 | 44.0 | 14.1 | 15.0 | 4.8 | 13.6 | 17.7 | 5.3 | 5.0 | 27.7 | 1.5 | 289.2 |
| 1974 | 175.2 | 46.4 | 14.1 | 13.8 | 4.5 | 14.6 | 15.9 | 4.7 | 5.0 | 27.7 | 1.6 | 283.8 |
| 1975 | 173.2 | 54.9 | 11.9 | 14.8 | 4.7 | 14.3 | 14.8 | 4.7 | 5.2 | 28.7 | 2.1 | 276.4 |
| 1976 | 165.5 | 58.6 | 11.9 | 15.8 | 4.3 | 15.7 | 15.0 | 4.7 | 5.1 | 27.5 | 2.2 | 270.0 |
| 1977 | 157.4 | 62.3 | 12.1 | 16.3 | 4.3 | 16.1 | 14.5 | 4.7 | 5.1 | 27.5 | 2.4 | 267.7 |
| 1978 | 152.6 | 65.6 | 11.7 | 15.8 | 4.4 | 17.0 | 13.9 | 4.7 | 5.1 | 27.3 | 2.6 | 272.6 |
| 1979 | 146.9 | 68.3 | 11.8 | 15.0 | 4.5 | 17.2 | 14.1 | 4.5 | 5.2 | 26.3 | 2.5 | 277.7 |
| 1980 | 140.6 | 71.8 | 11.8 | 14.4 | 4.5 | 17.6 | 13.3 | 4.5 | 5.7 | 26.5 | 2.6 | 272.4 |
| 1981 | 135.0 | 74.1 | 11.5 | 14.0 | 4.3 | 18.4 | 12.9 | 4.4 | 5.3 | 26.3 | 2.6 | 265.5 |
| 1982 | 130.5 | 75.6 | 11.0 | 13.6 | 4.6 | 20.1 | 12.7 | 4.2 | 5.6 | 26.4 | 2.7 | 265.2 |
| 1983 | 127.2 | 77.7 | 11.0 | 14.4 | 5.1 | 20.6 | 14.2 | 4.2 | 5.9 | 27.0 | 3.2 | 261.2 |
| 1984 | 122.6 | 80.7 | 11.9 | 15.2 | 5.0 | 21.7 | 14.1 | 4.2 | 6.4 | 27.1 | 3.6 | 260.9 |
| 1985[d] | 116.5 | 85.0 | 13.0 | 15.0 | 5.1 | 22.4 | 14.2 | 4.1 | 7.0 | 27.2 | 4.0 | 254.6 |

[a]Values are based on per capita sales figures.
[b]Values are based on per capita consumption figures.
[c]Values are based on civilian consumption only. Values include shell eggs and the appropriate shell-egg equivalent of dried and frozen eggs.
[d]Values are estimated for 1985.

SOURCE:  Adapted from K. Bunch and G. Simon, eds. 1985. Pp. 21, 22, and 25 in Food Consumption, Prices, and Expenditures, 1964–84. Statistical Bulletin 736, Economic Research Service, U.S. Department of Agriculture. Washington, D.C.: U.S. Government Printing Office.

whole milk to low-fat milk is most likely due to a combination of health concerns and taste preferences, since the per capita sales of skim milk have remained at about the same level for two decades. Bunch (1985) suggests that the food supply of fluid milk has declined due to demographic changes and competition from other beverages.

Yogurt is another dairy product that has increased tremendously in the food supply, particularly during the past 10 years. Between 1980 and 1985 it increased over 50 percent, between 1975 and 1985 it increased more than 90 percent, and between 1965 and 1985 it increased more than 1,200 percent. Nevertheless, per capita sales of yogurt account for little more than 1 percent of all dairy products. The amount of hard cheese in the food supply has also increased, by over 27 percent since 1980, by 95 percent between 1970 and 1985, and by more than 130 percent between 1965 and 1985. Ice cream, cottage cheese, and butter have remained around their 1970 levels.

### Dietary Survey Data

*NFCS (1977–1978).* The percentage of individuals using fluid milk decreased abruptly for those in their late teens and early twenties. Whereas 94 percent of males and 89 percent of females ages 15 to 18 drank milk at least once during the 3 survey days, only 78 percent of the males and 79 percent of the females ages 23 to 34 reported consuming milk. Average intake and serving size also dropped abruptly after age 18. Milk consumption for males was highest for 12- to 18-year-olds, who consumed an average of 19 ounces a day.

Women ages 35 to 50 drank the least amount of milk in the survey, averaging only 5 ounces per day. Twenty-eight percent of the women in this age group had not drunk milk on any of the 3 survey days. Males drank more milk than females in every age group.

Fifty-four percent of the survey respondents consumed eggs on at least 1 of the 3 survey days (Table 2–21). (Data are for eggs that are reported as a separate food and do not include quantities eaten as an ingredient in other foods.) In general, males had slightly higher intakes than females, averaging 37 grams per day compared to 24 grams for females. One large egg weighs approximately 50 grams. The survey data indicate that older adults eat eggs more frequently than do younger adults, although the intake per user is not as high. Twenty-four percent of males and 13 percent of females ages 65 and older ate eggs on all 3 of the survey days, compared with only 10 percent of the total population.

*CSFII (1985).* Women's intake of milk as a beverage and in dairy products has remained relatively constant between 1977 and 1985 (Table 2–22). The changes within the dairy category parallel those found in the food supply data. Total fluid milk intake declined 5 percent, but there was a substantial shift from whole milk, which was down 35 percent, to low-fat and skim milk, which was up 60 percent. Only about half of the women had drunk milk on the day surveyed (Behlen, 1986).

Cheese intake was up 6 percent from 1977 to 1985. This is much less of an increase than that indicated by the food supply data. However, a large proportion of cheese is consumed as an ingredient in mixed foods such as macaroni and cheese and in pizza, and in the CSFII, these foods would be included in the grain mixtures category. Similarly, cheese served on a hamburger or in a ham and cheese sandwich would be included in the meat mixtures category. Intake of meat mixtures and grain mixtures increased significantly from the previous survey. Therefore, the smaller increase in cheese intake in the CSFII is likely associated with the fact that more meat and grain mixtures are being eaten.

TABLE 2-21  Intake of Eggs

| Group and Age | Number of Survey Participants | Average Quantity/Eating Occasion[a] (g) | Consumption Level on: | | |
|---|---|---|---|---|---|
| | | | At Least 1 of 3 Days | Only 1 of 3 Days | 3 of 3 Days |
| Children | | | | | |
| <1 | 498 | 49 | 17.7 | 8.9 | 3.1 |
| 1–2 | 1,045 | 59 | 61.3 | 31.2 | 10.4 |
| 3–5 | 1,719 | 66 | 55.2 | 32.4 | 7.1 |
| 6–8 | 1,841 | 70 | 48.5 | 32.8 | 4.0 |
| Females | | | | | |
| 9–14 | 2,158 | 75 | 44.3 | 28.2 | 5.0 |
| 15–18 | 1,473 | 79 | 44.4 | 27.5 | 3.9 |
| 19–34 | 5,346 | 83 | 51.1 | 29.1 | 6.6 |
| 35–64 | 7,069 | 74 | 56.7 | 29.5 | 11.3 |
| 65–74 | 1,738 | 64 | 57.4 | 28.9 | 12.2 |
| 75+ | 993 | 63 | 57.4 | 29.5 | 13.7 |
| Males | | | | | |
| 9–14 | 2,089 | 85 | 49.1 | 31.2 | 5.4 |
| 15–18 | 1,394 | 101 | 52.3 | 27.0 | 9.6 |
| 19–34 | 3,928 | 105 | 54.8 | 27.3 | 10.9 |
| 35–64 | 4,929 | 93 | 62.0 | 27.1 | 16.9 |
| 65–74 | 1,118 | 81 | 66.7 | 25.6 | 21.9 |
| 75+ | 536 | 73 | 71.7 | 21.3 | 28.8 |
| Total | 37,874 | 82 | 54.3 | 28.6 | 10.3 |

[a]One large egg weighs 50 g.

SOURCE: E. M. Pao, K. H. Fleming, P. M. Guenther, and S. J. Mickle. 1982. Foods Commonly Eaten by Individuals: Amount Per Day and Per Eating Occasion. Pp. 44–45 in Home Economics. Report No. 44, Human Nutrition Information Service, U.S. Department of Agriculture. Washington, D.C.: U.S. Government Printing Office.

## Fats and Oils

### Food Supply Data (1965–1985)

Quantities of fats and oils in the food supply are measured by the manufacture of products such as shortening, margarine, and salad and cooking oils (Table 2–23). Data include all fats and oils except those that occur naturally in foods such as meats, milk and milk products, and nuts. Between 1965 and 1985, per capita disappearance of fats and oils increased 32 percent. Over the same time period, there was a shift from animal to vegetable sources, although this trend seems to have leveled off (Figure 2–3).

About 50 percent of fats and oils are used in processed foods such as baked goods, salad dressing, and potato and corn chips.

The remainder is used by restaurants and institutions or purchased in grocery stores for home use. Restaurant use of fats and oils increased 69 percent between 1969 and 1979, primarily because of the increase in the number of fast-food restaurants and other establishments serving fried foods like chicken, fish, and french fried potatoes (Bunch and Hazera, 1984). Although there is little information on changes since 1979, restaurant use of edible tallow for frying is primarily responsible for the increased use of animal fats since 1980 (Karen Bunch, USDA Economic Research Service, personal communication, 1986).

In 1985, butter, lard, and tallow accounted for 20 percent of the total use of fats and oils. About 4 pounds of lard and tallow per capita were used directly, either

TABLE 2-22 Milk, Milk Products, Eggs, Fats, and Oils: Trends in Consumption and Mean Intake

| Group and Age | Number of Study Participants | | Mean Intakes (g/day) | | Percentage of Study Participants | |
|---|---|---|---|---|---|---|
| | 1977 | 1985 | 1977 | 1985 | 1977 | 1985 |
| Children, 1–5 | 690 | 548 | | | | |
| Total milk and milk products | | | 403 | 428 | 92.6 | 95.0 |
| Total fluid milk | | | 357 | 381 | 87.7 | 89.2 |
| Whole | | | 260 | 228 | 65.4 | 53.6 |
| Low-fat and skim | | | 97 | 153 | 25.6 | 38.1 |
| Cheese | | | 8 | 11 | 21.3 | 31.2 |
| Cream and milk desserts | | | 20 | 19 | 21.3 | 24.4 |
| Yogurt | | | 1 | 5 | 0.4 | 4.5 |
| Eggs | | | 21 | 17 | 33.0 | 28.5 |
| Total fats and oils | | | 7 | 5 | 50.2 | 51.2 |
| Table fats | | | 4 | 3 | 39.0 | 40.0 |
| Salad dressings | | | 2 | 2 | 16.6 | 18.2 |
| Females, 19–50 | 2,228 | 1,503 | | | | |
| Total milk and milk products | | | 204 | 203 | 74.4 | 76.5 |
| Total fluid milk | | | 148 | 141 | 54.9 | 51.4 |
| Whole | | | 98 | 64 | 39.0 | 26.0 |
| Low-fat and skim | | | 48 | 77 | 16.1 | 26.1 |
| Cheese | | | 17 | 18 | 27.5 | 33.9 |
| Cream and milk desserts | | | 19 | 24 | 20.0 | 25.0 |
| Yogurt | | | 6 | 8 | 2.9 | 4.5 |
| Eggs | | | 25 | 18 | 29.3 | 24.3 |
| Total fats and oils | | | 14 | 16 | 61.2 | 63.9 |
| Table fats | | | 5 | 4 | 39.8 | 39.1 |
| Salad dressings | | | 8 | 11 | 32.5 | 36.4 |
| Males, 19–50 | 1,778 | 1,134 | | | | |
| Total milk and milk products | | | 278 | 287 | 73.5 | 73.3 |
| Total fluid milk | | | 215 | 205 | 55.9 | 48.0 |
| Whole | | | 156 | 117 | 44.0 | 27.2 |
| Low-fat and skim | | | 57 | 87 | 13.0 | 21.3 |
| Cheese | | | 16 | 17 | 26.0 | 33.0 |
| Cream and milk desserts | | | 27 | 35 | 21.4 | 23.3 |
| Yogurt | | | 3 | 3 | 1.4 | 1.9 |
| Eggs | | | 35 | 26 | 34.2 | 28.3 |
| Total fats and oils | | | 17 | 18 | 59.5 | 64.2 |
| Table fats | | | 8 | 7 | 43.1 | 41.3 |
| Salad dressings | | | 8 | 10 | 27.6 | 34.2 |

SOURCES: Adapted from U.S. Department of Agriculture. 1985. Pp. 12–13 and 18–19 in Women 19–50 Years and Their Children 1–5 Years, 1 Day, 1985. Nationwide Food Consumption Survey, Continuing Survey of Food Intakes by Individuals. Report 85-1, Human Nutrition Information Service. Hyattsville, Md.: U.S. Department of Agriculture. U.S. Department of Agriculture. 1986. Pp. 10–11 and 16–17 in Men 19–50 Years, 1 Day, 1985. Nationwide Food Consumption Survey, Continuing Survey of Food Intakes by Individuals. Report 85-3, Human Nutrition Information Service. Hyattsville, Md.: U.S. Department of Agriculture. See these reports for information on changes in methods and data bases that may affect differences in results between 1977 and 1985.

TABLE 2-23  Per Capita Disappearance of Separated Fats and Oils (edible weight in pounds)

| Year | Direct Use[a] Butter | Direct Use[a] Tallow | Direct Use[a] Lard | Margarine | Shortening | Salad and Cooking Oils | Other Edible Oils | Total Excluding Butter | Total Fat Content[b] Total | Total Fat Content[b] Animal | Total Fat Content[b] Vegetable | Total Product Weight |
|---|---|---|---|---|---|---|---|---|---|---|---|---|
| 1965 | 6.4 | | 6.3 | 9.8 | 14.2 | 12.5 | 1.6 | 44.4 | 47.7 | 16.4 | 31.3 | 50.8 |
| 1966 | 5.7 | | 5.5 | 10.6 | 16.0 | 12.7 | 2.4 | 47.1 | 49.6 | 15.4 | 34.2 | 52.9 |
| 1967 | 5.5 | | 5.3 | 10.5 | 15.9 | 12.7 | 2.4 | 47.3 | 49.1 | 15.7 | 33.4 | 52.3 |
| 1968 | 5.7 | | 5.5 | 10.7 | 16.3 | 13.5 | 2.4 | 48.4 | 51.0 | 16.4 | 34.6 | 54.1 |
| 1969 | 5.4 | | 5.0 | 10.7 | 17.0 | 14.2 | 2.3 | 49.3 | 51.6 | 14.6 | 37.0 | 54.7 |
| 1970 | 5.3 | | 4.6 | 10.8 | 17.3 | 15.4 | 2.3 | 50.5 | 52.6 | 14.1 | 38.5 | 55.8 |
| 1971 | 5.1 | | 4.2 | 10.9 | 16.8 | 15.6 | 2.3 | 49.9 | 51.8 | 14.4 | 37.4 | 55.0 |
| 1972 | 4.9 | | 3.7 | 11.1 | 17.6 | 16.8 | 2.3 | 51.7 | 53.4 | 13.3 | 40.1 | 56.6 |
| 1973 | 4.8 | | 3.3 | 11.1 | 17.1 | 17.7 | 2.6 | 51.7 | 53.3 | 11.6 | 41.7 | 56.5 |
| 1974 | 4.5 | | 3.2 | 11.1 | 16.9 | 18.1 | 1.7 | 50.9 | 52.3 | 11.9 | 40.5 | 55.4 |
| 1975 | 4.7 | | 2.8 | 11.1 | 17.0 | 17.8 | 2.0 | 50.7 | 52.3 | 10.3 | 41.9 | 55.5 |
| 1976 | 4.3 | | 2.6 | 12.0 | 17.8 | 19.5 | 2.0 | 53.9 | 54.9 | 9.7 | 45.2 | 58.2 |
| 1977 | 4.3 | | 2.2 | 11.4 | 17.3 | 19.1 | 1.9 | 52.0 | 53.2 | 10.2 | 42.9 | 56.3 |
| 1978 | 4.4 | | 2.1 | 11.3 | 17.9 | 20.1 | 2.0 | 53.5 | 54.7 | 10.5 | 44.2 | 57.9 |
| 1979 | 4.5 | 0.4 | 2.5 | 11.3 | 18.4 | 20.8 | 1.7 | 55.1 | 56.4 | 11.4 | 45.0 | 59.6 |
| 1980 | 4.5 | 1.1 | 2.6 | 11.4 | 18.2 | 21.2 | 1.5 | 56.0 | 57.2 | 12.3 | 44.9 | 60.4 |
| 1981 | 4.3 | 1.0 | 2.5 | 11.2 | 18.5 | 21.8 | 1.4 | 56.4 | 57.5 | 11.7 | 45.8 | 60.6 |
| 1982 | 4.3 | 1.3 | 2.5 | 11.1 | 18.6 | 21.8 | 1.6 | 57.0 | 58.2 | 11.3 | 46.8 | 61.3 |
| 1983 | 4.9 | 2.0 | 2.1 | 10.4 | 18.5 | 23.5 | 1.6 | 58.1 | 59.9 | 12.0 | 47.9 | 63.0 |
| 1984 | 4.9 | 1.7 | 2.1 | 10.4 | 21.3 | 19.8 | 1.7 | 56.9 | 58.7 | 12.4 | 46.3 | 61.8 |
| 1985 | 4.9 | 1.9 | 1.8 | 10.7 | 22.8 | 23.5 | 1.6 | 62.3 | 64.0 | 12.8 | 51.2 | 67.2 |

NOTE:  Values represent those for the total population, except for butter values, which are based on the civilian population.

[a]Direct use excludes use in some margarine, shortening, and nonfood products.

[b]Fat content of butter and margarine is 80 percent of the product's weight. For all other products, fat content and product's weight are the same. Totals may not add due to rounding.

SOURCE:  K. L. Bunch. 1987. P. 18 in Food Consumption, Prices, and Expenditures, 1985. Statistical Bulletin 749, Economic Research Service, U.S. Department of Agriculture. Washington, D.C.: U.S. Government Printing Office.

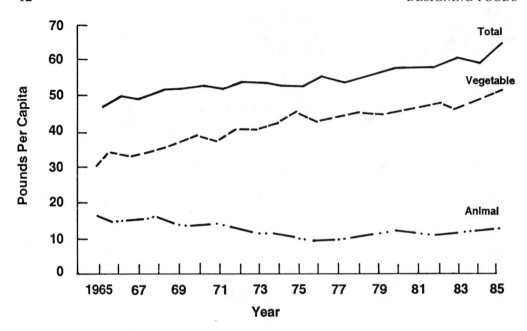

**FIGURE 2–3**  Total fat content of the food supply, 1985. Between 1965 and 1985 the total fat content of the food supply increased by about 34 percent. The shift from animal to vegetable sources has been even more dramatic: Fat from animal sources decreased 22 percent and fat from vegetable sources increased 64 percent during these 20 years. See also Table 2–23. Source: Adapted from K. L. Bunch, 1987. P. 18 in Food Consumption, Prices, and Expenditures, 1985. Statistical Bulletin 749, Economic Research Service, U.S. Department of Agriculture. Washington, D.C.: U.S. Government Printing Office.

by restaurants or consumers. Another 6 pounds were used to produce shortening and, to a lesser extent, margarine. Similarly, a variety of vegetable oils are used in the production of fat and oil products. Vegetable oils contain varying amounts of saturated and unsaturated fats, as shown in Table 2–8. Some vegetable oils, such as coconut and palm, actually contain as large a proportion (if not larger) of saturated fatty acids as tallow and lard.

Because these data are derived from estimates of production, they do not measure actual ingestion of fats and oils. Waste may be significant, especially for salad dressings and for fats and oils used in frying. Estimates of waste range from 2 percent for table spreads such as butter and margarine to 20 percent for salad oils and frying fats (Yan-

kelovich, Skelly and White, Inc., 1985). Some estimates of waste are as high as 30 percent for these products (U.S. Department of Agriculture, 1975).

### Dietary Survey Data

*NFCS (1977–1978).* It is difficult to measure intake of fats and oils (such as margarine or cooking oils) through a survey of individual diets because a large proportion of this fat is used in cooking or consumed in processed foods. Therefore, reported intake levels of fats and oils will be below the amounts actually consumed.

Intake of fats and oils reported in the NFCS ranged from 8 grams/day for children ages 1 to 11 to 16 grams/day for adults ages 19 to 64. Adult males ages 51 to 64 had the highest intake of all age groups, 21 grams/day. One tablespoon of butter or margarine weighs 13 grams; a tablespoon of salad oil weighs 11 grams.

*CSFII.* The trend in the food supply data toward increased use of fat and oil products was also reflected to some extent in food intakes measured by the CSFII. Again, these are fats and oils that are consumed directly or in processed foods rather than fats that occur naturally in foods. Women's intake of the fats and oils reported separately increased 14 percent between 1977 and 1985 because of a 38 percent increase in salad dressing use. Fats and oils consumed as ingredients in baked goods and mixed dishes, as seasoning, or absorbed during cooking are a part of the weight of the reported food. Since these amounts are expected to be substantial, surveys of individual intakes are not appropriate for measuring change in consumption of fats and oils.

## Special Studies

### Household Refuse Analysis Project

The Household Refuse Analysis Project at the University of Arizona attempted to estimate dietary patterns through recording label information from discarded food packages and analyzing food debris in household refuse. This project has collected data from six cities since 1977 (Rathje and Ho, 1987). Over a 7-year period from 1979 to 1985, the quantities of meat fat recorded from Tucson, Arizona, refuse indicated a trend toward greater discard of fat from meat cuts. From 1979 to 1982, the percentage of fat cut off red meats averaged between 3 and 10 percent; from 1983 to 1985 the discard percentage increased to 12 to 16 percent. Data from a retirement community in Arizona revealed that meat fat discard percentage rose from 13 percent in 1976 to 23 percent in 1985 (Rathje and Ho, 1987).

The other trend that was identified by this project is an overall decrease in the purchase of red meat with separable fat (for example, as retail cuts in the form of chops, steaks, and roasts) and an increase in the purchase of red meat with nonseparable fat (for example, ground beef, sausages, luncheon meats, hot dogs, and bacon). Convenience is cited as the most likely explanation for these seemingly contradictory trends; another possibility is that many consumers may not realize that the levels of fat present in ground beef, sausage, hot dogs, and bacon are substantially higher than those in closely trimmed retail cuts (Rathje and Ho, 1987).

### St. Joseph's University/American Meat Institute Study

Another estimate of the contribution of the fat present in red meat to the total fat content in the diet was made in a study for the American Meat Institute by the Academy of Food Marketing at St. Joseph's University (Stanton, 1987). Researchers substituted new nutrient composition data from *USDA Agriculture Handbook No. 8–13* for beef (U.S. Department of Agriculture, 1986) and *USDA Agriculture Handbook No. 8–10* for pork (U.S. Department of Agriculture, 1983) for the nutrient intake data from the 1977–1978 NFCS, made adjustments for the change in retail beef trim from 0.5 to 0.25 inch, and reestimated the number of individuals consuming the separable fat on meat. These adjustments resulted in an average total fat intake of 28 to 34 grams for males age 18 and older and 21 to 24 grams for females age 18 and older. The analysis indicated that with adjustments for these three factors, for males age 18 and older, there was a reduction in total fat intake of 11 to 12 percent and a reduction in grams of fat from meat of 28 to 29 percent; the reductions from previously reported NFCS estimates of fat consumption were comparable for females of the same ages.

## National Live Stock & Meat Board Study

The National Live Stock & Meat Board study (Breidenstein and Williams, 1987), which used per capita disappearance data and private consumer survey information, estimated the nutrient contribution of red meat to the diets of light, moderate, and heavy users of red meat. Researchers estimated that for moderate users, red meat contributes less than 12 percent of the calories from fat, of which about 4.5 percent is from saturated fat. In addition, red meat accounted for about 92 mg of the cholesterol and 526 mg of the sodium per day in the diets of moderate users. A summary of the study's findings is presented in Tables 2–18 and 2–19.

## REFERENCES

Behlen, P. 1986. Calcium in women's diets. Pp. 16–19 in National Food Review, NFR-34, U.S. Department of Agriculture, Economic Research Service. Washington, D.C.: U.S. Government Printing Office.

Breidenstein, B. C. and J. C. Williams. 1987. Contribution of Red Meat to the U.S. Diet. Chicago, Ill.: National Live Stock & Meat Board.

Bunch K. 1985. Whole milk is no longer the beverage of choice. Pp. 21–24 in National Food Review, NFR-29, Economic Research Service. Washington, D.C.: U.S. Department of Agriculture.

Bunch, K., and J. Hazera. 1984. Fats and Oils: Consumers Use More But Different Kinds. Pp. 18–21 in National Food Review, NFR-29, Economic Research Service. Washington, D.C.: U.S. Department of Agriculture.

Cheftel, J. C. 1977. Chemical and nutritional modifications of food proteins due to processing and storage. Pp. 401–445 in Food Proteins, J. R. Whitaker and S. R. Tannenbaum, eds. Westport, Conn.: AVI Press.

Grundy, S. M. 1986. Comparison of monounsaturated fatty acids and carbohydrates for lowering plasma cholesterol. N. Engl. J. Med. 314:745.

Hegsted, D. M., R. B. McGandy, M. L. Myer, and F. J. Stare. 1965. Quantitative effects of dietary fat on serum cholesterol in man. Am. J. Clin. Nutr. 17:281.

Keys, A., J. T. Anderson, and F. Grande. 1965. Serum cholesterol response to changes in the diet. IV. Particular saturated fatty acids in the diet. Metabolism 14:776.

Linkswiler, H. M. 1982. Importance of animal protein in human nutrition. P. 271 in Animal Products in Human Nutrition, D. C. Beitz and R. G. Hansen, eds. New York: Academic Press.

Love, J. 1982. Constituents of animal products that are affected by cooking and processing. Pp. 177–198 in Animal Products in Human Nutrition, D. C. Beitz and R. G. Hansen, eds. New York: Academic Press.

Pao, E. M., K. N. Flemming, P. M. Guenther, and S. J. Mickle. 1982. Foods commonly eaten by individuals: Amount per day and per eating occasion. Home Economics Report No. 44. Washington, D.C.: U.S. Department of Agriculture, Human Nutrition Information Service.

Rathje, W. L., and E. E. Ho. 1987. Meat fat madness: Conflicting patterns of meat fat consumption and their public health implications. J. Am. Dietet. Assoc. 87:1357.

Stanton, J. L. 1987. An Investigation of Fat Intake. Paper presented to the American Meat Institute, Washington, D.C., January.

Stucker, T., and K. Parham. 1984. Beef, pork, and poultry: Our changing consumption habits. Pp. 20–22 in National Food Review, NFR-25. U.S. Department of Agriculture, Economic Research Service. Washington, D.C.: U.S. Government Printing Office.

U.S. Department of Agriculture. 1975. Food Yields Summarized by Different Stages of Preparation. Agriculture Handbook No. 102, Agricultural Research Service. Washington, D.C.: U.S. Government Printing Office.

U.S. Department of Agriculture. 1983. Composition of Foods: Pork Products. Agriculture Handbook No. 8–10. Washington, D.C.: U.S. Government Printing Office.

U.S. Department of Agriculture. 1986. Composition of Foods: Beef Products. Agriculture Handbook No. 8–13. Washington, D.C.: U.S. Government Printing Office.

Yankelovich, Skelly and White, Inc. 1985. The Consumer Climate for Meat Products. Prepared for the American Meat Institute, Washington, D.C., and the National Live Stock & Meat Board, Chicago, Ill. New York: Yankelovich, Skelly and White, Inc.

# 3

# Target Levels and Current Dietary Patterns

## CALORIES

*Target: Caloric intake matched to individual needs and appropriate to achieve and maintain desirable body weight.*

All the national organizations issuing dietary guidelines include recommendations regarding caloric intake and body weight. The American Cancer Society (1984); the National Research Council's Committee on Diet, Nutrition, and Cancer (National Research Council, 1982); and the U.S. Senate Select Committee on Nutrition and Human Needs (1977) all advise a caloric intake that would avoid obesity. The American Heart Association (1986), the National Institutes of Health (1984b) consensus development conference statement, and the U.S. Department of Agriculture (USDA)/U.S. Department of Health and Human Services (DHHS) (1985) recommend caloric intake to maintain desirable body weight, while the National Research Council's Committee on Recommended Dietary Allowances (National Research Council, 1980) suggests a caloric intake adequate to meet individual needs based on sex, age, and level of phys-

ical activity. This committee accepts as a target level a caloric intake matched to individual needs and appropriate to achieve and maintain desirable body weight.

### Dietary Survey Data

Estimates of caloric intake from dietary survey data can be unreliable because respondents tend to underreport this variable (U.S. Department of Agriculture/U.S. Department of Health and Human Services, 1986). The Joint Nutrition Monitoring Evaluation Committee of the USDA and DHHS stated that "if reported diets represent usual food energy intakes and such a large proportion of the population is overweight, it must be concluded that many Americans are underactive" (U.S. Department of Agriculture/U.S. Department of Health and Human Services, 1986). The report *Promoting Health/Preventing Disease: Objectives for the Nation* (U.S. Public Health Service, 1980) recommended that by 1990, at least 60 percent of American adults ages 18 to 65 should participate in regular physical exercise; at present, this figure is only about 10 to 20 percent (Powell et al., 1985).

### Summary

Data from the 1976–1980 National Health and Nutrition Survey (NHANES) indicate that approximately 34 million U.S. adults are obese (body mass index ≥85th percentile), of which 12.4 million are severely obese (body mass index ≥95th percentile). The incidence of obesity varies widely according to age and sex, with black adults ages 45–54 having the highest incidence (61.2 percent for females and 41.4 percent for males) (Table 3-1). Childhood obesity is more difficult to estimate but may range from 4 to 14 percent among low-income populations (Table 3-2).

**TABLE 3-1** Obese Individuals, 1976–1980 (in percent)

| Group and Age | White | Black |
|---|---|---|
| Females | | |
| 25–34 | 17.9 | 33.5 |
| 35–44 | 24.8 | 40.8 |
| 45–54 | 29.9 | 61.2 |
| 55–64 | 34.8 | 59.4 |
| 65–74 | 36.5 | 60.8 |
| Males | | |
| 25–34 | 20.9 | 17.5 |
| 35–44 | 28.2 | 40.9 |
| 45–54 | 30.5 | 41.4 |
| 55–64 | 28.5 | 26.0 |
| 65–74 | 25.8 | 26.4 |
| Both sexes | | |
| (Age adjusted) | | |
| 25–74 | 27.2 | 41.1 |

NOTE: Obese is defined for men as a body mass index of ≥27.8 k/m², and for women as a body mass index of ≥27.3 k/m². These definitions are used because they represent the sex-specific 85th percentiles for persons 20 to 29 years of age in the 1976–1980 National Health and Nutrition Examination Survey.

SOURCE: Adapted from U.S. Department of Health and Human Services. 1985. P. 79 in Health United States, 1985. National Center for Health Statistics, DHHS Publication (PHS) 86-1232. Washington, D.C.: U.S. Government Printing Office.

**TABLE 3-2** Percentage of Low-Income Children Screened with Weight-for-Height Above the 95th Percentile, 31 States, United States, 1984

| Age and Group | Number Examined[a] | Weight-for-Height >95th Percentile |
|---|---|---|
| 0–11 months | | |
| White | 134,866 | 6.0 |
| Black | 68,502 | 8.8 |
| Hispanic | 30,595 | 7.0 |
| American Indian | 5,853 | 10.3 |
| Asian[b] | 3,310 | 8.5 |
| 12–23 months | | |
| White | 38,260 | 9.6 |
| Black | 26,087 | 11.3 |
| Hispanic | 5,435 | 12.4 |
| American Indian | 1,259 | 13.7 |
| Asian[b] | 973 | 7.4 |
| 2–5 years | | |
| White | 82,597 | 4.1 |
| Black | 53,675 | 5.3 |
| Hispanic | 10,014 | 7.5 |
| American Indian | 2,455 | 8.2 |
| Asian[b] | 1,791 | 3.9 |
| 6–9 years | | |
| White | 10,108 | 7.6 |
| Black | 7,836 | 5.6 |
| Hispanic | 417 | 12.2 |
| American Indian | 96 | Insufficient data |
| Asian[b] | 60 | Insufficient data |

NOTE: The Pediatric Nutrition Surveillance System, Centers for Disease Control, uses nutrition-related data collected by local health departments as part of the routine delivery of child health services. These data are the result of examinations of 610,439 new patients at 2,464 clinics in 31 states, the District of Columbia, and Puerto Rico. Anthropometric data on height, weight, and age are converted to percentiles of weight-for-height. These percentages represent the minimal number of children with obesity; these figures would be higher if moderate obesity were also included.

[a]The total does not equal 610,439 because of unknown or missing data for some variables and the exclusion of states with data errors.

[b]Data for Asians include data from an unknown number of recent Southeast Asian refugees.

SOURCE: Adapted from Centers for Disease Control. 1986. Annual summary 1984: reported morbidity and mortality in the United States. Morbidity Mortality Weekly Report, 32(54):105.

## TOTAL FAT AS PERCENTAGE OF CALORIES

*Target: Thirty percent or less of calories from fat for adults.*

Excesses of the first four nutrients identified by the Joint Nutrition Monitoring Evaluation Committee (JNMEC) (calories, total fat, saturated fatty acids, and cholesterol) have all been implicated, either directly or indirectly, in the etiology of cardiovascular disease. Despite a 2 percent annual decline in its prevalence since 1968, cardiovascular disease remains the leading cause of death in the United States (Centers for Disease Control, 1986a).

### Influence of Dietary Fats on Serum Lipid Levels

The type and amount of fat in the diet have become increasingly recognized as factors influencing nutritional status and overall health, as evidenced by numerous clinical studies (Grundy, 1986; O'Brien and Reiser, 1980; Reiser et al., 1985). It should be remembered that fat contributes about 9 calories/gram, more than twice as many as protein or carbohydrate (about 4 calories/gram each). In addition, different fatty acids of dietary fats can significantly alter serum lipid levels. In general, saturated fatty acids raise the serum cholesterol level (certain exceptions were discussed in Chapter 2). Furthermore, monounsaturated fatty acids have been shown to lower cholesterol levels relative to saturated fatty acids. The monounsaturated fatty acids produce reductions similar to those induced by polyunsaturated fatty acids (Becker et al., 1983; Mattson and Grundy, 1985). Recently, eicosopentaenoic and docosohexaenoic acids (found mainly in fish) have generated considerable scientific and public interest. Studies have shown that they may reduce platelet aggregation and lower serum triglyceride levels (Herold and Kinsella, 1986).

### Dietary Fat and Cancer

Some estimates indicate that nearly three-fourths of all cancers in the United States may be influenced by diet (Doll and Peto, 1981). Both animal experiments and epidemiological studies have shown an association between dietary fat and the incidence of cancer, particularly of the breast, prostate, and large bowel (Doll and Peto, 1981). The National Research Council's Committee on Diet, Nutrition, and Cancer cited that of all the dietary components it studied, "the combined epidemiological and experimental evidence is most suggestive for a causal relationship between fat intake and the occurrence of cancer" (National Research Council, 1982). It further concluded that epidemiological studies and animal experiments "provide convincing evidence that increasing the intake of total fat increases the incidence of cancer at certain sites, particularly the breast and colon, and, conversely, that the risk is lower with lower intakes of fat" (National Research Council, 1982).

### Dietary Guidelines for Total Fat Intake

All national health organizations agree that total dietary fat intake should be reduced by some or all members of the U.S. population (depending on how much fat they currently consume) to maintain health and optimal body weight and to reduce the risk of certain diseases, particularly cardiovascular disease and perhaps cancer. Several groups have qualified their recommendations, directing their advice to modify dietary fat intake to particular segments of the population. Other groups have focused their recommendations more generally. The National Research Council's Committee on Diet, Nutrition, and Cancer (National Research Council, 1982), a National Institutes of Health (1984b) consensus development conference statement, and the American Cancer Society (1984) have all recommended that fat intake not contribute more than 30 percent of total calories. Since 1968, the American Heart Association (1968, 1982, 1986) has recommended that 30 to 35 percent of total calories come from fat and has recently revised this recommendation to be less than 30 percent. Likewise, the National Research Council's Committee on Dietary Allowances (National Research Council, 1980) suggests a fat intake not to exceed 35 percent of calories, especially in diets of less than 2,000 total calories. The Committee on Nutrition of the American Academy of Pediatrics (1981) suggests that dietary fat not be restricted for children under 1 year of age; after this age, a decrease in the consumption of saturated fatty acids, cholesterol, and salt and an increased intake of polyunsaturated fatty acids should be followed with moderation. For the purposes of this report, the committee has accepted, for adults, the target level of 30 percent or less of calories from fat.

### Dietary Survey Data

The average percentage of calories from fat for the entire 1977–1978 National Food Consumption Survey (NFCS) population was 41 percent (U.S. Department of Agriculture/U.S. Department of Health and Human Services, 1986). This percentage is recognized as a high estimate for 1987 because of dietary changes that have occurred and the neglect by many respondents in the survey to report that fat on meat was not eaten. The 1977–1978 data imply an average need across the general population for an 11 percent reduction in the percentage of calories from fat, from the present 41 percent to the target level of 30 percent. While it is useful to note this as a general target level, it is important to focus on individual population subgroups, for which the 1977–1978 NFCS provides data. Some subgroups are at or near this 30 percent target level; others exceed it by a wide margin. Recommended alterations in eating

habits vary greatly, depending on how large a reduction is necessary. A summary of the distribution of individuals from the 1977–1978 NFCS by population subgroups and by percentage of calories from fat in the diet and the reductions needed to meet the target level are given in Table 3-3; comparable data from the 1985 Continuing Survey of Food Intake by Individuals (CSFII) are given in Table 3-4.

The percentage of calories from fat in 1985 was below the 41 percent level reported in the 1977–1978 survey, as evidenced by data from the 1985 CSFII. Among children ages 1 to 5, the percentage of calories from fat was 34 percent (U.S. Department of Agriculture, 1985). For women ages 19 to 50, the percentage of calories from fat was 37 percent; for men ages 19 to 50, the percentage of calories from fat was 36 percent (U.S. Department of Agriculture, 1985, 1986). The Nutrition Monitoring Division of the Human Nutrition Information Service within the USDA (U.S. Department of Agriculture, 1985) has suggested that some of the differences between 1977 and 1985 may have been due to changes in food selections, such as the shift from whole milk to low-fat milk, as well as to changes in the way data were collected (for example, more probing questions were asked about the intake of fat on meat and skin on poultry and the use of fat on vegetables).

### Summary

Data from the 1985 CSFII indicate that the average percentage of calories from fat for adults ages 19 to 50 was 36 to 37 percent, 6 to 7 percentage points above the 30 percent target level. For children ages 1 to 5, the percentage of calories from fat was 34 percent. Data from the 1985 CSFII indicate that 15 percent of children ages 1 to 5 and 12 percent of women ages 19 to 50 had diets meeting the target level (Table 3-4).

TABLE 3-3  Distribution (Percent) of Individuals by Percentage of Calories from Fat and Reductions Needed to Meet Target Level

| | Calories from Fat (%) | | | | |
|---|---|---|---|---|---|
| | Dietary Level: | Target Level ≤30 | >30 ≤40 | >40 ≤50 | >50 |
| Group and Age | Reduction Needed (Percentage Points) to Meet Target Level: | None | 0–10 | 10–20 | >20 |
| Children | | | | | |
| 1–2 | | 11 | 54 | 32 | 3 |
| 3–5 | | 9 | 57 | 32 | 2 |
| Females | | | | | |
| 19–22 | | 7 | 40 | 43 | 10 |
| 23–34 | | 6 | 38 | 46 | 10 |
| 35–50 | | 5 | 34 | 48 | 13 |
| Males | | | | | |
| 19–22 | | 5 | 39 | 47 | 9 |
| 23–34 | | 5 | 33 | 53 | 9 |
| 35–50 | | 4 | 30 | 52 | 14 |
| All (mean)[a] | | 6 | 41 | 45 | 8 |

NOTE:  The shaded column represents the target level and the percentage of individuals who met it.

[a]Mean for entire survey population (37,785 individuals).

SOURCE:  1977–1978 level of intake of percentage of calories from fat based on data from the 1977–1978 Nationwide Food Consumption Survey. Adapted from E. M. Pao and S. J. Mickle. 1981. Problem nutrients in the United States. Food Technol. 35:58–79.

TABLE 3-4  Distribution (Percent) of Women and Children by Percentage of Calories from Fat and Reductions Needed to Meet Target Level

| | Calories from Fat (%) | | | | |
|---|---|---|---|---|---|
| | Dietary Level: | Target Level ≤30 | >30 <40 | >40 <50 | >50 |
| Group and Age | Reduction Needed (Percentage Points) to Meet Target Level: | None | 0–10 | 10–20 | >20 |
| Children | | | | | |
| 1–3 | | 13 | 70 | 17 | 0 |
| 4–5 | | 17 | 67 | 16 | 0 |
| All (age 1–5) | | 15 | 69 | 16 | 0 |
| Females | | | | | |
| 19–34 | | 13 | 52 | 34 | 1 |
| 35–50 | | 12 | 52 | 34 | 2 |
| All (age 19–50) | | 12 | 52 | 34 | 2 |

NOTE:  The shaded column represents the target level and the percentage of individuals who met it.

SOURCE:  Adapted from Human Nutrition Information Service, U.S. Department of Agriculture, unpublished data on 4-day dietary intake, 1987.

## SATURATED, MONOUNSATURATED, AND POLYUNSATURATED FATTY ACIDS AS PERCENTAGE OF CALORIES

*Target: Ten percent or less of calories from saturated fatty acids, 10 percent or less of calories from polyunsaturated fatty acids, and 15 percent or less of calories from monounsaturated fatty acids for adults.*

"Eating extra saturated fat, high levels of cholesterol, and excess calories will increase blood cholesterol in many people. Of these, saturated fat has the greatest influence," states the USDA/DHHS (1985) Dietary Guidelines for Americans. Elevated serum cholesterol levels, a major cause of cardiovascular disease, have been strongly correlated to several dietary factors, including a high intake of calories, certain saturated fatty acids, and cholesterol. Genetics and environmental factors may also play an important role in the development of high serum cholesterol. The 1979 Surgeon General's report on health promotion and disease prevention, *Healthy People*, stated that "premature heart disease is unequivocally associated with elevated blood cholesterol . . . heart attacks are five times as frequent in men and women aged 35 to 44 who have cholesterol levels above 265 (mg per dl) as among those with levels below 220 (mg per dl). In general, the lower one's blood cholesterol level the less the likelihood of heart disease; the higher the cholesterol level the greater the risk" (Office of the Assistant Secretary for Health and the Surgeon General, 1979).

### Saturated Fatty Acids: Influence on Serum Lipid Levels

Saturated fatty acids are estimated to currently contribute about 13 percent of the total caloric intake of the average adult in the United States. These fatty acids, as a group, have been positively correlated with the prevalence of cardiovascular disease in many epidemiological studies (Hegsted et al., 1965; Keys, 1970; Stamler, 1979). Several specific saturated fatty acids have been shown to raise plasma levels of cholesterol and low-density lipoproteins, both of which are correlated with an increased risk of cardiovascular disease (Ahrens et al., 1957; Hegsted et al., 1965; Keys et al., 1965); lowering the level of saturated fatty acids in the diet will reduce the plasma cholesterol level (Hegsted et al., 1965; Keys et al., 1965).

Saturated fatty acids occur in both animal and plant fats. Particularly rich sources of saturated fatty acids from plants are coconut and palm oils. Animal fats contain saturated fatty acids of a wide range of chain lengths. Specific saturated fatty acids are believed to differ in their effects on plasma cholesterol. Three saturates—palmitic ($C_{16:0}$), myristic ($C_{14:0}$), and lauric ($C_{12:0}$) acids—have been shown to raise the plasma cholesterol level, while stearic acid ($C_{18:0}$), which is high in beef, lamb, and pork fat, apparently does not raise the plasma cholesterol level (Hegsted et al., 1965; Keys et al., 1965). The actions of the medium-chain fatty acids ($C_{8:0}$, $C_{10:0}$) on cholesterol levels are not well studied. As research confirms and refines the effects of stearic acid on the plasma cholesterol level, dietary recommendations may change to exclude this saturated fatty acid from the 10 percent caloric recommendation (Bonanome and Grundy, 1987).

### Dietary Guidelines for Fatty Acid Intake

A "reduction" in saturated fatty acid intake or "avoidance" of excessive intakes, without citing specific levels, has been recommended by the USDA and DHHS (U.S. Department of Agriculture/U.S. Department of Health and Human Services, 1985), the National Research Council's Committee on Recommended Dietary Allowances (National Research Council, 1980), and the Surgeon General (Office of the Assistant

Secretary for Health and the Surgeon General, 1979). Recommendations that intakes be reduced to less than 10 percent of total caloric intake have been made by the American Heart Association (1982) and a National Institutes of Health (1984b) consensus development conference statement; the U.S. Senate Select Committee on Nutrition and Human Needs (1977) suggested a range of 8 to 12 percent. This committee accepts, for adults, a target level of 10 percent or less of calories from saturated fatty acids.

Due to the unknown potential adverse effects of prolonged intakes of high levels of polyunsaturated fatty acids, the American Heart Association (1968) the National Institutes of Health (1984b), and the National Research Council's Committee on Dietary Allowances (National Research Council, 1980) have all cautioned against exceeding 10 percent of total calories from polyunsaturated fatty acids. This committee accepts, for adults, a target level of 10 percent or less of calories from polyunsaturated fatty acids.

The remainder of dietary fatty acids (15 percent of calories or less) should come from monounsaturated fatty acids, which are found in both animal and plant fats. The monoun-

saturated fatty acids have been shown in some studies to cause a lowering of serum cholesterol when exchanged for saturated fatty acids. They reduce low-density lipoprotein levels to about the same extent as do polyunsaturated fatty acids. There is no evidence that monounsaturates uniquely increase the risk for cancer. The committee accepts, for adults, a target level of 15 percent of calories or less from monounsaturated fatty acids.

### Dietary Survey Data

Data from the 1985 CSFII indicate that saturated fatty acids, as percentage of calories, average about 13.2 percent in the diets of adults ages 19 to 50 and 13.9 percent for children ages 1 to 5 (Table 3-5). Data on 4-day intakes for women and children indicate that 10 percent of women (ages 19 to 50) and 4 percent of children (ages 1 to 5) had diets that met the target level for percentage of calories from saturated fatty acids (Table 3-6). Comparable data are not available for men, but the trend is thought to be similar.

Data from the 1985 CSFII indicate that

TABLE 3-5 Calories from Fat and Fatty Acids, 1985 (in percent)

| Fat or Fatty Acid | Children at Age: | | | Females at Age: | | | Males at Age: | | |
|---|---|---|---|---|---|---|---|---|---|
| | 1–3 | 4–5 | All (1–5) | 19–34 | 35–50 | All (19–50) | 19–34 | 35–50 | All (19–50) |
| Total fat[a] | 34.3 | 34.4 | 34.3 | 36.2 | 37.2 | 36.6 | 35.3 | 37.6 | 36.4 |
| Saturated fatty acids[b] | 14.0 | 13.8 | 13.9 | 13.1 | 13.4 | 13.2 | 12.7 | 13.8 | 13.2 |
| Monounsaturated fatty acids | 12.3 | 12.6 | 12.4 | 13.3 | 13.7 | 13.5 | 13.5 | 14.2 | 13.8 |
| Polyunsaturated fatty acids | 5.4 | 5.5 | 5.5 | 7.2 | 7.5 | 7.3 | 6.7 | 7.0 | 6.8 |

[a]The value for the percentage of calories from total fat exeeds the value for the sum of the total saturated, monounsaturated, and polyunsaturated fatty acids by an amount equal to the value for glycerol and all other non-fatty lipid components.
[b]This category includes all types of saturated fatty acids, with carbon chain lengths from 6 to 18.

SOURCES: Adapted from U.S. Department of Agriculture. 1985. P. 49 in Women 19–50 Years and Their Children 1–5 Years, 1 Day. Nationwide Food Consumption Survey, Continuing Survey of Food Intakes by Individuals. Report 85-1, Human Nutrition Information Service. Hyattsville, Md.: U.S. Department of Agriculture. U.S. Department of Agriculture. 1986. P. 47 in Men 19–50 Years, 1 Day. Nationwide Food Consumption Survey, Continuing Survey of Food Intakes by Individuals. Report 85-3, Human Nutrition Information Service. Hyattsville, Md.: U.S. Department of Agriculture.

TABLE 3-6   Distribution (Percent) of Women and Children by Percentage of Calories from Saturated Fatty Acids and Reductions Needed to Meet Target Level

| | | Calories from Saturated Fatty Acids (%) | | | |
| | | Target Level | | | |
| | Dietary Level: | ≤10 | >10≤14 | ≥15≤19 | ≥20 |
| Group and Age | Reduction Needed (Percentage Points) to Meet Target Level: | None | 0–5 | 5–9 | ≥10 |
| Children | | | | | |
| 1–3 | | 6 | 59 | 35 | 1 |
| 4–5 | | 1 | 65 | 32 | 1 |
| All (age 1–5) | | 4 | 61 | 34 | 1 |
| Females | | | | | |
| 19–34 | | 9 | 55 | 35 | 1 |
| 35–50 | | 12 | 55 | 31 | 2 |
| All (age 19–50) | | 10 | 55 | 33 | 2 |

NOTE:   The shaded column represents the target level and the percentage of individuals who met it.

SOURCE:   Adapted from Human Nutrition Information Service, U.S. Department of Agriculture, unpublished data on 4-day dietary intake, 1987.

monounsaturated fatty acids accounted for 13.5 to 13.8 percent of calories in the diets of adults ages 19 to 50 and 12.6 percent in the diets of children ages 1 to 5 (Table 3-5). Data on 4-day intakes indicate that 74 to 80 percent of children ages 1 to 5 and 64 to 66 percent of women ages 19 to 50 had diets that met the target level of 15 percent or less of calories from monounsaturated fatty acids (Table 3-7). Comparable data for men are not available, but the trend is thought to be similar.

Data from the 1985 CSFII indicate that polyunsaturated fatty acids accounted for 6.8 to 7.3 percent of calories in the diets of adults ages 19 to 50 and 5.5 percent of calories in the diets of children ages 1 to 5 (Table 3-5). Four-day intake data indicate that 98 to 99 percent of children ages 1 to 5 and 85 to 87 percent of women ages 19 to 50 had diets that met the target level for 10 percent or less of calories from polyunsaturated fatty acids (Table 3-8).

### Summary

Data from the 1985 CSFII indicate that about 10 percent of women ages 19 to 50

and 4 percent of children ages 1 to 5 years had diets that met the target level for saturated fatty acids. Between 64 to 66 percent of women and 74 to 80 percent of children had diets that met the target level for monounsaturated fatty acids. About 98 to 99 percent of children and 86 percent of women met the target level for polyunsaturated fatty acids (Tables 3–6 through 3–8).

### CHOLESTEROL

*Target: Three hundred milligrams or less of cholesterol per day for adults.*

In some epidemiological studies, the risk of cardiovascular heart disease has been positively correlated to intakes of dietary cholesterol (Kannel et al., 1971; Shekelle et al., 1981). In one study, with intakes of up to about 400 mg/1,000 kcal, the plasma cholesterol response to dietary intakes of cholesterol was approximately linear: Each 1 mg/1,000 kcal resulted in a plasma cholesterol increase of about 0.1 mg/dl (Hegsted, 1986). Based on the results of that study, with a 2,500–kcal diet, an increase in dietary

TABLE 3-7  Distribution (Percent) of Women and Children by Percentage of Calories from Monounsaturated Fatty Acids and Reductions Needed to Meet Target Level

| | | Calories from Monounsaturated Fatty Acids (%) | | |
|---|---|---|---|---|
| | Dietary Level: | Target Level ≤15 | >15≤19 | ≥20 |
| Group and Age | Reduction Needed (Percentage Points) to Meet Target Level: | None | 0–5 | ≥5–10 |
| Children | | | | |
| 1–3 | | 80 | 20 | 0 |
| 4–5 | | 74 | 26 | 0 |
| All (age 1–5) | | 78 | 23 | 0 |
| Females | | | | |
| 19–34 | | 66 | 33 | 1 |
| 35–50 | | 64 | 34 | 2 |
| All (age 19–50) | | 65 | 34 | 1 |

NOTE:  The shaded column represents the target level and the percentage of individuals who met it.

SOURCE:  Adapted from Human Nutrition Information Service, U.S. Department of Agriculture, unpublished data on 4-day dietary intake, 1987.

cholesterol of 100 mg/day would be expected to increase the plasma levels by about 4 mg/dl. Likewise, a decrease in dietary cholesterol of 100 mg/day would decrease plasma levels by about 4 mg/dl.

## Dietary Guidelines for Cholesterol Intake

Reports from the USDA/DHHS (1985) and the Surgeon General (Office of the Assistant Secretary for Health and the Surgeon General, 1979) recommend a "reduction" in dietary intakes of cholesterol but do not cite precise levels. Organizations suggesting specific intakes include the U.S. Senate Select Committee on Nutrition and Human Needs (1977) (250 to 350 mg/day), the National Institutes of Health (1984b) consensus development conference statement (250 to 300 mg/day), and the American Heart Association (1986) (≤300 mg/day or 100 mg/1,000 kcal). Restriction of dietary cholesterol in children remains controversial, although a lowering of total dietary fat and an avoidance of obesity among this age group have been recognized as good preventive measures (Barness, 1986). This com-

mittee accepts, for adults, a target level for cholesterol of less than 300 mg/day.

## Dietary Survey Data

Data from the 1977–1978 NFCS indicate that the average cholesterol intake for the survey population was 385 mg/day, or 214 mg/1,000 kcal (U.S. Department of Agriculture/U.S. Department of Health and Human Services, 1986). Fifty-eight percent of the survey population had intakes greater than 300 mg of dietary cholesterol per day. The highest intakes were among 19- to 64-year-olds, with 78 percent of the males and 52 percent of the females consuming more than 300 mg/day. These data are summarized in Table 3–9. Data on cholesterol intakes from the 1985 CSFII are presented in Tables 3–10 and 3–11. About 77 percent of children ages 1 to 5 and 62 percent of women ages 19 to 50 had diets that met the target level of ≤300 mg/day.

## Summary

Data from the 1977–1978 NFCS indicate that about 52 percent of the survey popu-

TABLE 3-8   Distribution (Percent) of Women and Children by Percentage of Calories from Polyunsaturated Fatty Acids and Reductions Needed to Meet Target Level

| | | Calories from Polyunsaturated Fatty Acids (%) | | | |
|---|---|---|---|---|---|
| | Dietary Level: | Target Level ≤10 | >10≤14 | ≥15≤19 | ≥20 |
| Group and Age | Reduction Needed (Percentage Points) to Meet Target Level: | None | 0–5 | 5–9 | ≥10 |
| Children | | | | | |
| 1–3 | | 98 | 2 | 0 | 0 |
| 4–5 | | 99 | 1 | 0 | 0 |
| All (age 1–5) | | 98 | 2 | 0 | 0 |
| Females | | | | | |
| 19–34 | | 87 | 12 | 1 | 0 |
| 35–50 | | 85 | 15 | 0 | 0 |
| All (age 19–50) | | 86 | 14 | 1 | 0 |

NOTE:   The shaded column represents the target level and the percentage of individuals who met it.

SOURCE:   Adapted from Human Nutrition Information Service, U.S. Department of Agriculture, unpublished data on 4-day dietary intake, 1987.

lation had mean daily cholesterol intakes above 300 mg. This group included 78 percent of males ages 19 to 64 and 52 percent of females ages 19 to 64 years (Table 3–9). Dietary cholesterol intakes from the 1985 CSFII averaged 254 mg/day for children ages 1 to 5, 304 mg/day for women ages 19 to 50, and 439 mg/day for men ages 19 to 50 (Table 3–10). Nearly 77 percent of children ages 1 to 5 and 62 percent of women ages 19 to 50 from the 1985 CSFII consumed ≤300 mg of cholesterol per day (Table 3–11).

### CALCIUM

*Target: Calcium intake of the Recommended Dietary Allowance (RDA) for age and sex.*

### Dietary Guidelines

The National Institutes of Health consensus development conference statement on osteoporosis recommended adequate nutrition that included an elemental calcium intake of 1,000 to 1,500 mg/day for post-

TABLE 3-9   Mean Daily Cholesterol Intakes in Relation to Target Level

| | | % of Population with the Following Mean Intakes per Day (mg): | |
|---|---|---|---|
| Group and Age | Mean Intake (mg) | Target Level ≤300 | >300 |
| Children | | | |
| 1–8 | 289 | 61 | 39 |
| Females | | | |
| 9–18 | 328 | 51 | 49 |
| 19–64 | 345 | 48 | 52 |
| 65+ | 316 | 53 | 47 |
| Males | | | |
| 9–18 | 442 | 30 | 70 |
| 19–64 | 511 | 22 | 78 |
| 65+ | 461 | 29 | 71 |
| All | 385 | 42 | 58 |

NOTE:   The shaded column represents the target level and the percentage of individuals who met it.

SOURCE:   Adapted from U.S. Department of Agriculture/U.S. Department of Health and Human Services. 1986. P. 255 in Nutrition Monitoring in the United States: A Progress Report from the Joint Nutrition Monitoring Committee. DHHS Publication (PHS) 86-1255. Washington, D.C.: U.S. Government Printing Office.

TABLE 3-10   Mean Daily Cholesterol and Calorie Intakes, 1985

| Nutrient | Children at Age: | | | Females at Age: | | | Males at Age: | | |
|---|---|---|---|---|---|---|---|---|---|
| | 1–3 | 4–5 | All (1–5) | 19–34 | 35–50 | All (19–50) | 19–34 | 35–50 | All (19–50) |
| Calories (kcal) | 1,372 | 1,564 | 1,446 | 1,707 | 1,602 | 1,661 | 2,667 | 2,428 | 2,560 |
| Cholesterol (mg) | 247 | 266 | 254 | 306 | 302 | 304 | 443 | 427 | 435 |

SOURCES:  Adapted from the U.S. Department of Agriculture. 1985. Pp. 22 and 24 in Women 19–50 Years and Their Children 1–5 Years, 1 Day. Nationwide Food Consumption Survey, Continuing Survey of Food Intakes by Individuals. Report 85-1, Human Nutrition Information Service. Hyattsville, Md.: U.S. Department of Agriculture. U.S. Department of Agriculture. 1986. Pp. 20 and 22 in Men 19–50 Years, 1 Day. Nationwide Food Consumption Survey, Continuing Survey of Food Intakes by Individuals. Report 85-3, Human Nutrition Information Service. Hyattsville, Md.: U.S. Department of Agriculture.

menopausal women, as well as a program of modest weight-bearing exercise and estrogen replacement (National Institutes of Health, 1984a). The National Research Council's Committee on Dietary Allowances recommended calcium intakes of 800 mg/day for children ages 1 to 10 and adults ages 19 and older (National Research Council, 1980). For males and females ages 11 to 18, the recommended daily intake is 1,200 mg. For infants under 6 months, the RDA is 360 mg; for children ages 6 months to 1 year, the RDA is 540 mg. During pregnancy and lactation, an increase of 400 mg/day is recommended for women. This committee accepts as the target level the RDA for calcium for the various age and sex groups.

**Dietary Survey Data**

Data from the 1977–1978 NFCS indicate that about 42 percent of the survey population had calcium intakes below 70 percent of the RDA, and 26 percent had intakes between 70 and 100 percent of the RDA. These data are presented in Table 3–12. Table 3–13 compares calcium intakes from the 1977–1978 NFCS and the 1985 CSFII

TABLE 3-11   Distribution (Percent) of Women and Children by Cholesterol Intakes and Reduction Needed to Meet Target Level

| Group and Age | Cholesterol (mg) | | | |
|---|---|---|---|---|
| | Dietary Level: | Target Level ≤300 | >300≤400 | >400≤500 | >500 |
| | Reduction Needed (Percentage Points) to Meet Target Level: | None | <100 | 100–200 | >200 |
| Children | | | | | |
| 1–3 | | 80 | 11 | 7 | 2 |
| 4–5 | | 72 | 20 | 7 | 0 |
| All (age 1–5) | | 77 | 15 | 7 | 1 |
| Females | | | | | |
| 19–34 | | 62 | 20 | 11 | 8 |
| 35–50 | | 62 | 22 | 7 | 9 |
| All (age 19–50) | | 62 | 21 | 9 | 8 |

NOTE:   The shaded column represents the target level and the percentage of individuals who met it.

SOURCE:   Adapted from Human Nutrition Information Service, U.S. Department of Agriculture, unpublished data on 4-day dietary intake, 1987.

TABLE 3-12   Distribution (Percent) of Individuals by Calcium Intakes and Increases (as a percentage of RDA) Needed to Meet Target Level

| | Calcium (% RDA) | | |
| | Dietary Level: | Target Level 100 | ≥70<100 | <70 |
| Group and Age | Increase Needed (Percentage Points) to Meet Target Level: | None | 0–30 | >30 |
| --- | --- | --- | --- | --- |
| Children | | | | |
| <1 | | 81 | 14 | 5 |
| 1–8 | | 48 | 27 | 25 |
| Females | | | | |
| 9–18 | | 23 | 28 | 49 |
| 19–64 | | 19 | 23 | 58 |
| 65+ | | 18 | 26 | 56 |
| Males | | | | |
| 9–18 | | 42 | 29 | 29 |
| 19–64 | | 41 | 27 | 32 |
| 65+ | | 33 | 28 | 39 |
| All (mean) | | 32 | 26 | 42 |

NOTE:   The shaded column represents the target level and the percentage of individuals who met it.

SOURCE:   Adapted from U.S. Department of Agriculture/U.S. Department of Health and Human Services. 1986. P. 272 in Nutrition Monitoring in the United States: A Progress Report from the Joint Nutrition Monitoring Evaluation Committee. DHHS Publication (PHS) 86-1255. Washington, D.C.: U.S. Government Printing Office.

TABLE 3-13   Mean Daily Dietary Calcium Intakes for Individuals

| | Target Level, RDA (mg) | Total Intake (mg) | | mg/1,000 kcal | |
| Group and Age | | 1977 | 1985 | 1977 | 1985 |
| --- | --- | --- | --- | --- | --- |
| Children | | | | | |
| 1–3 | 800 | 717 | 824 | 602 | 622 |
| 4–5 | 800 | 728 | 864 | 498 | 564 |
| All (age 1–5) | 800 | 722 | 840 | 555 | 600 |
| Females | | | | | |
| 19–34 | 800 | 611 | 685 | 389 | 402 |
| 35–50 | 800 | 515 | 606 | 352 | 392 |
| All (age 19–50) | 800 | 570 | 651 | 374 | 398 |
| Males | | | | | |
| 19–34 | 800 | 871 | 975 | 364 | 366 |
| 35–50 | 800 | 736 | 849 | 315 | 353 |
| All (age 19–50) | 800 | 815 | 919 | 343 | 360 |

SOURCES:   Adapted from the U.S. Department of Agriculture. 1985. Pp. 23 and 46 in Women 19–50 Years and Their Children 1–5 Years, 1 Day. Nationwide Food Consumption Survey, Continuing Survey of Food Intakes by Individuals. Report 85-1, Human Nutrition Information Service. Hyattsville, Md.: U.S. Department of Agriculture. U.S. Department of Agriculture. 1986. Pp. 21 and 44 in Men 19–50 Years, 1 Day. Nationwide Food Consumption Survey, Continuing Survey of Food Intakes by Individuals. Report 85-3, Human Nutrition Information Service. Hyattsville, Md.: U.S. Department of Agriculture.

for men, women, and children. Average intakes as well as intakes per 1,000 kcal have increased for all three of these population groups. CSFII dietary levels of calcium averaged above the RDA for men and children and were about half the RDA for adult women.

Of interest in the 1977–1978 NFCS and the 1985 CSFII data are the percentage of individuals using vitamin and mineral supplements and how this figure has changed recently (Table 3–14). The percentage of children ages 1 to 3 using supplements has increased by about 20 percent and for children ages 4 to 5, by about 35 percent, with an overall increase for children ages 1 to 5 of about 26 percent. For women ages 19 to 34, there has been a 37 percent increase and for women ages 35 to 50, a 66 percent increase, for an overall increase among

TABLE 3-14   Use of Vitamin and Mineral Supplements

| Group and Age | Individuals Using (%) 1977 | Individuals Using (%) 1985 | Increase from 1977 to 1985 (%) |
|---|---|---|---|
| Children | | | |
| 1–3 | 50.8 | 60.7 | 19.5 |
| 4–5 | 43.2 | 58.5 | 35.4 |
| All (age 1–5) | 47.4 | 59.8 | 26.2 |
| Females | | | |
| 19–34 | 40.8 | 56.0 | 37.3 |
| 35–50 | 36.1 | 59.8 | 65.7 |
| All (age 19–50) | 38.9 | 57.6 | 48.1 |
| Males | | | |
| 19–34 | 25.0 | 42.5 | 70.0 |
| 35–50 | 28.7 | 47.9 | 66.9 |
| All (age 19–50) | 26.5 | 44.9 | 69.4 |

SOURCES: Adapted from the U.S. Department of Agriculture. 1985. P. 58 in Women 19–50 Years and Their Children 1–5 Years, 1 Day. Nationwide Food Consumption Survey, Continuing Survey of Food Intakes by Individuals. Report 85-1, Human Nutrition Information Service. Hyattsville, Md.: U.S. Department of Agriculture. U.S. Department of Agriculture. 1986. P. 56 in Men 19–50 Years, 1 Day. Nationwide Food Consumption Survey, Continuing Survey of Food Intakes by Individuals. Report 85-3, Human Nutrition Information Service. Hyattsville, Md.: U.S. Department of Agriculture.

women ages 19 to 50 of about 48 percent. For men ages 19 to 34, there has been a 70 percent increase, and for men ages 35 to 50, a 67 percent increase, for an overall increase among men ages 19 to 50 of about 69 percent.

### Summary

Data from the 1977–1978 NFCS indicate that 42 percent of the survey population have diets containing less than 70 percent of the RDA for calcium, including more than 50 percent of females age 19 and older. Another 26 percent of the survey population have diets containing from 70 to 100 percent of the RDA for calcium, including 31 percent of adolescents ages 9 to 18 (Table 3–12). Mean calcium intakes increased from the 1977–1978 NFCS to the 1985 CSFII for men, women, and children; but women's mean intakes still fell short of the RDA (Table 3–13). About three-fourths of the women did not meet 100 percent of the RDA; of this group, half did not achieve 70 percent of the RDA.

### IRON

*Target: Iron intake of the RDA for age and sex.*

### Definition and Prevalence of Iron-Deficiency Anemia

Iron deficiency is frequently cited as the most common single nutritional deficiency in the world and the cause of the most common form of childhood anemia in the United States (Dallman et al., 1984). Nutritional iron deficiency is caused by inadequate amounts of iron in the diet and can adversely affect health status, including a reduction in maximal work capacity, altered immune response, and, in children, behavioral abnormalities and a reduction in intellectual performance (Federation of American Societies for Experimental Biology, Life Sciences Research Office, 1984).

The NHANES II (1976–1980) data on iron status were analyzed by an expert scientific working group of the Life Sciences Research Office, Federation of American Societies for Experimental Biology (1984). The group's findings on the prevalence of impaired iron status are summarized in Table 3–15. It concluded that several population segments had relatively high prevalences of impaired iron status and warranted further consideration, including children ages 1 to 2, males ages 11 to 14, and females ages 15 to 44. It also concluded that the prevalence of impaired iron status was higher for blacks than for whites, was higher for persons below the defined poverty level than for those above it, and was associated with lower education level and, for women, higher parity.

A recent report from the Pediatric Nu-

trition Surveillance System of the Centers for Disease Control (1986b) indicated a decline in the prevalence of anemia among children enrolled in public nutrition and health programs during 1975 to 1985. The prevalence of anemia dropped from 7.8 percent in 1975 to 2.9 percent in 1985, with greater declines among children examined at follow-up visits as compared to those of the same age at initial visits. Vasquez-Seoane et al. (1985) have suggested that the decline was probably related to improvements in iron nutrition during infancy and childhood, due partly to participation in public nutrition and health programs.

Data on children from public health programs with hematocrit values below the 5th percentile are presented in Table 3–16. As with other indicators of poor nutritional status, the incidence of low hematocrits differs widely among age and ethnic groups.

TABLE 3-15   Prevalence of Impaired Iron Status, 1976–1980

| Group and Age | Estimated Range of Prevalence (%) |
| --- | --- |
| Children | |
| 1–2 | 9.2–9.4 |
| 3–4 | 3.6–5.5 |
| 5–10 | 3.2–4.5 |
| Females | |
| 11–14 | 2.7–6.1 |
| 15–19 | 2.5–14.2 |
| 20–44 | 4.0–9.6 |
| 45–64 | 3.8–4.8 |
| 65–74 | 2.7–3.7 |
| Males | |
| 11–14 | 3.5–12.1 |
| 15–19 | 0.1–0.9 |
| 20–44 | 0.6–0.8 |
| 45–64 | 1.9–2.0 |
| 65–74 | 1.8–3.6 |

SOURCE:   Federation of American Societies for Experimental Biology, Life Sciences Research Office. 1984. P. v in Assessment of the Iron Nutritional Status of the U.S. Population based on Data Collected in the Second National Health and Nutrition Examination Survey, 1976–1980, S. M. Pilch and F. R. Senti, eds. Bethesda, Md.: Life Sciences Research Office, Federation of American Societies for Experimental Biology.

## Dietary Guidelines for Iron Intake

The National Research Council's Committee on Dietary Allowances (National Research Council, 1980) recommends an iron intake of 10 mg/day for infants up to age 6 months, children ages 4 to 10, males 19 and older, and females 51 and older. It recommends an intake of 15 mg/day for children ages 6 months to 3 years, and an intake of 18 mg/day for males ages 11 to 18 and females ages 11 to 50. During pregnancy and lactation, it suggests a daily supplement of 30 to 60 mg of iron. This committee accepts as a target level the RDA for iron for the various age and sex groups.

## Dietary Survey Data

The data from the 1977–1978 NFCS indicate that approximately 33 percent of the survey population had iron intakes of less than 70 percent of the RDA, 23 percent had intakes between 70 and 100 percent of the RDA, and about 44 percent had intakes that met or exceeded the RDA (U.S. De-

TABLE 3-16   Percentage of Low-Income Children Screened with Hematocrit Values Below the 5th Percentile, 31 States, United States, 1984

| Age and Group | Number Examined[a] | Hematocrit <5th Percentile |
|---|---|---|
| 6–11 months | | |
| White | 21,278 | 7.0 |
| Black | 13,883 | 6.9 |
| Hispanic | 4,365 | 8.0 |
| American Indian | 967 | 7.9 |
| Asian[b] | 467 | 8.1 |
| 12–23 months | | |
| White | 31,960 | 6.3 |
| Black | 24,202 | 7.7 |
| Hispanic | 4,516 | 8.3 |
| American Indian | 1,153 | 5.8 |
| Asian[b] | 660 | 6.2 |
| 2–5 years | | |
| White | 66,485 | 7.6 |
| Black | 49,985 | 11.6 |
| Hispanic | 8,324 | 10.8 |
| American Indian | 2,234 | 6.8 |
| Asian[b] | 1,222 | 8.6 |
| 6–9 years | | |
| White | 10,355 | 3.8 |
| Black | 8,277 | 6.5 |
| Hispanic | 366 | 3.6 |
| American Indian | 103 | 2.9 |
| Asian[b] | 12 | Insufficient data |

NOTE: The Pediatric Nutrition Surveillance System, Centers for Disease Control, uses nutrition-related data collected by local health departments as part of the routine delivery of child health services. These data are the result of examinations of 610,439 new patients at 2,464 clinics in 31 states, the District of Columbia, and Puerto Rico. Hematocrit is the volume of red blood cells in whole blood.

[a]Total does not equal 610,439 because of unknown or missing data for some variables and the exclusion of states with data errors.
[b]Data for Asians include data from an unknown number of recent Southeast Asian refugees.

SOURCE: Adapted from Centers for Disease Control. 1986. Annual Summary 1984: reported morbidity and mortality in the United States. Morbidity Mortality Weekly Report 32 (54):107.

partment of Agriculture/U.S. Department of Health and Human Services, 1986). These data are summarized in Table 3–17. Groups with the lowest intakes are those previously described as having the highest prevalences of impaired iron status, including children to age 5, males ages 11 to 14, and females in their reproductive years, ages 15 to 50.

The most current dietary intake data on men, women, and children are presented and compared to data from the 1977–1978 NFCS in Table 3–18. Mean intakes for all three groups have increased somewhat from 1977 to 1985. For children, intakes per 1,000 kcal have also risen, but for men and women the figure has fallen.

TABLE 3-17   Distribution (Percent) of Individuals by Iron Intakes and Increases (as a pecentage of RDA) Needed to Meet Target Level

| | Iron (% RDA) | | | |
| | | Target Level | ≥70 | |
| | Dietary Level: | 100 | <100 | <70 |
| Group and Age | Increase Needed (Percentage Points) to Meet Target Level: | None | 0–30 | >30 |
| Children | | | | |
| <1 | | 58 | 12 | 30 |
| 1–8 | | 38 | 18 | 44 |
| Females | | | | |
| 9–18 | | 18 | 27 | 55 |
| 19–64 | | 18 | 26 | 56 |
| 65+ | | 53 | 34 | 13 |
| Males | | | | |
| 9–18 | | 36 | 38 | 26 |
| 19–64 | | 88 | 10 | 2 |
| 65+ | | 82 | 14 | 4 |
| All | | 44 | 23 | 33 |

NOTE:   The shaded column represents the target level and the percentage of individuals who met it.

SOURCE:   Adapted from U.S. Department of Agriculture/U.S. Department of Health and Human Services. 1986. P. 228 in Nutrition Monitoring in the United States: A Progress Report from the Joint Nutrition Monitoring Evaluation Committee. DHHS Publication (PHS) 86-1255. Washington, D.C.: U.S. Government Printing Office.

TABLE 3-18   Mean Daily Iron Intakes for Individuals

| Group and Age | Target Level, RDA (mg) | Total Intake (mg) | | mg/1,000 kcal | |
| | | 1977 | 1985 | 1977 | 1985 |
| Children | | | | | |
| 1–3 | 15 | 8.4 | 10.5 | 7.1 | 7.8 |
| 4–5 | 10 | 9.7 | 11.6 | 6.7 | 7.5 |
| All (age 1–5) | | 9.0 | 10.9 | 6.9 | 7.7 |
| Females | | | | | |
| 19–34 | 18 | 10.7 | 11.3 | 6.9 | 6.7 |
| 35–50 | 18 | 10.8 | 10.8 | 7.6 | 7.1 |
| All (age 19–50) | | 10.7 | 11.1 | 7.2 | 6.9 |
| Males | | | | | |
| 19–34 | 10 | 15.7 | 16.0 | 6.7 | 6.2 |
| 35–50 | 10 | 16.6 | 15.8 | 7.3 | 6.7 |
| All (age 19–50) | | 16.1 | 15.9 | 7.0 | 6.4 |

SOURCES:   Adapted from the U.S. Department of Agriculture. 1985. Pp. 23 and 46 in Women 19–50 Years and Their Children 1–5 Years, 1 Day. Nationwide Food Consumption Survey, Continuing Survey of Food Intakes by Individuals. Report 85-1, Human Nutrition Information Service. Hyattsville, Md.: U.S. Department of Agriculture. U.S. Department of Agriculture. 1986. Pp. 21 and 44 in Men 19–50 Years, 1 Day. Nationwide Food Consumption Survey, Continuing Survey of Food Intakes by Individuals. Report 85-3, Human Nutrition Information Service. Hyattsville, Md.: U.S. Department of Agriculture.

## Summary

Data from the 1977–1978 NFCS indicate that 33 percent of the survey population have diets containing less than 70 percent of the RDA, including more than 50 percent of females ages 9 to 64. Another 23 percent of the population have diets containing only 70 to 100 percent of the RDA for iron, including 38 percent of males and 27 percent of females ages 9 to 18 (Table 3–17). Although the mean dietary intakes of iron increased from 1977–1978 to 1985 for men, women, and children, they still averaged below the RDA for women (Table 3–18). About 95 percent of the women did not meet 100 percent of the RDA; of this group, three-fourths did not achieve 70 percent of the RDA.

## REFERENCES

Ahrens, E. H., Jr., W. Insull, Jr., R. Blomstrand, J. Hirsch, T. T. Tsaltas, and M. L. Peterson. 1957. The influence of dietary fats on serum-lipid levels in man. Lancet 1:943.

American Academy of Pediatrics, Committee on Nutrition. 1981. Nutritional aspects of obesity in infancy and childhood. Pediatrics 68:880.

American Cancer Society. 1984. Nutrition and cancer, cause and prevention. An American Cancer Society special report. Ca—A Cancer Journal for Clinicians 34(2):121–126.

American Heart Association. 1968. Diet and Heart Disease. Dallas, Tex.: American Heart Association.

American Heart Association. 1982. Rationale of the diet-heart statement of the American Heart Association. Report of the Nutrition Committee. Circulation 65:839A.

American Heart Association. 1986. Dietary guidelines for healthy adult Americans. Circulation 74:1465A.

Barness, L. A. 1986. Cholesterol and children. J. Am. Med. Assoc. 256:2871.

Becker, N., D. R. Illingworth, P. Alaupovic, W. E. Connor, and W. E. Sundberg. 1983. Effects of saturated, monounsaturated, and omega-6 polyunsaturated fatty acids on plasma lipids, lipoproteins, and apoproteins in humans. Am. J. Clin. Nutr. 37:355.

Bonanome, A., and S. Grundy. 1987. Stearic acid does not raise plasma cholesterol. Clin. Res. 35:365A.

Centers for Disease Control. 1986a. Epidemiologic notes and reports: Years of life lost from cardiovascular disease. Morbid. Mortal. Weekly Rep. 35(42):653–654.

Centers for Disease Control. 1986b. Current trends: Declining anemia prevalence among children enrolled in public nutrition and health programs, selected states, 1975 to 1985. Morbid. Mortal. Weekly Rep. 35(36):565–566.

Dallman, P. R., R. Yip, and C. Johnson. 1984. Prevalence and causes of anemia in the United States, 1976 to 1980. Am. J. Clin. Nutr. 39:437.

Doll, R., and R. Peto. 1981. The causes of cancer. Quantitative estimates of avoidable risks of cancer in the United States today. J. Natl. Cancer Inst. 66:1191.

Federation of American Societies for Experimental Biology, Life Sciences Research Office. 1984. Assessment of the Nutritional Status of the U.S. Population Based on Data Collected in the Second National Health and Nutrition Examination Survey, 1976–1980. Washington, D.C.: Federation of American Societies for Experimental Biology.

Grundy, S. M. 1986. Comparison of monounsaturated fatty acids and carbohydrates for lowering plasma cholesterol. N. Engl. J. Med. 314:745.

Hegsted, D. M. 1986. Serum cholesterol response to dietary cholesterol: A re-evaluation. Am. J. Clin. Nutr. 44:299.

Hegsted, D. M., R. B. McGandy, M. L. Myer, and F. J. Stare. 1965. Quantitative effects of dietary fat on serum cholesterol in man. Am. J. Clin. Nutr. 17:281.

Herold, P. M., and J. E. Kinsella. 1986. Fish oil consumption and decreased risk of cardiovascular disease: A comparison of findings from animal and human feeding trials. Am. J. Clin. Nutr. 43:566.

Kannel, W. B., W. P. Castelli, T. Gordon, and P. M. McNamara. 1971. Serum cholesterol lipoproteins and the risk of coronary heart disease. The Framingham Study. Ann. Intern. Med. 74:1.

Keys, A. 1970. Coronary heart disease in seven countries. Circulation 41(Suppl. 1):I-1–211.

Keys, A., J. T. Anderson, and F. Grande. 1965. Serum cholesterol response to changes in the diet. IV. Particular saturated fatty acids in the diet. Metabolism 14:776.

Mattson, F. H., and S. M. Grundy. 1985. Comparison of effects of dietary saturated, monounsaturated, and polyunsaturated fatty acids on plasma lipids and lipoproteins in man. J. Lipid Res. 26:194.

National Institutes of Health. 1984a. NIH Consensus Development Conference Statement on Osteoporosis. Vol. 5, No. 3. Washington, D.C.: National Institutes of Health.

National Institutes of Health. 1984b. NIH Consensus Development Statement on Lowering Blood Cholesterol to Prevent Heart Disease. Vol. 5, No. 7. Washington, D.C.: National Institutes of Health.

National Research Council. 1980. Recommended Dietary Allowances, 9th ed. Washington, D.C.: National Academy Press.

National Research Council. 1982. Diet, Nutrition, and Cancer. Washington, D.C.: National Academy Press.

O'Brien, B. C., and R. Reiser. 1980. Human plasma lipid responses to red meat, poultry, fish, and eggs. Am. J. Clin. Nutr. 33:2573.

Office of the Assistant Secretary for Health and the Surgeon General. 1979. Healthy People, the Surgeon General's Report on Health Promotion and Disease Prevention. DHEW (PHS) Publication No. 79–55071. Washington, D.C.: U.S. Public Health Service.

Powell, K. E., K. G. Spain, G. M. Christenson, and M. P. Mollenkamp. 1985. The status of the 1990 objectives for physical fitness and exercise. Public Health Rep. 100:180.

Reiser, R., J. L. Probstfield, and A. Silvers. 1985. Plasma lipid and lipoprotein response of humans to beef fat, coconut oil, and safflower oil. Am. J. Clin. Nutr. 42:190.

Shekelle, R. B., A. M. Shyrock, O. Paul, M. Lepper, J. Stamler, S. Liu, and W. J. Raynor. 1981. Diet, serum cholesterol and death from coronary heart disease. The Western Electric Study. N. Engl. J. Med. 304:65.

Stamler, J. 1979. Population studies. Pp. 25–88 in Nutrition, Lipids, and Coronary Disease: A Global View, R. I. Levy, B. M. Rifkind, B. H. Dennis, and N. Ernst, eds. New York: Raven Press.

U.S. Department of Agriculutre. 1985. P. 48 in Women 19–50 years and their children 1–5 years, 1 day, 1985. Nationwide Food Consumption Survey, Continuing Survey of Food Intakes by Individuals. Report 85–1, Human Nutrition Information Service. Hyattsville, Md.: U.S. Department of Agriculture.

U.S. Department of Agriculture. 1986. P. 46 in Men 19–50 years, 1 Day, 1985. Nationwide Food Consumption Survey, Continuing Survey of Food Intakes by Individuals. Report 85–3, Human Nutrition Information Service. Hyattsville, Md.: U.S. Department of Agriculture.

U.S. Department of Agriculture/U.S. Department of Health and Human Services. 1985. Nutrition and Your Health: Dietary Guidelines for Americans, 2nd ed. Home and Garden Bulletin No. 232. Washington, D.C.: U.S. Government Printing Office.

U.S. Department of Agriculture/U.S. Department of Health and Human Services. 1986. Nutrition Monitoring in the United States: A Progress Report from the Joint Nutrition Monitoring Evaluation Committee. DHHS Publication No. (PHS) 86–1255. Washington, D.C.: U.S. Government Printing Office.

U.S. Public Health Service. 1980. Promoting Health/Preventing Disease: Objectives for the Nation. Washington, D.C.: U.S. Public Health Service.

U.S. Senate Select Committee on Nutrition and Human Needs. 1977. Dietary goals for the U.S., 2nd ed., No. 052–070–04376–8. Washington, D.C.: U.S. Government Printing Office.

Vasquez-Seoane, P., R. Windom, and H. A. Pearson. 1985. Disappearance of iron-deficiency anemia in a high-risk infant population given supplemental iron. N. Engl. J. Med. 313:1239.

# 4

# Consumer Concerns and Animal Product Options

The combined sales of food and food products in stores and eating establishments in the United States totaled more than $389 billion in 1985—nearly 11 percent of the U.S. gross national product. (The U.S. gross national product in 1985 was $3.573 trillion in 1982 dollars.) Consumers spent more than $203.5 billion on food in grocery stores and supermarkets and another $185.6 billion in restaurants, school dining halls, and work cafeterias (National Restaurant Association, 1986; Supermarket Business, 1986a). In recent years, nutrition and health concerns have had an increasingly significant influence on the consumer's food choices, in both the at-home and away-from-home marketplaces. In response, food service establishments and grocery stores and supermarkets have begun to offer a wider variety of foods and food products that reflect changing consumer tastes and preferences.

## CHANGING CONSUMER ATTITUDES AND INDUSTRY RESPONSES

### General Trends

Several recent surveys have indicated that consumer behavior regarding food choices

is changing. From 1979 to 1980, the Economics and Statistics Service of the U.S. Department of Agriculture conducted a nationwide survey to obtain data linking consumer health and nutrition concerns with stated food use practices. The purpose of the survey was to provide information upon which to base future nutrition education programs (Jones and Weimer, 1981). About 28 percent of households making a change in food use for health or nutrition reasons cited a concern about fat intake; 23 percent were concerned about cholesterol; another 23 percent were trying to reduce salt intake or to control high blood pressure; and 43 percent wanted to lose weight.

More recent surveys confirm this continuing interest in the nutritional composition of foods and the diet as a whole. The 1986 consumer attitude and behavior survey conducted by the National Restaurant Association found that at least half of the respondents indicated that they were making a conscious decision to restrict the use of certain food components such as salt, sugar, fat, and cholesterol. About two-thirds indicated that they were including other types of nutritious foods in their diet, including those high in fiber, calcium, and starch. More than one-third either were on a special diet or had been on one during the previous year.

The 1986 edition of the Food Marketing Institute's *Trends: Consumer Attitudes & The Supermarket* reported that 93 percent of shoppers stated that they were concerned about the nutritional content of the food they ate, and 83 percent stated that the vitamin/mineral, salt, fat, cholesterol, or calorie content concerned them most (Food Marketing Institute, 1986). More than 4 out of 10 respondents considered cholesterol, fats, or salt in foods to be a serious health hazard.

## Consumer Behavior Away from Home

The Food Marketing Institute report also indicated that nearly three-fourths of the survey population was concerned about food ingredients when eating out. Two Gallup surveys, conducted for the National Restaurant Association in 1983 and 1986, concluded that consumers are changing their eating habits "by increasing their consumption of fruits, vegetables, or whole grains or by decreasing their consumption of refined sugar, animal fats, or salt." They revealed that 6 out of 10 consumers reported altering their at-home eating habits and 4 out of 10 were changing their away-from-home choices. The responses were very similar during both survey years, indicating that concern about nutrition has remained a strong influence and is not merely a passing fad.

The consumers surveyed for the National Restaurant Association stated that when dining in restaurants they were using less salt or no salt (23 percent), using less fat (20 percent), and avoiding fried foods (15 percent). Respondents were asked which of a list of various foods they were likely to try at a restaurant; the responses included lean meats (64 percent), broiled/baked fish or seafood (63 percent), poultry without skin (47 percent), and food cooked without salt (36 percent).

What consumers say they are doing and what they actually are doing do not always coincide, but in this instance the Gallup surveys confirmed consumer practice. The CREST (Consumer Reports on Eating Share Trends) Household Report, which evaluated menu changes from 1982 to 1985, indicated that the largest increases were in nonfried fish, main dish salads, rice, fruit, chicken, and Asian foods (CREST, 1986). The 1986 Gallup Organization's Survey of Restaurant Managers indicated that about one-third of the respondents mentioned more requests for lean meat, foods prepared without sauces and butter, and foods cooked without salt (Restaurants USA, 1986). New Restaurant Concepts, another National Restaurant Association survey conducted in 1985 and again in 1986, provides further evidence for this changing consumer behavior. It found that in 1986, 3 out of 10 consumers had patronized restaurants specializing in diet or light menu items, as compared to one-fourth in 1985.

## Response by Restaurateurs

In response to increasing concern about health and nutrition among consumers, many food service establishments have made changes in their menus or in their methods of preparation. In 1983, a report funded by the American Express Foundation described a series of innovative programs by restaurants geared toward preparing and promoting healthier foods (Public Voice for Food and Health Policy, 1983). It noted that restaurants emphasizing nutritious offerings almost always included a focus on freshness, simpler and lighter preparation, innovative use of menus, and varied promotional techniques, including publicized affiliation with health organizations and consumer groups.

The 1986 Gallup Survey of Restaurant Managers reported that 38 percent stated that they either featured a health or nutrition promotion or they planned to do so in the future. About one-third said they would honor requests for reduced-calorie salad dressings, low-fat or skim milk, or salt substitutes. Nearly three-fourths reported that they would alter preparation methods upon request. Nine out of 10 would serve sauce or salad dressing on the side, cook without salt, or substitute unsaturated for saturated fats upon request. Among those who would honor requests to alter cooking methods, 8 out of 10 would bake or broil a food rather than fry it and 6 out of 10 would remove the skin from poultry before cooking.

## Consumer Behavior in Grocery Stores and Supermarkets

According to the Food Marketing Institute's findings, consumers are concerned about the nutritional content of the food they buy, specifically its fat and cholesterol (30 percent), vitamin/mineral (22 percent), salt (20 percent), and calorie (11 percent) contents. Nearly half of all respondents indicated that they frequently checked food labels for protein and fat content, and more than a third avoided buying products that had no nutritional information. A Nielson report on consumer behavior cited three top motivators in the purchase of food items: taste, price, and healthfulness, with the order dependent on the circumstances (Carlson, 1983). It also estimated that about three-fourths of consumers were considering nutrition in their food purchasing decisions but that they would not buy a product more than once if the taste was not acceptable, even if it was cheaper and more healthful. Others have suggested that convenient preparation is the dominant theme among today's new products, with nutrition replacing price as the key consideration in many food purchase decisions (PF New Products Annual, 1986a).

In line with this attitude, sales of calorie- and portion-controlled frozen dinners hit an all-time high of $232 million in 1985, ac-counting for more than a third of all frozen food sales (PF New Products Annual, 1986b; Progressive Grocer, 1986a). In addition, 1985 sales of dietetic and low-calorie sauces and dressings increased nearly 10.5 percent, artificial sweeteners and sugar substitutes by 10.8 percent, and salt substitutes and low-sodium salt by almost 9 percent. Consumers are, in large part, putting into practice what they consider to be healthier eating habits. For example, the categories with the largest volume increases in dollar sales in 1985 included fresh and frozen poultry, fresh fruits and vegetables, fresh fish and seafood, and yogurt and fresh milk (Supermarket Business, 1986b). Yogurt sales alone increased 18.6 percent, bringing in nearly $1.6 billion. The categories experiencing the largest volume decreases in dollar sales further reflected consumer health perceptions: fresh and frozen beef, sugar, natural cheese, fresh and cured ham and pork, and bacon.

However, items like alcoholic coolers, frozen french toast and pancakes, and potato chips also enjoyed large increases in sales. Indeed, high-calorie, high-fat, premium foods were selling as well as some of the newer low-calorie, low-fat products. Langer (1985) has termed this phenomenon the "work out/pig out" paradox. Superpremium ice cream, such as Häagen-Dazs®, Frusen Glädjé®, and DoveBars®, contains 15 to 20 percent butterfat, as compared with 10 to 16 percent for traditional ice cream. Yet, sales of superpremium ice cream increased 20 percent in 1985 (Progressive Grocer, 1986b). Perhaps what we are seeing is actually an emerging new philosophy of nutrition: that a balanced diet can be achieved from a variety of foods—high-fat as well as low-fat—consumed over several days or even a week, compared with the more traditional thinking of three square meals a day.

The National Consumer Retail Beef Study, conducted jointly by Texas A&M University, the National Live Stock & Meat Board, and the National Cattlemen's Association, was an industry-wide program aimed at identifying consumer preferences for beef (Cross et al., 1986). It found that consumers considered price, fatness, and cholesterol as the three most important factors in the purchase of beef. Consumers perceived the closer or completely trimmed retail cuts of beef as being more appetizing, better tasting, and more nutritious (lower in cholesterol). Some consumers showed a clear purchase preference for the Good/Select grade (called Select in that study), even when it was priced higher than the Choice grade. A major recommendation of this study was to merchandise both grades of beef, each for its own strengths: Choice for its taste appeal and Good/Select for its leanness.

Another national survey of consumer opinions on issues regarding beef was the Farm Journal (1987) Beef Extra Survey of consumers, conducted in November 1986. A nationally representative sample of consumers was asked to identify which grade of beef had the least amount of fat; 56 percent said Prime, 16 percent said Choice, 3 percent said Good, 11 percent said Standard, and 14 percent indicated that they did not know. Fifty-eight percent of those surveyed stated that U.S. grades were helpful in making purchasing decisions. About one-third indicated that they had eaten less beef in 1986 than in 1985, and, of this group, 71 percent stated that they had done so for health reasons. Seventy-eight percent indicated that they would pay more for lower fat beef if it were available.

The American Meat Institute (1987) published the results of a survey conducted for Giant Food Inc. on consumer awareness, usage, and purchase patterns of a No-Roll (ungraded) beef equivalent to the Good/Select grade (Giant Lean™) versus beef of the Choice grade. Consumers purchasing Giant Lean™ ranked taste, healthfulness, value, nutrition, and leanness among the most important reasons for choosing this type of beef. Those who purchased Giant Lean™ also bought more beef, pork, lamb, veal, and fish than those who did not buy Giant Lean™. When asked which of four grades Giant Lean was, consumers answered Prime (34 percent), Choice (38 percent), Good (14 percent), and Standard (4 percent), with 9 percent answering that they did not know. This confirms previous research indicating that consumers are confused about grades.

## Response by Supermarkets

A number of supermarkets, grocery stores, and commodity organizations have developed consumer information programs to help the shopper identify the nutritional attributes of different food products. For example, Xtra Super Food Centers (Pompano, Florida), Giant Food Inc. (Washington, D.C.), and A&P Stores (Montvale, New Jersey) all have shelf-labeling programs that alert the consumer to foods that are low in calories, sodium, cholesterol, or fat. The National Dairy Board has a calcium education program that includes booklets keyed to different age groups and information about specific dairy products. Nutri-Facts™, a joint program of the Food Marketing Institute, the American Meat Institute, and the National Live Stock & Meat Board, provides point-of-purchase information about various cuts of meat.

Giant Food Inc. and Safeway Stores, Inc. have comprehensive nutrition education programs for their consumers, with printed recipes; brochures for special groups, such as the elderly, infants and toddlers, and pregnant women, and on different aspects of nutrition; point-of-purchase materials; advertising messages; and seasonal programs. Other food stores have developed unique consumer information programs; one example is Red Owl Stores (Hopkins, Minnesota). As a result of the university-based Minnesota Heart Health Project, Red Owl Stores instituted their Better Health with Lean Meat Program, which included identifying leaner cuts of meat with stickers bearing a red heart-shaped logo, printed recipes and brochures, cooking demonstrations, and a nutrition hotline.

As a direct result of the National Consumer Retail Beef Study's findings (Cross et. al., 1986), which were released in January 1986, several national and regional retail supermarket chains, including Kroger and Safeway, began closely trimming (0.25 inch) or completely trimming (no external fat) their retail cuts of beef. Meat packers, such as EXCEL Corporation, have reduced the level of external fat on their wholesale and subprimal cuts of beef. In addition, several organizations, including Public Voice for Food and Health Policy, the American Cancer Society, and the American Heart Association, petitioned the U.S. Department of Agriculture (USDA) to change the name of the Good grade to Select to improve its connotation for consumers. The American Meat Institute and the National Cattlemen's Association encouraged the USDA to make this change, and the department officially changed the name of the Good grade to Select, effective November 23, 1987.

One of the most visible responses by food retailers has been the growth of the service delicatessen, in-store bakery, fresh fish and seafood department, and salad bar, as well as the expansion in size and variety of the produce department. More than half of the nation's supermarkets have both a service delicatessen and an in-store bakery (Progressive Grocer, 1986d). In 1985, both these departments had increased sales by more than 12.5 percent over 1984, followed by fresh fish and seafood (10.8 percent) and produce (2.9 percent for vegetables, 5.8 percent for fruits) (Supermarket Business, 1986c).

## Consumer Behavior at Home

Several national surveys commissioned by the American Meat Institute and the National Live Stock & Meat Board indicate changing consumption patterns of meat and other animal products (Yankelovich, Skelly and White, Inc., 1985). These surveys found that households reported serving red meat less often and in smaller portions than in previous years. In addition, more households were serving poultry. Of the 30 percent of respondents who reported that their families had reduced red meat consumption, 40 percent reported that they had done so for health reasons. An additional 26 percent indicated that their red meat consumption had declined because there had been household changes affecting family meals, including fewer individuals eating or living at home, smaller meals, and eating out more often.

Several trends in food purchases reflect what consumers eat at home, how often they eat, how they prepare meals, and their changing food preferences. One-fourth of shoppers in the Food Marketing Institute's *Trends* report indicated that they frequently purchased delicatessen or carry-out food items; one-fifth often purchased items from the salad bar; 18 percent regularly bought food products designed especially for microwave cooking; and 14 percent consistently used fresh, partially prepared foods that required less at-home preparation time.

Similar trends were observed in grocery sales; for example, the service delicatessen ranked number one in 1985 as having the largest volume increase in dollar sales (Supermarket Business, 1986b). More than 40 percent of U.S. households already own microwave ovens, and this figure is expected to increase to 70 percent by the end of the decade (PF New Products Annual, 1986c). Ethnic foods, particularly Mexican, Italian, and Oriental, are becoming increasingly popular, as indicated by rising sales of burritos, chips, tortillas, salsas, and dips, as well as sauces and ethnic entrees. Among the best-selling frozen food items in 1985 were Italian dishes (sales up more than $96 million since 1984) and Oriental dishes (sales up more than $36 million since 1984) (Advertising Age, 1985).

Data from the 1985 Continuing Survey of Food Intake by Individuals (CSFII) indicate that individuals are eating more frequently throughout the day than they were at the time of the 1977–1978 National Food Consumption Survey (NFCS); these trends are presented in Table 4–1. For example, in 1977, about half of the adult respondents ages 19 to 50 reported eating three or fewer times per day and half reported eating four or more times per day. In 1985, this had changed to only about one-third reporting eating three or fewer times per day and two-thirds eating four or more times per day. The trend with young children ages 4 and 5 is even more dramatic; about 40 percent ate three or fewer times per day in 1977, compared to about 20 percent in 1985. Less than 60 percent of these children ate four or more times per day in 1977, compared to nearly 80 percent in 1985.

Food sales and surveys confirm data from the 1985 CSFII in that they reflect the trend toward "grazing"—snacking throughout the day—rather than eating the traditional three full meals. A recent national survey commissioned by the Condé Nast Package of Women reported that about one-third of women in the United States have abandoned regular eating habits in favor of snacking whenever they are hungry (Mark Clements Research/National Family Opinion Survey, 1985).

As stated earlier, trends in food choices are somewhat contradictory. Snack food sales increased more than 8 percent in 1985, totaling nearly $7.5 billion (Supermarket Business, 1986d). Within this category, fruit rolls and bars showed the largest percentage increase since 1984, up nearly 23 percent. Potato chip sales increased by more than 9 percent over 1984 figures, with more than twice the dollar sales (over $1.8 billion) of any other snack item. Sales of popcorn (packaged, unpopped), which is perceived as a healthy snack because of its low-calorie, high-fiber content, increased by more than 18.5 percent in 1985 for a total of nearly $400 million. The 17 brands of microwave popcorn and the 3 brands in the frozen food case are an interesting example of the combination of "healthful" food, the trend toward snacking as a meal, and microwave cooking (Progressive Grocer, 1986e).

Another irony of the grazing and health trends is the rise in candy and gum sales, up 3.7 percent for a total of nearly $9 billion in 1985 (Supermarket Business, 1986e). Of this figure, about $61 million (0.68 percent) was diet, low-calorie, or sugarless candy and gum. Chocolate bar sales, up 2.8 percent, accounted for over $2.6 billion in 1985. The largest percent increase was in the sale of chocolate-covered nuts, up more than 14

TABLE 4-1  Eating Occasions per Day (in percent)

| Eating Occasions Per Day | Children | | | | Females | | | | Males | | | |
|---|---|---|---|---|---|---|---|---|---|---|---|---|
| | 1–3 Years | | 4–5 Years | | 19–34 Years | | 35–50 Years | | 19–34 Years | | 35–50 Years | |
| | 1977 | 1985 | 1977 | 1985 | 1977 | 1985 | 1977 | 1985 | 1977 | 1985 | 1977 | 1985 |
| ≤3 | 33 | 15.3 | 40.7 | 20.4 | 52.4 | 33.3 | 47.5 | 31.8 | 51.3 | 39.0 | 47.1 | 30.7 |
| ≥4 | 67 | 84.7 | 59.3 | 79.6 | 47.6 | 66.7 | 52.5 | 68.2 | 48.7 | 61.0 | 52.9 | 69.3 |

SOURCES: Adapted from U.S. Department of Agriculture. 1985. P. 50 in Women 19–50 Years and Their Children 1–5 Years, 1 Day. Nationwide Food Consumption Survey, Continuing Survey of Food Intakes by Individuals. Report 85-1, Human Nutrition Information Service. Hyattsville, Md.: U.S. Department of Agriculture. U.S. Department of Agriculture. 1986. P. 48 in Men 19–50 Years, 1 Day. Nationwide Food Consumption Survey, Continuing Survey of Food Intakes by Individuals. Report 85-3, Human Nutrition Information Service. Hyattsville, Md.: U.S. Department of Agriculture.

percent since 1984. Per capita candy consumption has risen by 1 pound per year since 1982, to a total of 20 pounds per year in 1985 (Progressive Grocer, 1986f).

Sales of other foods also reflect the consumer's desire for smaller meals requiring less preparation, but consumers may not fully realize the quality of nutrition they may be trading for convenience. In-store bakeries ranked fourth in volume increases in dollar sales in 1985, with a 12.6 percent increase over 1984 figures (Supermarket Business, 1986b). Like the service delicatessen, the in-store bakery provides ready-to-eat products, convenience, and service. The interest in premium products is strong here, too: croissants have become a supermarket staple and account for $700 million in sales a year (Progressive Grocer, 1986g).

Frozen prepared (precooked) foods fit the consumer's preference for convenience, taste, and healthfulness, but often at a premium price. This category is the largest dollar segment in the frozen food section, and it is growing; sales increased by 8.3 percent in 1985, to a total of over $3.6 billion (Supermarket Business, 1986f). Frozen dinners had the largest increase in this category—10.3 percent over 1984 figures—generating more than $1.5 billion. Frozen pizza was second—up 4 percent, for a total exceeding $1 billion.

## OPTIONS IN THE MARKETPLACE

A key focus of the committee's work is to encourage the availability of animal products in the marketplace that could make it easier for consumers to comply with target levels of specific nutrients in their diets. These animal product options should be made available for consumers who have been advised to alter their diets by health professionals as well as for those who wish to change their eating habits on their own. To develop a sense of unmet needs, the committee surveyed products currently available. The committee sent written requests

for product information and nutritional composition to companies introducing new animal products between October 1985 and October 1986 that were lower in calories, fat, cholesterol, or saturated fatty acids or higher in calcium or iron. Between October and December 1986, the committee contacted 65 companies; 13 provided data on their new products. This information is presented in Tables 4–3 and 4–12. For many animal products, new or modified versions appear weekly that offer varying degrees of reduced calories, fat, sodium, or cholesterol at comparable prices.

The nutritional characteristics of both traditional and modified animal products are discussed in this section. Information is included on how well the nutritional composition of individual products matches the defined target levels of nutrients in the diet as a whole. The traditional and modified versions are compared in terms of differences in total caloric content; total fat, cholesterol, saturated fatty acids, and sodium contents; and vitamin and mineral composition. By comparing the nutritional content of individual foods in the diet, more flexibility can be gained in food selection and preparation. At the end of this chapter, these modified animal products are used in example diets for adult men and women.

### Milk and Milk Products

The dairy industry has been particularly responsive to consumer health needs and preferences. Table 4–2 gives the nutrient composition of many traditional dairy products, as well as some of the modified versions of these products. Milk and milk products are the main sources of calcium in the food supply and provide substantial amounts of high-quality protein, zinc, riboflavin, magnesium, and fortified vitamin D (Table 2–1). However, milk and milk products are also a major source of saturated fatty acids and cholesterol, nutrients identified as detrimental to the health of certain segments of

TABLE 4-2  Nutritional Composition of Selected Milk, Milk Products, and Eggs (in a 100 g, edible portion)

| Product | NDB No.[a] | Calories (kcal) | Protein (g) | Carbohydrate (g) | Total Fat (g) | SFA[b] (g) | Stearic Acid[c] ($C_{18:0}$) (g) | MFA[d] (g) | PUFA[e] (g) | Cholesterol (mg) | Calcium (mg) | Iron (mg) | Sodium (mg) |
|---|---|---|---|---|---|---|---|---|---|---|---|---|---|
| Milk | | | | | | | | | | | | | |
| 3.7% fat | 01-078 | 64 | 3.28 | 4.65 | 3.66 | 2.28 | 0.44 | 1.06 | 0.14 | 14 | 119 | 0.05 | 49 |
| 3.3% fat | 01-077 | 61 | 3.29 | 4.66 | 3.34 | 2.08 | 0.40 | 0.96 | 0.12 | 14 | 119 | 0.05 | 49 |
| 2% fat | 01-079 | 50 | 3.33 | 4.80 | 1.92 | 1.20 | 0.23 | 0.56 | 0.07 | 8 | 122 | 0.05 | 50 |
| 1% fat | 01-082 | 42 | 3.29 | 4.78 | 1.06 | 0.66 | 0.13 | 0.31 | 0.04 | 4 | 123 | 0.05 | 50 |
| Skim | 01-085 | 35 | 3.41 | 4.85 | 0.18 | 0.12 | 0.02 | 0.05 | 0.01 | 2 | 123 | 0.04 | 52 |
| Milk Products | | | | | | | | | | | | | |
| Cheese | | | | | | | | | | | | | |
| American, pasteurized | 01-042 | 375 | 22.15 | 1.60 | 31.25 | 19.69 | 3.80 | 8.95 | 0.99 | 94 | 616 | 0.39 | 1,430 |
| Cheddar | 01-009 | 403 | 24.90 | 1.28 | 33.14 | 21.09 | 4.01 | 9.39 | 0.94 | 105 | 721 | 0.68 | 620 |
| Cottage (2% fat) | 01-015 | 90 | 13.74 | 3.63 | 1.93 | 1.22 | 0.22 | 0.55 | 0.06 | 8 | 68 | 0.16 | 406 |
| Cottage (1% fat) | 01-016 | 72 | 12.39 | 2.72 | 1.02 | 0.64 | 0.12 | 0.29 | 0.03 | 4 | 61 | 0.14 | 406 |
| Creamed cottage | 01-012 | 103 | 12.49 | 2.68 | 4.51 | 2.85 | 0.52 | 1.28 | 0.14 | 15 | 60 | 0.14 | 405 |
| Monterey Jack | 01-025 | 373 | 24.48 | 0.68 | 30.28 | — | — | — | — | — | 746 | 0.72 | 536 |
| Mozzarella | 01-026 | 281 | 19.42 | 2.22 | 21.60 | 13.15 | 2.44 | 6.57 | 0.76 | 78 | 517 | 0.18 | 373 |
| Mozzarella, part skim | 01-028 | 254 | 24.26 | 2.77 | 15.92 | 10.11 | 1.94 | 4.51 | 0.47 | 58 | 646 | 0.22 | 466 |
| Ricotta | 01-036 | 174 | 11.26 | 3.04 | 12.98 | 8.30 | 1.28 | 3.63 | 0.38 | 51 | 207 | 0.38 | 84 |
| Ricotta, part skim | 01-037 | 138 | 11.39 | 5.14 | 7.91 | 4.93 | 0.87 | 2.31 | 0.26 | 31 | 272 | 0.44 | 125 |
| Swiss | 01-040 | 376 | 28.43 | 3.38 | 27.45 | 17.78 | 3.25 | 7.27 | 0.97 | 92 | 961 | 0.17 | 260 |

| | | | | | | | | | | | | |
|---|---|---|---|---|---|---|---|---|---|---|---|---|
| Ice cream | | | | | | | | | | | | |
| 16% fat | 01-062 | 236 | 2.79 | 21.59 | 16.00 | 9.96 | 1.94 | 4.62 | 0.59 | 59 | 102 | 0.07 | 73 |
| 10% fat | 01-061 | 202 | 3.61 | 23.85 | 10.77 | 6.70 | 1.30 | 3.11 | 0.40 | 45 | 132 | 0.09 | 87 |
| Ice milk, 4% fat | 01-064 | 140 | 3.94 | 22.11 | 4.30 | 2.68 | 0.52 | 1.24 | 0.16 | 14 | 134 | 0.14 | 80 |
| Yogurt | | | | | | | | | | | | |
| Plain, whole milk | 01-116 | 61 | 3.47 | 4.66 | 3.25 | 2.10 | 0.32 | 0.89 | 0.09 | 13 | 121 | 0.05 | 46 |
| Plain, skim milk | 01-118 | 56 | 5.73 | 7.68 | 0.18 | 0.12 | 0.02 | 0.05 | 0.01 | 2 | 199 | 0.09 | 76 |
| Fruit, low fat | 01-122 | 105 | 4.86 | 18.60 | 1.41 | 0.91 | 0.14 | 0.39 | 0.04 | 6 | 169 | 0.07 | 65 |
| Eggs, chicken, whole, poached | 01-131 | 157 | 12.09 | 1.20 | 11.10 | 3.33 | 0.85 | 4.44 | 1.44 | 545 | 57 | 2.08 | 293 |

NOTE: Dashes denote lack of reliable data for a constituent believed to be present in measurable amounts.

[a] Nutrient Data Bank Numbers (NDB No.) from Agriculture Handbook No. 8-1.
[b] Saturated fatty acids.
[c] Stearic acid ($C_{18:0}$) is a saturated fatty acid that, unlike other saturated fatty acids, does not raise the plasma cholesterol level.
[d] Monounsaturated fatty acids.
[e] Polyunsaturated fatty acids.

SOURCE: U.S. Department of Agriculture. 1976. Composition of Foods: Dairy and Egg Products. Agriculture Handbook No. 8-1. Washington, D.C.: U.S. Government Printing Office.

the population. In addition, milk and milk products uniquely contribute lactose to the diet, which some adults are unable to digest. Table 4–3 provides information on some of the most recently formulated milk and milk products, reduced in one or more of these components, and compares them to their traditional counterparts.

### Traditional Versus Modified Products

The change in the way fluid milk is sold today versus a few years ago provides a classic example of a successful industry response to changing consumer preferences. In 1975, low-fat and skim milk constituted 66.8 pounds of per capita sales; by 1985, this figure had risen to 98 pounds (Table 2–20). Yogurt is another example of a growing variety of products developed to meet consumer demand. Sales of yogurt in 1985 were nearly $1.6 billion, up more than 18 percent over the 1984 figure (Supermarket Business, 1986g).

As shown in Table 4–2, all the reduced-fat (modified) products offer more nutrients per 100 grams and, if comparably priced, offer more nutrients per dollar than do their traditional counterparts. A comparison of regular and low-fat fluid milks illustrates this difference. A change from 3.7 percent fat (whole) milk to 2 percent fat (low-fat) milk (which may represent a more acceptable alternative than skim milk for many people) offers a number of significant nutritional advantages: There is a 22 percent decrease in caloric content; a 48 percent decrease in both total fat and saturated fatty acid contents; a decrease of 43 percent in cholesterol content; increases in protein, vitamin A, the B vitamins, and calcium; and no significant change in all other minerals.

The most dramatic nutritional differences are seen in a change from fluid whole milk to skim milk. There is a 45 percent reduction in calories and a 95 percent reduction in both total fat and saturated fatty acid contents; cholesterol content drops 86 percent; the protein and vitamin A contents increase;

and all other nutrients remain about the same.

Modified versions of mozzarella and ricotta cheese are also available. A change from whole-milk to part-skim-milk mozzarella represents a 10 percent reduction in calories and a 25 percent decrease in total fat, saturated fatty acid, and cholesterol contents. All the B vitamins, as well as protein, iron, magnesium, phosphorus, vitamin A, potassium, and zinc, increase about 25 percent. In addition, the calcium content is increased around 25 percent in the part-skim-milk mozzarella; the product supplies 646 mg of calcium per 100 grams of cheese.

Changing from whole-milk to part-skim-milk ricotta has even more dramatic nutritional benefits for individuals seeking low-calorie and low-fat alternatives. The total caloric content is reduced 21 percent, and the total fat, saturated fatty acid, and cholesterol contents are decreased about 40 percent each. In addition, the sodium content is reduced by nearly half. Calcium content increases about 31 percent, with part-skim-milk ricotta providing 272 mg of calcium per 100 grams of cheese.

Ice cream is another dairy product for which industry has provided several options. The nutritional composition of ice creams with 16 or 10 percent fat and of ice milk with 4 percent fat are presented in Table 4–2. A change in ice cream from 16 percent fat to 10 percent fat results in a 14 percent decrease in calories, a 33 percent decrease in both total fat and saturated fatty acid contents, and a 21 percent decrease in cholesterol. A change from ice cream with 16 percent fat to ice milk with 4 percent fat represents much larger decreases in calories (41 percent) and total fat, saturated fatty acid, and cholesterol (73 to 76 percent each).

### Traditional Versus the Newest Formulations

The dairy industry has responded to the varied health needs of Americans and produced an array of new products to meet the nutritional and health requirements of different groups. For example, during 1986, at least 10 new milks appeared on the market, including milk extra-fortified with calcium (Vital 15™, by the California Milk Advisory Board, with 40 percent of the Recommended Dietary Allowance [RDA] per 8 ounces), promoted to meet the needs of the postmenopausal woman, and low-lactose/low-fat milk (LactAid®, with 70 percent less lactose and 1 percent fat), aimed at the adult segment of the population.

In 1985, a variety of nondairy, calcium-fortified products were introduced, including Tab® with Calcium by the Coca-Cola Company and calcium-fortified baking flours by Pillsbury and General Mills. During the past 12 months, at least four new kinds of sour cream have appeared, all with reduced calorie or fat content or both, and at least eight new types of ice cream or frozen dairy-based desserts have been introduced that are lower in fat and cholesterol than traditional versions.

Dozens of new cheeses have been marketed with modified proportions of fat, cholesterol, calcium, and sodium (see Tables 4–2 and 4–3). In nearly every case, the amount of fat and the cholesterol content have been reduced. Many of the newest products contain less sodium than their traditional counterparts, but may also have a lower calcium content. Nevertheless, the vast majority of these products still get 50 percent or more of their calories from fat. Many consumers assume that part skim means low fat, which it does not. However, these foods need not be eliminated from the diet, just used sparingly; other food selections lower in fat should be used more frequently to compensate.

## Fresh Beef

Beef is a nutrient-dense food especially rich in protein, the B vitamins, iron, and zinc. The nutrient composition of fresh, cooked beef differs by cut and grade and, to a lesser degree, by method of preparation,

since most fresh beef is cooked by broiling and roasting (dry heat) or braising (moist heat). The greatest variation occurs because of differing amounts of external and seam fat left on or in the cut during its retail preparation. In the home, the nutrient content of fresh beef depends directly on how much of the external and seam fat the consumer actually eats.

Most U.S. supermarkets carry the U.S. Choice grade of beef, a large number sell ungraded (No-Roll) beef, and a few carry U.S. Prime (almost always as an alternative gourmet item). A few supermarkets are selling Prime, Choice, and ungraded beef (largely Good/Select grade but actually a composite of Good/Select, Standard, Commercial, and Utility grades, plus Choice grade carcasses that are fatter than yield grade 3, plus occasional bullock and heiferette carcasses). Nutrient composition data for several cuts from each of three quality grades are presented in Table 4–4, along with data for ground beef of three fatness levels.

The following discussion describes the nutritional differences between cuts and grades of beef and how consideration of both factors can optimize selection of cuts to fit dietary and palatability needs of consumers.

### Options Between Grades

*Chuck Blade.* Even with a relatively fat cut of beef, such as chuck blade, grades differ substantially in the content of total fat and saturated fatty acids. For example, a cut of chuck blade from the Good/Select grade, braised, would have 13 percent less total fat and saturated fatty acids and 7 percent fewer calories than a cut of chuck blade from the Choice grade, also braised. The differences between the Prime and Good/Select grades are even greater. Prime is not universally available to the consumer at the retail level but is a frequent option in restaurants. The Good/Select grade is 19.5 percent lower in calories and has only two-thirds the fat and saturated fatty acids.

TABLE 4-3 Nutritional Composition of Traditional and Selected Newly Formulated Milk and Milk Products (100 g, edible portion)

| Product | Calories (kcal) | Protein (g) | Carbohydrate (g) | Total Fat (g) | Cholesterol (mg) | Calcium (mg) | Sodium (mg) |
|---|---|---|---|---|---|---|---|
| **Milk** | | | | | | | |
| 2% fat[a] | 50 | 3.3 | 4.8 | 1.9 | 8 | 122 | 50 |
| Nature's Calcium Plus[b] | 53 | 3.5 | 4.8 | 2.2 | NA | 219 | 57 |
| Pure Milk High Calcium[c] | 53 | 3.5 | 4.8 | 2.2 | NA | 306 | 57 |
| 1% fat[a] | 42 | 3.3 | 4.8 | 1.1 | 4 | 123 | 50 |
| CalciMilk™ Brand Calcium Added 1% Fat Milk[d] | 45 | 3.6 | 4.9 | 0.9 | NA | 223 | 58 |
| Lactaid® Brand 1% Fat Lactose Reduced Milk[d] | 44 | 3.5 | 4.8[l] | 0.9 | NA | 131 | 55 |
| Vital 15™ High Nutrient 1% Lowfat Milk[e] | 86 | 5.2 | 6.9 | 1.2 | 0.04 | 186 | 79 |
| **Cheese** | | | | | | | |
| American, pasteurized process[a] | 375 | 22.2 | 1.6 | 31.3 | 94 | 616 | 1,430 |
| Lactaid® Brand American Process Cheese Food[d] | 315 | 17.5 | 7.0 | 24.5 | NA | 350 | 1,190 |
| Light American Flavored Pasteurized Process Cheese Product[f] | 280 | 21.0 | 7.0 | 17.5 | NA | 700 | 1,330 |
| Light Low Cholesterol Lo Chol®[g] | 245 | 21.0 | 0.0 | 17.5 | 10.5 | 525 | 665 |
| Light n' Lively® American Flavored Pasteurized Process Cheese Product[f] | 245 | 21.0 | 7.0 | 14.0 | 52.5 | 700 | 1,050 |
| Lite-line® American Flavor Pasteurized Process Cheese Product[h] | 189 | 24.3 | 4.5 | 8.2 | 45 | 706 | 1,455 |
| Lite-line® Low Cholesterol Pasteurized Process Cheese Food Substitute American Flavor[h] | 316 | 18.5 | 7.6 | 23.5 | 20 | 464 | 1,525 |
| Cheddar[a] | 403 | 24.9 | 1.3 | 33.1 | 105 | 721 | 620 |
| Chedda-Jack™[g] | 315 | 24.5 | 3.5 | 24.5 | 84 | 700 | 350 |
| Light Natural Chedda-De Lite™[g] | 315 | 24.5 | 3.5 | 24.5 | 87.5 | 700 | 350 |
| Light Naturals Reduced Fat Cheddar Cheese[f] | 296 | 29.7 | 1.7 | 18.9 | 64 | 757 | 723 |
| Light n' Lively® Sharp Cheddar Flavor Pasteurized Process Cheese Product[f] | 245 | 21.0 | 7.0 | 14.0 | 52.5 | 700 | 1,120 |
| Lite-line® Sharp Cheddar Flavor Pasteurized Process Cheese Product[h] | 183 | 24.0 | 3.3 | 8.2 | 40 | 722 | 1,570 |
| Tendale® Cheddar Style Natural Cheese[i] | 252 | 29.3 | 1.3 | 14.9 | 42 | 945 | 616 |
| Monterey Jack[a] | 373 | 24.5 | 0.7 | 30.3 | NA | 746 | 536 |
| Light Natural Slim Jack™[g] | 315 | 21.0 | 3.5 | 24.5 | 80.5 | 525 | 315 |
| Light Naturals Reduced Fat Monterey Jack Cheese[f] | 298 | 29.8 | 1.4 | 19.3 | 66 | 765 | 568 |
| Lite-line® Monterey Jack Flavor Pasteurized Process Cheese Product[h] | 181 | 24.1 | 2.5 | 8.3 | 40 | 690 | 1,580 |

| | | | | | | | |
|---|---|---|---|---|---|---|---|
| Mozzarella[a] | 281 | 19.4 | 2.2 | 21.6 | 78.0 | 517 | 373 |
| Low Sodium, Low Moisture, Part Skim Mozzarella[g] | 280 | 28.0 | 3.5 | 17.5 | 52.5 | 700 | 315 |
| Polly-O® All Natural Lite™ Part Skim Mozzarella Cheese[j] | 246 | 24.5 | 3.5 | 14.0 | 52.5 | 350 | 700 |
| Muenster[a] | 368 | 23.4 | 1.1 | 30.0 | 96 | 717 | 628 |
| Light Natural Low Sodium Muenster[g] | 385 | 24.5 | 0.0 | 31.5 | 10.5 | 700 | 333 |
| Lite-line® Muenster Flavor Pasteurized Process Cheese Product[h] | 186 | 24.8 | 3.9 | 7.9 | 40 | 680 | 1,580 |
| Ricotta[a] | 174 | 11.3 | 3.0 | 13.0 | 51 | 490 | 84 |
| Polly-O® All Natural Lite™ Ricotta Cheese[j] | 140 | 12.3 | 5.3 | 7.0 | 26.3 | 350 | 114 |
| Swiss[a] | 376 | 28.4 | 3.4 | 27.5 | 92 | 961 | 260 |
| Light Natural No Salt Added Swiss Cheese[g] | 350 | 28.0 | 3.5 | 28.0 | 84 | 875 | 28 |
| Light Naturals Reduced Fat Swiss Cheese[f] | 305 | 33.5 | 2.0 | 18.1 | 74 | 1,150 | 187 |
| Light n' Lively® Swiss Flavored Pasteurized Process Cheese Product[h] | 245 | 21.0 | 7.0 | 14.0 | 52.5 | 700 | 980 |
| Lite-line® Swiss Flavor Pasteurized Process Cheese Product[h] | 183 | 24.1 | 3.8 | 7.9 | 40 | 706 | 1,165 |
| Ice Cream | | | | | | | |
| 16% fat[a] | 236 | 2.8 | 21.6 | 16.0 | 55 | 102 | 73 |
| Diabetic Ice Cream[k] | 190 | 4.0 | 21.0[k] | 10.0 | NA | NA | NA |
| Light n' Lively® Vanilla Flavored Ice Milk[f] | 158 | 5.1 | 25.3 | 4.2 | 10 | 189 | 83 |

NOTE: The shaded rows represent traditional versions of the listed milk and milk products. NA means that data were unavailable.

[a]Data are from the U.S. Department of Agriculture. 1976. Composition of Foods: Dairy and Egg Products. Agriculture Handbook No. 8-1. Washington, D.C.: U.S. Department of Agriculture.
[b]Data are from Dean Foods, Rockford, Ill.
[c]Data are from Pure Milk Co., Waco, Tex.
[d]Data are from Lactaid Inc., Pleasantville, N.J.
[e]Data are from the California Milk Advisory Board, Modesto, Calif.
[f]Data are from Kraft Inc., Glenview, Ill.
[g]Data are from N. Dorman & Company Inc., Syosset, N.Y.
[h]Data are from BORDEN, Inc., Columbus, Ohio.
[i]Data are from Associated Milk Producers, Inc., Madison Division, Madison, Wis.
[j]Data are from Pollio Dairy Products Corp., Mineola, N.Y.
[k]Data are from Dreyer's Grand Ice Cream, Oakland, Calif. Dreyer's Diabetic Ice Cream contains 7 g of lactose and 14 g of sorbitol (for a total of 21 g of carbohydrates) per 100 g.
[l]Lactaid® Brand 1% Fat Lactose Reduced Milk contains 1.3 g of lactose per 100 g of milk; unmodified milk contains 5.3 g of lactose per 100 g of unmodified milk.

TABLE 4-4  Nutritional Composition of Beef (100 g, separable lean only, edible portion)

| Cut and Grade | NDB No.[a] | Calories (kcal) | Protein (g) | Total Fat (g) | SFA[b] (g) | Stearic Acid[c] ($C_{18:0}$) (g) | MFA[d] (g) | PUFA[e] (g) | Cholesterol (mg) | Calcium (mg) | Iron (mg) | Sodium (mg) |
|---|---|---|---|---|---|---|---|---|---|---|---|---|
| Bottom round, braised | | | | | | | | | | | | |
| Prime | 13174 | 249 | 31.59 | 12.65 | 4.49 | 1.24 | 5.78 | 0.52 | 96 | 5 | 3.46 | 51 |
| Choice | 13170 | 225 | 31.59 | 9.96 | 3.54 | 0.98 | 4.55 | 0.41 | 96 | 5 | 3.46 | 51 |
| Good/Select | 13172 | 214 | 31.59 | 8.77 | 3.11 | 0.86 | 4.01 | 0.36 | 96 | 5 | 3.46 | 51 |
| Chuck arm, braised | | | | | | | | | | | | |
| Prime | 13048 | 261 | 33.02 | 13.36 | 5.07 | 1.58 | 5.82 | 0.54 | 101 | 9 | 3.79 | 66 |
| Choice | 13044 | 234 | 33.02 | 10.32 | 3.92 | 1.22 | 4.50 | 0.42 | 101 | 9 | 3.79 | 66 |
| Good/Select | 13046 | 222 | 33.02 | 8.97 | 3.40 | 1.06 | 3.91 | 0.36 | 101 | 9 | 3.79 | 66 |
| Chuck blade, braised | | | | | | | | | | | | |
| Prime | 13064 | 318 | 31.06 | 20.53 | 8.37 | 2.68 | 9.18 | 0.69 | 106 | 13 | 3.68 | 71 |
| Choice | 13060 | 275 | 31.06 | 15.80 | 6.44 | 2.06 | 7.06 | 0.53 | 106 | 13 | 3.68 | 71 |
| Good/Select | 13062 | 256 | 31.06 | 13.69 | 5.58 | 1.78 | 6.12 | 0.46 | 106 | 13 | 3.68 | 71 |
| Eye of round, roasted | | | | | | | | | | | | |
| Prime | 13190 | 198 | 28.99 | 8.25 | 3.16 | 0.91 | 3.63 | 0.29 | 69 | 5 | 1.95 | 62 |
| Choice | 13186 | 184 | 28.99 | 6.69 | 2.56 | 0.74 | 2.94 | 0.23 | 69 | 5 | 1.95 | 62 |
| Good/Select | 13188 | 178 | 28.99 | 5.99 | 2.29 | 0.66 | 2.63 | 0.21 | 69 | 5 | 1.95 | 62 |
| Ground beef, well done, broiled | | | | | | | | | | | | |
| Regular | 13313 | 292 | 27.20 | 19.46 | 7.65 | 2.30 | 8.52 | 0.73 | 101 | 12 | 2.74 | 93 |
| Lean | 13306 | 280 | 28.20 | 17.64 | 6.93 | 2.08 | 7.72 | 0.66 | 101 | 12 | 2.45 | 89 |
| Extra Lean | 13299 | 265 | 28.58 | 15.80 | 6.21 | 1.86 | 6.92 | 0.59 | 99 | 9 | 2.77 | 82 |

| | NDB No. | | | | | | | | | | | |
|---|---|---|---|---|---|---|---|---|---|---|---|---|
| Rib (6–12), broiled | | | | | | | | | | | | |
| Prime | 13093 | 280 | 26.03 | 18.70 | 7.97 | 2.51 | 8.25 | 0.56 | 82 | 10 | 2.52 | 69 |
| Choice | 13087 | 233 | 26.03 | 13.55 | 5.70 | 1.79 | 5.90 | 0.40 | 82 | 10 | 2.52 | 69 |
| Good/Select | 13090 | 213 | 26.03 | 11.27 | 4.80 | 1.51 | 4.97 | 0.34 | 82 | 10 | 2.52 | 69 |
| Tenderloin, broiled | | | | | | | | | | | | |
| Prime | 13259 | 232 | 28.25 | 12.36 | 4.83 | 1.62 | 4.81 | 0.49 | 84 | 7 | 3.58 | 63 |
| Choice | 13253 | 207 | 28.25 | 9.59 | 3.74 | 1.26 | 3.73 | 0.38 | 84 | 7 | 3.58 | 63 |
| Good/Select | 13256 | 196 | 28.25 | 8.35 | 3.26 | 1.09 | 3.25 | 0.33 | 84 | 7 | 3.58 | 63 |
| Tip round, roasted | | | | | | | | | | | | |
| Prime | 13206 | 213 | 28.71 | 10.06 | 3.69 | 1.15 | 4.14 | 0.41 | 81 | 5 | 2.94 | 65 |
| Choice | 13202 | 193 | 28.71 | 7.75 | 2.84 | 0.89 | 3.19 | 0.32 | 81 | 5 | 2.94 | 65 |
| Good/Select | 13204 | 183 | 28.71 | 6.72 | 2.46 | 0.77 | 2.77 | 0.27 | 81 | 5 | 2.94 | 65 |
| Top round, broiled | | | | | | | | | | | | |
| Prime | 13224 | 215 | 31.69 | 8.87 | 3.10 | 0.96 | 3.47 | 0.42 | 84 | 6 | 2.88 | 61 |
| Choice | 13219 | 194 | 31.69 | 6.45 | 2.26 | 0.70 | 2.53 | 0.30 | 84 | 6 | 2.88 | 61 |
| Good/Select | 13222 | 184 | 31.69 | 5.38 | 1.88 | 0.58 | 2.11 | 0.25 | 84 | 6 | 2.88 | 61 |

NOTE: Beef has no carbohydrates. USDA Prime, Choice, and Good/Select grades of beef are from animals less than 42 months of age. The grades differ by the amount of fat within muscle tissue (marbling). Prime grade contains a slightly abundant, moderately abundant, or abundant amount of marbling. Choice grade contains a small, modest, or moderate amount of marbling. Good/Select contains a slight amount of marbling.

[a]Nutrient Data Bank Numbers (NDB No.) from Agriculture Handbook No. 8-13.
[b]Saturated fatty acids.
[c]Stearic acid ($C_{18:0}$) is a saturated fatty acid that, unlike other saturated fatty acids, does not raise the plasma cholesterol level.
[d]Monounsaturated fatty acids.
[e]Polyunsaturated fatty acids.

SOURCE: U.S. Department of Agriculture. 1986. Composition of Foods: Beef Products. Agriculture Handbook No. 8-13. Washington, D.C.: U.S. Government Printing Office.

*Top Round.* Although this is a lean cut of beef, there are still some differences between grades. From Prime to Good/Select, there is a 14 percent difference in calories, a 39 percent difference in total fat content, and a 40 percent difference in saturated fatty acid content. Between Choice and Good/Select, the differences are smaller: 5 percent in calories and 17 percent in total fatty acid and saturated fatty acid contents.

*Ground Beef.* Many stores carry three types of ground beef, which differ in the percentage of total fat after cooking: regular (19.46 percent total fat), lean (17.64 percent total fat), and extra lean (15.80 percent total fat). Ground beef is an animal product with a high fat content; even extra lean ground beef gets more than 53 percent of its calories from fat and 21 percent from saturated fatty acids. Nevertheless, eating extra lean ground beef rather than regular ground beef does result in a 9 percent decrease in caloric content, a 10.5 percent decrease in calories from fat, and a 19 percent reduction in total fat and saturated fatty acid contents. A November 1987 revision of USDA-FSIS Policy Memo 070B has clarified the labeling of ground beef and hamburger as lean or extra lean (see Chapter 5).

Recent research has shown that the method of cooking affects percent yield and composition of ground beef patties over a wide range of fat levels (Berry and Leddy, 1984). It was found that the leaner formulations increased in fat percentage with cooking, while the fatter patties decreased in fat percentage with cooking. Of the six different cooking methods analyzed (electric broiling, charbroiling, roasting, convection heating, frying, and microwaving), microwaving produced cooked ground beef patties with the lowest fat and calorie contents.

### Options Between Cuts

*Bottom Round Versus Top Round.* Changing from one cut of beef to another similar, but leaner cut, still within the same grade, can provide substantial shifts in the proportions of nutrients. For example, within the Choice grade, top round has 14 percent fewer calories and 35 to 36 percent less total fat and saturated fatty acids than bottom round. Good/Select top round has 18 percent fewer total calories and 46 to 47 percent less total fat and saturated fatty acids than Choice bottom round.

*Chuck Blade Versus Chuck Arm.* Reductions in fat and calories can be seen in chuck arm versus chuck blade of the same grade. Fat and calories can also be reduced by choosing different cuts from different grades. For the Choice grade, chuck arm has 15 percent fewer calories and 35 to 39 percent less fat and saturated fatty acids than chuck blade. Good/Select chuck arm has 19 percent fewer total calories, 43 percent less total fat content, and 47 percent less saturated fatty acid than Choice chuck blade.

*Minimum-Maximum Intramuscular Fat Content.* Research at Texas A&M University has indicated that a minimum fat content in beef muscle of about 3 percent on an uncooked basis (equivalent to meat cuts that grade low Good/Select) is necessary for acceptable palatability and that no more than 7.3 percent fat (equivalent to meat cuts that grade high Choice) should be present to ensure nutritional merit. Based on these parameters, Figure 4–1 was developed to show the proposed "window of acceptability" for intramuscular fat content for meat products. The background data and research upon which this figure is based are presented in the paper by Savell and Cross (this volume).

*Nutrient Content of Leaner Beef.* A change to leaner beef would have multiple beneficial effects on the total diet, including a higher concentration of the B vitamins, iron, phosphorus, and zinc in the beef

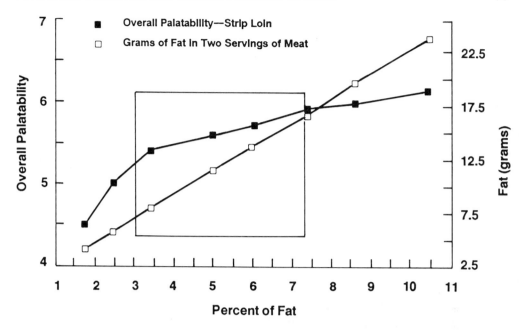

FIGURE 4–1 Window of acceptability for fat content of meat (palatability versus grams of fat, two servings). The window is based on a fat content range of 3.0 to 7.3 percent. This is equivalent to meat cuts that grade in the lower range of Good/Select (3.0 to 4.27 percent fat content) to those that grade in the high range of Choice (4.28 to 8.0 percent fat content). Source: Savell and Cross, this volume.

consumed. The riboflavin and iron content of beef ranges from about 10 to 20 percent of the RDA for 100 grams, with increased concentrations present in the leaner cuts. Niacin, phosphorus, and pyridoxine are also more concentrated in leaner tissue and average about 15 to 30 percent of the RDA per 100 grams. Leaner tissue contains much higher levels of both zinc and vitamin $B_{12}$, too, contributing between 36 and 68 percent of the RDA per 100 grams.

## Pork

A significant reduction of back fat and increased muscling (lean tissue) has occurred in the U.S. pig population since 1960. The grading system, genetic and nutritional effects on lean tissue composition, and options for the diet-conscious consumer are discussed in this section.

### Grading System for Pork

There are two USDA quality designations for swine and pork carcasses—acceptable, designated Grade U.S., and unacceptable, designated Grade U.S. Utility—and four cutability grades—Nos. 1, 2, 3, and 4. Grades are based on the interactions of back fat, carcass length or carcass weight, and muscling. U.S. No. 1 denotes the highest cutability (least fat), and U.S. No. 4 denotes the lowest cutability (most fat). The grading system has undergone several revisions (in 1955, 1968, and 1985) in response to improvements in leanness of swine and pork carcasses. Processors and packing companies who have grade and yield purchasing options have updated their grading criteria and price differentials in synchrony with the National Pork Producers Council's Pork Value program which recognizes the reduction in back fat and the increase in muscling of pigs that have occurred in the U.S. industry (National Pork Producers Council, 1982). This program encourages packers to pay for hogs based on lean yield. Table 4–5 presents data from three nationwide USDA surveys of barrow and gilt carcasses that show the changes in pork carcass composition (as evidenced by changes in USDA grades) that have occurred in the swine industry. A remarkable reduction in back fat and an increase in lean tissue (muscling) occurred in the market hog population from 1963 to 1983 (U.S. Department of Agriculture, 1963, 1983).

### Changes from 1963 to 1983

The leanness of retail cuts of pork improved markedly between 1963 and 1983. This is evident in Table 4–6, which compares lean and fat percentages for selected cuts for the years 1963 and 1983. Some of the differences in leanness or fatness shown can be accounted for by improvements in the leanness of market hogs during that period.

There appears to be little or no relationship between the amount of subcutaneous fat (back fat thickness) and the amount of intramuscular fat (marbling) in the market hog. The consensus is that genetic selection for back fat thickness and longissimus muscle intramuscular fat could be pursued independently with little influence of one on the other (Hays, 1968; Omtvedt, 1968).

The amount of dietary protein fed to growing-finishing swine greatly influences the fat content of the longissimus muscle (Hays, 1968; Wallace, 1968). For example, the ether-extractable (total lipid) content of the longissimus dorsi (loineye) muscle of market hogs fed a 12 percent crude protein diet averaged 16.3 percent, whereas that of swine fed a 16 percent crude protein diet averaged only 9.3 percent (dry matter basis). The energy concentration in the diet also influences the intramuscular fat level, as does limiting or restricting feed intake.

TABLE 4-5  Distribution of Barrow and Gilt Carcasses (in percent) Among Cutability Grades for Selected Years Using 1968 USDA Grading Standards

| Year Surveyed | Grade, U.S. No. | | | | |
|---|---|---|---|---|---|
| | 1 | 2 | 3 | 4 | Utility |
| 1960–1961 | | 33.0 | 38.8 | 25.9 | 2.2 |
| 1967–1968 | 8.1 | 42.1 | 35.7 | 12.2 | 1.8 |
| 1980 | 71.7 | 24.2 | 3.7 | 0.3 | 0.1 |

NOTE:  Grades are based on combinations of back fat, carcass length or carcass weight, and muscling. U.S. No. 1 denotes the highest cutability (least fat) and U.S. No. 4 denotes the least cutability (most fat). In terms of quality designation, utility means unacceptable. The 1960–1961 survey included 45,000 head; the 1967–1968 survey, 57,000 head; and the 1980 survey, 36,000 head.

SOURCES:  U.S. Department of Agriculture. 1969. Marketing Research Report No. 849. Economic Research Service. Washington, D.C.: U.S. Department of Agriculture. U.S. Department of Agriculture. 1982. ERS-675. Economic Research Service. Washington, D.C.: U.S. Department of Agriculture.

### Pork Quality Standards

The system of having only two USDA quality grades for pork—acceptable (Grade U.S.) and unacceptable (Grade U.S. Utility)—to predict differences in flavor, juiciness, and tenderness of the cooked product is not nearly as discriminating as the USDA grading system for beef. Pork grading standards have been proposed for wholesale cuts that would categorize the product by differences in color, structure, firmness, and degree of marbling in the lean tissue (University of Wisconsin, 1963). Some packing and processing companies use a quality grading system similar to that proposed by the Wisconsin Agricultural Experiment Station to segregate or identify fresh pork cuts and cured products. The branded hams that contain 5 percent or less fat are a good example. These hams are selected to meet strict color and intramuscular fat standards. Other examples of "quality" standardization are packaging, shelf life, and trim; quality standards also exist for the oven-ready or

TABLE 4-6  Comparison of Nutrient Composition Between 1963 and 1983 Market Hogs

| Cut | Year | kcal/100 g | Nutrient Composition (%) | |
|-----|------|-----------|--------------------------|---|
| | | | Protein | Fat |
| | | | *Separable lean* | |
| Boston, blade | 1963 | 180 | 18.0 | 11.4 |
| | 1983 | 165 | 19.0 | 9.3 |
| Ham | 1963 | 152 | 19.8 | 7.5 |
| | 1983 | 136 | 20.5 | 5.4 |
| Loin, whole | 1963 | 189 | 20.1 | 11.4 |
| | 1983 | 156 | 20.7 | 7.5 |
| Picnic | 1963 | 150 | 19.2 | 7.5 |
| | 1983 | 140 | 19.8 | 6.2 |

NOTE:  The 1963 data are based on an assumed distribution of 34, 40, and 25 percent of thin, medium, and fat pig types, respectively. For the 1983 data, 71.7 percent of the retail cuts were from U.S. Grade No. 1 carcasses; 24.2 percent from No. 2; and 3.7 percent from No. 3.

SOURCES:  U.S. Department of Agriculture. 1963. Composition of Foods: Raw, Processed, and Prepared. Agriculture Handbook No. 8. Washington, D.C.: U.S. Government Printing Office. U.S. Department of Agriculture. Marketing Research Report No. 849. 1969. Economic Research Service. Washington, D.C.: U.S. Department of Agriculture. U.S. Department of Agriculture. 1982. ERS-675. Economic Research Service. Washington, D.C.: U.S. Department of Agriculture. U.S. Department of Agriculture. 1983. Composition of Foods: Pork Products. Agriculture Handbook No. 8-10. Washington, D.C.: U.S. Government Printing Office.

microwave-ready fresh pork products that some companies with national distribution are now marketing (Allen and Pierson, 1986).

For the untrained consumer who is purchasing fresh pork products in the supermarket, there is no universal identification system to ensure that he or she is selecting a product that is low or moderately low in fat. Such a system could be very useful for those people who want to minimize their intake of fat and calories. If such an identification system were used, incentive would exist to significantly reduce fat content below the level listed in *USDA Handbook 8–10* for pork loin (U.S. Department of Agriculture, 1983). Research suggests that the longissimus dorsi muscle of the pork loin would have acceptable palatability if the intramuscular fat level was 3.5 to 4.5 percent on a fresh basis (Smith and Carpenter, 1976). When broiled, chops with 3.5 to 4.5 percent intramuscular fat would contain an estimated 6.7 to 8.5 percent fat, which is about one-half the fat content of the lean tissue of loin cuts listed in *USDA Handbook 8–10* (U.S. Department of Ag-

riculture, 1983). Recent research suggests that some pork carcasses may be as lean as 4.3 percent fat (K. J. Prusa, Iowa State University, personal communication, 1987). The nutritional composition of selected pork products is shown in Table 4–7.

### Summary

A quality grading system for pork cuts would help the consumer identify lean tissue with low, but acceptable, levels of intramuscular fat. With present technology, breeding and feeding programs could be developed immediately and implemented to ensure desirable levels of intramuscular fat in pork cuts. The alternative for the untrained, diet-conscious consumer is to select cuts of pork that are, on the average, lower in fat and cholesterol, as shown in the example diets presented at the end of this chapter.

### Lamb and Veal

Data from the food supply indicate that about 1.5 pounds of veal and 1.1 pounds of

TABLE 4-7  Nutritional Composition of Pork (100 g, separable lean only, edible portion)

| Cut | NDB No.[a] | Calories (kcal) | Protein (g) | Total Fat (g) | SFA[b] (g) | Stearic Acid[c] $(C_{18:0})$ (g) | MFA[d] (g) | PUFA[e] (g) | Cholesterol (mg) | Calcium (mg) | Iron (mg) | Sodium (mg) |
|---|---|---|---|---|---|---|---|---|---|---|---|---|
| Bacon, Canadian-style, grilled | 10131 | 185 | 24.24 | 8.44 | 2.84 | 0.88 | 4.04 | 0.81 | 58 | 10 | 0.82 | 1,546 |
| Bacon, fried | 10124 | 576 | 30.45 | 49.24 | 17.42 | 5.67 | 23.69 | 5.81 | 85 | 12 | 1.61 | 1,596 |
| Ham, cured, roasted (11% fat) | 10136 | 178 | 22.62 | 9.02 | 3.12 | 1.05 | 4.44 | 1.41 | 59 | 8 | 1.34 | 1,500 |
| Ham, extra lean, roasted (5% fat) | 10134 | 145 | 20.93 | 5.53 | 1.81 | 0.57 | 2.62 | 0.54 | 53 | 8 | 1.48 | 1,203 |
| Leg, whole, roasted | 10011 | 220 | 28.32 | 11.03 | 3.80 | 1.22 | 4.96 | 1.34 | 94 | 7 | 1.12 | 64 |
| Rump | 10015 | 221 | 29.14 | 10.66 | 3.67 | 1.18 | 4.79 | 1.29 | 96 | 7 | 1.14 | 65 |
| Shank | 10019 | 215 | 28.21 | 10.50 | 3.62 | 1.16 | 4.72 | 1.27 | 92 | 7 | 1.11 | 64 |
| Loin, blade, roasted | 10035 | 279 | 24.68 | 19.30 | 6.65 | 2.13 | 8.68 | 2.34 | 89 | 14 | 1.25 | 68 |
| Center, broiled | 10042 | 231 | 32.00 | 10.48 | 3.61 | 1.16 | 4.71 | 1.27 | 98 | 5 | 0.92 | 78 |
| Center rib, broiled | 10050 | 258 | 28.82 | 14.94 | 5.15 | 1.65 | 6.71 | 1.81 | 94 | 15 | 0.81 | 67 |
| Sirloin, roasted | 10059 | 236 | 27.49 | 13.17 | 4.54 | 1.45 | 5.92 | 1.60 | 90 | 10 | 1.09 | 62 |
| Tenderloin, roasted | 10061 | 166 | 28.79 | 4.81 | 1.66 | 0.53 | 2.16 | 0.58 | 93 | 9 | 1.54 | 67 |
| Whole, broiled | 10026 | 257 | 27.84 | 15.29 | 5.27 | 1.68 | 6.87 | 1.86 | 95 | 7 | 0.93 | 75 |
| Shoulder, whole, roasted | 10073 | 244 | 25.38 | 14.99 | 5.17 | 1.65 | 6.74 | 1.82 | 97 | 8 | 1.52 | 76 |
| Boston, blade, roasted | 10087 | 256 | 24.36 | 16.84 | 5.80 | 1.86 | 7.57 | 2.04 | 98 | 7 | 1.60 | 73 |
| Picnic arm, braised | 10078 | 248 | 32.26 | 12.21 | 4.21 | 1.35 | 5.49 | 1.48 | 114 | 8 | 1.95 | 102 |

NOTE:  Pork products in this table have no carbohydrates.

[a]Nutrient Data Bank Number (NDB No.) from Agriculture Handbook No. 8-10.
[b]Saturated fatty acids.
[c]Stearic acid $(C_{18:0})$ is a saturated fatty acid that, unlike other saturated fatty acids, does not raise the plasma cholesterol level.
[d]Monounsaturated fatty acids.
[e]Polyunsaturated fatty acids.

SOURCE:  U.S. Department of Agriculture. 1983. Composition of Foods: Pork Products. Agriculture Handbook No. 8-10. Washington, D.C.: U.S. Government Printing Office.

82

lamb are consumed per capita per year (Table 2–16). The primary differences between kinds of lamb and between kinds of veal with regard to composition of cuts are related to the ages at which they are slaughtered. (A versus B maturity for lamb; Bob veal versus Special Fed veal for bovine animals slaughtered at ages less than 3 months.) Tables 4–8 and 4–9 present the nutritional composition of a variety of cuts of two types of lamb and two types of veal, respectively.

### Lamb

Overall, cuts from older lambs (B maturity in Table 4–8—animals that were 8 to 9 months old at slaughter—versus A maturity—animals that were 4 to 4.5 months old at slaughter) have fewer calories and less total fat and cholesterol. For example, loin chops from B maturity lambs are 15 percent lower in fat and 5 percent lower in calories and cholesterol than loin chops from A maturity lambs; blade chops from B maturity lambs are 33 percent lower in fat, 16 percent lower in calories, and 12 percent lower in cholesterol than blade chops from A maturity lambs (Table 4–8).

### Veal

Bob veal, which is slaughtered at less than 4 weeks of age, tends to be lower in total fat and calories but higher in cholesterol than Special Fed veal, which is slaughtered at about 16 weeks of age. For example, a rib roast from Bob veal contains 64 percent less fat and 38 percent fewer calories but 10 percent more cholesterol than Special Fed veal. A Bob veal loin chop has 67 percent less fat and 24 percent fewer calories but 23 percent more cholesterol than a Special Fed veal loin chop (Table 4–9).

TABLE 4-8  Nutritional Composition of Cooked Lamb (100 g, separable lean only, edible portion)

| Cut | Age Group | Calories (kcal) | Protein (g) | Total Fat (g) | Cholesterol (mg) | Calcium (mg) | Iron (mg) | Sodium (mg) |
|---|---|---|---|---|---|---|---|---|
| Arm chop, braised | A | 277 | 35.97 | 13.81 | 119 | 21 | 2.2 | 72 |
|  | B | 280 | 35.18 | 14.36 | 124 | 30 | 3.2 | 79 |
| Blade chop, roasted | A | 229 | 26.71 | 12.79 | 96 | 23 | 1.6 | 94 |
|  | B | 197 | 25.79 | 9.65 | 86 | 25 | 2.0 | 82 |
| Foreshank, braised | A | 198 | 32.61 | 6.47 | 106 | 14 | 2.0 | 74 |
|  | B | 176 | 29.42 | 5.57 | 102 | 25 | 2.6 | 74 |
| Leg-shank, roasted | A | 184 | 28.42 | 7.00 | 95 | 7 | 1.9 | 63 |
|  | B | 176 | 27.84 | 6.35 | 79 | 9 | 2.2 | 69 |
| Leg-sirloin, roasted | A | 221 | 29.96 | 10.29 | 100 | 8 | 2.1 | 70 |
|  | B | 187 | 27.00 | 8.05 | 84 | 8 | 2.3 | 71 |
| Loin chop, broiled | A | 221 | 29.77 | 10.42 | 97 | 15 | 1.8 | 84 |
|  | B | 211 | 30.20 | 8.92 | 92 | 22 | 2.2 | 83 |
| Rib roast, roasted | A | 248 | 25.96 | 15.16 | 92 | 18 | 1.5 | 79 |
|  | B | 217 | 26.36 | 11.57 | 83 | 24 | 2.0 | 83 |

NOTE:  "A" animals were 4 to 4.5 months of age at slaughter and raised on shelled corn and mineral-vitamin pellets. "B" animals were 8 to 9 months of age at slaughter and raised on pasture supplemented with shelled corn and mineral-vitamin pellets. Most retail lamb in the United States is type B.

SOURCE:  K. Ono, B. W. Berry, H. K. Johnson, E. Russek, C. F. Parker, V. R. Cahill, and P. G. Althouse. 1984. Tables 2 and 5 in Nutrient composition of lamb of two age groups. J. Food Sci. 49:1233.

TABLE 4-9  Nutritional Composition of Cooked Veal (100 g, separable lean only, edible portion)

| Cut | Type of Veal | Calories (kcal) | Protein (g) | Total Fat (g) | Cholesterol (mg) | Calcium (mg) | Iron (mg) | Sodium (mg) |
|---|---|---|---|---|---|---|---|---|
| Arm steak, braised | B | 173 | 33.9 | 3.09 | 174 | 34.1 | 1.85 | 113 |
| | SFV | 206 | 36.1 | 5.73 | 152 | 29.6 | 1.33 | 86 |
| Blade steak, braised | B | 163 | 31.4 | 3.15 | 182 | 49.7 | 1.79 | 121 |
| | SFV | 204 | 32.9 | 7.06 | 154 | 38.5 | 1.41 | 98 |
| Cutlet, pan fried | B | 178 | 32.7 | 4.24 | 154 | 11.5 | 1.37 | 98 |
| | SFV | 184 | 33.3 | 4.69 | 120 | 6.2 | 0.79 | 73 |
| Loin chop, braised | B | 188 | 31.7 | 5.82 | 192 | 45.5 | 1.65 | 109 |
| | SFV | 233 | 33.9 | 9.74 | 148 | 29.2 | 1.00 | 79 |
| Rib roast, roasted | B | 134 | 25.0 | 2.98 | 142 | 24.0 | 1.16 | 124 |
| | SFV | 185 | 25.9 | 8.23 | 128 | 15.2 | 0.93 | 92 |
| Sirloin chop, braised | B | 178 | 32.8 | 4.16 | 186 | 27.6 | 1.79 | 97 |
| | SFV | 208 | 34.1 | 6.93 | 133 | 17.4 | 1.12 | 78 |

NOTE: "B" stands for Bob veal, which is from animals raised on maternal milk and slaughtered at less than 4 weeks of age (predominantly grade USDA Good/Select). "SFV" stands for special fed veal, which is from animals fed a special formulated liquid diet and slaughtered at about 16 weeks of age (predominantly grade USDA Choice). USDA Choice and Good/Select grades of beef are from animals less than 42 months of age. The grades differ by the amount of fat within muscle tissue (marbling). Choice grade contains a small, modest, or moderate amount of marbling. Good/Select contains a slight amount of marbling.

SOURCE: K. Ono, B. W. Berry, and L. W. Douglass. 1986. Table 2 in Nutrient composition of some fresh and cooked retail cuts of veal. J. Food Sci. 51C5:1352.

## Convenience Meats

The modified version of bologna is 39 percent lower in fat and has 21 percent fewer calories than the traditional version. A modified version of corned beef (Oscar Mayer Select Slices™) is 67 percent lower in fat and has 36 percent fewer calories but is 24 percent higher in sodium. The modified versions of pastrami are 76 to 92 percent lower in total fat and have 60 to 72 percent fewer calories than the traditional product but contain a comparable amount of sodium. Modified cooked ham is 36 to 50 percent lower in calories and 61 to 74 percent lower in fat than the traditional version.

Several modified versions of frankfurters are available, including chicken franks, turkey franks, and modified beef franks. Chicken franks are 18 percent lower in calories, 32 percent lower in total fat, and 54 percent lower in saturated fatty acids but have 34 percent more sodium than the traditional beef frank. Turkey franks and modified beef franks are 23 percent lower in calories and 39 percent lower in fat than the traditional beef franks.

## Poultry

Poultry makes substantial nutrient contributions to the food supply, particularly in terms of protein, niacin, and vitamin $B_6$. Like beef, the nutritional content can differ with the cut or part as well as by the method of preparation (Table 4–10). This latter factor is particularly important because chicken is so often batter-fried. Frying can increase the caloric content by nearly a third and double the amount of fat in the product in comparison with roasting or stewing.

### Chicken

The leg portion and other dark meat parts of chicken have higher fat and calorie con-

TABLE 4-10 Nutritional Composition of Poultry (100 g, edible portion)

| Part | NDB No.[a] | Calories (kcal) | Protein (g) | Carbohydrate (g) | Total Fat (g) | SFA[b] (g) | Stearic Acid[c] (C$_{18:0}$) (g) | MFA[d] (g) | PUFA[e] (g) | Cholesterol (mg) | Iron (mg) | Calcium (mg) | Sodium (mg) |
|---|---|---|---|---|---|---|---|---|---|---|---|---|---|
| Chicken, without skin | | | | | | | | | | | | | |
| Dark meat, roasted | 05045 | 205 | 27.37 | 0 | 9.73 | 2.66 | 0.63 | 3.56 | 2.26 | 93 | 1.33 | 15 | 93 |
| Light meat, roasted | 05041 | 173 | 30.91 | 0 | 4.51 | 1.27 | 0.32 | 1.54 | 0.98 | 85 | 1.06 | 15 | 77 |
| Chicken, with skin | | | | | | | | | | | | | |
| Breast | | | | | | | | | | | | | |
| Fried, batter-dipped | 05058 | 260 | 24.84 | 8.99 | 13.20 | 3.52 | 1.04 | 5.46 | 3.08 | 85 | 1.25 | 20 | 275 |
| Fried, flour-coated | 05059 | 222 | 31.84 | 1.64 | 8.87 | 2.45 | 0.58 | 3.50 | 1.96 | 89 | 1.19 | 16 | 76 |
| Roasted | 05060 | 197 | 29.80 | 0 | 7.78 | 2.19 | 0.45 | 3.03 | 1.66 | 84 | 1.07 | 14 | 71 |
| Stewed | 05061 | 184 | 27.39 | 0 | 7.42 | 2.08 | 0.42 | 2.90 | 1.58 | 75 | 0.92 | 13 | 62 |
| Leg | | | | | | | | | | | | | |
| Fried, batter-dipped | 05076 | 273 | 21.77 | 8.72 | 16.17 | 4.28 | 1.25 | 6.58 | 3.85 | 90 | 1.40 | 18 | 279 |
| Fried, flour-coated | 05077 | 254 | 26.84 | 2.50 | 14.43 | 3.90 | 0.95 | 5.68 | 3.33 | 94 | 1.43 | 13 | 88 |
| Duck, roasted | | | | | | | | | | | | | |
| Meat only | 05142 | 201 | 23.48 | 0 | 11.20 | 4.17 | 1.27 | 3.70 | 1.43 | 89 | 2.70 | 12 | 65 |
| Meat with skin | 05140 | 337 | 18.99 | 0 | 28.35 | 9.67 | 2.43 | 12.90 | 3.65 | 84 | 2.70 | 11 | 59 |
| Turkey, roasted | | | | | | | | | | | | | |
| Dark meat only | 05188 | 187 | 28.57 | 0 | 7.22 | 2.42 | 0.72 | 1.64 | 2.16 | 85 | 2.33 | 32 | 79 |
| Dark meat with skin | 05184 | 221 | 27.49 | 0 | 11.54 | 3.49 | 0.90 | 3.65 | 3.09 | 89 | 2.27 | 33 | 76 |
| Light meat only | 05186 | 157 | 29.90 | 0 | 3.22 | 1.03 | 0.31 | 0.56 | 0.86 | 69 | 1.35 | 19 | 64 |
| Light meat with skin | 05182 | 197 | 28.57 | 0 | 8.33 | 2.34 | 0.55 | 2.84 | 2.01 | 76 | 1.41 | 21 | 63 |

[a]Nutrient Data Bank Number (NDB No.) from Agriculture Handbook No. 8-5.
[b]Saturated fatty acids.
[c]Stearic acid (C$_{18:0}$) is a saturated fatty acid that, unlike other saturated fatty acids, does not raise the plasma cholesterol level.
[d]Monounsaturated fatty acids.
[e]Polyunsaturated fatty acids.

SOURCE: U.S. Department of Agriculture. 1979. Composition of Foods: Poultry Products. Agriculture Handbook No. 8-5. Washington, D.C.: U.S. Government Printing Office.

tents than equivalent amounts of chicken breast or other white meats. The method of cooking, particularly deep fat frying, adds to this difference. In comparing roasted poultry parts, a chicken breast is 15.1 percent lower in calories, about 42 percent lower in both total fat and saturated fatty acids, and 8.7 percent lower in cholesterol than a chicken leg. The vitamin and mineral contents of the breast and leg are about the same. A chicken breast that has been roasted, without batter, is 24 percent lower in calories, 41 percent lower in fat, and 37 percent lower in saturated fatty acids than one that has been batter-dipped and then fried.

### Turkey

Removal of the skin from roasted turkey before eating results in a dramatic reduction in caloric and fat contents. Roasted white meat without the skin is 20.3 percent lower in total calories, 61.3 percent lower in total fat, 56 percent lower in saturated fatty acids, and 9.2 percent lower in cholesterol than white meat with the skin intact. The levels of several micronutrients are increased, including niacin; pantothenic acid; vitamins $B_1$, $B_6$, and $B_{12}$; magnesium; phosphorus; and potassium. All other nutrients remain at about the same level.

Roasted dark meat without skin has about 50 percent more fat and about 16 percent more calories than roasted white meat without the skin. However, it is still 15.4 percent lower in calories, 37.4 percent lower in total fat, and 30.7 percent lower in saturated fatty acids than dark meat with the skin.

### Duck

Roasted duck without the skin is 40.4 percent lower in calories, 60.5 percent lower in total fat, and 56.9 percent lower in saturated fatty acids than roasted duck with the skin. The mineral contents, including zinc, potassium, magnesium, and phosphorus, are increased 25 to 40 percent each.

The increases in vitamin content are even greater, ranging from 33 to nearly 75 percent (for vitamin $B_{12}$).

### Fish, Shellfish, and Seafood

As a group, fish, shellfish, and seafood contribute substantial amounts of protein, niacin, and vitamin $B_{12}$ to the food supply (Table 2–1). In addition, their importance as a source of the omega-3 and omega-6 polyunsaturated fatty acids has only recently been appreciated. The nutritional composition of selected fish prepared by different methods is shown in Table 4–11. Like chicken, the nutritional composition of fish can be dramatically altered by the method of preparation, including the liquid in which it is canned.

### Steamed or Canned Fish Versus Fried Fish

In nearly every example, frying added considerably to the calorie, fat, and sodium contents of the seafood being compared. For example, the percentage of calories from fat doubled in some cases and quadrupled in others as a result of frying. The total fat content increased from 2- to 13-fold with frying, depending on the type of seafood.

### Canned with Oil Versus Water or Brine

Although the oil in canned seafood is usually drained before the seafood is eaten, a portion may still be consumed with the product, thereby influencing the ultimate calorie, fat, and sodium contents. Data for tuna fish canned in oil versus tuna canned in water or brine are given in Table 4–11. Canning in oil increases the total fat content by 200 to 500 percent compared with canning in water or brine. In addition, the calorie content is increased 37 to 38 percent by canning in oil.

TABLE 4-11  Nutritional Composition of Fish (100 g, separable lean only, edible portion)

| Product | Calories (kcal) | Protein (g) | Carbohydrate (g) | Total Fat (g) | SFA[a] (g) | Stearic Acid[b] (C$_{18:0}$) (g) | MFA[c] (g) | PUFA[d] (g) | Cholesterol (mg) | Calcium (mg) | Iron (mg) | Sodium (mg) |
|---|---|---|---|---|---|---|---|---|---|---|---|---|
| Crab, blue | | | | | | | | | | | | |
| Crab cake | 155 | 20.2 | 0.5 | 7.5 | 1.48 | 0.49 | 2.82 | 2.27 | 150 | 330 | 1.1 | 105 |
| Steamed | 102 | 20.2 | 0.0 | 1.8 | 0.23 | 0.06 | 0.28 | 0.68 | 100 | 104 | 0.9 | 279 |
| Haddock | | | | | | | | | | | | |
| Breaded-fried | 205 | 19.2 | 7.5 | 10.4 | 2.60 | 1.04 | 4.38 | 2.71 | 80 | 49 | 1.5 | 359 |
| Broiled | 112 | 24.2 | 0.0 | 0.9 | 0.17 | 0.04 | 0.15 | 0.31 | 74 | 42 | 1.3 | 87 |
| Halibut | | | | | | | | | | | | |
| Breaded-fried | 226 | 21.0 | 7.5 | 11.9 | 2.78 | 1.05 | 4.96 | 3.16 | 57 | 61 | 1.3 | 346 |
| Broiled | 140 | 26.7 | 0.0 | 2.9 | 0.42 | 0.06 | 0.97 | 0.94 | 41 | 60 | 0.8 | 69 |
| Oyster, eastern | | | | | | | | | | | | |
| Breaded-fried | 197 | 8.8 | 11.6 | 12.6 | 3.20 | 1.11 | 4.70 | 3.31 | 81 | 62 | 7.0 | 417 |
| Canned | 69 | 7.1 | 3.9 | 2.5 | 0.63 | 0.06 | 0.25 | 0.74 | 55 | 45 | 6.7 | 112 |
| Scallop | | | | | | | | | | | | |
| Breaded-fried | 215 | 18.1 | 10.1 | 10.9 | 2.67 | 1.06 | 4.50 | 2.86 | 61 | 42 | 0.8 | 464 |
| Steamed | 112 | 21.2 | 3.0 | 1.0 | 0.10 | 0.01 | 0.05 | 0.33 | 42 | 31 | 0.4 | 204 |
| Shrimp | | | | | | | | | | | | |
| Breaded-fried | 242 | 21.4 | 11.5 | 12.3 | 2.09 | 0.54 | 3.81 | 5.09 | 177 | 67 | 1.3 | 344 |
| Steamed | 99 | 20.9 | 0.0 | 1.1 | 0.29 | 0.10 | 0.20 | 0.44 | 195 | 39 | 3.1 | 224 |
| Surimi | 99 | 15.2 | 6.9 | 0.9 | 0.18 | 0.03 | 0.14 | 0.46 | 30 | 9 | 0.3 | 143 |
| Tuna | | | | | | | | | | | | |
| Light, oil pack | 199 | 29.1 | 0.0 | 8.2 | 1.53 | 0.09 | 2.95 | 2.89 | 65 | 8 | 1.4 | 354 |
| White, water pack | 136 | 26.7 | 0.0 | 2.5 | 0.65 | 0.10 | 0.65 | 0.92 | 56 | 20 | 0.6 | 392 |

[a]Saturated fatty acids.

[b]Stearic acid (C$_{18:0}$) is a saturated fatty acid that, unlike other saturated fatty acids, does not raise the plasma cholesterol level.

[c]Monounsaturated fatty acids.

[d]Polyunsaturated fatty acids.

SOURCE:  Human Nutrition Information Service, U.S. Department of Agriculture, unpublished data, 1987.

### Mixtures

One of the largest increases from the 1977–1978 NFCS to the 1985 CSFII was in the mixtures category: meat, fish, or poultry combined with sauces, grains, or other components of the diet. As discussed earlier in this report, animal products are being used more frequently as an ingredient in meals rather than as a separate entree. Table 4–12 (pages 90–91) gives the nutritional composition of selected frozen entrees. In 1985, frozen foods accounted for almost $14 billion in supermarket sales (Progressive Grocer, 1986c). This category ranked among the largest volume increases in dollar sales in 1985, rising 10.3 percent (Supermarket Business, 1986b). Sales of diet dinners rose 3 percent in 1985, hitting a new high of $232 million (Progressive Grocer, 1986a).

These products are aimed at meeting a variety of consumer needs; not only are they portion and calorie controlled, they are also convenient and easy to prepare. For these advantages, the consumer is often willing to pay the higher price charged for this type of product and to accept any trade-offs in nutritional quality. Although the calorie, fat, and cholesterol contents of the entrees listed in Table 4–12 are all well within the target levels defined previously, the sodium contents range from 1,700 to 5,200 mg/1,000 calories, depending on the entree chosen.

### USING ANIMAL PRODUCT OPTIONS TO MEET TARGET LEVELS OF NUTRIENTS IN THE DIET

There are numerous modified versions of traditional animal products in the marketplace that are readily available and comparatively priced. How these options can fit into the diet to meet target levels of nutrients is the topic of this section. Example menus for adult women, ages 23–50, and for adult men, ages 51 and older, illustrate the use of animal product options to replace traditional versions in the diet. These diets were calculated with Michael Jacobson's Nutrition Wizard™ software (copyright © 1986 by the Center for Science in the Public Interest); nutrient data from USDA's Home and Garden Bulletin *Nutritive Value of Foods* (U.S. Department of Agriculture, 1985) and USDA's Agriculture Handbooks *Dairy and Egg Products* (U.S. Department of Agriculture, 1976), *Poultry Products* (U.S. Department of Agriculture, 1979), *Pork Products* (U.S. Department of Agriculture, 1983), and *Beef Products* (U.S. Department of Agriculture, 1986).

### Adult Women, Ages 23–50

In this diet, lower fat, lower cholesterol milk and milk products are substituted for traditional high-fat versions. As shown in Tables 4–13 (pages 92–93) and 4–14 (page 93), low-fat (2 percent fat) milk was substituted for whole milk, low-fat yogurt for whole-milk yogurt, ice milk for ice cream, evaporated skim milk for light cream, imitation sour dressing for sour cream, and imitation mayonnaise for mayonnaise.

Lower fat meats are also used in the modified diet. Extra lean (5 percent fat) ham is substituted for regular ham (11 percent fat). A leaner cut of pork—tenderloin—is used in place of a higher fat version, Boston blade.

To make the calorie content of both diets comparable, an additional 0.5 ounce of breakfast cereal and an additional slice each of raisin bread and whole wheat toast was added to the modified diet.

These substitutions result in decreases in total fat (from 86 to 51 grams) and the percentage of calories from fat (from 38 to 23 percent). The percentage of calories from saturated fatty acids is also reduced (from 17 to 10 percent), and the percentage of calories from monounsaturated fatty acids and polyunsaturated fatty acids is lowered to within target levels. The cholesterol content is reduced to below the 300-mg target level. The calcium and iron contents are increased, and both exceed the RDA.

### Adult Men, Ages 51 or Older

Lower fat, lower cholesterol animal products are substituted in the modified diet for the adult male. As shown in Tables 4–15 (pages 94–95) and 4–16 (page 95), nonfat yogurt was substituted for whole-milk yogurt, reduced-calorie American cheese for regular American cheese, evaporated skim milk for light cream, and imitation whipped topping for whipped cream topping. Leaner ham and beef was used in the modified diet, as well as a lower fat cooking method for poultry. A lower fat dessert—angel food cake—was substituted for a high-fat version—pound cake.

The serving of oatmeal was increased from 1 cup to 1.5 cups, and graham crackers were added to the afternoon snack to bring the calorie content of the modified diet more in line with that of the traditional diet.

These changes resulted in decreases in total fat (from 102 to 55 grams) and the percentage of calories from fat (from 41 to 21 percent). The percentage of calories from saturated, monounsaturated, and polyunsaturated fatty acids were all lowered to within target levels, and the cholesterol content was reduced to below the 300-mg target level. Calcium and iron levels exceeded the targets in both traditional and modified diets for adult men.

These example diets demonstrate that it is possible to meet the target levels of nutrients using options currently available in the marketplace.

**TABLE 4-12** Nutritional Composition of Selected Calorie- and Portion-Controlled Frozen Entrees (100 g)

| Entree and Dinner | Calories (kcal) | Protein (g) | Carbohydrate (g) | Total Fat (g) | Cholesterol (mg) | Calcium (mg) | Iron (mg) | Sodium (mg) |
|---|---|---|---|---|---|---|---|---|
| Armour Classic® Lite | | | | | | | | |
| Beef Pepper Steak | 94 | 7.3 | 9.4 | 3.1 | 19.2 | 14 | 0.9 | 315 |
| Chicken Burgundy | 72 | 7.5 | 7.8 | 1.2 | 23.3 | 25 | 0.2 | 287 |
| Chicken Oriental | 84 | 8.7 | 9.1 | 1.4 | 26.2 | 14 | 0.3 | 255 |
| Filet of Cod Divan | 71 | 7.1 | 6.9 | 2.2 | 20.4 | 25 | 0.4 | 252 |
| Seafood Natural Herbs | 73 | 3.6 | 10.9 | 1.5 | 7.6 | 30 | 0.3 | 438 |
| Sliced Beef with Broccoli | 93 | 8.3 | 9.7 | 2.3 | 23.3 | 13 | 1.2 | 413 |
| Turkey Parmesan | 83 | 8.6 | 7.0 | 2.2 | 23.9 | 48 | 0.5 | 306 |
| Blue Star Foods Dining Lite® | | | | | | | | |
| Cod Fillets and Vegetables with Sauce | 70 | 8.4 | 4.5 | 2.4 | NA | 35 | 0.4 | 199 |
| Cheese Cannelloni with Tomato Sauce | 101 | 6.2 | 13.2 | 2.7 | NA | 136 | 0.7 | 385 |
| Chicken Aloha: Chicken & Sauce with Rice | 99 | 8.2 | 13.6 | 1.6 | NA | 16 | 0.3 | 416 |
| Chicken Chow Mein with Rice | 75 | 5.9 | 11.9 | 0.6 | NA | 6.3 | 0.6 | 450 |
| Glazed Chicken with Rice | 103 | 8.2 | 11.5 | 2.5 | NA | 8.2 | 0.6 | 395 |
| Oriental Pepper Steak with Rice | 102 | 8.3 | 12.5 | 2.7 | NA | 7.6 | 0.7 | 530 |
| Salisbury Steak with Creole Sauce | 81 | 8.1 | 5.2 | 3.0 | NA | 37 | 1.0 | 509 |

| Lean Cuisine® Brand (Stouffer Foods Corp.) | | | | | | | |
|---|---|---|---|---|---|---|---|
| Cheese Cannelloni with Tomato Sauce | 104 | 8.5 | 9.2 | 3.8 | 17.3 | 11.5 | 1.5 | 346 |
| Chicken à l'Orange with Almond Rice | 118 | 11.4 | 13.6 | 2.2 | 19.7 | 0.9 | 1.8 | 202 |
| Chicken Chow Mein with Rice | 77 | 4.9 | 11.0 | 1.5 | 7.7 | 0.6 | 1.8 | 356 |
| Glazed Chicken with Vegetable Rice | 111 | 10.7 | 9.5 | 3.3 | 22.6 | 0.8 | 1.6 | 309 |
| Filet of Fish Divan | 76 | 8.8 | 4.8 | 2.5 | 24.0 | 5.6 | 1.7 | 198 |
| Filet of Fish Jardiniere with Souffleed Potatoes | 87 | 9.3 | 5.6 | 3.1 | 31.2 | 6.2 | 0.6 | 261 |
| Oriental Beef with Vegetables and Rice | 110 | 8.1 | 12.2 | 3.3 | 14.2 | 0.8 | 4.1 | 467 |
| Turkey Dijon | 103 | 9.2 | 7.4 | 4.1 | 25.8 | 3.7 | 2.2 | 380 |
| Salisbury Steak with Italian Style Sauce and Vegetables | 100 | 9.2 | 5.2 | 4.8 | 35.0 | 5.5 | 5.5 | 258 |
| Le Menu® Light Style (Campbell Soup Co.) | | | | | | | |
| Beef A l'Orange | 101 | 8.4 | 10.8 | 2.8 | 19.4 | 2.1 | 5.2 | 210 |
| Chicken Cacciatore | 91 | 8.4 | 7.7 | 2.8 | 29.9 | 2.8 | 3.5 | 220 |
| Flounder vin Blanc | 77 | 5.9 | 9.1 | 1.7 | 24.6 | 2.8 | 5.2 | 230 |
| Glazed Chicken Breast | 84 | 9.8 | 6.6 | 1.7 | 24.6 | 2.1 | 5.2 | 260 |
| 3-Cheese Stuffed Shells | 98 | 5.3 | 12.9 | 2.8 | 7.0 | 5.2 | 5.2 | 260 |
| Turkey Divan | 98 | 7.3 | 9.1 | 3.1 | 14.1 | 3.5 | 5.2 | 290 |

NOTE: All nutritional composition data were converted into values per 100 g by using the following equivalents: 1 oz. = 28 g; 100 g = 3.5 oz. NA means data were unavailable.

SOURCE: Armour Food Co., Omaha, Nebr.; Blue Star Foods, Inc., Council Bluffs, Iowa; Campbell Soup Co., Camden, N.J.; Stouffer Foods Corp., Solon, Ohio.

TABLE 4-13   Application of Animal Product Options to Meet Target Levels of Nutrients for Women, Ages 23–50

| Eating Occasion | Traditional | Modified |
|---|---|---|
| Breakfast | Bran cereal | Bran cereal |
| | Whole milk (3.3% fat)* | Low-fat milk (2% fat)* |
| | Banana | Banana |
| | Raisin bread with butter | Raisin bread with butter |
| | Decaffeinated coffee with light cream* | Decaffeinated coffee with evaporated skim milk* |
| Lunch | Sandwich with | Sandwich with |
| | Ham (11% fat)* | Ham (5% fat, extra lean)* |
| | Swiss cheese | Swiss cheese |
| | Tomato and mayonnaise* | Tomato and imitation mayonnaise* |
| | Whole wheat toast | Whole wheat toast |
| | Fresh pear | Fresh pear |
| | Club soda | Club soda |
| Snack | Yogurt (whole milk)* | Yogurt (low-fat milk)* |
| | Bran muffin | Bran muffin |
| | Jam | Jam |
| Dinner | Pork, Boston, blade, roasted* | Pork, tenderloin, roasted* |
| | Baked potato with skin and sour cream* | Baked potato with skin and imitation sour dressing* |
| | Steamed asparagus | Steamed asparagus |
| | Cantaloupe with ice cream (10% fat)* | Cantaloupe with ice milk (4% fat)* |
| | Decaffeinated coffee with light cream* | Decaffeinated coffee with evaporated skim milk* |

| | Nutritional Composition | |
|---|---|---|
| Nutrients and Selected Target Levels | Traditional | Modified |
| Calories, 1,600–2,400 kcal | 2,033 | 2,013 |
| Protein, g | 82 | 100 |
| Carbohydrate, g | 255 | 320 |
| Fat, g ($\leq$ 30% kcal) | 86 (38% kcal) | 51 (23% kcal) |
| SFA[a] ($\leq$ 10% kcal) | 39 (17% kcal) | 23 (10% kcal) |
| MFA[b] ($\leq$ 15% kcal) | 27 (12% kcal) | 14 (6% kcal) |
| PUFA[c] ($\leq$ 10% kcal) | 13 (6% kcal) | 7 (3% kcal) |
| Cholesterol, less than 300 mg | 308 | 216 |
| Fiber, g | 30 | 36 |
| Calcium, 800 mg (100% RDA[d]) | 1,202 (150% RDA) | 1,503 (188% RDA) |
| Iron, 18 mg (100% RDA) | 15.4 (86% RDA) | 19.5 (108% RDA) |
| Sodium, mg | 2,384 | 2,693 |

NOTE:   Animal product options are marked with an asterisk. This diet was calculated with Michael Jacobson's Nutrition Wizard™ software (copyright © 1986 by the Center for Science in the Public Interest).

[a] Saturated fatty acids.
[b] Monounsaturated fatty acids.
[c] Polyunsaturated fatty acids.
[d] Recommended dietary allowance.

## TABLE 4-13 (Continued)

SOURCES: U.S. Department of Agriculture. 1976. Composition of Foods: Dairy and Egg Products. Agriculture Handbook No. 8-1. Washington, D.C.: U.S. Government Printing Office.

U.S. Department of Agriculture. 1979. Composition of Foods: Poultry Products. Agriculture Handbook No. 8-5. Washington, D.C.: U.S. Government Printing Office.

U.S. Department of Agriculture. 1981. Nutritive Value of Foods. Home and Garden Bulletin No. 72, Human Nutrition Information Service. Washington, D.C.: U.S. Government Printing Office.

U.S. Department of Agriculture. 1983. Composition of Foods: Pork Products. Agriculture Handbook No. 8-10. Washington, D.C.: U.S. Government Printing Office.

U.S. Department of Agriculture. 1986. Composition of Foods: Beef Products. Agriculture Handbook No. 8-13. Washington, D.C.: U.S. Government Printing Office.

## TABLE 4-14  Portion Changes in Traditional and Modified Diets for Women, Ages 23–50

| Eating Occasion | Traditional | Portion | Modified | Portion |
|---|---|---|---|---|
| Breakfast | Bran cereal | 1 oz | Bran cereal | 1.5 oz |
|  | Whole milk (3.3% fat) | 8 oz | Low-fat milk (2% fat) | 8 oz |
|  | Banana | 1 | Banana | 1 |
|  | Raisin bread with | 1 slice | Raisin bread with | 2 slices |
|  | butter | 1 pat | butter | 1 pat |
|  | Decaffeinated coffee with | 6 oz | Decaffeinated coffee with | 6 oz |
|  | light cream | 1 tsp | evaporated skim milk | 1 tsp |
| Lunch | Sandwich with |  | Sandwich with |  |
|  | Ham (11% fat) | 1.75 oz | Ham (5% fat) | 1.75 oz |
|  | Swiss cheese | 1 oz | Swiss cheese | 1 oz |
|  | Tomato | 1/2 | Tomato | 1/2 |
|  | Mayonnaise | 1 tbsp | Imitation mayonnaise | 1 tbsp |
|  | Whole wheat toast | 1 slice | Whole wheat toast | 2 slices |
|  | Fresh pear | 1 | Fresh pear | 1 |
|  | Club soda | 12 oz | Club soda | 12 oz |
| Snack | Yogurt (whole milk) | 8 oz | Yogurt (low-fat milk) | 8 oz |
|  | Bran muffin | 1 | Bran muffin | 1 |
|  | Jam | 1 tbsp | Jam | 1 tbsp |
| Dinner | Pork, Boston, blade | 3 oz | Pork, tenderloin | 3 oz |
|  | Baked potato with skin and | 1 | Baked potato with skin and | 1 |
|  | sour cream | 2 tbsp | imitation sour dressing | 2 tbsp |
|  | Steamed asparagus | 4 spears | Steamed asparagus | 4 spears |
|  | Cantaloupe with | 1/2 | Cantaloupe with | 1/2 |
|  | ice cream (10% fat) | 1/2 cup | ice milk (4% fat) | 1/2 cup |
|  | Decaffeinated coffee with | 6 oz | Decaffeinated coffee with | 6 oz |
|  | light cream | 1 tsp | evaporated skim milk | 1 tsp |

NOTE: This diet was calculated with Michael Jacobson's Nutrition Wizard™ software (copyright © 1986 by the Center for Science in the Public Interest).

SOURCES: U.S. Department of Agriculture. 1976. Composition of Foods: Dairy and Egg Products. Agriculture Handbook No. 8-1. Washington, D.C.: U.S. Government Printing Office.

U.S. Department of Agriculture. 1979. Composition of Foods: Poultry Products. Agriculture Handbook No. 8-5. Washington, D.C.: U.S. Government Printing Office.

U.S. Department of Agriculture. 1981. Nutritive Value of Foods. Home and Garden Bulletin No. 72, Human Nutrition Information Service. Washington, D.C.: U.S. Government Printing Office.

U.S. Department of Agriculture. 1983. Composition of Foods: Pork Products. Agriculture Handbook No. 8-10. Washington, D.C.: U.S. Government Printing Office.

U.S. Department of Agriculture. 1986. Composition of Foods: Beef Products. Agriculture Handbook No. 8-13. Washington, D.C.: U.S. Government Printing Office.

TABLE 4-15   Application of Animal Product Options to Meet Target Levels of Nutrients for Men, Ages 51 and Older

| Eating Occasion | Traditional | Modified |
|---|---|---|
| Breakfast | Oatmeal<br>Grapefruit juice<br>Cured ham (11% fat)*<br>Decaffeinated coffee with<br>  light cream* | Oatmeal<br>Grapefruit juice<br>Cured ham (5% fat)*<br>Decaffeinated coffee with evaporated<br>  skim milk* |
| Lunch | Chicken leg, batter-fried*<br>Baking powder biscuits with<br>  butter<br>Sliced tomatoes<br>Fresh peach<br>Club soda | Chicken breast, roasted*<br>Baking powder biscuits with<br>  butter<br>Sliced tomatoes<br>Fresh peach<br>Club soda |
| Snack | Yogurt (whole milk)*<br>Fresh strawberries | Yogurt (nonfat milk)*<br>Fresh strawberries<br>Graham crackers |
| Dinner | Beef, chuck, blade (Choice)*<br>Macaroni<br>American cheese*<br>Steamed broccoli<br>Pound cake* with whipped<br>  cream topping*<br>Decaffeinated coffee with<br>  light cream* | Beef, chuck, arm (Good/Select)*<br>Macaroni<br>American cheese (reduced calorie)*<br>Steamed broccoli<br>Angel food cake* with imitation<br>  whipped topping*<br>Decaffeinated coffee with evaporated<br>  skim milk* |

| | Nutritional Composition | |
|---|---|---|
| Nutrients and Selected Target Levels | Traditional | Modified |
| Calories, 2,000–2,800 kcal | 2,216 | 2,316 |
| Protein, g | 130 | 162 |
| Carbohydrate, g | 204 | 306 |
| Fat, g ($\leq$30% kcal) | 102 (41% kcal) | 55 (21% kcal) |
| SFA[a] ($\leq$10% kcal) | 41 (17% kcal) | 17.5 (7% kcal) |
| MFA[b] ($\leq$15% kcal) | 36 (15% kcal) | 18 (7% kcal) |
| PUFA[c] ($\leq$10% kcal) | 13 (5% kcal) | 9 (3% kcal) |
| Cholesterol, $\leq$300 mg | 418 | 269 |
| Fiber, g | 20 | 24 |
| Calcium, 800 mg (100% RDA[d]) | 1,314 (164% RDA) | 1,952 (244% RDA) |
| Iron, 10 mg (100% RDA) | 18.5 (185% RDA) | 21 (210% RDA) |
| Sodium, mg | 3,681 | 3,379 |

NOTE:   Animal product options are marked with an asterisk. This diet was calculated with Michael Jacobson's Nutrition Wizard™ software (copyright © 1986 by the Center for Science in the Public Interest).

[a] Saturated fatty acids.
[b] Monounsaturated fatty acids.
[c] Polyunsaturated fatty acids.
[d] Recommended dietary allowance.

SOURCES: U.S. Department of Agriculture. 1976. Composition of Foods: Dairy and Egg Products. Agriculture Handbook No. 8-1. Washington, D.C.: U.S. Government Printing Office.

TABLE 4-15  (*Continued*)

U.S. Department of Agriculture. 1979. Composition of Foods: Poultry Products. Agriculture Handbook No. 8-5. Washington, D.C.: U.S. Government Printing Office.
U.S. Department of Agriculture. 1981. Nutritive Value of Foods. Home and Garden Bulletin No. 72, Human Nutrition Information Service. Washington, D.C.: U.S. Government Printing Office.
U.S. Department of Agriculture. 1983. Composition of Foods: Pork Products. Agriculture Handbook No. 8-10. Washington, D.C.: U.S. Government Printing Office.
U.S. Department of Agriculture. 1986. Composition of Foods: Beef Products. Agriculture Handbook No. 8-13. Washington, D.C.: U.S. Government Printing Office.

TABLE 4-16  Portion Changes in Traditional and Modified Diets for Men, Ages 51 and Older

| Eating Occasion | Traditional | Portion | Modified | Portion |
|---|---|---|---|---|
| Breakfast | Oatmeal | 1 cup | Oatmeal | 1½ cups |
| | Grapefruit juice | 8 oz | Grapefruit juice | 8 oz |
| | Cured ham (11% fat) | 3.5 oz | Cured ham (5% fat) | 3.5 oz |
| | Decaffeinated coffee with | 6 oz | Decaffeinated coffee with | 6 oz |
| | light cream | 1 tbsp | evaporated skim milk | 1 tbsp |
| Lunch | Chicken leg, batter-fried | 3.5 oz | Chicken breast, roasted | 3.5 oz |
| | Baking powder biscuits with | 2 | Baking powder biscuits with | 2 |
| | butter | 1 pat | butter | 1 pat |
| | Sliced tomatoes | 1 | Sliced tomatoes | 1 |
| | Fresh peach | 1 | Fresh peach | 1 |
| | Club soda | 12 oz | Club soda | 12 oz |
| Snack | Yogurt (whole milk) | 8 oz | Yogurt (nonfat milk) | 8 oz |
| | Fresh strawberries | 1 cup | Fresh strawberries | 1 cup |
| | | | Graham crackers | 2 squares |
| Dinner | Beef, chuck, blade (Choice) | 3.5 oz | Beef, chuck, arm (Good/Select) | 3.5 oz |
| | Macaroni | 1 cup | Macaroni | 1 cup |
| | American cheese | 2 oz | American cheese (reduced calorie) | 2 oz |
| | Steamed broccoli | 2 spears | Steamed broccoli | 2 spears |
| | Pound cake with | 1 slice | Angel food cake with | 1 slice |
| | whipped cream topping | 2 tbsp | imitation whipped topping | 1 tbsp |
| | Decaffeinated coffee with | 6 oz | Decaffeinated coffee with | 6 oz |
| | light cream | 2 tbsp | evaporated skim milk | 2 tbsp |

NOTE:  This diet was calculated with Michael Jacobson's Nutrition Wizard™ software (copyright © 1986 by the Center for Science in the Public Interest).

SOURCES:  U.S. Department of Agriculture. 1976. Composition of Foods: Dairy and Egg Products. Agriculture Handbook No. 8-1. Washington, D.C.: U.S. Government Printing Office.
U.S. Department of Agriculture. 1979. Composition of Foods: Poultry Products. Agriculture Handbook No. 8-5. Washington, D.C.: U.S. Government Printing Office.
U.S. Department of Agriculture. 1981. Nutritive Value of Foods. Home and Garden Bulletin No. 72, Human Nutrition Information Service. Washington, D.C.: U.S. Government Printing Office.
U.S. Department of Agriculture. 1983. Composition of Foods: Pork Products. Agriculture Handbook No. 8-10. Washington, D.C.: U.S. Government Printing Office.
U.S. Department of Agriculture. 1986. Composition of Foods: Beef Products. Agriculture Handbook No. 8-13. Washington, D.C.: U.S. Government Printing Office.

## REFERENCES

Advertising Age. 1985. New products fatten '85 food-store sales. December 30, pp. 18–19.

Allen, J. W., and T. R. Pierson. 1986. Packaging has rising role in red meat's turnaround. Natl. Provisioner 195:6.

American Meat Institute. 1987. Giant Lean™ Awareness and Usage, Research Report to the Center for Meat Marketing Research, AMI. February. Photocopy.

Berry, B. W., and K. Leddy. 1984. Beef patty composition: Effects of fat content and cooking method. J. Am. Dietet. Assoc. 84:654.

Carlson, K. O. 1983. Natural foods—the consumer perspective. Presentation to the Flavor and Extract Manufacturers Association, October 21, 1983, Washington, D.C.

CREST (Consumer Reports on Eating Share Trends Household Report). 1986. Survey performed by GDR/CREST Enterprises, Parkridge, Ill., 1982 and 1985, as quoted in Foodservice Trends: Nutrition continues to affect restaurant choices. National Restaurant Association News. August, pp. 39–41.

Cross, H. R., J. W. Savell, R. E. Branson, D. S. Hale, J. J. Francis, J. W. Wise, and D. L. Wilkes. 1986. National Consumer Retail Beef Study. Final report to the Agricultural Marketing Service, U.S. Department of Agriculture, Washington, D.C.

Farm Journal. 1987. Beef Extra Survey. January, p. 26.

Food Marketing Institute. 1986. Trends: Consumer Attitudes and the Supermarket 1986. Washington, D.C.: Food Marketing Institute.

Hays, V. W. 1968. Nutritional management effects on performance and carcass measurements. Pp. 77–86 in The Pork Industry: Problems and Progress, D. G. Topel, ed. Ames: Iowa State University Press.

Jones, J. L., and J. Weimer. 1981. Perspective on Health-Related Food Choices. National Economics Division, Economics and Statistics Service, U.S. Department of Agriculture. Agricultural Outlook Conference. Session No. 26. Washington, D.C.

Langer, J. 1985. The workout/pigout paradox. Progressive Grocer. September, p. 10.

Mark Clements Research/National Family Opinion. 1985. Women and Food Survey. New York: Condé Nast.

National Pork Producers Council. 1982. The pork value approach—paying for value. Des Moines, Iowa: National Pork Producers Council.

National Restaurant Association. 1986. 1987 National Restaurant Association Foodservice Industry Forecast. National Restaurant Association, Washington, D.C.

Omtvedt, I. T. 1968. Some heritability characteristics and their importance in a selection program. Pp.

128–135 in The Pork Industry: Problems and Progress, D. G. Topel, ed. Ames: Iowa State University Press.

PF New Products Annual. 1986a. The new product parade continues. September, pp. 10–20.

PF New Products Annual. 1986b. September, p. 14.

PF New Products Annual. 1986c. September, p. 12.

Progressive Grocer. 1986a. Supermarket sales manual: New players in the losing game. July, pp. 99–102.

Progressive Grocer. 1986b. Ice cream: The cream also rises. July, p. 115.

Progressive Grocer. 1986c. Frozen foods: The big squeeze. July, p. 105.

Progressive Grocer. 1986d. Deli: A switch in product mix. July, pp. 43–44, 95.

Progressive Grocer. 1986e. Snacks: Sales still snappy. July, pp. 147–148.

Progressive Grocer. 1986f. Candy and gum: It's not just kid stuff. July, pp. 61–62.

Progressive Grocer. 1986g. Bakery foods: A category on the rise. July, pp. 43–44.

Public Voice for Food and Health Policy. 1983. Nutrition and the American restaurant: A report on nutritious food offerings and consumer information programs. Washington, D.C.: Public Voice for Food and Health Policy.

Restaurants USA. 1986. Foodservice trends: Operators responding to consumer nutrition concerns. August, pp. 39–41.

Smith, G. C., and Z. L. Carpenter. 1976. Eating quality of meat animal products and their fat content. Pp. 147–183 in Fat Content and Composition of Animal Products. Washington, D.C.: National Academy Press.

Supermarket Business. 1986a. 39th Annual Consumer Expenditures Study. September, p. 75.

Supermarket Business. 1986b. September, p. 69.

Supermarket Business. 1986c. September, pp. 79, 81, 83.

Supermarket Business. 1986d. September, p. 88.

Supermarket Business. 1986e. September, p. 85.

Supermarket Business. 1986f. September, p. 81.

Supermarket Business. 1986g. September, p. 79.

University of Wisconsin. 1963. Pork Quality Standards. Wisconsin Agricultural Experiment Station. Special Bulletin No. 9.

U.S. Department of Agriculture. 1963. Composition of Foods. Agriculture Handbook No. 8. Washington, D.C.: U.S. Government Printing Office.

U.S. Department of Agriculture. 1976. Composition of Foods: Dairy and Egg Products. Agriculture Handbook No. 8-1. Washington, D.C.: U.S. Government Printing Office.

U.S. Department of Agriculture. 1979. Composition of Foods: Poultry Products. Agriculture Handbook No. 8-5. Washington, D.C.: U.S. Government Printing Office.

U.S. Department of Agriculture. 1983. Composition of Foods: Pork Products. Agriculture Handbook No. 8-10. Washington, D.C.: U.S. Government Printing Office.

U.S. Department of Agriculture. 1985. Nutritive Value of Foods. Home and Garden Bulletin No. 72. Washington, D.C.: U.S. Government Printing Office.

U.S. Department of Agriculture. 1986. Composition of Foods: Beef Products. Agriculture Handbook No. 8-13. Washington, D.C.: U.S. Government Printing Office.

Wallace, H. D. 1968. Nutritional and management effects on muscle characteristics and quality. Pp. 128–135 in The Pork Industry: Problems and Progress, D. G. Topel, ed. Ames: Iowa State University Press.

Yankelovich, Skelly and White, Inc. 1985. The Consumer Climate for Meat Products. Prepared for the American Meat Institute, Washington, D.C., and the National Live Stock & Meat Board, Chicago, Ill. New York: Yankelovich, Skelly and White, Inc.

# 5

## Policies Affecting the Marketplace

The animal products industry has been remarkably responsive to consumer demand considering its inherent biological and technological constraints. In the animal products industry in general, and in the meat industry in particular, "high quality" has historically been associated with high fat content. Meat producers have responded over the years to the market signals they have received by breeding and feeding for fatter animals. But this has changed dramatically in recent years as more information has become available linking diet and health. We have every reason to believe that producers will be equally responsive to this new situation, producing leaner animals and developing leaner products, given market signals reflecting informed consumer choice.

The industry has, for the most part, already recognized that consumers are changing their dietary habits, especially to reduce fat intake. Producers, processors, and retailers are developing innovative responses to this new environment. Beef and pork producers, in particular, have taken important steps in this direction that should be further encouraged by developing marketplace signals that provide reinforcement and by eliminating the policy constraints that inhibit constructive responses. Specifically, the committee is encouraged that—

• Consumers are taking an active interest in planning their diets and monitoring their own health status;

• The percentage of calories in the diet from animal sources of fat is declining, and total fat and the percentage of total calories from fat in individual diets appear to be declining also; and

• A variety of initiatives within the private sector are well under way to reduce the fat content of animal products, increase their nutritional value, and present the consumer with better, clearer information about the nutrient content of these products.

The committee is discouraged that—

• Consumers in most purchase situations cannot obtain the necessary nutrition information they need to make informed choices to meet their individual needs;

• Despite demonstrated general consumer interest in less fat in food products, the national food supply continues to show annual increases in total fat content. Market forces based more on consumer preference for convenience and taste than on nutritional merit continue to dominate the food system; and

• Although the private sector has taken the initiative in providing nutrition information at points of purchase and is providing a greater choice of animal products with less fat, salt, and cholesterol, these efforts lack coordination across the food sectors, lack standardization, suffer from impeding government policies, and are based on minimal research as to how to best shape the food and food marketing system to the nutritional interests of the consumer. In short, the initiatives are purposeful but not clearly focused.

In the face of tremendous strides in scientific knowledge, changing consumer preferences, and a responsive industry, the overall federal role in the food system appears disjointed, sometimes functioning at cross-purposes. Moreover, tremendous scientific and technological opportunities to produce even better food products appear within reach. Yet many poorly focused government programs and policies continue without recognition of the new priorities.

A principal finding of the committee is that public policies influence consumer choice. And new policies are needed to further encourage the positive trends now evident both among consumers and throughout the animal products industry. Committee objectives include providing consumers with the opportunity to exercise personal choice in the marketplace, encouraging the development of a range of products consistent with those choices, and ensuring sufficient consumer education and information to make those choices "informed decisions."

**PRODUCTION POLICIES**

Since producers have always been responsive to the markets, much of the im-

provement in animal products at the production level will flow from the incentives produced by the policy changes recommended in this chapter. However, progress can also be made at the initiative of individual producers.

The starting point is a recognition by producers and their industry associations that they need to understand marketplace trends and the role of foods in a healthy diet. This involves a basic knowledge of nutrition and an understanding of the way consumers are modifying their dietary practices. Without this, the proper positioning of animal products for the marketplace of the near future will be difficult, if not impossible.

Production policies can affect the levels of fat, cholesterol, and other nutrients in animal products. Technologies are already available to produce foods that are lower in fat and cholesterol by applying appropriate feeding programs and slaughtering animals at optimal ages. Further progress can be made through breeding and selection. A detailed discussion of these technological options is provided in the appended papers.

The committee recommends a commitment on the part of producers to understand the role of foods in a healthy diet and to implement the appropriate feeding, breeding, and selection programs to produce feed animals consistent with this role.

**GRADES**

It is essential that producers be given the proper economic incentives to reinforce the progress they have made in meeting the demands of today's marketplace. Grading is basic to the marketing and pricing processes, but the current U.S. grading system deters the production of lean red meat.

The U.S. Department of Agriculture (USDA) grades for carcasses of red meat animals are based on estimations of the relative quality (flavor, juiciness, and tenderness) of the meat when cooked and on relative cutability (yield of trimmed cuts from the carcass). Nomenclature for the grading systems is not identical for beef, pork, and lamb; but, in general, words like Prime and Choice are used to indicate quality and numbers are used to indicate cutability. The wholesomeness of the meat and freedom from disease ensured by USDA inspection do not relate to grade but rather are determined prior to grading.

The main determinant used in the quality grading of carcasses of red meat animals is the amount of intramuscular fat. The higher the fat content of the muscles, the higher the quality grade, because marbling improves the chances of the meat being flavorful, juicy, and tender when cooked. The main determinant for yield grading of carcasses is the lean to fat ratio. The higher the fat content of the carcass in the form of external, seam, and body cavity fat deposits, the lower the yield grade. Higher yield grades (higher fat) are denoted by higher numbers.

In 1984, 65.1 percent of steer and heifer beef (53.5 percent of total beef) in the U.S. federally inspected slaughter was officially graded and stamped. Of that, 3 percent was Prime, 93 percent was Choice, and 4 percent was Good/Select. In that same year, 3 percent was yield grade 1, 42 percent was yield grade 2, 49 percent was yield grade 3, and 5 percent was yield grade 4. Of the 12 billion pounds of red meat (beef, lamb, calf, and veal) that was officially graded and stamped in 1984, more than 90 percent was beef.

Essentially all beef and lamb carcasses are presented to USDA officials for grading, but packers seldom allow rolling of the carcasses with the official grade stamp unless the carcasses qualify as Prime or Choice and as 1, 2, or 3 yield grades. Thus, the ungraded carcasses are brought together under the term No-Roll for marketing as a single carcass type. This ungraded 47.5 percent of the beef slaughter in 1984 contained beef ranging in quality from high Good/Select to

the bottom of the Canner grade, but the majority consisted of the ungraded 35.9 percent of the steer and heifer beef, most of which would have graded Good/Select or Standard. Assuming that the No-Roll steer and heifer beef all would grade Good/Select, then the steer and heifer quality grades in the market for 1984 were 2 percent Prime, 62 percent Choice, and 36 percent Good/Select.

Over the years, the lower quality grade names of Good/Select, Standard, and Utility have come to signify inferior quality, although they are often leaner, a factor sidestepped to some extent with the unofficial No-Roll designation. All the current grade terms designating quality levels are meaningless in the supermarket, however, where the average consumer is confused about grade names, often equating Choice or Prime with low fat content. Prime and Choice have meaning only in the context of the specialty restaurant business, where the focus continues to be primarily on optimal tenderness, juiciness, and flavor.

It is USDA policy that grading of red meat can only be done in the carcass form to ensure that grading decisions are accurate and consistent. Therefore, grading is provided only at the point of slaughter. Once the meat has been cut and packaged for sale, its equivalent carcass grade cannot be determined.

For beef, the quality grades and the yield grades are said to be coupled; that is, neither grade can be assigned without simultaneously assigning the other grade. The grading systems are uncoupled for lamb carcasses. In practice, lamb carcasses are seldom yield-graded because the industry has not chosen to use yield grades in the trading process.

The committee considered the extent to which the current quality grading system is a deterrent to increasing the leanness of red meat animals. There is no question that it does encourage overfattening of both lambs and cattle, but not swine. (The pork grading system is not hierarchical and is not used by the industry in the same way as the quality grading system for beef or lambs.)

The current grading system for cattle provides ample incentive to cause overfeeding to the point of obesity in the hope of achieving the Choice or Prime grade, and a premium price. Statistics indicate that 64 percent of the steer and heifer beef achieves these grades, and the incentive promotes addition of fat to No-Roll steers and heifers. In fact, this incentive pushes the system beyond the level of fatness necessary for consumer acceptability, which is a Slight degree of marbling—3 to 4 percent intramuscular fat in the Good/Select grade (Savell and Cross, this volume). Increasing fatness to the level required for a carcass to grade Choice requires an overall increase in carcass fat. While a significant amount of that excess fat can be trimmed, the increase in intramuscular fat cannot, and there is the risk that the trimmed fat will be reintroduced into the food supply at some later point.

Lambs can attain fatness levels sufficient to grade Choice or Prime without ever having been fed grain, so overfeeding to achieve a certain quality grade almost never occurs.

The greatest incentive to overfeeding and excessive fattening of both cattle and lambs has been the use of dressing percentage (weight of the carcass as a percentage of live weight) in the current pricing system whereby packers pay more for animals that have a higher dressing percentage. To increase dressing percentage, cattle and lamb feeders overfeed and overfatten their animals. The push for fattening to increase dressing percentages has persisted only because wholesalers and retailers have tolerated the additional fat knowing that it is considered by the consumer to be an indicator of "quality." Now that consumer tastes are changing in favor of leaner products and the retailers are responding rapidly with quarter-inch fat trim, this impetus will no longer exist. There is, in addition, enough genetic variability

among animals that types of cattle can be identified that will deposit marbling in the muscles sufficient to qualify for the Choice and Prime grades without depositing excessive quantities of subcutaneous, intermuscular, or kidney-pelvic fat.

In fact, market incentives are already beginning to reverse this overfattening trend. The committee therefore believes that complete restructuring of the grading system is not necessary and agrees with the conclusions drawn by the National Cattlemen's Association, Beef Grading Subcommittee (1986), which state that—

- Consumers want lean beef regardless of USDA quality grade;
- Changing the USDA beef quality grading standards is not a prerequisite for producing leaner beef;
- The retail consumer market is segmented between those who place emphasis on taste and a high degree of marbling and those who place greater emphasis on leanness;
- Combining the Choice and Good/Select grades into one grade would reduce the industry's ability to market beef effectively to those two consumer segments; and
- Any attempt to change the USDA beef quality grading standards would be interpreted by consumers as negative.

The committee supports the recent name change of the Good grade to Select and recommends consideration of guidelines for trimming fat on the slaughter floor.

### Renaming the Good Grade

In the wake of the 1985 National Consumer Retail Beef study (Cross et al., 1986), the Public Voice for Food and Health Policy (1986) petitioned the USDA to replace the word *Good* with the word *Select* as a grade name for beef carcasses having a Slight amount of marbling (3.0 to 4.3 percent fat in the longissimus dorsi muscle). It argued that "the consumer in search of leaner beef at the supermarket is not assisted by the federal grades" and concluded that such a change in nomenclature—although one purely of semantics—would be in the best interest of all concerned.

The name substitution would not discourage the consumption of leaner beef and might, if properly promoted, allow consumers to find a grade of beef with very low intramuscular fat content. The appeal of the word Select to consumers was demonstrated in the National Consumer Retail Beef study and in a subsequent study conducted by the American Meat Institute; Select was perceived to have a more positive connotation than Good by individuals in focus-group discussions (Schroeter Research Services, 1986; Yankelovich, Skelly and White, Inc., 1985).

On March 4, 1987, the USDA issued a formal proposal in the *Federal Register* to "rename the US Good grade as US Select." The proposal states that the proposed changes would "provide the industry with an opportunity, through the use of a more positive grade name, for improved marketing of beef with less marbling than Prime or Choice," and "also provide consumers who desire beef having the attributes of Select with an officially graded product as an alternative to the Prime and Choice grades." The proposed rule change was accepted and became effective November 23, 1987 (U.S. Department of Agriculture, 1987).

### Trimming Fat on the Slaughter Floor

There is no doubt that the production of lean products in line with consumer tastes and preferences is in the interest of the entire meat industry. In the long run, this involves giving producers the appropriate price signals to encourage production of leaner animals. In the short run, it involves removing excess fat from products. It makes economic sense to do this as early as possible in the fabrication process to minimize transportation costs and to encourage efficient use of by-products.

In late 1986, the American Meat Institute (AMI) took the position that the trimming of external fat to one-quarter inch, as initiated by retailers, was desirable. It also stated that the most efficient place to accomplish most fat removal was the slaughter floor. AMI suggested that this hot-fat trimming (removing subcutaneous fat immediately after slaughter) would—

- Remove dressing percentage as a price-determining factor in purchases of live cattle,
- Discourage overfeeding and overfattening of cattle,
- Allow for removal of excess fat at a point where its value is highest, and
- Make possible payment to producers of the highest prices for the leanest cattle.

If excess external fat is removed on the slaughter floor and cattlemen are paid only for the remaining carcass weight, there would be no incentive to overfatten cattle.

Beef is now graded after the carcasses have been chilled. Because yield grades and quality grades are currently coupled for beef, carcasses that are trimmed prior to presentation for grading cannot be accurately yield graded and so are ineligible for quality grading. This has led to a recent proposal to uncouple yield and quality grading.

Although removal of excess external (subcutaneous) fat on the slaughter floor clearly appears to be a step forward, there is a danger that the uncoupling of the current grading system could result in some excessively fat carcasses going undetected through the hot-fat trimming process. Carcasses that would previously have been identified as yield grade 4 could be more difficult to detect; those carcasses would produce wholesale cuts with a higher degree of intermuscular (seam) fat than desired by the retailer and consumer. Since only 4 to 5 percent of all beef carcasses now officially graded are of yield grades 4 or 5 and since hot-fat trimming would discourage further production of these overfat animals, this problem can be overcome.

The committee recommends that procedures to allow hot-fat trimming on the slaughter floor be given serious consideration. This could be accomplished by a change in official grade standards allowing for uncoupling of yield and quality grades for those carcasses moving through a hot-fat trim process. This change would allow packers who wish to hot-fat trim to have the carcasses quality-graded, and permit packers who wish to continue assigning both yield and quality grades under the present system without hot-fat trimming to do so. A further improvement could be made by extending the uncoupling to No-Roll carcasses that could then be yield-graded. At present, because of the coupling of yield and quality grades, No-Roll carcasses are not graded at all. These two changes would encourage an orderly movement toward efficiencies in the system without precluding continuation of current practices.

Before uncoupling is effected, the committee recommends that the USDA investigate methods (for example, ultrasound) for making reliable determinations of USDA yield grades on the untrimmed carcass so that yield grade 4 and 5 carcasses can be detected and treated differently (for example, muscle-boned to remove seam fat) from yield grade 1, 2, and 3 carcasses. The lean to fat ratio in the meat as it would be cut for retail use is important to both retailer and consumer. A rapid and economical method for determining yield grade, the proportion of lean to fat tissue in carcasses, or both would make removal of fat on the slaughter floor feasible without yield grade uncertainty and without the risk of excessive seam fat in wholesale or retail cuts.

These suggestions may not be long-term solutions. Success in the long run will be indicated by shifts in the amounts of target nutrients in the food supply. New monitoring protocols are needed to assess whether policy implementations are achieving target goals. If they are not, restructuring of the grading system should be considered.

## Options to the Present System

The committee was presented with alternatives to the present grading system. The ones showing the most promise for effecting improvements in the nutritional characteristics of animal products were those that abandoned descriptive terms alluding to subjective aspects of quality in favor of alphanumerical systems to objectively relate the most important quality characteristics of the product. The most practical example of the use and efficacy of such a system is the Canadian approach to beef grading. In 1972, Canada changed its beef grading system to counter the economic bias toward fat. The letters A through E denote increasing animal maturity and, presumably, toughness. The numbers 1 through 4 denote levels of fatness. The A-1 grade denotes carcasses from young, lean beef; the E-4 grade signifies carcasses from old, fat bulls or stags. Prices have varied with the interplay of demand for levels of maturity and fat.

Before 1972, the Canadian grading system matched that used in the United States and Choice grade cattle dominated the market (65 percent). Since the grading change, the market has become dominated by A-1 and A-2 type cattle, most closely associated with the U.S. Good grade, and it is these types that bring premium prices. The arguments against the Canadian system are that it does not detect economically important variations in yield, and total grading costs increase as the grade becomes essential to marketing. Although the grading system is not compulsory, 100 percent of carcasses are graded.

The Canadian grading system at this time is not, in the view of the committee, the ideal system. It does, however, demonstrate that a grading system can profoundly affect the factors for change targeted by the committee. The USDA, together with the private sector, should continue to explore a structure of the U.S. grading system that would present a full range of options to consumers and bring the U.S. food supply more in line with the targets recommended. The question is still open as to whether the defined target levels of nutrients can be met within the present grading system.

## LABELING AND STANDARDS OF IDENTITY

Proper market signals and information are just as important to consumers as they are to producers. Information on the label or as conveyed by standards of identity is a basic starting point for consumers wishing to exercise informed choice in the marketplace.

Food labels and standards have been a matter of controversy for nearly a century. USDA personnel review every meat and poultry product label before it can be used and require an ingredient statement even if the product is covered by a standard of identity. In 1985, 134,000 labels were approved and 19,000 were disapproved. The Food and Drug Administration (FDA) does not review labels, nor does it require ingredient statements for standardized foods.

Currently, the Food, Drug and Cosmetic Act and the Federal Meat Inspection Act leave it to the USDA or FDA to determine whether a standard of identity is needed to protect the public. The USDA has standards of identity that set specific requirements for a food's composition.

The most formal procedure for changing the rules for labeling or standards of identity is the issuance of a new regulation. New regulations are typically published in the *Federal Register* followed by a comment period and sometimes a public hearing. The USDA can avoid formal regulation changes by issuing policy memos to make modest

changes in policy, which it does about 25 times each year. These are also published in the *Federal Register* but only as a matter of public information. The USDA considers policy memos to be interpretations of regulations. But because the memos do not have the same legal status as formal regulations, it is not always clear that they supersede state or local regulations for the product in question.

A recent proposed rule was published by the FDA in the November 25, 1986, edition of the *Federal Register* (U.S. Department of Health and Human Services, 1986). The rule would set forth definitions for the terms *cholesterol free, low cholesterol,* and *cholesterol reduced* in the labeling of food products.

### Cholesterol Labeling

Dietary cholesterol is present only in animal products. It is now widely accepted that a number of Americans should probably reduce their cholesterol intake. However, current FDA regulations are restrictive as to the inclusion of cholesterol information on product labels. The proposed rule mentioned above would "encourage the voluntary declaration of cholesterol and fatty acid contents on labeling to assist individuals in lowering their intake of these substances should they so desire, as well as to assist those individuals who have been medically directed to modify their intake."

The committee agrees with the FDA that regulations restricting truthful and nonmisleading information are not in the consumer's best interest. The committee therefore recommends that cholesterol labeling be encouraged through adoption of either the currently proposed rule or one very similar in context and purpose.

### Controlling Use of the Terms *Natural* and *Lite*

The committee evaluated the trend toward promotion of red meat products labeled *Natural* and *Light* or *Lite*. Exact implications of such claims are in the purview of the Standards and Labeling Division of the USDA, Food Safety and Inspection Service (FSIS).

The term *Natural* is being promoted by some elements of the industry as representing meat from animals that have not been exposed to drugs, growth promoters, hormones, antibiotics, pesticides, or feed additives. It is being used by others to represent animals that are reared in open spaces or on the range as opposed to feedlots and that are fed forages or roughages instead of grains. However, these usages are not codified in state or federal regulations. The committee therefore recommends that use of the term Natural for meat products be standardized in a manner similar to the current FDA effort to standardize use of the terms to be used in cholesterol labeling. However, care must be taken not to imply that meat from animals otherwise designated is somehow unnatural and thus unhealthy. This would be wholly inappropriate and misleading.

In addition, the terms *Light*, *Lite*, and *Lean* are being used in an inappropriate manner by some elements of the food industry to imply superiority in leanness when such may not be the case. USDA-FSIS Policy Memos 071A and 070B state that the terms Lean and Low Fat can be used only on products containing no more than 10 percent fat. Extra Lean may be used only for those products that contain no more than 5 percent fat except for ground beef and hamburger. Light, Lite, Leaner, and Lower Fat can be used only on products that contain at least 25 percent less fat than the majority of such products in the marketplace. Prior to issuance of these memoranda, fat claims such as these could be used interchangeably on meat and poultry products containing 25 percent less fat than a comparable product and on products containing no more than 10 percent fat. Enforcement of these two policy memos

began on April 1, 1987 and November 18, 1987, respectively. The impact of this new use of terminology should be assessed to determine whether the original intent is being met.

The committee is concerned that these descriptive adjectives are used for red meat products at the retail level, even though the verification of relative leanness is made at the carcass level. This can result in erroneous designations because retail cuts from a lean carcass can—depending on the extent of trimming—be either fat or lean after the meat is fabricated at the time of presentation to the consumer. The committee recommends that the USDA restrict use of such terminology to products in the form that would be presented to the consumer. In other words, certification of the relative leanness of carcasses should not simply be carried over from the carcass level to the retail cut as is now often done. Use of this descriptive terminology at the retail level should require some objective standard for verification of leanness of the cut itself.

**Standards of Identity**

Standards of identity are an established range of mandatory ingredients for certain foods, such as catsup, mayonnaise, frankfurters, and bologna, that do not have to appear on the product label. Food science and technology and most of the food industry as we know it today did not exist at the time when most standards of identity, legislation, and regulations were first promulgated. Several additional laws and regulations have been enacted or amended over the last two decades to further protect and inform consumers on the issues of food additives, pesticides, and nutrition labeling.

Standards of identity specifications for some animal products are so restrictive that replacing the high-fat or high-cholesterol components of foods with nonfat or low-fat ingredients is impossible. For example, hot dogs can contain no more that 10 percent added water, thereby restricting the manufacturer's ability to produce a lower fat product. Low-fat and low-sodium cheeses have no standards of identity and cannot legally be called cheese. There is little agreement as to the consumer perception of standards of identity modifiers such as Low, Lite, and Lean. Still pending is AMI's Oct. 1984 petition to USDA for light sausages, containing 25 percent less fat.

The committee recommends that all federal standards of identity regulations be made consistent and reduced in number. Particular attention should be given to eliminating all specific ingredient and manufacturing process restrictions beyond those minimally necessary to maintain the recognized characteristics of each standardized food and to enhancing industry's ability to produce and market new low-fat and low-sodium products. This recommendation is made in view of the lack of uniformity in the promulgation and enforcement of standards of identity, the presence of additional new regulations to protect consumers, the mature nature of the food industry, and the great advances in food science and technology made since standards of identity were first developed.

### POINT-OF-PURCHASE INFORMATION

The creation of a wide range of marketplace options allows consumers maximum flexibility in matching products to their own dietary and life-style needs. However, for the system to work effectively, shoppers must have the information needed to make informed choices. Nutrition labeling is an important step in this direction, but additional information available at the point of purchase should also be encouraged. General nutrition information and dietary guidelines are important, but many people find it difficult to bridge the gap from general nutrition guidelines to specific product choices when shopping for food. Point-of-purchase materials—for example, pamphlets and information tags on products—

could help consumers actually apply the principles of good nutrition.

Point-of-purchase information could also play an important role in helping consumers understand the new low-fat products. Some low-fat products may look different from the traditional products consumers are accustomed to seeing in the store. All are likely to require some modification in cooking procedures because they usually require more careful preparation than do their traditional counterparts.

The market has already demonstrated an ability to respond to shopper information needs with a variety of innovative programs such as in-store brochures, shelf tags indicating nutritional attributes of specific products, and the Meat Nutri-Facts™ program. However, inconsistent and needlessly complex government regulations discourage the use of point-of-purchase materials. This situation can and should be corrected.

FDA regulations currently allow for point-of-purchase information programs that present factual nutrition information without subjective comment. But approval is difficult to obtain, and these programs are treated as experimental with no guarantee that they will be continued after a limited trial period.

Both the FDA and USDA have broad statutory authority to regulate nutrition information. In addition, the Federal Trade Commission (FTC) has the authority to regulate nutrition information presented in advertising. The FTC and the FDA have entered into a Memorandum of Understanding that restricts the initiation of dual proceedings to highly unusual situations in order to avoid duplication of work. This leaves the FDA with jurisdictional primacy over nutritional information in most cases.

The FDA considers point-of-purchase information to include nutrition claims made through labeling. Therefore, to the extent that such programs make any nutrition information available about specific products, those products must bear complete nutrition labeling. This interpretation follows the Food, Drug and Cosmetic Act (FDCA), which defines labeling as "all labels and other written, printed, or graphic matter (1) upon any article or any of its containers or wrappers or (2) accompanying such article" (21 USC §321 [m] [1976]). It is the FDA's view that to highlight one or more nutritional attributes of a particular product and not provide a complete nutritional profile is to misbrand in violation of the FDCA.

The USDA exerts statutory authority over meat and poultry products. The USDA and FDA differ in their approach in two important respects. First, the statutes administered by the USDA do not explicitly require that products bear complete nutrition labeling whenever any nutrition information is provided. Second, the USDA has not adopted rigid nutrition information labeling regulations. Therefore, the USDA is far more flexible in its approach to the regulation of nutrition information programs.

Since most of the nutrition information programs currently being pursued by food retailers involve predominantly FDA-regulated products, the USDA's approach is of limited usefulness. However, the innovation possible under this approach has been amply demonstrated. The most notable example is the Meat Nutri-Facts™ program developed jointly by the Food Marketing Institute, the American Meat Institute, and the National Live Stock & Meat Board.

The Meat Nutri-Facts™ program introduced in May 1985 presents factual nutrient data about fresh meat products by using placard-style graphics at the point of purchase, on-pack stickers that give calorie information, recipes for low-calorie meals, and supplementary informational materials available in the stores. At present, more than 9,000 supermarkets across the United States are participating in this program.

In September 1986, the American Dietetic Association awarded Meat Nutri-Facts™ its President's Circle Nutrition Education Award for "excellence in providing scientif-ically sound nutrition education to the public." The award has been given only once before, to the National Dairy Council in 1983.

Although this program presents only factual information without subjective claim, the nutrient information carried on the placards is not complete or set forth in the format established by FDA regulations and stickers attached to packages give calorie information only. For all these reasons, the program is not in compliance with FDA regulations. Similar difficulties surround the creation of innovative programs that would display factual information on the shelf for other products under FDA regulation. The agency has provided an impractical alternative, but one that could be modified to eliminate the problem.

In 1983, the FDA amended its regulations to permit food retailers to engage in labeling experiments even for products not bearing complete nutrition information on their labels (21 CFR Part 101.108 [1985]). These exemption regulations, despite their intended flexibility, remain highly restrictive in that they require that a company undertake such a program in an experimental mode limited to a specific geographic area and time period. The application is to include information regarding the dates on which the experiment will begin and end and on which a written report or analysis of the experimental data will be submitted to the FDA. Furthermore, such an experimental program must receive the FDA's approval before it can begin. At least one retail food chain experienced a delay of several years before receiving the necessary permission to start.

The reality of the current situation is that few food retailers are willing to undertake the development of innovative point-of-purchase information programs in the face of the FDA's uncertain bureaucratic process. The committee therefore recommends that the FDA make available permanent exemptions for such programs as quickly as possible in light of the continued growth of point-of-purchase nutrition information programs, the popularity of these programs with customers, and the demonstrated willingness of retailers and processors to make information available beyond that now supplied on labels. This could easily be done by publishing specific guidelines for providing factual nutrition data presented without subjective judgment or comment. This would remove the rigidity of receiving prior approval for a program that will evolve in form and content as customer reaction is obtained, as well as the uncertainty of being able to continue the program once the investment has been made in program development and customer education. Indeed, this would be a great step forward in encouraging development of the kind of point-of-purchase information consistent with the doctrine of informed consumer choice.

Restaurants are also beginning to participate in modified point-of-purchase nutrition information programs, particularly those chains with fixed menus. But current practices minimize consumer exposure to this information. Generally, consumers must either ask for the material or otherwise make special efforts to obtain it. Unlike the efforts of supermarkets, these informational programs seldom become an integral part of a restaurant's advertising program or a direct factor in customer purchases.

Until restaurants use the information directly as an inducement to consumers to make choices between food products, these programs are not likely to shape demand significantly on the basis of nutritional quality. Still, true point-of-purchase nutrition information at these outlets could have a tremendous impact on the quality of the American diet for two reasons. First, fast-food restaurants provide an ever-increasing share of the calories in the average consumer's diet. Second, they tend to use large amounts of fat in their food. The committee recommends that restaurants be encouraged to provide meaningful and readily accessible point-of-purchase nutrition information to their customers.

## SOURCES OF DATA

As point-of-purchase nutrition information programs are developed that reach beyond the information currently supplied on package labels, an easily accessible source of credible data is essential. Product manufacturers obviously have access to data on their own products. Providers of point-of-purchase nutrition information do not. They must rely on nutrition information provided in public data banks or supplied voluntarily by the manufacturers. Several data banks currently exist with overlapping jurisdictions and conflicting formats. The two most notable are those of the USDA and the FDA.

The committee recommends that all government food data banks be consolidated under a common oversight body with consistent procedures and formats. Any decisions made in consolidating the data base should involve food retailers and processors, who can ensure that the end product will meet the needs of the marketplace.

### Serving Sizes

Users of public data bases must rely on the serving sizes indicated in the data bases. As a result, point-of-purchase nutrition information programs are often criticized for selecting an inappropriate serving size, even though no alternative may have been available. There is a current controversy as to whether serving sizes should conform to amounts commonly eaten or to amounts consistent with dietary guidelines. For example, should the serving size for meat products be the 3-ounce serving recommended by health professionals, or should it reflect the larger serving size more commonly found in today's diets?

The committee recommends that the establishment of a consolidated data base be accompanied by the establishment of standards for serving sizes and a mechanism for reviewing those serving sizes periodically.

### Advertising and Promotion

Probably no policy issue has received more attention from regulators, consumer advocacy groups, and food manufacturers than claims that a particular food or food product promotes health or prevents disease. Aside from the fact that such claims may initiate mandatory nutrition labeling, the major problem appears to be satisfactory documentation of their validity.

The high level of public awareness of nutrition information is the result primarily of consumer education and the availability of product alternatives in the marketplace rather than specific health claims in advertising. Consumers appear to have a general idea of desirable calorie and cholesterol consumption levels and, given a choice, will exercise their options without considering specific health claims by food manufacturers.

The committee recommends that industry give serious consideration to developing advertising and promotional guidelines that restrict or eliminate the use of misleading claims and claims that specific foods can cure, or prevent, disease.

### GOVERNMENT'S ROLE IN NUTRITION EDUCATION

Government has a dual role to play in nutrition education. It must communicate clear and accurate nutrition information to consumers and communicate the latest in scientific information and marketplace trends to producers.

One of the problems in nutrition education is that misinformation often passes for scientific fact, particularly in the popular press. In addition, inconsistent recommendations can be issued by different agencies within the federal government; target nutrient levels serve as an example. Because of the many conflicting claims and counterclaims made in the field of nutrition, government agencies play a vital role in establishing the basic facts for consumers and producers. Organizations such as the Food and Nutrition Board of the National Research Council and the American Heart Association translate research into practical information for use by nutrition educators. The Food and Nutrition Board's Recommended Dietary Allowances, which are widely used around the world, are an example of this process. USDA's Extension Service provides a nationwide nutrition education system that connects nutrition and agricultural concerns. Through its vast network of nutrition professionals, educators, scientists, and consumer groups, it can effectively communicate to targeted audiences. The committee recommends that the various government agencies make every effort to reach consensus positions that would enable them to speak with one voice on nutrition and health issues.

Although much remains to be done, a great deal of progress has already been made in nutrition education. Unfortunately, as the popular image of animal fat has changed, so has the image of nonfat animal products. To a large extent, animal products of all kinds serve in the minds of American consumers as proxies for fat. Consequently, consumers tend not to make distinctions important to their dietary health.

The committee strongly cautions consumers not to reduce fat consumption simply by avoiding all animal products or only animal products. This could dangerously widen the current maldistribution of essential nutrients, particularly by keeping certain nutrients from segments of the population already deficient in them. This is especially true for women, who are typically deficient in calcium and who should not eliminate dairy products from their diets, and for young children and women of childbearing age who are typically deficient in iron and thus should not eliminate red meat from their diets.

Lowering the fat content of the diet by

selecting leaner meats and lower fat milk products actually enriches the concentrations of desired nutrients like protein, calcium, iron, and B vitamins. Without careful analysis of added fats and oils in substituted nonanimal products, a person can easily fail to make any reduction in the total calories derived from fats and simultaneously produce deficiencies in many essential nutrients.

The committee recommends a coordinated effort by the government to dispel the dietary misinformation present among consumers by communicating the following basic information:

• Animal fats contain a variety of fatty acids. Like plant fats, some fatty acids are saturated and some are unsaturated. On the average, most animal fats have a higher percentage of saturated fatty acids than do plant fats;

• Not all fatty acids are harmful in the diet;

• For many consumers, the separated animal fats and oils (butter, salad dressings, cooking oils, and fats and oils added to fabricated foods such as bakery goods, chocolate bars, and potato chips) are important contributors to the total fat content in the diet;

• The amount of intramuscular fat in the Good/Select grade of beef allows use of this grade in diets designed with target levels of under 30 percent for total calories from fat. White meats are also useful in such diets. Both are rich sources of protein, bioavailable iron, B vitamins, and zinc;

• We do not yet understand all the advantages or disadvantages associated with animal products and their effects on human health; and

• The technology exists to further improve the nutritional composition of animal products.

One basic piece of information essential to dietary recommendations is the level of fat consumed by the typical American. In the past, government data sources may have inaccurately estimated this amount, particularly for animal fat. Attempts are currently under way by the USDA to improve dietary survey methodologies to more accurately reflect actual intake. The committee commends this and recommends that the food disappearance data also be modified to better reflect actual use. In addition, the government should take steps to more accurately distinguish and monitor the fatty acid composition of fats in the diet. The committee also recommends that the USDA obtain data on the fat content of partially trimmed meats and, if possible, on the percentage of consumers who trim their meats completely, partially, or not at all. The committee encourages coordinated efforts among the various government agencies and industry to deliver consumer information at the point of purchase. The most recent example of a program of this type is the "Eat for Health" program developed by Giant Foods Inc., a regional supermarket chain in the Washington, D.C.–Baltimore, Maryland, area, and the National Cancer Institute of the U.S. Department of Health and Human Services. This is a 2-year experimental program to promote changes in shopping behavior by informing customers about nutrition, health, and the relationship between diet and certain types of cancer. It consists of customer information bulletins, in-store signs and shelf labels, and media support.

Other joint information programs have been undertaken with manufacturers and retailers by agencies such as the FDA; the National Heart, Lung, and Blood Institute; and the American Heart Association. These programs combine the expertise of government and private industry and should be encouraged where appropriate.

## INTEGRATED RESEARCH AND EDUCATION PROGRAMS

There is a pressing need for more balanced coordination among all the appropriate disciplines in issues relating to food, nutrition, and public health. Fragmentation of effort often leads to inefficiencies, waste, inertia, and duplication of effort and prevents development of the necessary tools for assessing and responding to structural changes in the food system.

A major policy issue emerging from the committee's deliberations is the need to promote a total food systems approach to all aspects of animal and plant agriculture. Integration should include food production, processing and fabrication, storage, distribution and marketing, nutrient supply, health and safety factors, and the extent of consumer options. There are four basic components to a total systems approach, each carrying equal weight:

- Biological and physical sciences;
- Social and behavioral sciences;
- Economics and commerce; and
- Public health, ecology, safety, law, epidemiology, and biometry.

A systems approach is basic to a better understanding of consumer and producer behaviors and the need for consumer-directed options in the marketplace. The national goal of optimum health is consistent with the producer's goal of a robust animal agriculture and the consumer's interest in a healthy economy that provides a wide range of food product alternatives. A systems approach does not call for more diverse data, but rather for less data—better selected to facilitate understanding of the total system.

The committee recommends that all research pertaining to animal agriculture take a full systems approach whenever possible. This extends to the expenditure of funds raised by producer groups through check-off programs. Check-off programs include a per-head fee assessed when animals are slaughtered. The organizations charged with collecting check-off funds use the money for special programs such as research or education. There is a temptation to spend such funds solely on advertising and promotion, but this tactic misses the opportunity to

focus producer attention on the changing consumer marketplace. In addition, failure to devote appropriate funding to research might result in lost opportunities to develop science and technology designed to improve leanness, reduce the saturated fatty acid content, lower cholesterol, and increase the quantities of desirable nutrients such as zinc, iron, calcium, and B vitamins in meat products.

Producer groups that have supported research projects along with their promotional programs are to be commended. This activity should be encouraged. The committee recommends that producer check-off programs include regular funding for total systems research as it pertains to specific products.

## REGULATIONS AND BIOTECHNOLOGY

The committee urges an evaluation of government policies that may impede the implementation of new technologies. It is imperative that the United States maintain the high quality and safety standards associated with its foods and food products. However, research and development initiatives are being inhibited in the public and private sectors because of overly stringent regulations and an unwillingness to accept research data from other countries. The committee encourages a responsive regulatory policy that does not inhibit creativity or innovation.

Hesitation in the approval of new food ingredients (for example, blood proteins), food labels, or standards of identity; excessive testing and development requirements that force companies to develop and market new agricultural products in foreign countries; and requirements that mandate full testing of new applications of products even though they have met quality and safety standards when used in other situations will all have major influences in the United States.

After more than 2 years of work by 18 federal agencies, the final part of the "Coordinated Framework for the Regulation of Biotechnology" was published in the *Federal Register* on June 26 (Office of Science and Technology Policy, 1986). These policy guidelines are based on generally accepted scientific principles and provide a rational basis for regulation. The guidelines are now being used by the National Institutes of Health (NIH), FDA, USDA, U.S. Environmental Protection Agency (EPA), and others.

A Biotechnology Science Coordinating Committee (BSCC) has been formed that includes the Commissioner of the FDA, the Director of the NIH, the Assistant Secretary of the USDA, the Assistant Administrators of the EPA for Pesticides and Toxic Substances and Research and Development, and the Assistant Director of the National Science Foundation for Biological, Behavioral and Social Sciences. The BSCC focuses on scientific questions and acts to coordinate agency interaction.

The committee commends the agencies for developing this interdisciplinary approach to science and regulation and urges a dynamic interaction of the agencies and the scientific community.

### RECOMMENDATIONS

Recommendations are made in the following areas.

### Production Policies

The starting point for change is a recognition by producers and industry associations of the need to understand marketplace trends and the role of foods in a healthy diet. The committee recommends a commitment on the part of producers to understand how diet relates to health and to implement appropriate feeding, breeding, and selection programs.

### Grades

The committee supports the recent change in the name of the Good grade of beef to

Select. The objective is to provide a term that would encourage the consumption of leaner beef. The change, which became effective November 23, 1987, will provide the industry with an opportunity to improve marketing of beef with less marbling than is found in Prime or Choice.

The committee recommends that procedures to allow hot-fat trimming on the slaughter floor also be considered. A change in official USDA grade standards would allow for uncoupling of yield and quality grades that would enable packers who wish to hot-fat trim on the slaughter floor to still have carcasses quality-graded while permitting packers who wish to continue the present practice of assigning both quality and yield grades to do so.

Before uncoupling is effected, the committee recommends that the USDA investigate methods such as ultrasound that can reliably detect carcasses of yield grades 4 and 5 so that they can be treated differently from yield grade 1, 2, and 3 carcasses. The lean to fat ratio in the meat as it would be prepared for retail display is important to both retailer and consumer. A rapid and economical method for determining yield grade and the proportion of lean to fat tissue in carcasses would make removal of fat on the slaughter floor feasible without yield grade uncertainty and with less risk of excessive seam fat in wholesale or retail cuts.

The USDA should monitor the effects of both these recommendations and of industry initiatives to lower the amounts of fat, saturated fatty acids of animal origin, and cholesterol in the food supply. Options to restructure the grading system should be established so that target goals can be met without undue delay.

### Labeling and Standards of Identity

The committee agrees with the FDA that regulations restricting truthful and nonmisleading information are not in the consumer's best interest. It therefore recommends that cholesterol labeling be encouraged either through adoption of the currently proposed rule (U.S. Department of Health and Human Services, 1986) or of one very similar in context and purpose.

The committee recommends that use of the term Natural for meat products be standardized in a manner similar to the current FDA effort to standardize the use of terms to be used in cholesterol labeling. However, in standardizing the term, care should be taken that use of the term Natural not connote that meat from animals otherwise designated is somehow unnatural and thus unhealthy.

The committee recommends that the USDA restrict use of the words Light, Lite, or Lean to products in the form that would be presented to the consumer. Furthermore, use of this descriptive terminology on retail cuts should require some objective standard for the cut itself.

## Point-of-Purchase Information

The creation of a wide range of marketplace options allows consumers maximum flexibility in matching products to their dietary and life-style needs. However, for the system to work effectively, shoppers must have the information needed for informed choice. Nutrition labeling is an important step in this direction, but additional information available at the point of purchase is also encouraged.

The committee recommends that the FDA make available permanent exemptions for point-of-purchase information programs as quickly as possible. This could easily be done by publishing specific guidelines for providing factual nutrition data presented without subjective judgment or comment. The committee also recommends that restaurants be encouraged to provide meaningful and readily accessible point-of-purchase information for their customers.

## Sources of Data

The committee believes that all government food data banks should be consolidated under a common oversight body with consistent procedures and formats. Food retailers and processors should be involved to share their experience with data banks and to ensure that the end product will meet the needs of the marketplace. The committee further recommends that the establishment of a consolidated data base be accompanied by the establishment of standards for serving sizes together with a mechanism for reviewing those serving sizes periodically.

## Advertising and Promotion

Probably no policy issue has received more attention from regulators, consumer advocacy groups, and food manufacturers than claims that certain foods can promote health or prevent disease. The committee recommends that industry seriously consider developing advertising and promotional guidelines that restrict or eliminate the use of misleading claims and claims that specific foods can cure or prevent disease.

## Government's Role in Nutrition Education

Government has a dual role to play in nutrition education. It must communicate nutrition information to consumers and relay the latest in scientific information and marketplace trends to producers.

One of the problems in nutrition education is that misinformation often passes for scientific fact. Because of the many conflicting claims made in the field of nutrition, government agencies play a vital role in establishing the basic facts for both consumers and producers. The Extension Service of the USDA provides a nationwide nutrition education system that connects nutrition and agricultural concerns. Through its vast network of nutrition professionals, educators, scientists, and consumer groups, it can effectively communicate to targeted audiences.

The committee recommends that the various government agencies make every effort to reach consensus on nutrition and health issues. The committee further recommends a coordinated effort by government to dispel the dietary misinformation held by consumers.

The level of fat consumption by the typical American is essential to any dietary recommendation. It is clear that current government data overestimate the amount of fat consumed that is of animal origin, particularly from red meat products. The committee recommends that the USDA modify the food disappearance data to reflect more accurately consumption of animal products. The committee also encourages coordinated efforts between the various government agencies and industry to deliver nutrition information at the point of purchase.

## Integrated Research and Education Programs

The committee recommends that all research pertaining to animal agriculture take a systems approach whenever possible. This also pertains to the expenditure of funds raised by producer groups through check-off programs. Those producer groups that have already supported research projects are to be commended. Such activity should be encouraged, with consideration given to integrating activities under the oversight of an appropriate body like the land-grant university system. The committee further recommends that producer check-off programs include regular funding for total systems research as it relates to specific products.

## Regulations and Biotechnology

The committee urges that government policies that could inhibit the implementa-

tion of new technologies be evaluated. It is imperative that the United States maintain the high quality and safety standards associated with its foods and food products, but research and development initiatives are currently being impeded in the public and private sectors because of overly stringent regulations and an unwillingness to accept research data from other countries. The committee encourages a responsive regulatory policy that does not inhibit creativity or innovation.

## REFERENCES

Cross, H. R., J. W. Savell, R. E. Branson, D. S. Hale, J. J. Francis, J. W. Wise, and D. L. Wilkes. 1986. National Consumer Retail Beef Study. Final report to the Agricultural Marketing Service, U.S. Department of Agriculture, Washington, D.C.

National Cattlemen's Association, Beef Grading Subcommittee. 1986. Consensus Report on Topics Related to Beef Quality Grading. Denver, Colo.: National Cattlemen's Association.

Office of Science and Technology Policy. 1986. Coordinated Framework for Regulation of Biotechnology. Federal Register 51(123):23302–23393.

Public Voice for Food and Health Policy. 1986. Citizen petition to change the name of the "Good" federal beef grade to reflect that it is leaner than "Prime" or "Choice." Before the U.S. Department of Agriculture, Agricultural Marketing Service, May 6.

Schroeter Research Services. 1986. Beef grades—consumer attitudes. Focus groups conducted for the Center for Beef Marketing Research, American Meat Institute. Weston, Conn.: Schroeter Research Service.

U.S. Department of Agriculture. 1987. Standards for Grades of Slaughter Cattle and Standards for Grades of Carcass Beef. Federal Register 52(184):35679–35683.

U.S. Department of Health and Human Services. 1986. Food Labeling; Definitions of Cholesterol Free, Low Cholesterol, and Reduced Cholesterol. Federal Register 51(227):42584–42593.

Yankelovich, Skelly and White, Inc. 1985. Laboratory Test Market Study of Fresh Beef Products. Report to the Texas Agricultural Experiment Station, the Texas A&M University System. New York: Yankelovich, Skelly and White, Inc.

# 6

# Existing Technological Options and Future Research Needs

## THE NEED TO MODIFY THE NUTRITIONAL ATTRIBUTES OF ANIMAL PRODUCTS

Research on food-producing animals has led to decreased production costs, improved product quality, and advances in understanding human biological needs. Figure 6–1 provides a schematic illustration of some of the interactions that occur between livestock research and production, animal products, life-styles, and human health. It is important to note that all interactions occur in both directions. In fact, the committee's major purpose is an example of this—namely, to determine what technological options can be used to alter animal products to enhance human nutrition.

The following questions must be taken into consideration:

- What components of animal products are important to human nutrition and health?
- What components of animal products can be altered with current technologies or through additional research?
- What effect does altering the components of animal products have on shelf life, visual appeal, flavor, texture, safety, nutrient content, and stability of different retail products?
- Is there sufficient consumer demand to justify the research and product development efforts necessary to generate new products?
- Are there standards of identity or regulatory aspects that preclude or seriously impede the development of new or altered animal products?

The last question is of particular importance, for in addition to health-related and marketplace needs, there must also be in place the appropriate technology and regulations needed to develop wholesome, nutritious, and palatable products.

The marketplace is changing in relation to consumer needs and the variety of food products that can be selected. Each year, about 6,000 to 8,000 "new" products appear that are either newly packaged, newly formulated, or newly fabricated. Many are in direct response to consumer concern about the link between nutrition and diet. The wide variety of different dairy products on the market reflects this.

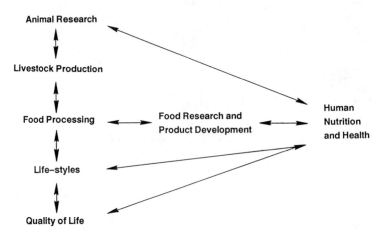

**FIGURE 6–1** Schematic of interactions among animal, food, and human dimensions affecting human health.

It seems likely that animal products or their components will be increasingly altered, fractionated, and formulated to address consumer needs and market opportunities, but this will require additional inputs in research and technology as well as reexamination of some current regulatory policies such as standards of identity.

It is important to recognize who does research on animal products and how it is funded. Food product development can be divided into three distinct phases. First, the components of the food ingredient or raw material (such as an agricultural commodity) must be described. It may be desirable to separate these components for uses in other applications. In this case, the processes for separation and reformulation must be developed, and the characteristics of and potential applications for the individual components must be determined. Second, it must be determined how the various components interact to give the food product its different characteristics. Finally, the commodity, its individual components, or a partially modified product must be converted into a retail product that is wholesome, palatable, and in demand. In addition, the product must have a reasonable shelf life, conform to all labeling and regulatory standards, and, ideally, be nutritious.

The first part of this research is usually conducted by the public sector—university or U.S. Department of Agriculture (USDA) laboratories. Likewise, much of the second phase is done in the public sector, but, depending on the need and the product, a significant amount may be done in the private sector (for instance, by a food industry firm). Some of the technologies developed will be patented to protect investments since the food product per se is generally not patentable. The third dimension is primarily the responsibility of the private sector, mainly because of the market orientation of these firms.

A variety of sources fund these research phases. Typical sources include—

• State and federal government funding of agricultural experiment stations (all three phases);
• Commodity check-off funds (all three phases);
• Competitive government agency grants (limited amount in the first and second phases);
• Industry-funded public research (first and second phases); and
• Private industry, in-house research and development (primarily the second and third phases).

All these research efforts would benefit somewhat from a more systematic approach, especially in terms of product development. There is also a need to better coordinate work between the public and private sectors. A systems approach based on major topic areas, such as animal products, would help link some of the public and private sector programs that are contributing to similar goals.

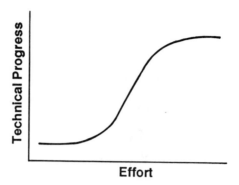

## CURRENT STATUS OF TECHNOLOGY MANAGEMENT

Before identifying potentially useful changes in technology, the maturity of the technologies currently in use must be examined. A tool commonly used for this purpose in strategic planning and technology forecasting is the S-curve, shown in Figure 6–2 (Becker and Speltz, 1986).

In a young technology (few agricultural production technologies are young), extensive long-term research is needed to produce technical progress. As the technology grows, significant advances can be made with smaller and smaller increments of effort. But as technology matures, each effort produces smaller and smaller increments of progress. This is illustrated by the top curve in the figure. At the midpoint of the curve, research productivity declines (see the bottom curve in the figure) and the research manager must decide whether sufficient gains can be made to justify continued effort (research resources) or whether a new technology must be discovered, developed, or perfected to ensure continued technical progress and product growth or acceptance.

As an example, if one uses a performance index for the modern broiler chicken that includes reproductive capacity, hatchability, growth rate, feed conversion, body composition, and the like and plots that index against time, an S-curve like that shown in Figure 6-3 might be constructed (hypothetically, since it is difficult to accurately reconstruct an index). The technolo-

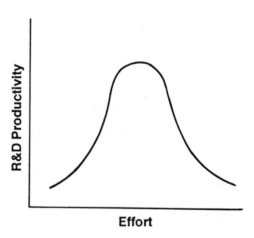

FIGURE 6–2 The S-curve of technical progress versus effort. As technology matures, each effort produces smaller increments of progress (top curve); at the midpoint of the curve, research productivity declines (bottom curve). Source: R. H. Becker, and L. M. Speltz. 1986. Working the S-curve: Making more explicit forecasts. Res. Manage. 29:21.

gies involved in shifting this index included nutrition, genetics, disease resistance and control, and management; but it is clear that some new technology was needed during the late 1960s or early 1970s. In fact, a new technology (dotted line in the figure) was being developed—recombinant DNA technology—but it was largely ignored by poultry scientists and other animal scientists and is only now, in the late 1980s, appearing on the food production scene.

The research recommendations discussed in this section should be useful to research

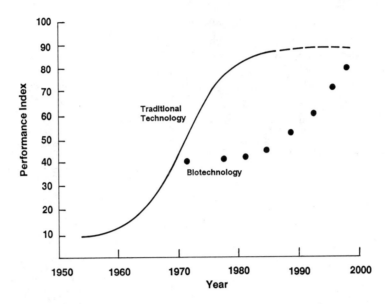

FIGURE 6–3  A hypothetical S-curve for broiler chicken growth performance. Source: R. H. Becker, and L. M. Speltz. 1986. Working the S-curve: Making more explicit forecasts. Res. Manage. 29:21.

administrators in selecting the most appropriate technological options for improving the nutritional attributes of animal products.

## ASSESSING CURRENT AND FUTURE TECHNOLOGIES

The committee organized two workshops to assess (1) the knowledge that is currently available and that can be implemented immediately to modify the composition of animals and animal products and (2) the new technologies that may eventually be useful for modifying the composition of animals and animal products. Both workshops were held at the National Academy of Sciences' Woods Hole Study Center during summer 1986.

The objective of the first workshop was to document current knowledge related to the measurement of intact body and carcass composition; the influence of genetics, nutrition, and management on the composition of animal food products; and the influence of processing technology on the composition of foods made from animal products. The second workshop was convened to identify new technologies offering promise for increasing the nutritional quality of animal products. Special emphasis was given to identifying those technologies that influence growth—particularly the repartitioning of fat to muscle.

Papers presented at these workshops appear in the Appendix and are cited throughout this chapter.

## TARGET LEVELS OF NUTRIENTS AND RELATED RESEARCH PRIORITIES

### Determining the Level of Fat in Live Animals and Carcasses

More than 30 techniques exist to estimate live animal and carcass composition. Equipment costs range from $1 to over $1 million (Topel and Kauffman, this volume). For commercial use, accuracy must be considered as well as cost and practicality. Research is needed to improve certain methods and to make them less expensive and more practical. Economic imperatives to use these techniques are also necessary. This calls for marketing incentives that favor trim, muscular animals, which, at present, are receiving only minor premiums in the marketplace.

There is considerable variation in body composition among animals of the same species and between different species, depending on growth stage, nutritional history, and genetic base. Pork and beef carcasses average 30 to 35 percent fat and 35 to 50 percent muscle (Topel and Kauffman, this volume). Increased muscularity should become important to the livestock industry as consumer demand for leaner animals increases and economic pressures mount in favor of more efficient livestock production.

Many indirect methods of varying degrees of complexity are available to estimate body fat. Most of the methods have been validated for predictability and precision by other indirect methods but rarely by direct carcass analysis of an animal. Therefore, the final choice of an indirect method ultimately depends on cost, the objective of the measurement, and the physical conditions under which the method is to be used.

### Survey of Methods

Older methods of determining fat levels include linear measurement of live animals and carcasses and the back fat probe for live animals. Linear measurement is not satisfactory for live animals but does provide good (though not excellent) information about carcasses. The back fat probe is reasonably accurate, easy to standardize and use, and inexpensive; but it is slow for large numbers of animals. While the back fat probe is considered commercially practical at this time, it is not widely used (Topel and Kauffman, this volume).

Other simple techniques include the reflectance probe, live weight, and visual assessment. The reflectance probe is widely used in Europe but not in the United States. It is simple and fast and also indicates some meat quality characteristics. Growth curves developed from the live weight of animals can be used to estimate body composition, if genetic history is known. However, the correlation of live weight with fatness can also be influenced by feeding, environment, health status, and digestive tract contents. Visual assessment and subjective evaluation is the most common technique used to estimate composition, but because of difficulties in distinguishing muscle from fat, it is of limited value (Topel and Kauffman, this volume).

Newer methods of fat measurement use sophisticated physical and chemical technologies. Ultrasonic measurement is based on the principle that high-frequency sound waves pass through tissue but are reflected back at the interface between two different types of tissue. Time variations for return of reflected signals measure distances between tissue boundaries. Of the many nondestructive evaluation techniques, ultrasound may have the greatest immediate practical potential (Topel and Kauffman, this volume).

Video image analysis could replace or supplement subjective visual assessment for grading carcasses. The technique uses a video camera to create an image that is then processed by an analog/digital converter and analyzed by a computer. While application is not simple, its benefits point toward future adoption by the U.S. beef industry (Topel and Kauffman, this volume).

Whole-body potassium counting of a live animal relies on the direct relation of potassium to lean body mass and its indirect relation to fat. It is a useful research tool, but the bulky and expensive equipment and the time required, as well as some uncertainties in measurement, restrict commercial application (Topel and Kauffman, this volume).

Body density methods treat the body as a two-component system—fatty tissue and fat-free body—each component having a different and constant density. The proportions of the components are estimated from the density of the whole body. Problems arise in measuring the volume of live animals, and the method is slow; therefore, its use is limited mostly to research (Topel and Kauffman, this volume).

The Anyl-ray technique utilizes x-ray attenuation as an index of tissue fatness and is used commercially for ground meat. The tissue-sawdust technique for frozen carcasses is used only as a research tool. Dilution techniques introduce a known amount of tracer that becomes uniformly distributed in the body's water; when equilibrium is reached, the tracer's concentration is measured. Soluble, short-lived radioactive gas tracers are halogenated gases with an affinity for fatty tissue. The amount of these gases taken up is used in research to estimate body composition. Urea dilution may be applicable to both research and industry (Topel and Kauffman, this volume).

Computerized tomography (CT) presents body areas by computed synthesis of an image from x-ray transmission data. The CT scan is widely used in human medicine and has great potential as a research tool and also in genetic selection of breeding stock. European researchers have adopted computerized tomography faster than Americans (Topel and Kauffman, this volume).

In nuclear magnetic resonance (NMR) imaging, strong magnetic fields and pulsed radio waves induce resonance of protons within the body; these protons return to their original orientation in a measured time and an image is produced. NMR is being used in human medicine and has great potential for application to the livestock industry, but it is expensive and complex (Topel and Kauffman, this volume).

Near-infrared reflectance is currently used to predict the composition of plant materials and may be adapted for analysis of carcass composition. It is simple and inexpensive,

but research is needed to develop it for commercial use (Topel and Kauffman, this volume).

Total body electrical conductivity (TOBEC) utilizes the principle that muscle conducts electricity more readily than fat because of its higher water and electrolyte contents. In practice, the animal is surrounded by a coil to which a current is applied, generating an electromagnetic field. The animal absorbs heat energy, perturbing the field. The loss of energy detected in the coil measures the animal's conductive mass. The theoretical basis of TOBEC has been confirmed, and the method has been applied to both human and animal subjects. TOBEC technology is promising, but more research is needed to determine its accuracy (Boileau, this volume).

## Influencing the Level of Fat in the Growing Animal

An animal's body composition results from its cumulative growth. Altering the proportion of fat to lean therefore requires regulation and modification of growth. Lipid composition presents the greatest source of muscle tissue variation (Allen, this volume). The primary lipid fraction contributing to this variation is the triglyceride fraction that is stored in adipocytes within the muscle. These deposits are commonly referred to as marbling, and within the range of marbling found in the longissimus dorsi muscle of beef, the ether-extractable lipid (primarily triglyceride) varies from 1.77 to 10.42 percent (mean values for marbling scores) on a wet tissue weight basis (Savell et al., 1986).

In the present and near future, the most promising approach to enhancing the rate and efficiency of muscle growth (increasing lean tissue, decreasing fat tissue) is the administration of recombinant hormones (Allen, this volume). Recombinant growth hormone has been shown to have impressive effects on growth, feed efficiency, and carcass composition in pigs (Etherton, this volume). Research has also shown that recombinant-derived bovine growth hormone dramatically increases milk production and mammary growth in dairy cattle (Gorewit, this volume). Transgenic animals, whose genes are transmittable to subsequent generations, may have a place in livestock production systems, although reproduction has suffered in some early studies (Hammer, et al., 1985). It may also be possible to construct and perpetuate important hormone genes that can be regulated at will by coupling them to promoters that can be turned on or off at critical periods through nutritional, pharmacological, or environmental manipulation (Allen, this volume).

Technologies can be used to reduce fat deposition in the growing animal, which should facilitate production of animals with the appropriate amount of fat, thereby precluding the need for extensive trimming of fat from carcasses after slaughter. The contributions of genetics, nutrition, and management to fat reduction in cattle, swine, poultry, and milk products are reviewed next.

## Cattle

Efficient production of palatable lean beef must be a primary objective of the beef industry if it is to maintain its competitive position over the long term. Traditionally, production of lean beef has been increased by breeding cattle of a larger frame size. These cattle produce beef that contains more protein and less fat than the beef produced by earlier-maturing (smaller frame size) strains or by breeds that were favored in the past (Byers, Cross, and Schelling, this volume). However, it would be cost-effective to modify cattle growth so that lean beef could be produced regardless of the animal's frame size. In the future, genetic engineering may be applied to this problem, but for now, growth management

strategies offer immediate application. These require scientific knowledge of genetics, nutrition, and growth regulation.

An animal's genetics establishes the patterns, limits, and types of growth that can be obtained. Nutrition affects the rate of deposition of fat and protein in the growing animal. As the growth rate increases, the proportion of protein decreases while the proportion of fat increases. Thus, animals managed in deferred feeding programs will be leaner at any slaughter weight and will also be heavier when typical slaughter end points are reached (Byers, Cross, and Schelling, this volume).

Integrated growth management programs seek to regulate growth by synchronizing nutrient supplies and nutrient needs to support the type of growth desired. The use of growth hormones, growth hormone releasing factors, beta-adrenergic agonists, and immunization strategies to remove negative feedback on growth may later prove useful in these programs (Schelling and Byers, this volume). For the present, anabolic implants are effective as growth promoters, shifting nutrients from fat deposition to protein accretion and also enhancing growth rates (Byers, Cross, and Schelling, this volume).

Current technologies to optimize tissue growth include synchronization of nutrition with the animal's needs for protein growth, continuous delivery of repartitioning agents in all phases of growth from birth to slaughter, and use of intact male animals, which provide leaner cuts than do cows or castrated bulls (Byers, Cross, and Schelling, this volume). Desired results are reduction of fat deposition; generation of leaner beef through production rather than trimming; maintenance of desirable beef quality, flavor, and taste; and establishment of beef as a "lean" product. Research programs should be targeted to yield beef products that meet consumer preferences, to implement available technology, and to develop new technologies that allow more precise regulation of growth in animals to meet market needs.

### Swine

Dramatic changes in swine carcass composition have occurred during the past 15 years of genetic selection, yielding the modern lean-type hog. More options are available to further reduce back fat and increase muscling such as breeding, nutrition, management, and endocrinology (Speer, this volume).

The percentage of fat in market hogs differs among sex classes with intact males (boars) being lowest, females (gilts) intermediate, and castrates (barrows) highest. The percentage of fat also varies with weight; above 90 kg, lean generally plateaus and fat increases. Nutrition has some influence; increasing protein intake can reduce fat deposition, while increasing fat intake has the opposite effect. Restriction of the animal's overall feed intake increases the proportion of lean tissue in the carcass. In addition, the fatty acid composition of dietary fats directly correlates with fat deposition in the animal. Thus, increasing the percentage of unsaturated fatty acids in the pig's diet will cause an increase in unsaturated fatty acids in the carcass tissue (Speer, this volume).

A number of hormones can be administered to improve carcass composition in favor of lean tissue, including methyltestosterone, epinephrine, and the beta-adrenergic agonists (Speer, this volume). Porcine somatotropin, administered by daily injection, has been shown to improve daily gain, feed efficiency, and carcass measurements (Etherton, this volume). It can now be manufactured in large quantities via genetically engineered bacteria, thus expanding possibilities for its field application.

A new application of immunology to swine production may come from recent work on immunization against androstene steroids (those compounds that cause boar or sex

odor in the meat). Other potential applications might result from research showing that immunization of lambs against somatostatin can improve growth and that immunization of rats against differentiation of preadipocytes into fat cells can result in a 30 percent reduction in carcass fat (Speer, this volume). This last technique has been extended experimentally to sheep, and theoretically could be applied to any species, including swine, cattle, and poultry.

Overall, a number of options are currently available to the producer to change carcass composition in the market hog, and several other experimental products or procedures hold promise for reducing fatness and increasing muscularity. However, the pork industry requires guidance on desirable levels of fat in lean tissue to ensure consumer acceptance of its products.

### Poultry

Fat content varies in dressed, ready-to-cook broilers. As the percentage of fat increases, the percentage of protein, minerals, and vitamins decreases. Thus, the fat content of poultry affects its nutritional value more than does any other factor. Broilers currently have 2 to 3 percent of their live body weight as abdominal fat, which is often discarded before cooking. The total body fat of broilers ranges from 15 to 20 percent of live weight and is mostly subcutaneous. Muscle fat varies less than skin or abdominal fat (Gyles, this volume), but intramuscular fat is higher in red muscle (leg and thighs) than in white muscle (breast).

Several genetic options exist to reduce fat in broilers. Strain selection against fat is practiced commercially. Candidate breeders can be chosen on the basis of fat content of spent dams, but this method is not currently used. Selection for improved feed efficiency is effective both in reducing fat deposition and in improving growth and carcass yield and is widely used in the poultry industry. Selection directed against very-low-density-lipoproteins in sera reduces final carcass fat and is used to some extent in the poultry industry (Gyles, this volume).

Nutrition options are considered short term and palliative compared with genetic solutions, but many nutritional components can be manipulated to reduce fat content in poultry. Changing the energy to protein ratio in favor of protein; attention to protein quality in feed; restricting feed intake during early life or, alternatively, shortly before marketing; and formulating special feeds for males versus females to precisely meet nutritional requirements can all reduce final carcass fat percentage. In addition, the type of dietary fat determines the chemical composition of carcass fat: a diet rich in unsaturated fatty acids results in an increased proportion of unsaturated fatty acids in the carcass (Gyles, this volume).

Management options include marketing broilers at younger ages and at a smaller size and weight to reduce fatness, growing males and females separately to address their different feed requirements, and allowing marketing of younger females and older males (Gyles, this volume).

The most practical of these options to reduce fatness, subject to the needs of a particular poultry organization, may be *genetic*—strain selection against abdominal fat, selection against very-low-density lipoproteins in blood sera, and selection for improved feed efficiency—and *nutritional*—manipulation of the energy to protein ratio and restriction of feed energy shortly before marketing.

## Milk

Milk fat, lactose, and proteins are synthesized in the mammary gland cells from precursors absorbed from the blood. They are released in the milk by apocrine, merocrine, or holocrine secretion. Many physiological and environmental factors can influence milk secretion; among those related to increases in yield are increased body weight, advancing age, increased level of nutrition, fall or winter calving, and moderate or cool environmental temperatures (Gorewit, this volume).

Fat content in milk can vary, subject to a variety of factors. Natural variation among breeds of dairy cows ranges from 3.4 to 5.6 percent milk fat (Bonner, 1974). Total milk yield and percentage composition of milk constituents have a negative genetic correlation, making it difficult to breed to improve both traits simultaneously (Linn, this volume). Milk fat and protein content are positively correlated (Bonner, 1974); thus, genetic selection for lowered fat content should also decrease protein content. Current dairy industry incentives are geared toward the maximum production of milk that contains the maximum content of both fat and protein.

During a normal lactation of the dairy cow, the milk yield starts at a high level, peaks 3 to 6 weeks after calving, and then gradually declines toward the end of lactation (Gorewit, this volume). Milk fat and protein percentages are inversely related to milk yield (Gorewit, this volume); in addition milk fat percentage can be affected by environment/management and health/physiology. Variations occur with stage of lactation, season, and the milking process. Mastitis can also affect fat content, as can hormones. However, one of the most important means for causing variation appears to be diet (Linn, this volume).

Cows can be made to produce milk with a lowered fat content by feeding on a high-concentrate/low-roughage diet (Gorewit, this volume). This diet also increases the proportion of unsaturated fatty acids in the milk. However, high-concentrate/low-roughage diets can cause health problems in cows, notably rumenitis and liver abscesses, and therefore have not been used commercially. It has been shown, though, that milk fat percentage can be lowered from the normal 3.5 percent to 1.0 percent in severe cases of "milk fat depression" (Linn, this volume).

Other dietary changes can also cause milk fat depression, including heat-treated or pelleted feeds, the physical form of the feed, the amount of dietary fat, and the lushness of pasture. However, high-grain/low-roughage is the most important type of fat-depressing diet (Bonner, 1974). It may speed up nutrient passage, allowing less time for absorption of milk fat precursors, and alter rumen fermentation to increase the proportion of propionate, causing changes in physiological pathways that lead to decreased milk fat synthesis. Furthermore, insulin levels may rise, inhibiting mobilization of fat from adipose tissue (Bonner, 1974; Linn, this volume). Little research has been performed on the long-term health effects of fat-depressing diets in cows.

Dietary fats themselves can alter milk fat composition. They can appear in milk fat without being changed during digestion and absorption, or they can be hydrogenated by rumen microorganisms or dehydrogenated before their incorporation into milk fat. They can also affect lipid metabolism in the animal. It is possible to increase the proportion of polyunsaturated fatty acids in milk fat by increasing their proportion in dietary fat through the use of oilseed supplements (Linn, this volume). A variety of dairy products have been test manufactured from such milk. However, increased polyunsaturated fatty acids reduce shelf life via faster oxidation, which also changes product flavor, aroma, and color. There are conflicting reports on the direction of change in total milk fat content when the proportion of polyunsaturated fatty acids in the diet is increased.

## Altering the Level of Fat in Animal Products

Various processing technologies exist that can alter the fat level or change fat composition in animal products. Whether these will be used commercially depends on such factors as product safety, economics of manufacture, storage life, and effects on sensory characteristics and product identity, as well as on government regulations and consumer preferences.

### Processed Beef, Lamb, and Pork

Commercial production of "95 percent fat-free" hams has been a notable success. The technique of "restructuring" a product probably represents the ultimate in fat reduction, since muscle with all visible surface and seam fat removed still contains about 0.5 to 5.0 percent fat as intramuscular fat and extractable intra- and intercellular lipids (Rust, this volume).

The commonly accepted level of 25 to 30 percent fat in cooked sausage is difficult to reduce without causing the meat to have a rubbery, tough texture. This can be offset by added water, but current USDA regulations restrict this practice (Rust, this volume). It might be better to regulate sausage composition based on minimum protein instead of the current fat and water maximums.

It is also possible to substitute a nonbinding protein for some of the fat in sausage. For instance, 10 percent cooked pork skins can be substituted for 10 percent pork fat in dry sausage. USDA labeling requirements for identifying "mechanically separated meat" may discourage processors from adopting this technology and using this product because of fear of consumer resistance (Rust, this volume).

Fat can be modified in processed meat products by substituting vegetable fats and oils for animal fat. For example, vegetable oil preemulsified with milk proteins can be substituted for two-thirds of the animal fat in bologna. Stabilized preemulsions can be used to reduce visible fat in meat products. However, current USDA labeling requirements prevent commercial applications of either of these procedures.

## Poultry

Poultry products have a relatively high nutrient to calorie ratio. Even so, poultry meat is the current focus of fat-reduction technologies seeking to increase preference for poultry in the consumer market. Between 1965 and 1985, per capita U.S. poultry consumption increased 72 percent; however, this reflected a 54 percent decrease in whole poultry consumption and a 575 percent increase in further processed poultry consumption. Three-quarters of the poultry consumed in 1985 was cut up or further processed (Mast and Clouser, this volume). Thus, the growth potential in this industry lies in increasing the demand for poultry convenience foods rather than increasing purchases of whole birds.

The fat content of skinless, uncooked poultry is low, ranging from 1.6 to 4.9 percent, depending on the type of bird and the type of meat (light versus dark). These amounts of fat increase four- to sevenfold for meat with the skin intact (Mast and Clouser, this volume). As with most other meats (beef, veal, pork), less than half of the fatty acids in poultry are saturated, but the proportion of polyunsaturated to saturated fatty acids is higher in poultry than in other meats. When total lipids are decreased in poultry, the proportion of phospholipids and cholesterol rises and the proportion of triglycerides decreases. There is slightly more cholesterol and a higher overall fat content in dark versus light meat because of the fat depots between muscles. The depot fat, however, has more triglycerides than does the intramuscular fat (Mast and Clouser, this volume).

Consumption of fat from poultry has increased more than threefold since the early 1900s. While this mainly reflects an overall increase in poultry consumption, chicken (80 percent of the poultry consumed) has been higher in fat since the 1960s owing to changes in breeding and feeding (Mast and Clouser, this volume). The demand for larger and faster growing birds has led to production of carcasses with 10 to 15 percent more fat, most of which lies in the bird's abdominal fat pad. The fat pad averages 40 grams and is 2.5 percent of total carcass weight and 10 percent of total body fat. Consumers remove it before cooking; now processors are removing it prior to marketing. Current poultry production practice necessitates removal of excess carcass fat at the processing level, thereby increasing costs to both processors and consumers.

Poultry frankfurters contain 18 to 22 percent fat versus the 25 to 30 percent fat found in beef and pork franks. Some producers have lowered the fat content of poultry franks to 13 to 16 percent by using mechanically deboned poultry from the breast and neck sections, which contain less fat than the backs or legs (Mast and Clouser, this volume). However, as with low-fat beef and pork franks, such products tend to be rubbery, tough, and less acceptable to consumers.

Fat can also be reduced in fried poultry products. The four standard cooking methods for battered and breaded, fried commercial products all yield a final meat with similar fat content. Breaded chicken products with reduced fat and caloric content can be manufactured, however, by removing the skin from the meat prior to breading and then hot-air cooking instead of deep fat frying (which reduces fat by 23 to 31 percent and calories by 13 to 15 percent), for a total caloric decrease of 42 to 65 percent and a final fat content of 27 percent of total calories (versus 60 percent in conventional cooking) (Mast and Clouser, this volume). Such cooking systems are likely to become widely used as consumer demand accelerates for processed poultry products with lower calories and fat.

## Dairy Products

There is an increasing demand for low-fat milk products, which are derived by processing whole milk. Processing technologies can also be used to exploit surplus milk fat and to separate and concentrate it for the manufacture of other dairy products.

The cheese-making process concentrates the protein and fat components of milk, reduces the water, and eliminates the carbohydrate. The whey derived from cheese manufacture can be further processed to concentrate the highly nutritional proteins lactalbumin and lactoglobulin. Ultrafiltration is now being used to concentrate whey proteins, to manufacture cheese base for further processing, and to concentrate milk fat and protein for other cheese manufacture (Hettinga, this volume). Ultrafiltration is a high-pressure microfiltration process that selectively segregates components of various molecular weights. Milk-processing membranes have been developed with varying pore sizes to retain fat and protein while letting lactose, water, and salts pass through.

While the United States has a surplus of butterfat, it is still relatively expensive and therefore often substituted for, rather than used in, food formulation.

## Methods of Altering Cholesterol Levels in Animal Products

### Milk

The concentration of cholesterol in bovine milk ranges between 10 and 15 mg/100 ml, or 0.2 to 0.4 percent of total milk lipid. Milk cholesterol is 95 percent unesterified; the balance is esterified to long-chain, usually saturated, fatty acids. Seventy-five percent of milk cholesterol is dissolved in milk fat, 10 percent is in the fat globule membrane, and 15 percent is in the skim milk (Hettinga, this volume). The effects of commercial processing on the concentrations and distribution of milk cholesterol are poorly defined, but this information is needed so that technologies can be applied to decrease the cholesterol content of milk.

A cholesterol reductase from species of *Eubacterium* might have use in converting milk cholesterol into coprostanol and cholestanol, which are poorly (or not at all) absorbed by humans. Supercritical carbon dioxide extraction also holds promise for reducing the level of cholesterol in milk. However, it will be necessary to penetrate the milk fat globules, which contain most of the cholesterol, without destroying the globules themselves (Hettinga, this volume). In general, supercritical fluid extraction works by penetrating the structure of a material to be separated, dissolving soluble components, and carrying them away. Advantages of this method compared with conventional extraction techniques include reduced energy costs, higher yields, lower operating temperatures (yielding better quality products), and elimination of explosive or toxic solvents. At present, this technology is too expensive and its technical feasibility for removing lipids and cholesterol is questionable.

### Eggs

Annual egg consumption has declined consistently since the 1940s, from 400 to 260 eggs per capita (Mast and Clouser, this volume). This is largely attributable to health concerns about cholesterol, which is present at the level of 545 mg/100 grams of whole egg, or about 270 mg per large egg. Much past research focused on how to reduce egg cholesterol by altering hens' diets or by genetic selection; these approaches met with varying degrees of success (or failure). Overall, the nutrient composition of eggs has not changed greatly in response to modern industry practices.

Eggs from hens fed the usual commercial diets differ little in the amount of cholesterol they contain. While unusual diets can increase or decrease cholesterol, they also tend to have deleterious effects on the nutritional value of the egg or the hen's performance. Drugs added to hens' diets can reduce cholesterol in eggs, but they have harmful side effects (Gyles, this volume).

Cholesterol in eggs is not affected by age of the hen, cage versus floor management, strain of commercial layer, or geographic location of feed source. Eggs from meat-type hens, turkeys, ducks, and quails contain greater concentrations of cholesterol than chicken eggs; however, the former are rarely consumed in the United States (Gyles, this volume).

Reducing cholesterol in eggs through genetic selection would be desirable, but to date, increases have been obtained only through breeding. Furthermore, some experiments indicate that when the level of cholesterol per egg decreases, so does the number of eggs laid (Gyles, this volume).

The alternative is to modify the egg yolk after the egg is laid, but only processed eggs (about 13 percent of all eggs now consumed) are amenable to such tactics. Approaches have included dilution of whole liquid egg with egg white and removal of portions of the yolk lipids and cholesterol with "solvents" to reduce the cholesterol content of the final product, and complete removal of the yolk and replacement with a substitute "yolk" made from vegetable oils and other ingredients to produce a cholesterol-free product. Numerous U.S. patents have been obtained toward these ends, nine of which are discussed in detail by Mast and Clouser (this volume).

Supercritical fluid extraction, which may be able to selectively extract cholesterol without removing the polar lipids that are responsible for functional and sensory properties in egg products, might be an alternative to solvent extraction. Supercritical fluid extraction utilizes the high-density/low-viscosity properties of supercritical fluids, which are gases subjected to high pressures at temperatures above their critical point. Supercritical fluids can readily diffuse into and out of foods, thereby increasing extrac-tion efficiency. By varying the fluid's density through changes in pressure, its solubility can be adjusted to preferentially extract certain components of interest. To date, this technology has not been used on eggs or egg products. However, research is under way to extract cholesterol from the egg yolk with supercritical carbon dioxide at various temperatures and pressures (Mast and Clouser, this volume).

### Poultry, Beef, Veal, Pork, and Lamb

The cholesterol content of muscle tissue varies less than the lipid content and has been found to be fairly constant across and within maturity groups (Stromer et al., 1966), among yield grades (Rhee et al., 1982), and across breed type and nutritional background (Eichhorn et al., 1986). It is possible to find variation in the cholesterol content of meat, however, because adipose tissue tends to have a different concentration of cholesterol than muscle (Allen, this volume). Consequently, differences in the amount of subcutaneous or intermuscular fat consumed with the lean portion can alter cholesterol intake. It has been calculated that 37 to 56 percent of the cholesterol in a cooked rib steak of beef originates from subcutaneous and intermuscular adipose tissue (Rhee et al., 1982). It is possible that supercritical fluid extraction could be adapted to remove cholesterol from meat products.

### Methods To Alter Sodium Levels in Animal Products

Salt is an important ingredient in many food-processing techniques. However, diets containing no added salt already provide 1.0 to 1.8 grams of sodium a day, which clearly exceeds the daily requirement of 0.5 to 1.0 grams. When salt added by consumers in cooking and at the table is considered, per capita daily consumption exceeds 3.6

grams. This does not include salt consumption due to the ingestion of processed foods, which can be substantial.

### Meat Products

Salt (sodium chloride) has three major functions in a meat product: preservation, promotion of binding properties in proteins, and flavoring.

Salt is important in preserving dry-cured meats (for example, hams and certain sausages); in fact, some research points to an increased danger of toxins arising if salt in cured meats is lowered beyond a certain point. Yet, no minimum effective salt levels have been set. Clearly, it is necessary to achieve a brine concentration sufficient to inhibit growth of molds, yeasts, and microbial pathogens. Research on salt/citrate/ phosphate interactions and their effects on pathogens is needed (Rust, this volume).

The role of salt in protein-binding properties is twofold. First, it extracts salt-soluble myofibrillar proteins that then encapsulate fat particles to create a stable "emulsion" or meat batter. Second, it promotes swelling of these proteins, which exposes more bonding sites for water. These properties are needed to produce stable sausages (Rust, this volume).

The flavor preference for sodium chloride is an acquired taste. Consumers in general have reduced their sodium intake, and the meat industry has responded by lowering the sodium content of many of their products. Other chlorides can be substituted, but many present flavor problems. For instance, potassium chloride has a bitter flavor and can be substituted successfully for sodium chloride only at or below the 25 percent level. Furthermore, the health effects of added dietary potassium are still unknown (Rust, this volume). On the other hand, flavoring agents such as spices can be used to enhance flavor in place of sodium chloride.

Alkaline phosphates can be combined with sodium chloride to enhance sodium function in low-sodium products. Generally, though, these phosphates are mostly the sodium salts; hence, actual sodium reduction is minimal. Use of a number of alkaline potassium phosphates is allowed under USDA-Food Safety and Inspection Service (FSIS) regulations, including dipotassium phosphate, monopotassium phosphate, potassium tripolyphosphate, and potassium pyrophosphate. Their use is limited, however, by solubility problems, lower functionality than their sodium counterparts, and the potassium flavor problem (Rust, this volume).

### Poultry Products

Processing of poultry can influence the sodium content of the meat. Immersion chilling and hot-deboning both leach sodium from the tissue, the latter to a greater degree (Mast and Clouser, this volume). Further processing of poultry into various manufactured products can also increase its sodium content.

Sodium can be lowered in processed products by replacing some or all of the sodium chloride with calcium chloride, magnesium chloride, or potassium chloride. In poultry frankfurters, for example, 35 percent of the sodium chloride can be replaced by potassium chloride without adverse effects on flavor. On the other hand, magnesium chloride at this level causes off-flavors (Mast and Clouser, this volume).

Enzymatic modification could partially alleviate the need for salt in processed poultry products, but spices would have to be added to compensate for changes in flavor. Phosphate combined with salt can also serve to produce acceptable low-salt products. Currently, poultry frankfurters average 2.2 percent sodium chloride, or 860 mg of sodium/100 grams of meat. This level could be reduced to 1.5 percent sodium (590 mg/100 grams) by adding phosphate or even 0.5 percent sodium (197 mg/100 grams)

## Milk

The salt system in milk appears to be regulated by the synthesis of carbohydrates, casein, and citrate and by leakage of blood constituents into milk. Sodium is present mainly as free ions in the diffusible fraction. Its total measured level in milk is 0.6 mg/liter; mastitis increases this level. A nutritional regimen for the cow that includes sodium bicarbonate lowers the sodium content of milk because it lowers plasma sodium. Overall, however, genetics, health, and nutrition have minimal effects on milk's sodium content (Linn, this volume). Most of the salt in dairy products is added during processing, as in the manufacturing of cheese.

### Methods To Alter Calcium Levels in Animal Products

#### Milk

Calcium is secreted by the Golgi apparatus. Average levels of calcium in milk are 30 mmol/liter, but vary slightly with breed of dairy cattle and stage of lactation. Levels decline with mastitis. Nutrition of dairy cattle has little effect on calcium content (Linn, this volume).

Milk is a particularly good source of calcium. Its absorption and utilization by humans is facilitated by the presence of vitamin D, obtained from sunlight or fortified into the milk itself (Hettinga, this volume). Milk can be further fortified by the addition of extra calcium. Most milk products, especially cheese, are rich sources of bioavailable calcium.

#### Eggs and Poultry

Two large eggs (about 100 grams total) contain about 57 grams of calcium (Table 4-2). This is at least twice the calcium content

of poultry flesh, although storage causes small increases in the calcium content of poultry meat due to leaching of calcium from the bones into the muscle. Cooking does not significantly affect the calcium content of poultry, but processing options can increase the calcium content of such products as poultry bologna and frankfurters (Mast and Clouser, this volume). For example, turkey and chicken frankfurters can contain 88 to 104 mg of calcium.

### Methods To Alter Iron Levels in Animal Products

#### Milk

Iron is present in milk at low levels, approximately 0.05 mg/100 grams. It is bound to lactoferrins, transferrins, casein, fat globules, and xanthine oxidase (Linn, this volume). Its concentration is not affected by the cow's diet (Hettinga, this volume).

Unfortified cow's milk is a poor source of iron. Only 10 to 12 percent of the iron present in cows' milk can be absorbed by human infants, in contrast to the 50 percent absorbability of the iron in human milk. But if cow's milk is fortified with iron sulfate or iron gluconate, infants can absorb up to four times the iron they normally get from human milk. Iron-fortified milk offers the opportunity to enrich the diets of infants, children, adolescents, and pregnant women, all of whom are at risk for iron deficiency.

Fortification must use chelated iron to ensure initial transfer to the phosphoserine groups of casein; this ligand exchange reaction protects iron from reactive milk lipids and promotes effective utilization of this element (Hettinga, this volume).

#### Eggs and Poultry

Two large eggs (100 grams total) contain about 2.08 mg of iron, while 100 grams of poultry flesh (light meat, roasted) contain

1.06 mg of iron (Table 4-10). Slightly higher values are present in processed poultry products made from mechanically deboned poultry (Mast and Clouser, this volume).

Poultry giblets—heart, gizzard, and liver—are rich sources of iron. Giblets are underutilized in the United States because of their undesirable texture and functional protein characteristics. These shortcomings may be improved, though, by chemical, enzymatic, and physical agents (Mast and Clouser, this volume). The technique with the best potential is acylation—the addition of chemical groups to the functional groups on amino acid side chains.

### Beef, Veal, Pork, and Lamb

These animal products contain substantial amounts of heme iron from the hemoglobin and myoglobin present in the tissues. Heme iron is unaffected by other components in the diet, resulting in consistently high absorption rates. The iron content of beef ranges from about 2.0 to 3.8 mg/100 grams; for pork it is 0.8 to 2.0 mg/100 grams; for lamb it is 1.5 to 3.2 mg/100 grams; and for veal it is 0.9 to 1.9 mg/100 grams (see the composition tables in Chapter 4).

The blood from these animals would provide a concentrated, bioavailable source of heme iron, but it is rarely used in the formulation of human food products in the United States. Blood is, however, used in nonfood products such as fertilizers and feed additives. Mast and Clouser (this volume) suggest that blood is not used in foods for humans in the United States because the consumer has an unfavorable image of blood as a food ingredient.

### RECOMMENDATIONS

Pre- and postharvest technologies provide insights into options that are currently available for reducing the fat content of animal products. Even though some of these are now being applied, others have not yet been adopted because of high costs, lack of demand, product-labeling standards, or, in some cases, the quality stability of such products in the marketplace. These problems must be addressed by both basic and applied research. In addition, other pre- and postharvest areas of research have been identified that hold promise for reducing the fat content of animal products.

The more that is known about the basic biology of factors controlling the partitioning of nutrients into protein or fat in animals, the higher the probability of changing these processes through genetic or metabolic manipulation. Just as animal biology is advancing, so is our understanding of food science and the postharvest research needs. These research advances are the basis for improved and new foods composed of or containing animal products.

The following research recommendations suggest areas that could lead to useful new technologies for addressing the reduction of fat or salt in animal products.

### Preharvest Technology

• *Recommendation* Develop technologies for determining carcass fat content. Current methods are time-consuming, costly, or not sufficiently accurate.

• *Recommendation* Alter lean to fat ratios of meat and fat content in milk through breeding, nutrition, and management. These methods have long been used in response to market incentives and can result in changes that range from slow to quite rapid.

• *Recommendation* Alter the fatty acid composition of meat, milk, and eggs through dietary or genetic manipulation. Although this is more difficult to do in ruminants, it can be accomplished at additional cost. In nonruminants, carcass fat readily reflects the dietary fatty acid pattern. A major limitation is that shelf life of animal products is decreased if the fatty acid profile is shifted too far toward the polyunsaturated fatty acids.

• *Recommendation* Improve methodologies for determining the fat and protein contents of live animals and carcasses. Rapid, accurate, and cost-effective methodologies would greatly enhance industry's ability to determine animal or carcass composition and thus be of great economic value. Such technology would also be useful for measuring human body composition and for making humans more aware of the relationship of obesity to diet and health.

• *Recommendation* Identify cellular and molecular mechanisms that control partitioning of feed nutrients into meat, milk, and eggs. It is well known that livestock species display considerable genetic variability in their abilities to convert feedstuffs into muscle, fat, milk, and eggs. To fully utilize the tools of biotechnology, much more information is needed about the exact genes and cellular or molecular mechanisms that contribute to this genetic variation. With this information, the probability of being able to optimize favorable responses through bioregulation or genetic engineering will be greatly enhanced.

• *Recommendation* Determine the extent of genetic variation in the cholesterol content of meat, milk, and eggs. Without this information, it is not possible to know whether genetic selection or engineering could be used to develop lower cholesterol animal products. In addition, more research is needed on the metabolism of cholesterol in the tissues and on the quantity of cholesterol that is essential to the function of the cell or organelle. This research need exists for both animals and humans.

• *Recommendation* Determine whether oxidative rancidity of animal products can be reduced through special feeding or management of animals. Some research indicates that feeding vitamin E to nonruminants decreases the rate of oxidative rancidity in their meat products. More research is needed to determine whether other natural or approved synthetic antioxidants are beneficial in extending product shelf life.

• *Recommendation* Develop more cost-effective methods for producing low-fat animal products by integrated production management systems. Systems analysis is an effective method for examining the multitude of biological, physical, and economic factors that influence the cost-effectiveness of programs and processes for reducing or altering fat in animal products.

• *Recommendation* Expand research in the area of reproductive physiology that would permit rapid selection and propagation of genetically or metabolically superior animals. Examples include sexing semen and embryos, splitting embryos, and gene insertion and gene expression.

## Post-Harvest Technology

Postharvest technologies to reduce fat in animal products can be used quite satisfactorily in many situations. However, these technologies are not without costs and are usually associated with some change in product characteristics such as texture, flavor, or shelf life. In addition—depending on the product and the changes—a variety of regulatory and labeling issues must also be addressed.

• *Recommendation* Use physical methods to reduce fat at the earliest possible stage in processing. Some such methods are being used extensively, including trimming meat, centrifuging milk, and separating egg yolks and whites. Low-fat milk and meat products are examples of the results that can be achieved. Furthermore, use of such procedures would create by-products of lower economic value that could be used effectively in food or, preferably, nonfood products. The recommendations made in Chapter 5 to allow hot-fat trimming on the slaughter floor and to change the USDA grade standards to allow for uncoupling of yield and quality grades are in concert with this recommendation.

• *Recommendation* Simulate the textural and sensory properties of fat by using nonfat or low-fat ingredients. Certain polysaccharides and proteins might be useful for this purpose and could produce satisfactory results in a number of products if labeling standards were more flexible.

• *Recommendation* Adopt standards of identity that reflect today's technology and consumer needs. In some instances standards are too restrictive, and even though a technology exists that could be used to improve a product, it cannot be applied because of current regulations.

• *Recommendation* Reduce oxidative rancidity to extend product shelf life. The occurrence of oxidative rancidity is one of the most serious limitations to adequate shelf life and optimal palatability of many animal products. Use of certain packaging technologies and approved antioxidants and control of certain processing variables help minimize this problem in some, but not all, products. For example, skim milk and fresh pork sausage have shortened shelf lives because of the incidence of oxidative rancidity.

• *Recommendation* Use fat substitution to alter the fatty acid composition of processed animal products (that is, to increase the proportion of unsaturated fatty acids). However, the potential for increasing the susceptibility to oxidative rancidity when the fatty acid profile is shifted too far toward unsaturated fatty acids must be considered and controlled.

• *Recommendation* Improve methodologies for the analysis of fat and sensory and other quality characteristics of animal products. Rapid, accurate, and cost-effective analyses are important to the production and monitoring of a variety of food characteristics.

• *Recommendation* Utilize molecular genetics and other biotechnologies to improve fermentation processes that are important in the manufacture of animal products such as cheese, yogurt, and sausage.

For example, the newest technologies could be used to generate new microorganisms that could reduce the cholesterol content of the end product.

• *Recommendation* Determine how selective extraction of saturated fats and cholesterol can be used to reduce these components in animal products. The use of supercritical carbon dioxide as an extractant shows promise for this purpose.

• *Recommendation* Search for ways to safely and organoleptically reduce or replace sodium in manufactured animal products. Sodium chloride plays a critical role in delaying microbial growth, providing flavor, and contributing to the functional characteristics of many processed products. Therefore, it should not be reduced or replaced without serious consideration of the consequences or until a satisfactory replacement for sodium chloride is found for use in products such as cheese and sausage.

## REFERENCES

Becker, R. H., and L. M. Speltz. 1986. Working the S-curve: Making more explicit forecasts. Res. Manage. 29:21.

Bonner, J. M. 1974. Effects of 1,3–Butanediol in Cows with Milk Fat Depression. Ph.D. dissertation. Iowa State University, Ames.

Eichhorn, J. M., L. J. Coleman, and E. J. Wakayama. 1986. Effects of breed type and restricted versus ad libitum feeding on fatty acid composition and cholesterol content of muscle and adipose tissue from mature bovine females. J. Anim. Sci. 63:781.

Hammer, R. E., R. L. Brinster, and R. D. Palmiter. 1985. Use of gene transfer to increase animal growth. Cold Spring Harbor Symp. Quant. Biol. 50:379.

Rhee, K. S., T. R. Dutson, and G. C. Smith. 1982. Effect of changes in intermuscular and subcutaneous fat levels on cholesterol content of raw and cooked beef steaks. J. Food Sci. 47:1638.

Savell, J. W., H. R. Cross, and G. C. Smith. 1986. Percentage ether extractable fat and moisture content of beef longissimus muscle as related to USDA marbling score. J. Food Sci. 51:838.

Stromer, M. H., D. E. Goll, and J. H. Roberts. 1966. Cholesterol in subcutaneous and intramuscular lipid depots from bovine carcasses of different maturity and fatness. J. Anim. Sci. 25:1145.

# APPENDIX

# Hormonal Regulation of Growth

F. C. LEUNG

Animal growth is a complex physiological process regulated by the endocrine system (Figure 1), which also mediates the effects of nutritional, environmental, and genetic factors in animals. To enhance growth and improve feed conversion efficiency in agricultural animals, scientists must understand the roles of hormones (peptide and steroid) and peptide growth factors in these processes and identify the limiting factors so that these processes can be modulated.

The hormones that affect growth in animals are growth hormone, insulin, thyroid hormones, glucocorticoids, prolactin, and gonadal steroids (androgens and estrogens). Their role in growth and development has traditionally been investigated by examining the effect of hormone deprivation after organ ablation; the effects of excess amounts of hormones can be observed by administering the hormones to animals in vivo.

Growth hormone (GH) is generally believed to be the most important hormone affecting growth and development. Clinical observations show that GH deficiency in children results in dwarfism and that excess GH results in acromegaly and gigantism (Underwood and Van Wyk, 1981). This has

led to the assumption that an increase in the circulating concentration of GH would result in faster growth. This hypothesis has been confirmed by the gene insertion technique. Palmiter et al. (1983) produced transgenic mice by direct injection of cloned rat GH or human GH recombinant DNA, ligated with a mouse metallothionein promoter, into the pronuclei of fertilized eggs. Transgenic mice that carried the extra GH gene, and that therefore had high circulating concentrations of GH, grew to twice the size of their control littermates. Hammer et al. (1984) also used this technique to correct dwarfism in a strain of "Little" mice, which are deficient in GH; the transgenic mice grew even larger than normal mice.

Injected GH has been reported to improve the growth rate and feed conversion efficiency of normal pigs (Chung et al., 1985; Machlin, 1972), calves (Brumby, 1959), and lambs (Wagner and Veenhuizen, 1978). Administration of GH to dairy cows reportedly increases the efficiency of milk production (see the papers by Gorewit and Linn in this volume), and in pigs and lambs shifts carcass composition from fat toward protein and moisture (Chung et al., 1985;

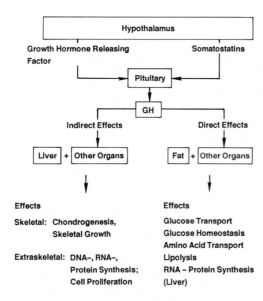

**FIGURE 1**  Regulation and effects of growth hormone.

Machlin, 1972; Wagner and Veenhuizen, 1978). The effects of exogenous GH on growth in fish (salmon and trout) and chickens have recently been reported by Kawauchi et al. (1986) and Leung et al. (1986b). However, responses in these animals were much less marked than those observed in transgenic mice.

To investigate the impact of increased circulating GH concentration on growth and feed efficiency, Leung et al. (1986b) used various experimental approaches to manipulate the endocrine systems of chicks. A discussion of their methodologies and results follows.

### THE INFLUENCE OF GH ON GROWTH

Pituitary GH synthesis and reaction are generally believed to be regulated by the hypothalamic releasing factor, GH releasing factor (GRF) and inhibiting factor, and somatotropin releasing/inhibiting factor. In avian species, a third hypothalamic factor, thyrotropin releasing hormone (TRH), which stimulates thyrotropin stimulating hormone

at the pituitary level, is also a potent GH releaser (Harvey et al., 1978). In contrast to mammalian species, where there is only one GH releasing factor, avian species appear to have two. It is widely thought that the lipolytic effect of GH is direct but that somatomedin-C (SM-C) mediates the growth response of GH (Chawla et al., 1983; Underwood and Van Wyk, 1981). There is also evidence that GH may act directly in the tibia to promote bone growth (Isaksson et al., 1982; Russell and Spencer, 1985). The various experimental methods used to elevate serum concentrations of GH are listed in Table 1.

### Effects of Chicken GH on Body Weight Gain in Chickens

Large quantities of chicken pituitary GH were purified to examine its effect on growth (Leung et al., 1986b). The purified chicken GH (cGH), which was biologically active in the rat tibia bioassay, gave a dose-dependent response parallel to that of the bovine GH standard. The amino acid composition of cGH was similar to that of mammalian GH, and particle-sequencing analysis of cGH showed 79 percent homology with bovine GH. Four-week-old Hubbard × Hubbard broiler cockerels were used in all experiments. Thirty-six birds were individually caged in a temperature- and light-controlled

**TABLE 1**  Methods for Elevating Serum Concentration of Growth Hormone

1. Treat with GH.

2. Treat with GRF for TRH.

3. Increase secretion of endogenous GRF or TRH by control of neuroregulators.

4. Decrease secretion or action of endogenous somatomedin releasing/inhibiting factor.

5. Increase secretion of endogenous GRF or GH by inserting multiple copies of their structural genes, linked to an appropriate promoter, into the chicken genome.

room; they were randomly divided into four treatment groups of nine birds each, with food and water available ad libitum.

The purified cGH was dissolved in physiological saline and given daily by intravenous injection via the brachial vein at concentrations of 5, 10, and 50 μg/bird in 100-μl volumes. Body weight and feed consumption were recorded twice weekly for 2 weeks. At the end of the experiment, birds were killed, defeathered, and ground in a meat grinder. Tissues were analyzed by New Jersey Feed Laboratory, Inc. (Plainsfield, N.J.), for moisture, protein, and fat content, according to the procedure recommended by the Association of Official Analytical Chemists.

Birds that received 5 μg of cGH daily showed significant weight gains (20.6 and 13.5 percent over control birds) on days 3 and 6, respectively. Birds that received 10 μg of cGH also showed significant weight gains over control birds after 3 and 6 days of treatment (19.6 and 11.3 percent, respectively). Birds that received 50 μg of cGH showed an improvement in weight gain over control birds, but the increase was not statistically significant. Overall, the increase in body weight gain seemed to be transient, so that the stimulating effect of cGH was diminished by the end of the experiment. There was no difference in the effect of feed conversion efficiency on carcass composition between cGH-treated and control birds.

## Effects of Human Pancreatic GRF and TRH on Body Weight Gain in Chickens

Chicken hypothalamic GRF has not yet been isolated and purified, but a synthetic human pancreatic GRF (hpGRF) has been shown to be active in stimulating cGH release in chickens both in vivo and in vitro (Leung and Taylor, 1983; Scanes et al., 1984). In addition, TRH, which is a hypothalamic peptide, has been shown to stimulate cGH release in vivo. The objective of the studies described below was to determine the effect of hypothalamic peptides on growth in chickens.

Four-week-old Hubbard × Hubbard broiler cockerels were used in all experiments. In the hpGRF experiment, birds were individually caged and randomly distributed into four treatment groups of nine birds each. In the TRH experiment, birds were individually caged and randomly divided into four treatment groups of 8 to 10 birds. All birds were housed in a temperature- and light-controlled room (25°C; 14 hours of light, 10 hours of darkness) and provided with food and water ad libitum. Food consumption and weight were recorded twice weekly for 2 weeks. At the end of the experiment, birds were killed and defeathered, and carcass composition was analyzed as described in the previous section. The hpGRF$_{44}$ (Bachem, Torrance, Calif.) and TRH (Beckman, Palo Alto, Calif.) were dissolved in physiological saline and injected via the brachial vein at concentrations of 0.1, 1.0, or 10.0 μg/bird in a 100-μl volume. Control birds received 100 μl of a saline solution.

Birds that received 0.1 μg of hpGRF daily showed a significant increase in body weight gain early on, but that soon diminished. The similarly transient stimulating effect of cGH and hpGRF on body weight gain suggests that hpGRF is also mediated through pituitary GH.

Birds that received 1.0 or 10.0 μg of TRH daily showed significant increases in body weight compared to controls. In contrast to the effect of hpGRF, the growth response to TRH injections was not transient (Leung et al., 1984c). The difference between the effects of the two hormones is probably due to the additional stimulation of thyroid hormone by TRH. Thyroid hormones (triiodothyronine [T$_3$] and thyroxine [T$_4$]) have been shown to influence body weight gain in chickens (Leung et al., 1985).

### Somatomedin-C

The growth activity of GH is believed to be mediated by SM-C growth factor, generated mainly in the liver. Somatomedin-C is GH-dependent, and purified SM-C has been shown to stimulate body weight gain in both hypophysectomized and intact rats (Hizuka et al., 1986; Schoenle et al., 1982). Since chicken SM-C has not been isolated and purified, a human SM-C radioimmunoassay (RIA) was used to measure serum immunoreactive SM-C when purified cGH was injected into 4-week-old cockerels (Leung et al., 1986b). Purified cGH did not affect weight or incorporation of $^3$H-proline or $^{35}SO_4$ in 9- to 10-day-old chicken embryo cartilage cultured in vitro, but purified human SM-C had a significant effect (Burch et al., 1985). Thus, it seems that the growth promotion axis of hypothalamic GRF-pituitary GH-hepatic SM-C in chickens is similar to that in mammals, but investigation of the biological effects of purified chicken GRF and chicken SM-C is needed to validate this hypothesis.

### Growth Hormone Receptor

Hormone-receptor interaction is the first step in hormone action, but receptor physiology has only recently been given attention. Many human diseases are known to result from receptor defects, but the biological significance of the receptor is only beginning to be recognized. For example, analysis of the amino acid and nucleotide sequences of purified epidermal growth factor receptor (EGF-R) has enabled scientists to link the structure-function relationships of oncogenes (v-*erbB*) and EGF-R (Downward et al., 1984). Although there is no structural analysis (amino acid response) for the GH receptor as yet, its eventual determination will lead to an understanding of the molecular basis of GH action.

Leung et al. (1984a) demonstrated a specific hepatic GH receptor in chickens and observed paradoxically high blood concentrations of GH, as measured by a homologous cGH RIA (Leung et al., 1984b), in sex-linked dwarf chickens (Lilburn et al., 1986). These chickens grew to less than half the size of normal chickens, leading Leung et al. (1984a) to examine GH receptor binding in the same strain. There was a significant decrease in hepatic receptor binding at 6, 8, and 20 weeks of age compared to that of normal, fast-growing broiler chickens (Leung et al., 1987). Huybrechts et al. (1985) reported that sex-linked dwarf chickens also had significantly lower circulating immunoreactive SM-C concentrations compared to those of normal birds. And Leung et al. (1984a) observed that sex-linked dwarf chickens had significantly higher hepatic (IGF-I) receptor binding.

These observations may provide evidence that dwarfism is sex-linked and may be due to a defect in the GH receptor. Based on preliminary results, we believe that GH receptors may be the limiting factor in the growth promoter axis in chickens. For example, normal Leghorn chickens, which grow at a much slower rate than broiler chickens, possess significantly fewer GH receptors than broiler chickens (Leung et al., 1987). However, that hypothesis does not agree with data reported for mammalian species. Growth hormone has been shown to maintain its own receptors in rat adipocytes and to up-regulate its hepatic receptors (Baxter and Zaltsman, 1984). Recently, Chung and Etherton (1986) reported that the number of hepatic GH receptors is increased in pigs that have received GH injections. The method of regulating GH receptors in other agricultural animals is not known. However, if GH up-regulates its receptors at the target tissue, it is logical to assume that an increase in circulating GH would result in an amplified biological response to GH.

### Gene Insertion

The technology for introducing foreign genes into mammalian embryos forms the basis of a powerful approach for studying gene regulation and the genetic basis of development (Palmiter and Brinster, 1985). A dramatic growth increase in transgenic mice from eggs that were microinjected with a metallothionein GH foreign gene suggests that this technology could be valuable for agricultural applications. Indeed, Hammer et al. (1985) successfully introduced foreign genes into the genes of rabbits, sheep, and pigs by microinjecting eggs, using mouse metallothionein-human GH recombinant DNA. The foreign DNA was integrated and expressed in transgenic rabbits and pigs. Thomas E. Wagner (Ohio University, personal communication, 1986) also successfully introduced foreign genes in pigs by microinjection. Leung and co-workers have attempted to directly inject foreign DNA into the blastoderm of freshly laid eggs with recombinant DNA technology (unpublished data). And Souza et al. (1984) used the retroviral approach in introducing foreign genes into chickens.

Kopchick et al. (1985) constructed a recombinant DNA (pbGH-4) that is an avian retroviral long-terminal repeat (LTR), ligated to the structural bovine GH (bGH) gene. This recombinant DNA is biologically active in a transient eukaryotic expression assay system. When this recombinant DNA was totally integrated into a mouse fibroblast cell line, mature bGH was expressed and secreted into the culture medium. Leung et al. (1986a) purified and characterized the recombinant bGH from culture medium and showed that the recombinant bGH possesses the same physiochemical and physical properties as native pituitary bGH. This recombinant bGH DNA was then introduced into the germinal disk of the freshly laid egg by opening a window in the egg and injecting various amounts of DNA in circular or linear form with a micropipette. Only seven of the chicks that hatched from the 3,000 injected eggs had measurable circulating immunoreactive bGH. When serum samples were measured with both a homologous cGH RIA and a bGH RIA, the cross-reactivity of purified cGH and bGH in the RIA was less than 5 percent. The expression of bGH was transient; no detectable immunoreactive bGH was present after 10 weeks of age. All the chickens were killed or crossed after sexual maturity. Tissue DNA was analyzed by dot blot and Southern gel assays. No measurable immunoreactive bGH was detected by RIA from seven samples collected from first-generation offspring. It appears, therefore, that this method is inefficient. In addition, since the germinal disk in freshly laid eggs consists of at least 500 to 1,000 cells, even if the foreign DNA is integrated in the host cell genome it is unlikely that the foreign DNA will enter the germ line.

Use of a retroviral vector to introduce foreign genes into chicken genes provides an alternative experimental approach. Indeed, Souza et al. (1984) generated a recombinant retrovirus by cloning chicken GH cDNA into a modified Rous sarcoma virus Schmiedt-Ruspin A genome in which the sac gene was entirely deleted. Recombinant infectious virus that expresses cGH was generated to infect 9-day-old chick embryos. Subsequently born chicks expressed circulating concentrations of cGH that were two- to threefold higher than those of normal birds. In addition, the birds were uremic. Salter et al. (1986) obtained similar results using a different retroviral vector. These results suggest that the retroviral approach may be more effective than direct injection of foreign DNA in introducing foreign genes into the germ line of chickens.

## CONCLUSIONS AND FUTURE DIRECTIONS

Our preliminary information that the GH receptor, rather than GH itself, may be the limiting factor in the growth production axis in chickens opens up new research directions. Pituitary GH has been purified from many agricultural animals, and antibodies to these preparations have also been generated for RIA. Somatomedin-C has been purified only from humans and rodents (Spencer et al., 1983); with recombinant DNA technology, scientists should be able to clone the SM-C gene and express synthetic recombinant SM-C using prokaryotic and eukaryotic cell expression systems. Only then can the biological activities of SM-C in agricultural animals be determined. The techniques for inserting foreign DNA into genes by microinjection into the pronucleus of fertilized eggs have been successful in agricultural animals (Hammer et al., 1986), and the retroviral vector approach in chickens is also promising. However, further research is needed to determine which genes are most desirable for use in gene insertion, define the sites of integration, and attain the fine control for expressing the exogenous genes that is necessary to make such technology useful to agriculture.

## ACKNOWLEDGMENTS

I am grateful for the collaboration of Drs. John Kopchick, Jim Smith, H. Chen, and Mike Lilburn and for the expert assistance of J. Taylor, A. Van Iderstine, C. A. Ball, K. N. Ngiam-Rilling, B. Goggins, C. I. Rosenblum, R. Malavarca, E. Mills, and F. Macks. I also thank M. E. Mericka and H. B. Crow for typing this manuscript and D. L. Felton for her expert editing.

## REFERENCES

Baxter, R. C., and Z. Zaltsman. 1984. Induction of hepatic receptors for growth hormone (GH) and prolactin by GH infusion is sex dependent. Endocrinology 115:2009.

Brumby, P. J. 1959. The influence of growth hormone on growth in young cattle. N.Z. J. Agric. Res. 2:683.

Burch, W. M., G. Corda, J. J. Kopchick, and F. C. Leung. 1985. Homologous and heterologous growth hormones fail to stimulate avian cartilage growth in vitro. J. Clin. Endocrinol. Metab. 60:747.

Chawla, R. K., J. S. Parks, and D. Rudman. 1983. Structural variants of human growth hormone: Biochemical, genetic and clinical respects. Annu. Rev. Med. 34:519.

Chung, C. S., and T. D. Etherton. 1986. Characteri-

zation of porcine growth hormone (pGH) binding to porcine liver microsomes: Chronic administration of pGH induces pGH binding. Endocrinology 119:780.

Chung, C. S., T. D. Etherton, and J. P. Wiggins. 1985. Stimulation of swine growth by porcine growth hormone. J. Anim. Sci. 60:118.

Downward, J., Y. Yarden, E. Mayes, G. Scarce, N. Totty, P. Stockwell, A. Ullrich, J. Schlessinger, and M. D. Waterfield. 1984. Close similarity of epidermal growth factor receptor and v-erb-B oncogene protein sequences. Nature 307:521.

Hammer, R. E., R. D. Palmiter, and R. L. Brinster. 1984. Partial correction of murine hereditary growth disorder by germ-like incorporation of a new gene. Nature 311:65.

Hammer, R. E., V. G. Pursel, C. E. Rexroad, R. J. Wall, D. J. Bolt, K. M. Ebert, R. D. Palmiter, and R. L. Brinster. 1985. Production of transgenic rabbits, sheep and pigs by microinjection. Nature 315:680.

Hammer, R. E., V. G. Pursel, C. E. Rexroad, R. J. Wall, D. J. Bolt, R. D. Palmiter, and R. L. Brinster. 1986. Genetic engineering of mammalian embryos. J. Anim. Sci. 63:269.

Harvey, S., C. G. Scanes, N. J. Bolton, and A. Chadwick. 1978. Effect of thyrotropin-releasing hormone (TRH) and somatostatin (GH-RIH) on growth hormone and prolactin secretion in vitro and in vivo in the domestic fowl (*Gallus domesticus*). Neuroendocrinology 26:249.

Hizuka, N., K. Takano, K. Asakawa, M. Miyakawa, I. Tanaka, R. Harikawa, and K. Shizume. 1986. Insulin-like growth factor I stimulates growth in normal growing rats in vivo. In Proceedings of the 68th Annual Endocrine Society Meeting, June 25–27, 1986, Anaheim, Calif. Bethesda, Md.: Endocrine Society.

Huybrechts, L. M., D. B. King, T. J. Lauterio, J. Marsh, and C. G. Scanes. 1985. Plasma concentrations of somatomedin-C in hypophysectomized, dwarf and intact growing domestic fowl as determined by heterologous radioimmunoassay. J. Endocrinol. 104:233.

Isaksson, O. G. P., J.-O. Jansson, and I. A. M. Gause. 1982. Growth hormone stimulates longitudinal bone growth directly. Science 216:1237.

Kawauchi, H., S. M. Ama, A. Yasuda, K. Yamaguchi, K. Shirahata, J. Kubota, and T. Hirano. 1986. Isolation and characterization of chum salmon growth hormone. Arch. Biochem. Biophys. 244:542.

Kopchick, J. J., R. Malavarca, T. Livelli, and F. C. Leung. 1985. Use of avian retroviral-bovine growth hormone DNA recombinants to direct expression of bovine growth hormone by cultured fibroblasts. DNA 4:23.

Leung, F. C., and J. E. Taylor. 1983. In vivo and in vitro stimulation of growth hormone release in chickens by synthetic human pancreatic growth hormone releasing factor (hpGRF). Endocrinology 113:1913.

Leung, F. C., J. Gillett, M. S. Lilburn, and J. Kopchick. 1984a. Analysis of growth hormone receptors and genes in sex-linked dwarf chickens. J. Steroid Biochem. 20:1557.

Leung, F. C., J. E. Taylor, S. L. Steelman, C. D. Bennett, J. A. Rodkey, R. A. Long, R. Serio, R. M. Weppelman, and G. Olson. 1984b. Purification and properties of chicken growth hormone and the development of a homologous radioimmunoassay. Comp. Endocrinol. 56:389.

Leung, F. C., J. E. Taylor, and A. Van Iderstine. 1984c. Thyrotropin-releasing hormone stimulates body weight gain and increases thyroid hormones and growth hormone in plasma of cockerels. Endocrinology 115:736.

Leung, F. C., J. E. Taylor, and A. Van Iderstine. 1985. Effects of dietary thyroid hormones on growth, plasma $T_3$, $T_4$ and growth hormone in normal and hypothyroid chickens. Gen. Comp. Endocrinol. 59:91.

Leung, F. C., B. Jones, S. L. Steelman, C. I. Rosenblum, and J. J. Kopchick. 1986a. Purification and physiochemical properties of a recombinant bovine growth hormone produced by cultured murine fibroblasts. Fndocrinology 119:1489.

Leung, F. C., J. E. Taylor, S. Wien, and A. Van Iderstine. 1986b. Purified chicken growth hormone (cGH) and a human pancreatic growth hormone releasing factor (hpGRF) increased body weight gain in chickens. Endocrinology 118:1961.

Leung, F. C., W. J. Styles, C. R. Rosenblum, M. S. Lilburn, and J. A. Marsh. 1987. Diminished hepatic growth hormone receptor bindings in sex-linked dwarf broiler and Leghorn chickens. Proc. Soc. Exp. Biol. Med. 184:234.

Lilburn, M. S., K. N. Ngiam-Rilling, J. H. Smith, and F. C. Leung. 1986. The relationship between age and circulating concentrations of triiodothyronine ($T_3$), thyroxine ($T_4$), and growth hormone in commercial meat strain chickens. Proc. Soc. Exp. Biol. Med. 182:336.

Machlin, L. J. 1972. Effect of porcine growth hormone on growth and carcass composition of the pig. J. Anim. Sci. 35:794.

Palmiter, R. D., and R. L. Brinster. 1985. Transgenic mice. Cell 41:343.

Palmiter, R. D., G. Norstedt, R. E. Gelines, R. E. Hammer, and R. L. Brinster. 1983. Metallothionein-human GH fusion genes stimulated growth of mice. Science 222:809.

Russell, S. M., and E. M. Spencer. 1985. Local injections of human or rat growth hormone or of purified human somatomedin-C stimulate unilateral tibial epiphyseal growth in hypophysectomized rats. Endocrinology 116:2563.

Salter, D. W., E. J. Smith, S. H. Hughes, S. E. Wright, A. M. Fadly, R. L. Witter, and L. B. Crittenden. 1986. Gene insertion into the chicken germ line by retroviruses. Poultry Sci. 65:1445.

Scanes, C. G., R. V. Carsia, T. J. Lauterio, L. Huybrechts, J. Rivier, and W. Vale. 1984. Synthetic human pancreatic growth hormone releasing factor (GRF) stimulates growth hormone secretion in the domestic fowl (Gallus domesticus). Life Sci. 34:1127.

Schoenle, E., J. Zapf, R. E. Humbel, and E. R. Froesch. 1982. Insulin-like growth factor I stimulates growth in hypophysectomized rats. Nature 296:252.

Souza, L. M., T. C. Boone, D. Murdock, K. Langley, J. Wypych, D. Fenton, S. Johnson, P. H. Lai, R. Everette, R. Y. Hsu, and R. Bosselman. 1984. Application of recombinant DNA technologies to studies on chicken growth hormone. Exp. Zool. 232:465.

Spencer, E. M., M. Ross, and B. Smith. 1983. The identity of human insulin-like growth factors I and II with somatomedins C and A and homology with rat IGF I and II. Proceedings of a Symposium on Insulin-Like Growth Factors/Somatomedins, Nairobi, Kenya, November 13–15, 1982. Berlin: Walter de Gruyter.

Underwood, L. E., and J. J. Van Wyk. 1981. Hormones in normal and aberrant growth. P. 1149 in Textbook of Endocrinology, R. H. Williams, ed. Philadelphia: W. B. Saunders.

Wagner, J. F., and E. L. Veenhuizen. 1978. Growth performance, carcass deposition and plasma hormone levels in wether lambs when treated with growth hormone and thyroprotein. J. Anim. Sci. 45:397.

# Muscle Cell Growth and Development

RONALD E. ALLEN

Skeletal muscle from domestic animals is a major source of high-quality protein in the human diet. Past technological advances in production of animal muscle protein have been based on empirical and fundamental biological research. Future technological advances, however, are less likely to occur unless research is firmly grounded in the basic biology of muscle and animal growth. The primary function of this paper is to review information about the structure and composition of muscle, muscle differentiation and development, and key elements of protein metabolism as they relate to muscle growth. It also describes current areas of active research interest and speculates on applications of new research knowledge and future research needs.

## MUSCLE CELL STRUCTURE AND COMPOSITION

The differentiated muscle cell in postnatal muscle is the muscle fiber, a highly specialized, long, cylindrical cell that can range in diameter from 10 to 100 μm and in length from millimeters up to many centimeters. The primary differences in fibers of different

species are fiber length and number of fibers per muscle. Each fiber is surrounded by a 7.5- to 10-nm-thick plasmalemma, called the sarcolemma. The sarcolemma is a lipid bilayer like the cell membranes of other cells and has a lipid composition of roughly 60 percent protein, 20 percent phospholipid, and 20 percent cholesterol. Surrounding the sarcolemma is the basal lamina, or basement membrane. This somewhat amorphous structure, 50 to 70 nm thick, is composed of mucopolysaccharides and collagen (types III and V). The cell membrane of muscle has a specialized structure—the motor endplate—which accommodates interaction with an axon from a motoneuron. In addition, the membrane maintains an electrical potential that is propagated from the motor endplate, down the membrane, and finally into the cell by a complex set of invaginations that form the transverse tubular system.

Muscle fibers contain the major organelles present in most cells. The most striking difference between muscle cells and the majority of other cells is their multinucleated nature. Depending on its size, an individual fiber may contain hundreds of nuclei. They are found just beneath the sarcolemma and seem to be randomly distributed along the length of the fiber. Mitochondria are present between the contractile elements of muscle; their concentration varies with the metabolic activity of the particular fiber. Ribosomes are dispersed within the cytoplasm, but very few are associated with endoplasmic reticulum, primarily because muscle fibers synthesize few secreted proteins. The endoplasmic reticulum in muscle has formed a specialized set of membrane structures called the sarcoplasmic reticulum. The primary function of this structure is regulation of free calcium ion concentration. When free calcium ion concentration is maintained below approximately 0.1 μM, contraction does not occur. But when the membrane is depolarized, the action potential reaches the interior of the cell through the transverse tubular system, calcium is released from the sarcoplasmic reticulum, the concentration approaches 1 μM, and contraction is activated. Lysosomes are not readily seen in muscle fibers, although lysosomal enzymes are present. The lysosomes are most likely sequestered in the sarcoplasmic reticulum.

By far the most unique subcellular aspect of muscle fibers is the contractile machinery, the myofibril. This is an aggregation of 12 to 14 proteins into highly organized contractile threads that are insoluble at the ionic strength of the cytoplasm in muscle cells. It is noteworthy that this specialized set of proteins constitutes about 55 percent of the total protein in muscle. Consequently, many developmental studies of muscle have focused on myofibrillar protein gene expression and synthesis, which are discussed later in this paper.

Myofibrils are composed of two main classes of filaments: thick filaments and thin filaments. Thick filaments measure approximately 15 nm by 1,500 nm. The major protein in thick filaments is myosin, which has the active site that hydrolyzes adenosine triphosphate (ATP) and the site that binds to actin in the thin filament. The thin filament is roughly 6 nm by 1,000 nm and is composed of actin, which forms the beaded backbone of the filament, and tropomyosin and troponin, which perform regulatory functions. At one end, thin filaments insert into a protein lattice called the Z-line; at the other end, they overlay with thick filaments in a hexagonal array. Additional small-diameter filament systems are present within myofibrils to provide an elastic component. Also, an intermediate-diameter filament system, found outside the periphery of the myofibril, links adjacent myofibrils and maintains their contractile units in register. Specific details of the ultrastructure of myofibrils and the biochemical properties of this interdigitating array of filaments can be found in Goll et al. (1984).

These features of muscle cells are common to all skeletal muscle fibers, but specific fibers have differentiated somewhat depending on their purpose. Some populations of fibers are primarily responsible for rapid contractions on an intermittent basis, while others have slower contraction speed and sustain contractile activity over extended periods of time. Muscle fiber types have been described extensively in many species; and their biochemical, physiological, and morphological differences are significant to problems of muscle growth and meat quality. A generalized scheme for describing fiber types classifies them on the basis of their contraction speed and on the energy metabolism pathways primarily used to provide energy for contraction. Peter et al. (1972) provided one of the most descriptive classification systems by grouping fibers into three general categories. Fibers that were dependent on oxidative metabolism and had slower contraction speeds were classified as slow-twitch, oxidative fibers (SO). Fibers with faster contraction times that were dependent on anaerobic, or glycolytic, energy metabolism pathways were termed fast-twitch, glycolytic fibers (FG). A third broad category contained fast-twitch fibers that had glycolytic metabolic capabilities but also a significant capacity for oxidative metabolism; these were termed fast-twitch, oxidative-glycolytic fibers (FOG).

Contraction speed is correlated with myosin adenosine triphosphatase (ATPase) activity and, therefore, with the particular myosin isozymes synthesized by the fiber. Other myofibrillar protein isoform variations may also be associated with contractile properties. The complexity and degree of development of the sarcoplasmic reticulum, t-tubule system, and neuromuscular junctions have all been associated with contraction speed and fiber class. As expected, mitochondrial content and glycolytic enzyme content vary among fiber types, as do energy substrates such as glycogen and triglyceride. Aspects of fiber type variation that affect muscle growth include the notable differences in fiber size that generally correlate with muscle fiber type. SO fibers are smaller in diameter than FG fibers, and FOG fibers tend to be intermediate in size. Smaller fiber diameters may facilitate efficient gas exchange in oxidative fibers. In addition, SO fibers tend to have higher nuclei concentrations and, therefore, lower protein concentrations per nucleus. Satellite cell frequency, however, is reportedly higher for SO fibers (Kelly, 1978b). Because individual muscles vary in fiber type composition, factors that differentially affect the development or growth of specific fiber types can result in alterations in muscle mass (for example, the transition from FG to FOG that can accompany aerobic conditioning). Reductions in fiber diameter and, consequently, muscle mass would be expected. Alterations in gene expression and in quantitative aspects of protein metabolism that are responsible for such fiber type transitions are poorly understood.

Chemical composition of muscle tissue can be quite variable, and the primary source of variation is intramuscular adipose tissue. It is clear that most of the variation in major constituents is minimized when expressed on a fat-free basis. Some compositional variation can be found in association with aging, but, in general, it is attributable to changes in moisture content. Skeletal muscle from very young animals has a high moisture content that decreases with maturity. As a result, protein concentration increases with maturity. Subtle changes in other constituents, such as glycogen, can vary among muscles and species, but these differences may not have major nutritional significance when considering the composition of muscle as a food.

The primary lipid fraction contributing to muscle tissue variation is triglyceride, which is stored in adipocytes within the muscle. These depositions are commonly referred to as marbling, and within the range of marbling found in the longissimus muscle of beef, the ether-extractable lipid (primarily triglyceride) varies from 1.77 to 10.42 percent on a wet weight basis (Savell et al., 1986).

Cholesterol content, on the other hand, is less variable. This can best be understood in light of its role in muscle tissue. Cholesterol is an integral part of cell membranes, mainly the plasma membrane. On a tissue basis across maturity groups and marbling contents within maturity groups, cholesterol content of beef muscle does not vary (Stromer et al., 1966). In addition, the amount of cholesterol per gram of whole steak was not significantly different among the five yield grades examined by Rhee et al. (1982). Furthermore, neither breed type nor nutritional background affected cholesterol content of lean muscle tissue in beef cows (Eichhorn et al., 1986). It is possible to find variation in cholesterol content of meat, however, because adipose tissue tends to have a higher cholesterol concentration than do muscle fibers. Consequently, variations in the amount of subcutaneous or intermuscular fat consumed with the lean portion can alter cholesterol intake. It has been calculated that 37 to 56 percent of the cholesterol in a cooked rib steak of beef originates from subcutaneous and intermuscular adipose tissue (Rhee et al., 1982).

In looking only at muscle cells, however, significant variations in cholesterol content have not been seen, even among most of the species used for muscle foods (Reiser, 1975; Watt and Merrill, 1963). This is also true for the amino acid composition of muscle. The majority of muscle cell proteins are myofibrillar and are very highly conserved across species. In addressing topics such as alteration of tissue composition to enhance nutritional quality, it is important to keep in mind that the biology of the animal or tissue must come first. Our ability to manipulate cells in animals has both physiological limits and ramifications.

## MUSCLE FIBER DEVELOPMENT

### Prenatal Development

Myogenesis originates in cells of the embryonic mesoderm and apparently follows a similar course in all species examined. Perhaps the most detailed descriptions come from studies of human (Hauschka, 1974) and chick (White et al., 1975) embryo development. In the human, no apparent organization is noted in the limb mesoderm on day 28 of development, but by day 43 loose connective tissue cell regions and compact myogenic cell regions are visible. By day 45 the first small multinucleated myotubes (the precursors of muscle fibers) have formed; by day 50 the general organization of major muscles and bones is essentially complete. Beyond this point, the rate of muscle histogenesis occurs at different rates between and within individual muscles. In the gastrocnemius on day 62, well-developed, myofibril-containing muscle fibers are present, but the majority of cells are still mononucleated. This population decreases to about 50 percent of the total by day 72, while fibers increase two- to threefold. During the next 2 weeks, fiber formation proceeds

rapidly, with the percentage of mononucleated cells diminishing to 20 percent by day 95 and further decreasing to the point that only a few single cells persist in association with fibers by day 146.

In other vertebrate species, comparable developmental patterns are discernible. One striking observation in rat and chick muscle is the development of two populations of fibers (Kelly and Zacks, 1969; McLennan, 1983). The "primary fibers" develop early and are surrounded by closely associated mononucleated cells. In the chick embryo, "secondary fiber" formation proceeds rapidly after about 12 days of development until most of the mononucleated cell population is exhausted and fiber formation is complete. This occurs before hatching in the chick and before birth in most mammals. A similar biphasic developmental pattern has been documented in fetal lamb skeletal muscle (Ashmore et al., 1972). In general, fiber formation is complete near the time of birth.

The study of myogenesis focuses on the muscle development process and has centered around efforts to unravel myogenic lineages and the mechanisms responsible for alterations in the synthetic programs of muscle cells that lead to the formation of fibers and the expression of muscle-specific cell characteristics. One of the most important initial observations on the mechanisms of myogenesis came from a series of experiments reported by Stockdale and Holtzer (1961) that directly demonstrate that multinucleated myotubes arise from the fusion of mononucleated myogenic cells (myoblasts). Furthermore, only mononucleated cells have the ability to proliferate; the nuclei in myotubes cannot replicate their DNA and divide. Consequently, the transition from a proliferating myoblast to a nonproliferating myotube that can synthesize muscle-specific macromolecules represents the terminal step in muscle differentiation.

There now appear to be several different

types of myogenic cells that are actively proliferating and differentiating during specific periods of development. Their collective developmental patterns are responsible for the general pattern of muscle histogenesis. At least two broad types and four subtypes of myogenic cells have been identified by White et al. (1975), based on the in vitro morphology and medium requirements of cloned myogenic cells from various stages of embryo development. One general type is the early muscle-colony-forming cell, which predominates in early development; the colonies are noted for having small, thick myotubes with few nuclei. In contrast, the predominant form of myogenic cells in later periods of development form colonies in vitro that are extensively fused and contain large myotubes with many nuclei; these are the late muscle-colony-forming cells. Miller and Stockdale (1986) have identified four types of myogenic cells based on the presence of specific isoforms of the myosin heavy chains present in early and late muscle-colony-forming cells.

Early and late classes of cells appear to be distinct, since they can maintain their class-specific characteristic when subcloned up to five times, until proliferative senescence (Rutz and Hauschka, 1982). Additional experiments reported by Seed and Hauschka (1984) have shown that transplanting limb buds at various stages results in the absence of late myogenic cells in the transplant, even though the early class of muscle-colony-forming cells was present. The late class apparently migrates into the limb bud from the somite at a later stage than the early class and, furthermore, does not appear to descend from the early class, in agreement with the previous in vitro experiments (Rutz and Hauschka, 1982). The appearance of early and late muscle-colony-forming cells appears to correlate well with the anatomical appearance of primary and secondary fibers that are formed during development. Different myogenic classes of cells are further implicated in the

formation of primary and secondary fibers because the in vivo formation of secondary fibers is nerve-dependent (McLennan, 1983), as is the in vitro development of fibers from one of the later muscle-colony-forming types (Bonner and Adams, 1982).

An additional class of myogenic cells, or branch of the myogenic lineage, is the satellite cell, which is discussed further in the subsection on postnatal development.

As mentioned previously, a striking transition takes place in muscle development with the differentiation of mononucleated myoblasts into multinucleated myofibers. This terminal step in differentiation is accompanied by the cessation of proliferation and the expression of genes responsible for the muscle phenotype. For many years, there were two general theories to explain myogenesis. The first postulated that a major reorganization in gene expression took place in specific mitotic cycles, and the resultant daughter cells had protein synthesis capabilities that differed from those of the mother cell. This special cell cycle was referred to as a "quantal" cell cycle (Holtzer and Bischoff, 1970). This theory has now been expanded to hypothesize that a fixed number of cell divisions occur between the stem cell compartment to the terminally differentiated, fusion-competent myoblast compartment (Quinn et al., 1984). Key to this description of myogenesis is the "commitment" step of myoblasts to withdraw from the cell cycle, fuse, and initiate the synthesis of muscle-specific proteins.

In contrast, a second theory of myogenesis (Buckley and Konigsberg, 1974) was based on a model that predicted that myoblasts remaining in the $G_1$ phase of the cell cycle had an increasing probability of fusion that resulted in permanent withdrawal from the cell cycle and the initiation of muscle protein synthesis. The probability of remaining in the cell cycle or fusing depended on the presence or absence of environmental factors that stimulate these activities. In this model, withdrawal from the cycle and initiation of muscle gene expression was thought to be the result of the fusion process itself.

A current, and more likely, explanation encompasses elements of both the original theories. It appears that during the early part of the $G_1$ phase of the cell cycle, proliferating myoblasts have the option of continuing to proliferate or of differentiating and fusing into myotubes (Nadal-Ginard, 1978). The commitment to withdraw from the cell cycle is made before fusion, not as a result of fusion. This commitment, however, depends on the presence of growth-stimulating factors in the environment (probably mitogens) that keep myoblasts in the cell cycle. For many years, it appeared that withdrawal from the cell cycle, fusion, and expression of the muscle phenotype were coupled events; recent experiments with a temperature-sensitive mutant of the muscle cell line L6E9 have cast doubts on the obligatory relationship of these events. In experiments with wild-type and mutant L6E9 myoblasts, Nguyen et al. (1983) demonstrated that muscle-specific isoforms of certain myofibrillar proteins could be induced in the mutant cells under conditions that did not permit commitment to withdrawal from the cell cycle. In fact, these cells could be stimulated to reenter the cell cycle even after induction of myofibrillar protein synthesis. Additional experimentation with wild-type L6E9 myoblasts arrested in a low-calcium medium indicated that induction of myofibrillar protein synthesis occurred in cells that could subsequently be stimulated to synthesize DNA and divide. Reentry into the cell cycle, however, resulted in a rapid cessation of myofibrillar protein synthesis and degradation of existing muscle-specific messenger RNAs (Nadal-Ginard et al., 1984). Similar experiments were reported with primary cultures of quail embryo muscle that were arrested in a low-calcium medium (Devlin and Konigsberg, 1983). Apparently, induction of the gene expression transitions leading to the muscle phenotype can be uncoupled from permanent withdrawal from the cell cycle. In normal muscle development, however, the commitment to withdraw from the cell cycle and the induction of the muscle phenotype are closely correlated and occur simultaneously.

The in vivo signals that affect the commitment decision made by myoblasts during fetal development and myofiber formation have not been identified. One class of protein growth factors, the fibroblast growth factor (FGF), has been shown to be mitogenic for myoblasts in culture and can reduce the tendency to differentiate (Allen et al., 1984; Gospodarowicz et al., 1976; Linkhart et al., 1981). A second growth factor, transforming growth factor beta (TGF-β), is a very potent inhibitor of myoblast differentiation and could be responsible for regulating myogenic cell activities in vivo (Florini et al., 1986). In contrast to the two inhibitors of differentiation, the insulin-like growth factors have been reported to stimulate myoblast proliferation and differentiation in culture (Ewton and Florini, 1980, 1981). The means by which these two antagonistic processes can be stimulated by the same hormone, however, has not been completely clarified. In general, the activities of the growth factors and hormones in embryonic muscle development have yet to be verified in vivo.

Although the specific regulatory agents involved in stimulating differentiation have not been thoroughly documented, many of the gene transitions that occur in association with the terminal step in muscle cell differentiation have been reported (Young and Allen, 1979). From the standpoint of gene regulation, some of the interesting events center around the contractile proteins. The major myofibrillar proteins are synthesized in a coordinate fashion shortly after fusion (Devlin and Emerson, 1978, 1979). These events seemed relatively straightforward, until it became possible to examine them in greater molecular detail. It now appears that there are a series of subtle transitions in expression of specific skeletal muscle isoforms of individual proteins during the in vivo and in vitro development of muscle (reviewed by Caplan et al., 1983). The actin that is first synthesized after myoblast differentiation is of the alpha isoform, but it is alpha-cardiac actin and not alpha-skeletal actin. The transition from alpha-cardiac to alpha-skeletal actin occurs as the myotube matures (Bains et al., 1984; Paterson and Eldridge, 1984). Similarly, myosin light chains and heavy chains (Bandman et al., 1982; Crow et al., 1983; Gauthier et al., 1982; Lowey et al., 1983; Lyons et al., 1983; Whalen et al., 1978) progress through isoform transitions that include fetal, neonatal, and, finally, adult isoforms of the subunits of these proteins. These transitions occur in vivo and are also recapitulated in regenerating muscle (Marechal et al., 1984). Regulators of this developmental scheme have not been elucidated; however, innervation and load-bearing functions may be involved in the feedback that is responsible for alterations in gene expression (Hoffman et al., 1985; Rubinstein and Kelly, 1978).

The environmental factors that regulate the synthesis of specific isoforms and the rate at which these proteins are accumulated are not specifically known, but the mechanisms will be resolved in the near future because genes for these proteins are being studied in detail (reviewed by Robbins et al., 1986; Young et al., 1986). For example, the regulation of alpha-skeletal actin may depend on the DNA sequence in regions of the gene preceding the 5'-untranslated part of the message-coding region (Bergsma et al., 1986; Hu et al., 1986; Melloul et al., 1984). It has been suggested that "transacting" factors in the cytoplasm of myogenic cells interact with nuclear genes to activate their expression (Chiu and Blau, 1984), but the nature of these factors has not been described. In the case of myosin, thyroid hormone may be involved in myosin heavy-chain synthesis (Butler-Brown et al., 1986; Gambke and Rubinstein, 1984; Izumo et

al., 1986). The chemical mediators of the effect of activity level (Brevet et al., 1976; Hoffman et al., 1985) and neurogenic influences (Rubinstein and Kelly, 1978) remain undefined. Detailed information about the structure of important muscle-specific genes, including identification of regulatory sequences, will open the door to studies that are critical to understanding quantitative aspects of muscle protein synthesis regulation, one of the key problems in animal growth research.

## Postnatal Development

Understanding the regulation of postnatal muscle growth requires an appreciation of the cellular events underlying the process. Postnatal muscle growth is frequently considered to be due to muscle fiber hypertrophy, in contrast to prenatal muscle growth. This assumption stems from the documented fact that muscle fiber number does not increase dramatically after birth in most animals; consequently, increases in size must be due to hypertrophy (reviewed by Goldspink, 1972; Swatland, 1976).

Although postnatal muscle growth is often thought of in terms of fiber hypertrophy, and not hyperplasia, proliferation and differentiation of myogenic cells are central to the process of postnatal muscle growth. For example, Winick and Noble (1966) demonstrated an 8.5-fold increase in rat muscle DNA from 21 to 133 days of age, corresponding to an 88 percent increase in muscle DNA. Moreover, the relationship between DNA accretion and muscle growth was more firmly established by the findings of Moss (1968) and Swatland (1977), which demonstrated that muscle fiber diameter in growing chicken and pig muscle, respectively, is directly related to the total number of muscle fiber nuclei. Additional studies supporting these results have been reviewed by Allen et al. (1979) and continue to appear regularly in the literature.

Consistent with the point of view that

myogenic cell proliferation is critical to the attainment of maximum muscle mass in livestock are studies involving strains of swine that differ in muscle growth potential (Harbison et al., 1976; Powell and Aberle, 1981) and growth studies in cattle (Trenkle et al., 1978). Of the biochemical parameters evaluated in these experiments, DNA accretion and protein/DNA ratios were most intimately related to muscle growth. In addition, the most rapid period of DNA accretion coincided with the most rapid period of muscle growth. The cumulative evidence presented by these and other studies suggests that most muscle fiber DNA found in mature muscle is accumulated postnatally, and the accretion of DNA in muscle is a key factor in regulating muscle growth.

The idea that muscle fiber number is constant beyond the neonatal period had been accepted for years, as had the notion that nuclei within muscle fibers do not replicate their DNA or divide. However, these observations were clearly inconsistent with the large increases in DNA occurring in postnatal muscle. This is explained by the role of satellite cells, the small mononucleated cells that reside between the sarcolemma and basement membrane of muscle fibers (Mauro, 1961). These cells have the ability to proliferate, differentiate, and fuse into adjacent fibers (Moss and Leblond, 1971), which results in the addition of the satellite cell nucleus to the muscle fiber.

Satellite cells are only discernible at the electron microscope level because they look like normal myonuclei that are located adjacent to the sarcolemma inside the fiber. Satellite cells are evenly distributed across the surface of muscle fibers, except for an increased density around the neuromuscular junction (Gibson and Schultz, 1983; Kelly, 1978a). In normal adult muscle from many species, the cells generally make up only a small fraction of the total nuclei associated with fibers, usually ranging from

2 percent to less than 10 percent (Allbrook et al., 1971; Cardasis and Cooper, 1975; Schultz, 1974; Snow, 1977) and varying from one type of fiber and muscle to another; slow-twitch fibers often have a higher percentage of satellite cells than do fast-twitch fibers (Gibson and Schultz, 1983; Kelly, 1978b). Also, there seems to be a greater percentage present in muscles of very young animals and a smaller percentage in muscles of old animals; this is particularly evident in fast-twitch muscle fibers (Gibson and Schultz, 1983).

The myogenic potential of satellite cells and their ability to synthesize DNA, divide, and fuse into existing fibers was established by Moss and Leblond (1971). Their myogenic properties were further documented by isolating mononucleated cells from minced muscle digests (Bischoff, 1974) or by isolating individual muscle fibers (Bischoff, 1975; Konigsberg et al., 1975) and monitoring the division of mononucleated cells in culture. Not only did these mononucleated cells divide but they eventually fused to form multinucleated myotubes. Myotubes formed by satellite cells in vitro synthesize muscle-specific proteins and spontaneously contract in culture (Allen et al., 1980; Cossu et al., 1980).

Although qualitatively they resemble embryonic myogenic cells, satellite cells may well be a separate type of myogenic cell. Cossu et al. (1980) first noted major differences in the morphology of the two, and Allen et al. (1982) found that myotubes derived from satellite cells were only able to synthesize one-third to one-half as much alpha-actin as myotubes formed from neonatal rat muscle. Cossu et al. (1983, 1985) also demonstrated that satellite cells and embryonic myogenic cells responded differently to a tumor promoter, 12-O-tetradecanoylphorbol-13-acetate (TPA). TPA did not stimulate division or inhibit differentiation of satellite cells, as it did with myogenic cells of embryonic origin. Therefore, factors that stimulate the proliferation or differentiation of embryonic myogenic cells may or may not have the same effect on satellite cells.

Even though the importance of satellite cells to muscle regeneration and normal growth has been appreciated for some time, details of their regulation are only now beginning to emerge. The stimulatory effect of five different growth factors and hormones and the inhibitory effect of one growth factor on satellite cell proliferation have been documented in vitro (Allen, 1986; Allen et al., 1984; Dodson et al., 1985). Three of these proteins are insulin-like growth factors I and II (IGF-I and IGF-II) and insulin (Dodson et al., 1985). These proteins are members of the same gene family and share high degrees of sequence homology (Klapper et al., 1983; Marquardt and Todaro, 1981; Rinderknecht and Humbel, 1978). Insulin is active only at supraphysiological concentrations, which has been explained in terms of its action as an IGF-I analog. Both IGFs (commonly referred to as somatomedins) stimulate satellite cell proliferation at concentrations well within the physiological range. The significance of the IGFs—particularly IGF-I—lies in their relationship to growth hormone. IGF-I mediates the growth hormone signal at the target cell level. Consequently, in vitro data directly link the action of the IGFs to an authentic target cell in postnatal skeletal muscle.

Two additional growth factors active in promoting satellite cell proliferation are the basic (Allen et al., 1984) and acidic (R. E. Allen, University of Arizona, unpublished data) forms of fibroblast growth factor. Unlike the IGFs, however, the basic form of FGF only stimulates proliferation and actually inhibits differentiation. Unfortunately, the physiological role of FGFs or similar proteins has not been established. FGFs have been isolated from a variety of cells and tissues; brain and pituitary tissue are the two most commonly used sources for purification (Gospodarowicz et al., 1976).

It is particularly noteworthy that similar protein fractions have been isolated from skeletal muscle (Kardami et al., 1985) and from peritoneal macrophages (Baird et al., 1985). The observations that this growth factor is not freely circulating but can be found in a variety of cells and tissues make it a reasonable candidate for an autocrine or paracrine hormone. This concept may have particular importance in regulation of skeletal muscle regeneration and work-induced hypertrophy, where a local signaling mechanism would seem to be necessary. Insights into the molecular mechanisms of FGF action are sparse, although receptors have been identified (Olwin and Hauschka, 1986). The possible role of FGF or FGF-like proteins as local signals for myogenic cell proliferation is an interesting concept that should be addressed.

Satellite cell culture systems have also been used to evaluate the response of satellite cells to growth hormone, prolactin, luteinizing hormone, thyroid stimulating hormone, epidermal growth factor, platelet-derived growth factor, and nerve growth factor. None of these proteins had the ability to stimulate satellite cell growth in vitro (Allen et al., 1986).

As mentioned previously, an inhibitor of satellite cell proliferation and differentiation has been identified: transforming growth factor beta (TGF-β). In vitro, very low concentrations of TGF-β (≤0.5 ng/ml) can affect both processes (Allen, 1986). This factor is interesting because it can be found in many cell types and has a variety of effects on their functions. It can be either stimulatory or inhibitory, depending on cell type and the presence of other growth factors (Moses et al., 1985). TGF-β apparently is identical to the differentiation inhibitor described by Evinger-Hodges et al. (1982) and Florini et al. (1986).

In summary, it appears that satellite cell activity can be controlled by several protein hormones/growth factors, and it may be the interplay of these factors that determines the state of the cell (quiescence, proliferation, or differentiation). Nutritional and environmental factors that influence muscle fiber DNA accretion in postnatal muscle may be mediated through one or more of these proteins.

## MUSCLE FIBER PROTEIN METABOLISM

Muscle protein metabolism encompasses a broad range of cellular activities, many of which are integral parts of energy metabolism in the whole animal. Most notable among these biochemical processes are the deamination of amino acids and the utilization of the carbon skeletons for energy production; supplying amino acids to the liver for gluconeogenesis is another important function. These aspects of muscle protein metabolism are obviously critical to the physiology of the animal, but they are not necessarily directly related to muscle growth. Consequently, this discussion dwells on two broad growth-related processes in muscle: protein synthesis and protein degradation. The quantitative balance between these two activities determines the net accumulation of protein in muscle.

A fundamental concept that has been widely appreciated only within the past decade or so is the fact that muscle protein is in a constant state of flux. Protein is constantly being degraded. It would not be out of the ordinary, for example, to experience a 5 to 10 percent rate of degradation of protein per day. To maintain muscle mass, the muscle would have to synthesize an amount of protein equivalent to 5 to 10 percent of its protein content on a daily basis. The ramifications of this are enormous when one considers the energetic costs of synthesizing one peptide bond and the total number of peptide bonds that must be degraded and resynthesized per day. It is easy to understand why protein turnover represents a significant factor in the "maintenance" energy requirements of an animal.

It is also easy to see how the efficiency of growth or production could be enhanced if protein turnover could be altered in a favorable way.

A number of studies have demonstrated the balance between protein synthesis and degradation in domestic animals, laboratory animals, and humans and have revealed a general trend: In growing animals, synthesis and degradation rates are elevated with synthesis rate exceeding degradation rate; as maturity is approached, both synthesis and degradation rates decrease and ultimately reach a low and equal rate. With only minor variations, these trends have been observed in cattle, chickens, and laboratory animals (Lewis et al., 1984; MacDonald and Swick, 1981; McCarthy et al., 1983; Millward and Waterlow, 1978; Millward et al., 1976).

Certain metabolic hormones influence protein turnover; glucocorticoids, for example, cause muscle atrophy by depressing synthesis and degradation (McGrath and Goldspink, 1982). Synthesis rate is apparently depressed to a greater extent than degradation rate. Insulin, on the other hand, causes net accretion of protein, primarily by affecting synthesis rate (Tischler, 1981), and generally antagonizes the glucocorticoid effect on synthesis and degradation (Tomas et al., 1984). Thyroid hormone, T3, can increase degradation rate, but this modulation tends to follow the rate of synthesis (Millward, 1985), so there is a minimal change in protein accretion. Metabolites such as branched-chain amino acids or the keto acids of these amino acids may also be involved in depressing degradation (Mitch and Clark, 1984; Tischler et al., 1982). The integrated response of muscle to the interplay of metabolites and metabolic hormones is not completely understood but represents an important feature of muscle protein accretion regulation.

In addition to the homeostatic regulation of protein turnover, relative rates of synthesis and degradation are altered during growth. Thus far, the only growth-related hormones that have been implicated in regulating protein degradation are the insulin-like growth factors, the somatomedins. Most of the work in this area has been conducted in vitro, where potent inhibitory effects have been observed (Ballard et al., 1986; Janeczko and Etlinger, 1984). The involvement is somewhat perplexing, since rapid growth rates in young animals are accompanied by increased rates of degradation, not decreased degradation. This point of contention, however, may be related to the in vitro assay system; the key element in the observation may be the decrease in degradation rate relative to synthesis rate.

Several physiological conditions have been shown to affect the rates of synthesis and degradation in skeletal muscle. Included among these are physical influences such as muscle stretching, which leads to hypertrophy (Goldspink, 1978; Summers et al., 1985). In vitro muscle stretching decreases protein degradation (Baracos and Goldberg, 1985). Inflammation, fever, and burns also have a dramatic effect by accelerating protein turnover (Goldberg et al., 1984); the common denominator in these observations and in the stretch-induced alteration in turnover may be calcium metabolism. In vitro, an influx of calcium into cells increases protein degradation (Silver and Etlinger, 1985). Furthermore, the calcium-induced elevation in degradation is of nonlysosomal origin (Furuno and Goldberg, 1986), as evidenced by the failure of lysosomal protease inhibitors to inhibit this calcium-induced response.

At present, an inadequate mechanistic understanding of the biochemical details of protein synthesis and degradation—especially degradation—is blocking progress in research on the regulation of these processes. Nutritional/physiological experimentation has provided an important descriptive base, but future progress depends on cellular and molecular details. As mentioned previously, new information on the regulation of myofibrillar protein isoform tran-

sitions and the structure and regulation of genes encoding these proteins will have a dramatic impact on our view of muscle protein synthesis regulation. Molecular details of the interaction of key hormones or their second messengers with myofibrillar protein genes should be forthcoming within the next decade.

It is traditionally assumed that lysosomal enzymes are responsible for intracellular protein degradation. These proteases are contained in lysosomes and are active at acidic pH. Several different proteases are grouped in this class and called cathepsins. Not all cathepsins are able to cleave peptide bonds in myofibrillar proteins; only cathepsins $B_1$, D, H, and L have been found in muscle and are active on myofibrillar protein substrates (see Goll et al., 1983). A problem with attributing myofibrillar protein degradation in skeletal muscle to catheptic proteases is the fact that myofibrils or myofilaments have not been observed in lysosomal structures in muscle. Nor have lysosome-like organelles been observed in association with myofibrils. In addition, treatment of cells with lysosomal enzyme inhibitors failed to suppress calcium-induced protein degradation (Furuno and Goldberg, 1986). Although it has been possible in some cases to show correlations between lysosomal enzyme activity and protein degradation, the cause-and-effect relationship has not been proved.

A more likely mechanism for explaining myofibrillar protein degradation begins with the action of nonlysosomal cytoplasmic proteases that selectively cleave certain myofibrillar proteins, resulting in the disassembly of filaments in the myofibril (Dayton et al., 1975). Individual myofibrillar proteins or fragments of these proteins can then be taken up by lysosomes and degraded to individual amino acids. If such a scheme is accurate, one of the rate-limiting steps in the process would be the initial degradation steps accomplished by nonlysosomal proteases. Recent evidence suggests that activation of calcium-induced and injury-induced protein degradation in muscle does not involve a lysosomal mechanism (Furuno and Goldberg, 1986).

A couple of strong candidates have been suggested for this degradation role, the first of which is the calcium-dependent neutral protease described by Dayton et al. (1976). This protease, with a molecular weight of 110,000 daltons, is located inside skeletal muscle cells, as well as many other cell types, and is active at neutral pH. In skeletal muscle cells, it is found in the sarcoplasm and not in lysosomal structures or other intracellular membrane-bound organelles. The specificity of this protease is somewhat limited in that it generally cleaves only one or a few peptide bonds in a protein. In the myofibril, the proteins affected are troponin-T, troponin-I, tropomyosin, C-protein, filamin, desmin, the Z-line structure, and possibly titin (Goll et al., 1983). Many of these proteins have regulatory and structural significance. Note, however, that the primary proteins in the myofibril—actin and myosin—are apparently not hydrolyzed by this protease.

Although the regulatory details of this protease have not been elucidated, it is clear that calcium ions and a free sulfhydryl group are required for activity. It is also accepted that two forms of the protease exist, one that requires millimolar concentrations of calcium and another that only requires micromolar concentrations for activity. These are distinctly different proteins that share a high degree of sequence homology. The active sites of these proteins are similar to those of papain, and the calcium-binding regions are similar to those of calmodulin (Emori et al., 1986). To add to the complexity of the system, an inhibitor of these proteases is also found in skeletal muscle. The physiological regulation of these different forms of the enzyme and inhibitor is not clear, but it may be crucial to an understanding of protein degradation and turnover.

Other soluble proteases may also be important components of the myofibril degradation process. Several alkaline or neutral proteases have the ability to hydrolyze actin or myosin, but most of these are not found in muscle cells. Perhaps the degradative system understood in greatest detail is an ATP-dependent protease system (Hershko and Ciechanover, 1982), which is found in many cells but has been most extensively studied in reticulocytes. This system is composed of a small, heat-stable protein called ubiquitin (because of its presence in a highly conserved form in most cells) that interacts with an activating enzyme in an ATP-dependent process to ultimately form a covalent isopeptide bond between the carboxyl group of the C-terminal glycine residue of ubiquitin and an epsilon amino group of a lysine on the target protein. The covalent attachment of ubiquitin is thought to target the protein for protease attack. The proteases responsible are ill-defined, but the end products are peptides and a released ubiquitin that can recycle. This system could be responsible for identifying proteins that were damaged structurally or otherwise inactivated. Other protease systems requiring ATP may also be present in cells, but their characterization is far from complete. The primary problems with proposed roles for these ATP-dependent proteolytic systems in muscle protein degradation are the lack of detailed information about the specificity of these systems for muscle proteins and the presence and location of these systems in muscle cells.

During normal growth and in many metabolic states, rates of synthesis and degradation tend to move in tandem. Even during fasting, degradation is depressed and not increased, presumably to spare protein. These observations suggest that during normal growth, protein synthesis may represent the primary site of regulation, and degradation may follow (Millward, 1985). It is virtually impossible to tie together endocrine and nutritional influences on animal protein degradation and the subcellular events that mediate these effects because of the present gap that exists between our knowledge of the cellular and biochemical mechanisms involved in skeletal muscle protein degradation and the whole animal and tissue level descriptions of the process. This does not eliminate the possibility of targeting degradation as a site for muscle growth regulation, but it makes it difficult to devise strategies to manipulate protein degradation to enhance the efficiency of muscle growth in meat animals.

## STRATEGIES FOR REGULATING MUSCLE DEVELOPMENT AND GROWTH IN MEAT-PRODUCING ANIMALS

Significant research areas that can be layered over the muscle-specific problem are the integration of metabolism during growth and the manner in which tissue growth is coordinated within the animal. These topics are more general and, at face value, more pertinent to altering efficiency of protein accretion and the composition of the product than are the studies of specific cellular and biochemical events in developing and growing muscle. But progress in these areas can only proceed as rapidly as progress toward a mechanistic understanding of muscle growth.

Establishing muscle cellularity, in its broadest sense, involves prenatal fiber development and nuclear accretion during postnatal growth. Fiber development is the result of myogenesis that takes place in the developing embryo or fetus. The final event in this cascade of proliferation and differentiation is the fusion of myoblasts into multinucleated myotubes that mature into fibers. Currently, hormones and growth factors that stimulate and inhibit the proliferative and differentiative events in myogenic cells are being identified, but the factors that regulate the number of fibers that are formed from a given cohort of myoblasts have not been considered experimentally. It may be that innervation plays a key role in establishing fiber number and

organization in muscle, since innervation is required to sustain fibers. For many years, it has been accepted that major differences in muscle mass in mature animals can be attributed in large part to differences in fiber number. Consequently, alterations in fiber number during late prenatal life would likely result in differences in muscularity. At present, however, there is probably insufficient mechanistic detail to suggest specific approaches. A critical question in this regard is whether it is advisable to increase muscularity prenatally; in cattle, for example, increased management problems associated with dystocia could offset any advantages due to increased muscle growth potential. In swine or poultry, this problem may not be so acute.

Cellularity could conceivably be altered by nuclear accretion postnatally without reproductive problems. Again, we are beginning to understand more about the activation, proliferation, and differentiation of satellite cells, although specific physiological regulators have not yet been confirmed. Assuming that satellite cell activity could be altered and nuclear accretion in fibers could be influenced, satellite cells may be more receptive to manipulation efforts during certain periods of growth than others. Early postnatal growth is the time of greatest satellite cell activity and would correspond to the period of greatest sensitivity to hormones and growth factors. On the other hand, later phases of growth are marked by decreasing nuclear accretion rate; therefore, stimulating additional satellite cell proliferation and differentiation could result in an extension of the rapid muscle growth phase that is normally associated with muscle growth in younger animals.

Affecting changes in muscle growth by altering protein metabolism has been the most commonly considered avenue, primarily because of the erroneous assumption that cellularity does not change after birth. During normal growth, synthesis and degradation tend to move in parallel, with synthesis rate exceeding degradation rate. Consequently, accelerated growth rate is accompanied by an accelerated degradation rate; hence, there is no increase in efficiency of protein accretion. Because these processes seem to be coupled, Millward (1985) suggested that manipulating synthesis may be the most reasonable way to affect protein accretion. Specific alterations in synthesis await increased knowledge of the mechanisms of muscle protein gene regulation and the elucidation of hormones or other external signals, such as electrical stimulation or stretch, that modulate the expression of these genes.

Likewise, strategies for manipulating degradation rate in muscle will not progress beyond the empirical stage without a mechanistic understanding of the proteases involved and their regulation. Protein degradation is, however, an attractive target for postnatal growth manipulation. If degradation rate could be decreased, net rate of protein accretion would be accelerated and less energy would be expended on resynthesizing degraded protein.

To illustrate that the present level of cellular and molecular understanding of important regulatory events is grossly inadequate and, indeed, limiting, consider some current growth-manipulating techniques. Take three growth-altering treatments: growth hormone (GH), steroid hormones and their analogs, and beta-adrenergic agonists. With all three, scientists are still dependent on information that is often one or two decades old, or on empirical observations, the biology of which is still not fully understood. In these cases current biology is not leading the way to new applications; rather, new applications are leading basic biological investigation.

Let us begin with GH. Direct administration of GH to domestic meat animals was first reported in pigs by Truman and Andrews (1955), Henricson and Ullberg (1960), and Machlin (1972). Later, Chung et al. (1985) also reported direct administration of

GH to pigs. Dramatic increases in muscle growth in GH-treated pigs (Etherton et al., 1986) could be the result of action at several sites, such as adipose tissue, where GH could be having an antilipogenic effect. If energy is not stored in adipose tissue, it may be more available for growth. It is also possible that when growth processes are stimulated, they demand more energy than do adipose tissue triglyceride storage activities. GH could also be having part of its effect by stimulating higher levels of somatomedins that are, in turn, stimulating satellite cells. Arguments can be made for increased muscle growth as a result of nuclear accretion and subsequent protein accumulation directed by new nuclei. Another plausible alternative may be somatomedin-mediated depression of muscle protein degradation. Or, the net effect could be due to a combination of the above. The point is that it is application that is leading scientists to undertake basic biological research.

Next consider the steroid hormones and their analogs. Studies that were mostly empirical in nature gave us diethylstilbestrol. Its application has come and gone from agriculture, yet we still do not know its precise mode of action. Even the action of testosterone on muscle growth is unclear. Trenbolone acetate (TBA) is another example—it stimulates growth, but again, the mechanism is unknown. In terms of the biological events responsible for muscle growth, it must either directly or indirectly stimulate nuclear accretion, stimulate protein synthesis, or decrease protein degradation. At least one report suggests that protein synthesis is depressed but that protein degradation is depressed to a greater extent, thus leading to a net increase in rate of protein accretion as well as in efficiency of protein gain (Vernon and Buttery, 1976). This in vivo study was not able to address the direct or indirect nature of the action of TBA. In vitro studies are limited; however, TBA does not appear to have a direct effect on protein degradation in L6 muscle cells in culture (Ballard and Francis, 1983).

Another example of application leading basic investigation concerns a class of agents that has received a great deal of attention in recent years, the beta-adrenergic agonists. One of these—clenbuterol—was originally designed as a respiratory drug but was subsequently shown to have a stimulatory effect on rat growth. Since then, it has been used to stimulate growth and feed efficiency in poultry, sheep, and cattle (Baker et al., 1984; Dalrymple et al., 1984; Ricks et al., 1984). A great deal of effort is currently being devoted to understanding how it works. An obvious site of action would be as a lipolytic agent for adipose tissue; however, this alone could not explain the extreme muscle hypertrophy observed in sheep (Beermann et al., 1986). Recently, Kim et al. (1986) reported that the major effect appeared to be on hypertrophy of fast-twitch muscle fibers and that muscle DNA concentration actually decreased in the cimaterol-treated group. Beermann, however, indicated that a significant increase in DNA content was noted in 12-week studies with sheep but that DNA content increased after muscle hypertrophy (D. H. Beermann, personal communication, 1986). In another report, cimaterol was demonstrated to have an inhibitory effect on protein degradation in cultured myotubes from a rat muscle cell line (Forsberg and Merrill, 1986). Evidently, the beta-adrenergic agonists may have multiple sites of action, especially for protein degradation and adipose tissue metabolism, but this conclusion remains highly speculative.

These examples of a few of the most interesting agents currently being investigated for use in stimulating muscle growth not only demonstrate that application is leading investigation, they also provide striking demonstrations that muscle growth in meat animals can be manipulated to increase protein production and decrease triglyceride deposition beyond the normal physiological limits of a particular animal.

They also suggest that the muscle growth processes mentioned earlier—protein synthesis and degradation and pre- and postnatal muscle cellularity alterations—represent legitimate targets for growth-regulating strategies.

In the future, several approaches may be used to enhance rate and efficiency of muscle growth, but for now the most promising are administration of recombinant hormones. As indicated, recombinant GH has been shown to have impressive stimulatory effects on growth, feed efficiency, and carcass composition in pigs. Other hormones will surely be investigated in a similar manner. Based on recent research in muscle development, somatomedin-C/IGF-I is a logical choice for such application. New growth factors or combinations of growth factors that affect muscle development, such as fibroblast growth factor and IGF-II, are also candidates.

At present, GH administration entails regular injections during later stages in postnatal life. In a second generation of studies, researchers may wish to effect a permanent change in the cellularity of the animal, such as increased fiber number or myonuclei content. In contrast to approaches that are designed primarily to alter protein metabolism, cellular/developmental changes may only require acute treatments during early, critical stages of development. Therefore, the need for costly, labor-intensive administration schemes could be eliminated, as would potential questions about the presence of drug residues in the final product.

At another level of sophistication, transgenic animals may have a place in livestock production systems. Growth has already been accelerated in transgenic mice carrying a metallothionein-human growth hormone fusion gene (Palmiter et al., 1982) and in mice expressing the metallothionein-human growth hormone releasing factor minigene (Hammer et al., 1985). In addition, these genes have been shown to be transmittable to subsequent generations, although reproduction suffered in some of the initial studies (Hammer et al., 1985). These techniques will undoubtedly be applied in large domestic animals to produce new germplasm. Furthermore, it may be possible to construct and perpetuate the genes of important hormones that can be regulated by coupling the genes to promoters that can be turned on or off at critical periods through nutritional, pharmacological, or environmental manipulation. These approaches will obviously require a more detailed description of the significant regulatory events in muscle growth and the important factors that mediate these events so that appropriate molecular targets can be selected.

## CONCLUSIONS

Major obstacles exist. New fundamental knowledge of cellular and molecular mechanisms of growth is desperately needed. Technical advances are also needed in the area of delivery systems for effectively administering exogenous agents at specific times and in appropriate amounts. Of critical importance are practical means for targeting the delivery of agents to specific tissues. It is conceivable that a factor could have a beneficial effect on one tissue or organ and a detrimental effect on another. This may be a major impediment to the application of certain hormones or growth factors. Technical advances are still needed in gene transfer and gene construct technology, but progress is occurring rapidly. These are only a few of the problem areas that need to be addressed.

Advances in the production of nutritious muscle protein foods will probably not come by altering the cellular composition of a muscle fiber. Membrane systems and myofibrillar proteins in muscle are highly conserved and may not be amenable to efforts to inflict gross alterations that would provide a more desirable balance of amino acids or reduced cholesterol content. An approach

to improving the nutritional attributes of meat products that holds greater promise is one that attempts to reduce the amount of adipose tissue associated with meat products while maintaining palatability. Great advances can be made in the efficient production of muscle protein by providing a growing knowledge base in biology, by rapidly adopting new scientific technologies, and by fostering innovative applied research.

## REFERENCES

Allbrook, D. B., M. F. Han, and A. E. Hellmuth. 1971. Population of muscle satellite cells in relation to age and mitotic activity. Pathology 3:233–243.

Allen, R. E. 1986. Transforming growth factor-beta inhibits the IGF-I-induced proliferation and differentiation of skeletal muscle satellite cells. J. Cell Biol. 103(5):120a.

Allen, R. E., R. A. Merkel, and R. B. Young. 1979. Cellular aspects of muscle growth. Myogenic cell proliferation. J. Anim. Sci. 49(1):115–127.

Allen, R. E., P. K. McAllister, and K. C. Masak. 1980. Myogenic potential of satellite cells in skeletal muscle of old rats. Mech. Age. Dev. 13:105–109.

Allen, R. E., P. K. McAllister, K. C. Masak, and G. R. Anderson. 1982. Influence of age on accumulation of α-actin in satellite-cell-derived myotubes in vitro. Mech. Age. Dev. 18:89–95.

Allen, R. E., M. V. Dodson, and L. S. Luiten. 1984. Regulation of skeletal muscle satellite cell proliferation by bovine pituitary fibroblast growth factor. Exp. Cell Res. 152:154–160.

Allen, R. E., M. V. Dodson, L. K. Boxhorn, S. L. Davis, and K. L. Hossner. 1986. Satellite cell proliferation in response to pituitary hormones. J. Anim. Sci. 62:1596–1601.

Ashmore, C. R., D. W. Robinson, P. Rattray, and L. Doerr. 1972. Biphasic development of muscle fibers in the fetal lamb. Exp. Neurol. 37(2):241–255.

Bains, W., P. Ponte, H. Blau, and L. Kedes. 1984. Cardiac actin is the major actin gene product in skeletal muscle cell differentiation in vitro. Mol. Cell. Biol. 4:1449–1453.

Baird, A., P. Mormede, and P. Böhlen. 1985. Immunoreactive fibroblast growth factor in cells of peritoneal exudate suggests its identity with macrophage-derived growth factor. Biochem. Biophys. Res. Commun. 126:358–364.

Baker, P. K., R. H. Dalrymple, D. L. Ingle, and C. A. Ricks. 1984. Use of a β-adrenergic agonist to alter muscle and fat deposition in lambs. J. Anim. Sci. 59:1256–1261.

Ballard, F. J., and G. L. Francis. 1983. Effects of

anabolic agents on protein breakdown in L6 myoblasts. Biochem. J. 210:243–249.

Ballard, F. J., L. C. Read, G. L. Francis, C. J. Bagley, and J. C. Wallace. 1986. Binding properties and biological potencies of insulin-like growth factors in L6 myoblasts. Biochem. J. 233:223–230.

Bandman, E., R. Matsuda, and R. C. Strohman. 1982. Developmental appearance of myosin heavy and light chain isoforms in vivo and in vitro in chicken skeletal muscle. Dev. Biol. 93:508–518.

Baracos, V. E., and A. L. Goldberg. 1985. $Ca^{2+}$, interleukin-1 and failure to maintain normal length stimulate protein degradation in isolated skeletal muscle. Pp. 603–605 in Intracellular Protein Catabolism, E. A. Khaviallah, J. S. Bond, and J. W. C. Bird (eds.). New York: Alan R. Liss.

Beermann, D. H., D. E. Hogue, V. K. Fishell, R. H. Dalrymple, and C. A. Ricks. 1986. Effects of cimaterol and fishmeal on performance, carcass characteristics and skeletal muscle growth in lambs. J. Anim. Sci. 62:370–380.

Bergsma, D. J., J. M. Grichnik, L. M. A. Gossett, and R. J. Schwartz. 1986. Delimitation and characterization of cis-acting DNA sequences required for the regulated expression and transcriptional control of the chicken skeletal α-actin gene. Mol. Cell. Biol. 6:2462–2475.

Bischoff, R. 1974. Enzymatic liberation of myogenic cells from adult rat muscle. Anat. Rec. 180:645–662.

Bischoff, R. 1975. Regeneration of single skeletal muscle fibers in vitro. Anat. Rec. 182:215–236.

Bonner, P. H., and T. R. Adams. 1982. Neural induction of chick myoblast differentiation in culture. Dev. Biol. 90:175–184.

Brevet, A., E. Pinto, J. Peacock, and F. E. Stockdale. 1976. Myosin synthesis increased by electrical stimulation of skeletal muscle cell cultures. Science 193:1152–1154.

Buckley, P. A., and I. R. Konigsberg. 1974. Myogenic fusion and the duration of the post-mitotic gap ($G_1$). Dev. Biol. 37:193–212.

Butler-Brown, G. S., G. S. Cambon, C. Laurent, G. Prulier, M. Toutant, S. Watkins, and R. G. Whalen. 1986. Control of myosin isoenzyme transitions by thyroid hormone in the dwarf mouse strain. J. Physiol. 377:93.

Caplan, A. I., M. Y. Fiszman, and H. M. Eppenberger. 1983. Molecular and cell isoforms during development. Science 221:921–927.

Cardasis, C. A., and G. W. Cooper. 1975. An analysis of nuclear numbers in individual muscle fibers during differentiation and growth. A satellite cell-muscle fiber growth unit. J. Exp. Zool. 191(3):347–358.

Chiu, C. P., and H. M. Blau. 1984. Reprogramming cell differentiation in the absence of DNA synthesis. Cell 37:879–887.

Chung, C. S., T. D. Etherton, and J. P. Wiggins.

1985. Stimulation of swine growth by porcine growth hormone. J. Anim. Sci. 60(1):118–130.

Cossu, G., B. Zani, M. Colletta, M. Bouche, M. Pacifici, and M. Molinaro. 1980. In vitro differentiation of satellite cells isolated from normal and dystrophic mammalian muscles. A comparison with embryonic myogenic cells. Cell Differ. 9:357–368.

Cossu, G., M. Molinaro, and M. Pacifici. 1983. Differential response of satellite cells and embryonic myoblasts to a tumor promoter. Dev. Biol. 98:520–524.

Cossu, G., P. Cicinelli, C. Fieri, M. Coletta, and M. Monlinaro. 1985. Emergence of TPA-resistant 'Satellite' cells during muscle histogenesis of human limb. Exp. Cell Res. 160:403–411.

Crow, M. T., P. S. Olson, and F. E. Stockdale. 1983. Myosin light-chain expression during avian muscle development. J. Cell Biol. 96:736–744.

Dalrymple, R. H., C. A. Ricks, P. K. Baker, J. M. Pensak, P. E. Gingher, and D. L. Ingle. 1984. Use of the beta-agonist clenbuterol to alter carcass composition in poultry. Poultry Sci. 63:2376–2383.

Dayton, W. R., D. E. Goll, M. H. Stromer, W. J. Reville, M. G. Zeece, and R. M. Robson. 1975. Some properties of a $Ca^{++}$-activated protease that may be involved in myofibrillar protein turnover. Pp. 551–577 in Proteases and Biological Control, E. Reich, D. B. Rifkin, and E. Shaw (eds.). Cold Spring Harbor, N.Y.: Cold Spring Harbor Laboratory.

Dayton, W. R., D. E. Goll, M. G. Zeece, R. M. Robson, and W. J. Reville. 1976. A $Ca^{2+}$-activated protease possibly involved in myofibrillar protein turnover. Purification from porcine muscle. Biochemistry 15:2150–2158.

Devlin, R. B., and C. P. Emerson, Jr. 1978. Coordinate regulation of contractile protein synthesis during myoblast differentiation. Cell 13:599–611.

Devlin, R. B., and C. P. Emerson, Jr. 1979. Coordinate accumulation of contractile protein mRNAs during myoblast differentiation. Dev. Biol. 69:202–216.

Devlin, B. H., and I. R. Konigsberg. 1983. Reentry into the cell cycle of differentiated skeletal myocytes. Dev. Biol. 95:175–192.

Dodson, M. V., R. E. Allen, and K. L. Hossner. 1985. Ovine somatomedin, multiplication-stimulating activity, and insulin promote skeletal muscle satellite cell proliferation in vitro. Endocrinology 117:2357–2363.

Eichhorn, J. M., L. J. Coleman, E. J. Wakayama, G. J. Blomquist, D. M. Bailey, and T. G. Jenkins. 1986. Effects of breed type and restricted versus ad libitum feeding on fatty acid composition and cholesterol content of muscle and adipose tissue from mature bovine females. J. Anim. Sci. 63:781–794.

Emori, Y., H. Kawasaki, H. Sugihara, S. Imajoh, S. Kawashima, and K. Suzuki. 1986. Isolation and sequence analyses of cDNA clones for the large subunits of two isozymes of rabbit calcium-dependent protease. J. Biol. Chem. 261:9465–9471.

Etherton, T. D., C. M. Evock, C. S. Chung, P. E. Walton, M. N. Sillence, K. A. Magri, and R. E. Ivy. 1986. Stimulation of pig growth performance by long-term treatment with pituitary porcine growth hormone (pGH) and a recombinant pGH. J. Anim. Sci. 63:219 (Abstr.).

Evinger-Hodges, M. J., D. Z. Ewton, S. C. Seifert, and J. R. Florini. 1982. Inhibition of myoblast differentiation in vitro by a protein isolated from liver cell medium. J. Cell Biol. 93:395–401.

Ewton, D. Z., and J. R. Florini. 1980. Relative effects of the somatomedins, multiplication-stimulating activity, and growth hormone on myoblasts and myotubes in culture. Endocrinology 106:577–583.

Ewton, D. Z., and J. R. Florini. 1981. Effects of the somatomedins and insulin on myoblast differentiation in vitro. Dev. Biol. 86:31–39.

Florini, J. R., A. B. Roberts, D. Z. Ewton, S. L. Falen, K. C. Flanders, and M. B. Sporn. 1986. Transforming growth factor-β. A very potent inhibitor of myoblast differentiation, identical to the differentiation inhibitor secreted by buffalo rat liver cells. J. Biol. Chem. 261:16509–16513.

Forsberg, N. E., and G. Merrill. 1986. Effects of cimaterol on protein synthesis and degradation in monolayer culture of rat and mouse myoblasts. J. Anim. Sci. 63:222 (Abstr.).

Furuno, K., and A. L. Goldberg. 1986. The activation of protein degradation in muscle by $Ca^{2+}$ or muscle injury does not involve a lysosomal mechanism. Biochem. J. 237:859–864.

Gambke, B., and N. A. Rubinstein. 1984. A monoclonal antibody to the embryonic myosin heavy chain of rat skeletal muscle. J. Biol. Chem. 259:12092–12100.

Gauthier, G. F., S. Lowey, P. A. Benfield, and A. W. Hobbs. 1982. Distribution and properties of myosin isozymes in developing avian and mammalian skeletal muscle fibers. J. Cell Biol. 92:471–484.

Gibson, M. C., and E. Schultz. 1983. Age-related differences in absolute numbers of skeletal muscle satellite cells. Muscle Nerve 6:574–580.

Goldberg, A. L., V. Baracos, P. Rodemann, L. Warman, and C. Dinarello. 1984. Control of protein degradation in muscle by prostaglandins, $Ca^{2+}$, and leukocytic pyrogen (interleukin 1). Proc. Fed. Am. Soc. Exp. Biol. 43:1301–1306.

Goldspink, G. 1972. Postembryonic growth and differentiation of striated muscle. P. 179 in The Structure and Function of Muscle, Vol. 1, 2nd Ed., G. H. Bourne (ed.). New York: Academic Press.

Goldspink, D. F. 1978. The influence of passive stretch on the growth and protein turnover of the denervated extensor digitorum longus muscle. Biochem. J. 174:595–602.

Goll, D. E., Y. Otsuka, P. A. Nagainis, J. D. Shannon, S. K. Sathe, and M. Muguruma. 1983. Role of muscle proteinases in maintenance of muscle integrity and mass. J. Food Biochem. 7:137–177.

Goll, D. E., R. M. Robson, and M. H. Stromer. 1984. Skeletal muscle, nervous system, temperature regulation, and special senses. Pp. 548–580 in Dukes' Physiology of Domestic Animals, 10th Ed., M. J. Swenson (ed.). Ithaca, N.Y.: Cornell University Press.

Gospodarowicz, D., J. Weseman, J. S. Moran, and J. Lindstrom. 1976. Effect of fibroblast growth factor on the division and fusion of bovine myoblasts. J. Cell Biol. 70:395–405.

Hammer, R. E., R. L. Brinster, and R. D. Palmiter. 1985. Use of gene transfer to increase animal growth. Cold Spring Harbor Symp. Quant. Biol. 50:379–387.

Harbison, S. A., D. E. Goll, F. C. Parrish, V. Wang, and E. A. Kline. 1976. Muscle growth in two genetically different lines of swine. Growth 40:253–283.

Hauschka, S. D. 1974. Clonal analysis of vertebrate myogenesis. III. Developmental changes in the muscle-colony-forming cells of the human fetal limb. Dev. Biol. 37:345–368.

Henricson, B., and S. Ullberg. 1960. Effects of pig growth hormone on pigs. J. Anim. Sci. 19:1002.

Hershko, A., and A. Ciechanover. 1982. Mechanisms of intracellular protein breakdown. Annu. Rev. Biochem. 51:335–364.

Hoffman, R. K., B. Gambke, L. W. Stephenson, and N. A. Rubinstein. 1985. Myosin transitions in chronic stimulation do not involve embryonic isozymes. Muscle Nerve 8:796–805.

Holtzer, H., and R. Bischoff. 1970. Mitosis and myogenesis. Pp. 29–51 in Physiology and Biochemistry of Muscle as a Food, Vol. 2, E. J. Briskey, R. G. Cassens, and B. B. Marsh (eds.). Madison: University of Wisconsin Press.

Hu, M. C. T., S. B. Sharp, and N. Davidson. 1986. The complete sequence of the mouse skeletal α-actin gene reveals several conserved and inverted repeat sequences outside of the protein-coding region. Mol. Cell. Biol. 6:15–25.

Izumo, S., B. Nadal-Ginard, and V. Mahdavi. 1986. All members of the MHC multigene family respond to thyroid hormone in a highly tissue-specific manner. Science 231:597–600.

Janeczko, R. A., and J. D. Etlinger. 1984. Inhibition of intracellular proteolysis in muscle cultures by multiplication-stimulating activity. Comparison of effects of multiplication-stimulating activity and insulin on proteolysis, protein synthesis, amino acid uptake, and sugar transport. J. Biol. Chem. 259:6292–6297.

Kardami, E., D. Spector, and R. C. Strohman. 1985. Myogenic growth factor present in skeletal muscle is purified by heparin-affinity chromatography. Proc. Natl. Acad. Sci. USA 82:8044–8047.

Kelly, A. M. 1978a. Perisynaptic satellite cells in the developing and mature rat soleus muscle. Anat. Rec. 190:891–904.

Kelly, A. M. 1978b. Satellite cells and myofiber growth in the rat soleus and extensor digitorum longus muscles. Dev. Biol. 65:1–10.

Kelly, A. M., and S. I. Zacks. 1969. The histogenesis of rat intercostal muscle. J. Cell Biol. 42:135–153.

Kim, Y. S., Y. B. Lee, C. R. Ashmore, and R. H. Dalrymple. 1986. Effect of the repartitioning agent, cimaterol (CL 263,780), on growth, carcass characteristics and skeletal muscle cellularity of lambs. J. Anim. Sci. 63:221 (Abstr.).

Klapper, D. G., M. E. Svoboda, and J. J. Van Wyk. 1983. Sequence analysis of somatomedin-C. Confirmation of identity with insulin-like growth factor I. Endocrinology 112:2215–2217.

Konigsberg, U. R., B. H. Lipton, and I. R. Konigsberg. 1975. The regenerative response of single mature muscle fibers. Dev. Biol. 45:260–275.

Lewis, S. E. M., F. J. Kelly, and D. F. Goldspink. 1984. Pre- and post-natal growth and protein turnover in smooth muscle, heart and slow- and fast-twitch skeletal muscles of the rat. Biochem. J. 217:517–526.

Linkhart, T. A., C. H. Clegg, and S. D. Hauschka. 1981. Myogenic differentiation in permanent clonal mouse myoblast cell lines: Regulation by macromolecular growth factors in the culture medium. Dev. Biol. 86:19–30.

Lowey, S., P. A. Benfield, D. D. LeBlanc, and G. S. Waller. 1983. Myosin isozymes in avian skeletal muscles. I. Sequential expression of myosin isozymes in developing chicken pectoralis muscles. J. Mus. Res. Cell Motil. 4:695–716.

Lyons, G. E., J. Haselgrove, A. M. Kelly, and N. A. Rubinstein. 1983. Myosin transitions in developing fast and slow muscles of the rat hindlimb. Differentiation 25:168–175.

MacDonald, M. L., and R. W. Swick. 1981. The effect of protein depletion and repletion on muscle-protein turnover in the chick. Biochem. J. 194:811–819.

Machlin, L. J. 1972. Effect of porcine growth hormone on growth and carcass composition of the pig. J. Anim. Sci. 35(4):794.

Marechal, G., K. Schwartz, G. Beckers-Bleukx, and E. Ghins. 1984. Isozymes of myosin in growing and regenerating rat muscles. Eur. J. Biochem. 138:421–428.

Marquardt, H., and G. J. Todaro. 1981. Purification and primary structure of a polypeptide with multiplication-stimulating activity from rat liver cell cultures. Homology with human insulin-like growth factor II. J. Biol. Chem. 256:6859–6865.

Mauro, A. 1961. Satellite cell of skeletal muscle fibers. J. Biophys. Biochem. Cytol. 9:493–495.

McCarthy, F. D., W. G. Bergen, and D. R. Hawkins. 1983. Muscle protein turnover in cattle of differing genetic backgrounds as measured by urinary Nτ-methylhistidine excretion. J. Nutr. 113:2455–2463.

McGrath, J. A., and D. F. Goldspink. 1982. Glucocorticoid action on protein synthesis and protein breakdown in isolated skeletal muscles. Biochem. J. 206:641–645.

McLennan, I. S. 1983. Neural dependence and independence of myotube production in chicken hindlimb muscles. Dev. Biol. 98:287–294.

Melloul, D., B. Aloni, J. Calvo, D. Yaffe, and U. Nudel. 1984. Developmentally regulated expression of chimeric genes containing muscle actin DNA sequences in transfected myogenic cells. Eur. Mol. Biol. Org. J. 3:983–990.

Miller, J. B., and F. E. Stockdale. 1986. Developmental origins of skeletal muscle fibers. Clonal analysis of myogenic cell lineages based on expression of fast and slow myosin heavy chains. Proc. Natl. Acad. Sci. USA 83:3860–3864.

Millward, D. J. 1985. The physiological regulation of proteolysis in muscle. Biochem. Soc. Trans. 13:1023–1026.

Millward, D. J., and J. C. Waterlow. 1978. Effect of nutrition on protein turnover in skeletal muscle. Fed. Proc. 37:2283–2290.

Millward, D. J., P. J. Garlick, D. O. Nnanyelugo, and J. C. Waterlow. 1976. The relative importance of muscle protein synthesis and breakdown in the regulation of muscle mass. Biochem. J. 156:185–188.

Mitch, W. E., and A. S. Clark. 1984. Specificity of the effects of leucine and its metabolites on protein degradation in skeletal muscle. Biochem. J. 222:579–586.

Moses, H. L., R. F. Tucker, E. B. Leof, R. J. Coffey, Jr., J. Halper, and G. D. Shipley. 1985. Type-β transforming growth factor is a growth stimulator and a growth inhibitor. Pp. 65–71 in Cancer Cells 3/Growth Factors and Transformation, J. Feramisco, B. Ozanne, and C. Stiles (eds.). Cold Spring Harbor, N.Y.: Cold Spring Harbor Laboratory.

Moss, F. P. 1968. The relationship between the dimensions of the fibres and the number of nuclei during normal growth of skeletal muscle in the domestic fowl. Am. J. Anat. 122:555–564.

Moss, F. P., and C. P. Leblond. 1971. Satellite cells as the source of nuclei in muscles of growing rats. Anat. Rec. 170:421–436.

Nadal-Ginard, B. 1978. Commitment, fusion and biochemical differentiation of a myogenic cell line in the absence of DNA synthesis. Cell 15:855–864.

Nadal-Ginard, B., H. T. Nguyen, and V. Mahdavi. 1984. Induction of muscle-specific genes in the absence of commitment is reversible. Exp. Biol. Med. 9:250–259.

Nguyen, G. T., R. M. Medford, and B. Nadal-Ginard. 1983. Reversibility of muscle differentiation in the absence of commitment. Analysis of a myogenic cell line temperature-sensitive for commitment. Cell 34:281–293.

Olwin, B. B., and S. D. Hauschka. 1986. Identification of the fibroblast growth factor receptor of Swiss 3T3 cells and mouse skeletal muscle myoblasts. Biochemistry 25:3487–3492.

Palmiter, R. D., R. L. Brinster, R. E. Hammer, M. E. Trumbauer, M. G. Rosenfeld, N. C. Birnberg, and R. M. Evans. 1982. Dramatic growth of mice that develop from eggs microinjected with metallothionein-growth hormone fusion genes. Nature 300:611–614.

Paterson, B. M., and J. D. Eldridge. 1984. α-Cardiac actin is the major sarcomeric isoform expressed in embryonic avian skeletal muscle. Science 224:1436–1438.

Peter, J. B., R. J. Barnard, V. R. Edgerton, C. A. Gillespie, and K. E. Stempel. 1972. Metabolic profiles of three fiber types of skeletal muscle in guinea pigs and rabbits. Biochemistry 11:2627–2633.

Powell, S. E., and E. D. Aberle. 1981. Skeletal muscle and adipose tissue cellularity in runt and normal birth weight swine. J. Anim. Sci. 52:748–756.

Quinn, L. S., M. Nameroff, and H. Holtzer. 1984. Age-dependent changes in myogenic precursor cell compartment sizes. Exp. Cell Res. 154:65–82.

Reiser, R. 1975. Fat has less cholesterol than lean. J. Nutr. 105:15–16.

Rhee, K. S., T. R. Dutson, and G. C. Smith. 1982. Effect of changes in intermuscular and subcutaneous fat levels on cholesterol content of raw and cooked beef steaks. J. Food Sci. 47:1638–1642.

Ricks, C. A., R. H. Dalrymple, P. K. Baker, and D. L. Ingle. 1984. Use of a β-agonist to alter fat and muscle deposition in steers. J. Anim. Sci. 59:1247–1255.

Rinderknecht, E., and R. E. Humbel. 1978. Primary structure of human insulin-like growth factor II. FEBS 89:283–286.

Robbins, J., T. Horan, J. Gulick, and K. Kropp. 1986. The chicken myosin heavy chain family. J. Biol. Chem. 261:6606–6612.

Rubinstein, N. A., and A. M. Kelly. 1978. Myogenic and neurogenic contributions to the development of fast and slow twitch muscles in the rat. Dev. Biol. 62:473–485.

Rutz, R., and S. Hauschka. 1982. Clonal analysis of vertebrate myogenesis. VII. Heritability of muscle colony type through sequential subclonal passages in vitro. Dev. Biol. 91:103–110.

Savell, J. W., H. R. Cross, and G. C. Smith. 1986. Percentage ether extractable fat and moisture content of beef longissimus muscle as related to USDA marbling score. J. Food Sci. 51:838–840.

Schultz, E. 1974. A quantitative study of the satellite cell population in postnatal mouse lumbrical muscle. Anat. Rec. 180:589–596.

Seed, J., and S. D. Hauschka. 1984. Temporal separation of the migration of distinct myogenic precursor populations into the developing chick wing bud. Dev. Biol. 106:389–393.

Silver, G., and J. D. Etlinger. 1985. Regulation of myofibrillar accumulation in chick muscle cultures. Evidence for the involvement of calcium and lysosomes in non-uniform turnover of contractile proteins. J. Cell Biol. 101:2383–2391.

Snow, M. H. 1977. Myogenic cell formation in regenerating rat skeletal muscle injured by mincing. II. An autoradiographic study. Anat. Rec. 188:201–218.

Stockdale, F. E., and H. Holtzer. 1961. DNA synthesis and myogenesis. Exp. Cell Res. 24:508–520.

Stromer, M. H., D. E. Goll, and J. H. Roberts. 1966. Cholesterol in subcutaneous and intramuscular lipid depots from bovine carcasses of different maturity and fatness. J. Anim. Sci. 25:1145–1147.

Summers, P. J., C. R. Ashmore, Y. B. Lee, and S. Ellis. 1985. Stretch-induced growth in chicken wing muscles. Role of soluble growth-promoting factors. J. Cell. Physiol. 125:288–294.

Swatland, H. J. 1976. Recent research on postnatal muscle development in swine. Proc. Recip. Meat Conf. 29:86–103.

Swatland, H. J. 1977. Accumulation of myofiber nuclei in pigs with normal and arrested development. J. Anim. Sci. 44:759–764.

Tischler, M. E. 1981. Hormonal regulation of protein degradation in skeletal and cardiac muscle. Life Sci. 28:2569–2576.

Tischler, M. E., M. Desautels, and A. L. Goldberg. 1982. Does leucine, leucyl-tRNA, or some metabolite of leucine regulate protein synthesis and degradation in skeletal and cardiac muscle? J. Biol. Chem. 257:1613–1621.

Tomas, F. M., J. Murray, and L. M. Jones. 1984. Interactive effects of insulin and corticosterone on myofibrillar protein turnover in rats as determined by N-methylhistidine excretion. Biochem. J. 220:469–479.

Trenkle, A., D. L. DeWitt, and D. G. Topel. 1978. Influence of age, nutrition and genotype on carcass traits and cellular development of the M. Longissimus of cattle. J. Anim. Sci. 46:1597–1603.

Truman, E. J., and F. N. Andrews. 1955. Some effects of purified anterior pituitary growth hormone on swine. J. Anim. Sci. 14:7.

Vernon, B. G., and P. J. Buttery. 1976. Protein turnover in rats treated with trienbolone acetate. Br. J. Nutr. 36:575–579.

Watt, B. K., and A. L. Merrill. 1963. Composition of foods—raw, processed, prepared. In USDA Agricultural Handbook 8. Washington, D.C.: U.S. Department of Agriculture.

Whalen, R. G., G. S. Butler-Browne, and F. Gros. 1978. Identification of a novel form of myosin light chain present in embryonic muscle tissue and cultured muscle cells. J. Mol. Biol. 126:415–431.

White, N. K., P. H. Bonner, D. R. Nelson, and S. D. Hauschka. 1975. Clonal analysis of vertebrate myogenesis. IV. Medium-dependent classification of colony forming cells. Dev. Biol. 44:346–361.

Winick, M., and A. Nobel. 1966. Cellular response in rats during malnutrition at various ages. J. Nutr. 89:300–306.

Young, R. B., and R. E. Allen. 1979. Transitions in gene activity during development of muscle fibers. J. Anim. Sci. 48:837–852.

Young, R. B., D. M. Moriarity, and C. E. McGee. 1986. Structural analysis of myosin genes using recombinant DNA techniques. J. Anim. Sci. 63:259–268.

# The Role of Growth Hormone in Fat Mobilization

H. MAURICE GOODMAN

Around 1931, several papers appeared in both the English and German literature suggesting that the pituitary gland contained a fat mobilizing or fat metabolism substance (Anselmino and Hoffman, 1931; Burn and Ling, 1929, 1930). The first indication that growth hormone might be that substance came from Lee and Shaffer (1934), who showed, by analysis of carcass composition, that animals treated with a pituitary preparation rich in growth-promoting activity had less fat than untreated animals and that the composition of the growth that ensued largely favored the accumulation of protein.

Rats treated with highly purified growth hormone had considerably less body fat than did control rats; growth hormone favored the deposition of more protein and less fat (Li et al., 1949). The decrease in the proportion of fat seen in rats treated with growth hormone reflects a decrease in the amount of lipid stored in the adipose tissue (Goodman, 1963).

This decrease in adipose mass could be the result of changes in several aspects of lipid metabolism. For example, there was a decrease in fat synthesized within the tissue, as well as a decrease in the deposition of fat synthesized in the liver or consumed in the diet. There was also an increase in mobilization of fat from the adipose tissue. These data suggest that adipose tissue might be a target tissue for growth hormone.

The fat cell readily stores preformed fat that enters by way of the gut or is synthesized in the liver. In addition, it can synthesize fat from glucose or amino acids. Lipid is stored in adipose tissue in the form of triglyceride, which is a triester composed of three molecules of long-chain fatty acids per molecule of glycerol. Stored lipids can be mobilized from the fat cell to meet the energy needs of muscle and other tissues. Fat leaves the adipose cell in the form of free fatty acids (FFAs) after cleavage of the three ester bonds of the triglyceride. FFAs released from adipose tissue can be consumed directly by muscle. It appears that muscle takes up FFAs from the circulation in proportion to the amount that is there (Armstrong et al., 1961), although muscle may not immediately burn all the FFAs extracted from the circulation. In addition, muscle and other tissues consume the carbons of fatty acids after conversion of FFAs to ketone bodies in the liver. Thus, regulation of lipid storage, mobilization, and oxidation is really determined by events that take place at the level of the fat cell. The glycerol released along with the FFAs travels to the liver, where it can serve as a substrate for gluconeogenesis.

Growth hormone might act in several ways to decrease the amount of fat in adipose tissue. It might promote fatty acid mobilization and thereby oxidation, or it might decrease fatty acid synthesis. Either would be consistent with previous reports, in which growth hormone was reported to decrease the respiratory quotient (the ratio of $CO_2$ produced to oxygen consumed) (Astwood, 1955; DeBodo and Altszuler, 1957; Ketterer et al., 1957). To determine whether growth hormone decreased carbohydrate utilization and fatty acid synthesis in adipose tissue, Goodman (1968b) injected hypophysectomized rats with growth hormone. At various times thereafter, the epididymal fat was removed, divided into segments, and incubated in vitro along with various radioactive substrates. In tissue segments from animals that were treated with growth hormone 3.5 hours earlier, there was a decrease in the utilization of glucose both in terms of its oxidation to $CO_2$ and its conversion to fatty acids. Oxidation of pyruvate and fructose and the incorporation of their carbons into long-chain fatty acids were similarly reduced. Thus, growth hormone, even as early as 3.5 hours after injection, decreased the conversion of carbohydrate to fat. Therefore, one of the ways in which growth hormone decreases carcass fat is to decrease the synthesis of triglycerides in adipose tissue. The rat is one species that relies heavily on its adipose tissue for synthesis of long-chain fatty acids. In other species, the liver is the principal site of lipogenesis; thus, it is reasonable to expect a similar effect of growth hormone on the liver.

Another way in which growth hormone may decrease the content of lipid in adipose tissue is by promoting fatty acid release. Goodman and Knobil (1959) treated intact and hypophysectomized rhesus monkeys with growth hormone at 8:00 a.m., immediately after removing food from their cages. Blood samples were obtained from the femoral vein at various times during the day. In the control animals, plasma concentrations of FFAs increased about fourfold in 8 hours. When these animals were given 50 μg of simian growth hormone per kilogram of body weight, FFA concentrations increased even more rapidly and were significantly higher at 4 and 8 hours. Similar results were obtained in hypophysectomized animals, except that the rate of mobilization of FFAs in the untreated monkeys was significantly lower than normal.

Two important points are illustrated by these experiments. First, the effects of growth hormone are slow to appear and last for a long time. Second, animals must be fasted for this effect of growth hormone to be seen. When FFAs were measured in monkeys or rats that were allowed to eat during the experiment, the effects of growth hormone on fat mobilization were small and difficult to show. This is largely because there are many other influences, in addition to growth hormone, that affect fat and carbohydrate metabolism. Certainly insulin, and also glucose, have very marked effects on the release of FFAs from adipose tissue. This has complicated studies of the actions of growth hormone and has contributed to the controversy over whether growth hormone is a lipolytic agent.

It therefore appears that in order to see a growth hormone effect, some other signal that operates simultaneously is needed for fatty acid mobilization (Goodman and Schwartz, 1974). Growth hormone appears to enhance the efficacy of other signals for lipolysis. Because energy metabolism is governed by redundant control systems in the intact animal, compensatory adjustments that can be made when we disrupt the system may mask the actions of a hormone such as growth hormone that does not have very large effects in the short time span of an experiment. The effects of growth hormone may be relatively small and slow to develop and dissipate, but even small changes can be quite meaningful over a long period of time.

Fat is stored in adipose tissue in the form of triglycerides, which are synthesized continuously from fatty acids, and alpha-glycerol phosphate, which is derived from glucose. Triglycerides, in turn, are broken down by an enzyme, the hormone-sensitive lipase, which is dependent on cyclic adenosine monophosphate (cyclic AMP) (Steinberg and Huttunen, 1972) and stimulated primarily by epinephrine and to a lesser extent by a wide variety of other hormones. The activity of this enzyme is probably the major rate-determining factor in lipolysis and involves the splitting off of the first fatty acid molecule from the triglyceride. The cycle of lipolysis and esterification appears to be ongoing. Growth hormone can change the rate of fatty acid mobilization in two ways—either by accelerating lipolysis, which would make the cycle spin faster, or by slowing reesterification, which would increase the fraction of fatty acids escaping from the cell.

As mentioned, growth hormone decreases glucose utilization in fat. In order for fatty acids to be incorporated into triglyceride, alpha-glycerol phosphate must be present. The glycerol that is released in lipolysis cannot be reutilized in adipose tissue, which is almost totally devoid of the enzyme glycerol kinase (Margolis and Vaughan, 1962). Hence, all free glycerol produced by lipolysis escapes from the fat cell. Therefore, the rate of glycerol release can be used as an index of the rate of lipolysis. The fatty acids that are liberated in this process can be either recycled or released as FFAs. In fact, if adipose tissue were studied in vitro, it would be seen that only a very small fraction of the fatty acids that are released by lipolysis actually get out of the tissue. If there were no reesterification, the ratio of FFAs to glycerol released from the tissue ought to be 3:1. Actually, it is usually closer to 1:1, or perhaps less, suggesting that at least two-thirds of the fatty acids produced by lipase activity are normally reconverted to triglyceride. If reesterification were blocked, there would be potential for tripling the release of FFAs without changing the speed of the cycle. This can be accomplished just by limiting the rate of alpha-glycerophosphate production. Certainly this is one of the important effects that growth hormone has on adipose tissue, and it follows directly from limiting glucose metabolism.

Because of the reciprocal relationship between glucose and fatty acid metabolism, virtually anything that interferes with glucose metabolism is reflected in increased fatty acid mobilization. Thus, how an experiment is conducted very much influences the results, and such variables as time of last feeding and amount fed may be crucial. This was made quite clear by Goodman and Knobil's (1959) studies on the effects of growth hormone on plasma FFAs in monkeys. Growth hormone readily produced an increase in plasma concentrations of FFAs when given to animals that were accustomed to eating ad libitum until the time of hormone administration. When the same protocol of giving growth hormone immediately upon removal of food was used with monkeys that were accustomed to eating only one meal a day, no such effect was seen. Growth hormone increased FFAs in these animals only when given at the end of a 24-hour fast. It appeared that in these animals, which were accustomed to a nearly 24-hour interval between meals, removal of food at the time of hormone administration was not a sufficient stimulus to activate fasting responses.

Hormones acting at the surface of the adipocyte activate adenylate cyclase by a receptor-driven mechanism that is discussed in more detail later. Adenylate cyclase catalyzes the conversion of adenosine triphosphate to cyclic AMP, which binds to the cyclic AMP-dependent protein kinase enzyme complex and releases free catalytic units that catalyze the transfer of the terminal phosphate group of adenosine triphosphate to the lipase (Steinberg, 1976). It appears that the hormone-sensitive lipase is an 84,000-dalton protein that is converted from an inactive to an active enzyme by phosphorylation of a single serine residue (Stralfors et al., 1984). Presumably there is also a phosphatase that restores the enzyme to its inactive dephospho-form. This cycle appears to be responsible for all known hormone stimulation of the lipolytic process. The reaction is very rapid, and the physiologically important hormone that activates the lipase is epinephrine. The effects of growth hormone are presumably expressed through the same enzyme. Before discussing growth hormone, however, the effects of epinephrine, which are typical of the other lipolytic hormones and therefore color expectations for the effects of growth hormone, should be examined.

Birnbaum and Goodman (1977) incubated segments of adipose tissue from normal rats in bicarbonate buffer in the presence or absence of epinephrine. To obtain frequent measurements of glycerol production, the tissue segments were transferred to a fresh medium every 5 minutes. The amount of glycerol that was released into the medium during each of those 5-minute intervals was measured with a sensitive enzymatic assay. Again, glycerol production served as an indicator of how fast the lipolytic cycle was turning. Within just a few minutes, epinephrine increased glycerol production about fivefold. This effect persisted as long as the hormone was present, and dissipated within minutes after removing epinephrine.

Growth hormone has been shown to be among the most potent hormones in causing an increase in FFAs in vivo and is the only pituitary hormone to produce such an effect (Goodman and Knobil, 1959). Yet when growth hormone was added to adipose tissue in vitro, very little or no effect was seen.

Initially, investigators looked for the same rapidly activated lipolysis resulting with epinephrine, or at least for some effect in the first hour of incubation—a time when growth hormone has absolutely no lipolytic effect (Goodman and Schwartz, 1974). Even when tissues were incubated for 3 or 4 hours, growth hormone did not do very much by itself. Studies by Fain and colleagues expanded on some earlier findings of an apparent interaction of growth hormone and adrenal hormones (Fain et al., 1965) and produced the first convincing in vitro lipolytic results with growth hormone. They showed that when adrenal glucocorticoid hormones were added along with growth hormone, a lipolytic effect of growth hormone was obtained but that the response had a built-in delay. Goodman and Knobil's (1959) in vivo studies found that the effects of growth hormone take a couple of hours to develop. In fact, if one allows enough time and examines lipolysis in the presence of some other agents, particularly glucocorticoids, lipolytic effects of growth hormone are obtained with reasonable consistency.

Goodman et al. (1986) transferred segments of normal epididymal fat to a fresh medium every hour. Tissues were incubated with a small amount (0.1 µg/ml) of dexamethasone, a synthetic glucocorticoid, and 1 µg/ml of bovine growth hormone. During the first hour, the rate of glycerol production in the absence of hormones and the rate in the presence of growth hormone and steroid were the same. No effect of the combination of growth hormone and dexamethasone was seen until the end of the second hour. The effect was initially small, but it gradually increased during the third and fourth hours, when it was relatively large. Neither growth hormone nor dexamethasone alone had any effect. The underlying mechanisms for the actions of glucocorticoid and growth hormone are not yet established. Their effects require the synthesis of new proteins and ribonucleic acid (Fain, 1967; Fain and Saperstein, 1970), but the nature of those proteins is not yet defined. Part of the effect of glucocorticoid may be mediated by induction of an inhibitor of the activity of the enzyme phospholipase A2, which releases the arachidonic acid precursor of prostaglandins from membrane phospholipids (Flower and Blackwell, 1979). It is unlikely, however, that this action can explain all the effects of glucocorticoids on adipose tissue. The effects of growth hormone may also involve protein synthesis, but the nature of the induced proteins is unknown.

In a slightly different experimental situation, Goodman (1968a) studied adipose tissue of hypophysectomized animals to determine whether there was an absolute dependence on the steroid. Dexamethasone was replaced with theophylline, which, at the time of these experiments, was thought to act solely by inhibiting cyclic nucleotide phosphodiesterase and thereby allowing cyclic AMP to accumulate. It now appears that theophylline has at least one other effect: blocking the adenosine receptor (Londos et al., 1978), which may account for its lipolytic activity. Tissues were incubated in Krebs Ringer bicarbonate buffer and transferred to a fresh medium every hour; theophylline (0.3 mg/ml) was always present. The lipolytic effect of growth hormone was seen only after a lag period of 1 hour. The standard errors were always about 10 percent at the mean, and the response to growth hormone was always statistically significant by the second hour after hormone addition. Curiously, the effect of growth hormone seen in the presence of theophylline was not blocked with inhibitors of RNA or protein synthesis (Goodman, 1968b).

Using this model to study the reversibility of the lipolytic action of growth hormone, Goodman (1981) added neutralizing antibodies at various times after growth hormone and measured glycerol production each hour. In the control tissues, glycerol production was highest in the first hour and then declined very rapidly. In the presence of growth hormone, the initial rapid rate of lipolysis was sustained as long as the hormone was present. With the antiserum alone, or with growth hormone plus antiserum added at zero time, there was a similar, rapid decline in glycerol production after the first hour. When antiserum was added 1 or 2 hours after growth hormone, the high lipolytic rate was maintained for at least 1 hour and then declined to the same level as the control, whereas when growth hormone was added without antiserum, the initial high lipolytic rate persisted throughout the experiment. These results provide a further illustration that actions of growth hormone are slow in onset and dissipate slowly and, in this respect, are very different from the effects of epinephrine.

Goodman et al. (1986) next investigated the concentration dependency of the lipolytic response by using bovine growth hormone prepared by Dr. Martin Sonnenberg of the Memorial Sloan Kettering Institute in New York City. Tissues from normal rats were preincubated for 3 hours with dexamethasone, and the various concentrations of growth hormone and lipolysis were measured in the fourth hour (Goodman and Grichting, 1983). Significant effects were obtained with $\geq 3$ ng/ml, but in many experiments significant effects were seen with 1 ng/ml, and sometimes a maximum effect was observed at around 10 ng/ml. This is an extremely sensitive response. The protocol adopted, which takes into account the glycerol released only in the fourth hour, provides more sensitive conditions for showing the lipolytic effect than simply measuring glycerol released over the entire 4 hours. When glycerol release is measured over the entire 4 hours, the hormonal effect is partially obscured by the low rate of glycerol production during the rather long lag period. When only that narrow window of just the fourth hour is observed, when the response is largest, it is more likely that a lipolytic effect will be detected.

The magnitude of the lipolytic effect of growth hormone was compared with that of epinephrine (Goodman and Grichting, 1983). In this experiment, the concentration response range was narrow, and a maximum lipolytic effect of growth hormone was obtained with 3 ng/ml. Growth hormone increased glycerol production about twofold, from 1.5 to 4 $\mu$M/g of tissue per hour, whereas 100 ng/ml of epinephrine, which is a submaximal concentration, increased glycerol production sixfold, to 9 $\mu$M/g per hour. The response could not be increased beyond 4 $\mu$M/g per hour by adding more growth hormone, even though the tissues had ample capacity for a more rapid rate of lipolysis.

Exposure of tissues of hypophysectomized rats to growth hormone in the presence of theophylline yields a similar concentration/response relationship (Goodman et al., 1986). In this case, the maximum response to growth hormone was seen at a concentration of about 10–30 ng/ml. The response was significant and almost maximal at 3 ng/ml. Once again, lipolysis was measured only in the fourth hour of incubation.

In comparing the concentration of growth hormone needed for lipolysis to the concentration of growth hormone circulating in rat blood, it is evident that maximum stimulation of lipolysis usually occurs at the low end of the range found in blood. The data of Tannenbaum et al. (1976) illustrate a peculiar ultradian secretory pattern in the rat, in which every 3.5 hours there is a burst of growth hormone secretion. The rat rarely has a growth hormone concentration lower than 50 ng/ml. Yet, a maximum lipolytic effect is often seen at around 10 ng/ml. If the in vitro data are in any way representative of in vivo events, it is difficult to see how growth hormone could be an activator or signal for increased fatty acid mobilization, because increased lipolysis is seen at concentrations that are as low or lower than the usually prevailing concentrations in blood. It is likely, therefore, that growth hormone acts as a facilitator or potentiator of the effects of other agents,

such as epinephrine, which are the primary signals for fatty acid mobilization. Growth hormone might act as a gain control, being a regulator only in the sense that it increases or decreases responsiveness to other signals.

The effects of growth hormone on lipolysis are multiple. Goodman (1968a) investigated growth hormone in adipose tissue from normal rats and from hypophysectomized rats that were either untreated or given growth hormone for 2 days. In normal tissues, glycerol production was nearly doubled in 4 hours of incubation with growth hormone and dexamethasone. The control tissues released less fatty acid than glycerol, instead of the theoretical threefold-greater amount of fatty acids. Most of the fatty acid that was formed was reconverted to triglyceride. In the presence of growth hormone and dexamethasone, the ratio of glycerol to fatty acid production decreased from about 4 to about 1.2. Thus, growth hormone and dexamethasone increased fatty acid mobilization in at least two ways: (1) by increasing glycerol production and (2) by decreasing the amount of fatty acids reconverted to triglyceride. In contrast to its effects in the presence of theophylline, growth hormone had no effect on lipolysis when examined in the presence of dexamethasone in tissues of hypophysectomized rats. Treatment of the rats with growth hormone for 2 days, but not 1 day, enabled the tissues of hypophysectomized rats to respond when growth hormone and dexamethasone were later added in vitro. It appears that growth hormone has some long-term effect on the lipolytic system that takes days to develop. That effect is distinct from the shorter term stimulation of lipolysis, which requires an hour or two, and both, in turn, are different from the lipolytic effects that growth hormone produces in tissues of hypophysectomized rats when theophylline is present. In conclusion, there are multiple effects of growth hormone on adipose tissue that are ultimately reflected in increased lipolysis. Also, it is evident that the effects of growth hormone are expressed in increased fatty acid release as well as increased glycerol release.

In adipose tissue obtained from hypophysectomized rats, the lipolytic response to epinephrine is severely curtailed (Goodman, 1970). Hypophysectomy grossly decreases the sensitivity of these tissues to virtually any lipolytic agent. The hypophysectomized rat obviously lacks more than just growth hormone. At least two other hormones that are related to pituitary secretions are also involved in maintaining responsiveness of the lipolytic apparatus (Goodman, 1970): thyroid hormone and adrenal glucocorticoid. The effects of growth hormone and dexamethasone on the response to epinephrine were examined by Goodman (1969). Eight segments of adipose tissue were taken from each of eight hypophysectomized rats and preincubated for 3 hours. Two segments from each rat were incubated without any hormone, two were incubated only with dexamethasone, two with only growth hormone, and two with a combination of growth hormone and dexamethasone. The tissues were then transferred to a fresh medium for incubation in the fourth hour in the presence or absence of a test dose of 0.01 μg/ml epinephrine. Tissues pretreated for 3 hours with dexamethasone produced an almost threefold increase in the response to the test dose of epinephrine. Preincubation with growth hormone alone had little or no effect, but when growth hormone was added along with dexamethasone in the 3-hour preincubation period, there was a significant increase above the response evoked by epinephrine in the presence of dexamethasone alone. Thus, growth hormone clearly increased the lipolytic effects of another agent, and this response also required glucocorticoid.

In an effort to pinpoint where within the lipolytic cycle growth hormone may be working, epinephrine was replaced in the previous protocol with dibutyryl cyclic AMP,

which is an analog of cyclic AMP that readily penetrates fat cells (Goodman, 1969). Neither dexamethasone nor growth hormone alone or in combination increased the lipolytic response to dibutyryl cyclic AMP. This suggests that the potentiating effects of growth hormone and dexamethasone on lipolysis are more likely related to cyclic AMP formation than to cyclic AMP action.

Receptor-mediated generation of cyclic AMP is complex, and there are many sites at which growth hormone might have an effect. It appears that in adipose tissue, and other tissues as well, the cyclic AMP-generating system is under the control of both stimulatory and inhibitory agents. Stimulatory agents such as epinephrine act through beta-adrenergic receptors. Inhibitory agents include catecholamines (which might affect alpha-2 receptors in some species), the prostaglandins, and adenosine. Both prostaglandin and adenosine seem to be formed in adipose tissue by endogenous mechanisms (Schwabe et al., 1973; Shaw and Ramwell, 1968). Experimentally, it can be shown that the activity of adenylate cyclase under "resting conditions" represents a balance determined by the combined influence of inhibitory and stimulatory agents. What is called resting or basal activity actually represents the preponderance of inhibitory influences that keep the system shut down (Kather et al., 1985).

The prostaglandins seem to be important endogenous inhibitors of lipolysis and adenylate cyclase (Steinberg et al., 1964). Along with the recognition that one of the major effects of glucocorticoid hormones in vivo is to inhibit the release of arachidonic acid from phospholipids in cell membranes (Flower and Blackwell, 1979) arose the possibility that dexamethasone may promote lipolysis by blocking prostaglandin formation. Arachidonate is the precursor for prostaglandins. Therefore, Goodman et al. (1986) attempted to determine whether indomethacin, which is an inhibitor of the conversion of arachidonic acid to prostaglandin (Vane,

1971), might mimic the effect of dexamethasone in the lipolytic system described above. Using the same protocol, tissues were preincubated with 50 μg/ml indomethacin, dexamethasone, or growth hormone. Neither dexamethasone alone nor growth hormone alone had much effect on lipolysis. The combination of dexamethasone and growth hormone significantly increased lipolysis, as did the combination of indomethacin and growth hormone. At least in this experiment, indomethacin and dexamethasone seemed to have a similar effect, suggesting that at least part of the effect of dexamethasone on lipolysis in response to epinephrine or growth hormone may be to block prostaglandin formation. This, in turn, somehow allows growth hormone, wherever it might be acting in the lipolytic system, to express its effects. Thus, when tissues were exposed to both agents, lipolysis was evident even though neither indomethacin nor growth hormone alone had much of a lipolytic effect. It is not certain that all the effects of dexamethasone can be explained in this way.

The other prominent endogenous inhibitory agent in adipose tissue is adenosine, which is released from fat cells by the breakdown of cyclic AMP. Therefore, Goodman et al. (1986) used adenosine deaminase to eliminate the endogenous adenosine produced during the experiment. The effects of adenosine are most clearly shown in isolated adipocytes, rather than tissue segments; but with at least some preparations of adenosine deaminase, these effects can be demonstrated in tissue segments as well. Tissue segments rather than isolated cells were studied, largely because segments are easier to study and introduce fewer artifacts. Tissues were preincubated for 3 hours in the presence or absence of adenosine deaminase and hormones, and lipolysis was examined in the fourth hour. Acceleration of adenosine destruction increased glycerol production in a manner that is probably analogous to what has been seen with theophylline, which seems to block the adenosine receptor (Londos et al., 1978). Again, growth hormone alone had very little effect, but when added along with adenosine deaminase, a substantial lipolytic effect was observed. Thus, it appears that there are two antilipolytic agents present in the tissue, at least in vitro, and that these agents contribute to the low basal activity of lipase. Presumably, they are also present in vivo. During incubation in vitro, spontaneous production of prostaglandins and adenosine appear to inhibit lipolysis; growth hormone and glucocorticoids apparently relieve that inhibition.

To gain insight into how endogenous inhibitors might interact with the cyclic AMP-generating system, the regulation of adenylate cyclase should be looked at in more detail. The catalytic component responsible for conversion of ATP to cyclic AMP relates to the receptors for stimulatory or inhibitory hormones by way of two other proteins, called G-proteins, because they bind guanine nucleotides (Spiegel et al., 1985). For stimulatory input, the recognition subunit of the receptor complex communicates with the catalytic unit by way of the stimulatory guanine nucleotide binding protein ($G_s$), which somehow activates adenylate cyclase. Inhibitory effects appear to be mediated in a similar fashion through an inhibitory subunit ($G_i$). The inhibitory and stimulatory subunits can be examined by taking advantage of the fact that certain bacterial toxins specifically affect these subunits. When plasma membranes are incubated in the presence of cholera toxin and $^{32}$P-labeled NAD (nicotinamide-adenine dinucleotide), there is a marked increase in the incorporation of $^{32}$P into $G_s$, reflecting NAD ribosylation of the stimulatory subunit. Ribosylation of $G_s$ in intact cells results in irreversible activation of adenylate cyclase. Pertussis toxin catalyzes the NAD ribosylation of the inhibitory subunit, which irreversibly inactivates $G_i$ and, in intact cells, blocks all inhibitory input to adenylate cyclase (Spiegel et al., 1985).

The effects of pertussis toxin on lipolysis in normal adipose tissue were examined (Goodman et al., 1986). Tissue segments were preincubated with the toxin for 3 hours, and lipolysis was measured in the fourth hour. The intense lipolysis seen when the inhibitory influence was removed in the absence of an activator of adenylate cyclase substantiates the idea that adenylate cyclase is under powerful inhibitory control under basal conditions. When that inhibitory control is removed, activation of lipolysis is as profound as when a strong lipolytic agent is added.

One possible site of action of growth hormone could be on the linkage of the recognition subunits for either excitatory or inhibitory signals to the adenylate cyclase catalytic subunit. Incubating adipocyte plasma membranes with excess NAD, guanosine triphosphate, and toxin (that is, conditions in which the subunit is limiting), gives some idea of whether these inhibitory or stimulatory guanine nucleotide-binding subunits are subject to change as a result of hormonal treatment. Membranes prepared from adipocytes of hypophysectomized or normal rats and from hypophysectomized rats treated with growth hormone 3 hours earlier were incubated with $^{32}$P-labeled NAD and cholera toxin or a mixture of cholera toxin and pertussis toxin (Goodman et al., 1986). The membranes were then dissolved in sodium dodecyl sulfate and subjected to electrophoresis on slabs of polyacrylamide gel. NAD-ribosylated proteins were visualized by autoradiography. When cholera toxin was present alone, two bands with apparent molecular weights of about 45,000 and 53,000 daltons appeared and were of about equal intensity regardless of whether the membranes were obtained from normal rats, hypophysectomized rats, or hypophysectomized rats treated with growth hormone. The band at 45,000 daltons is thought to be the alpha-subunit of the $G_s$ protein. When pertussis toxin was present, another band (molecular weight, 41,000 daltons)

appeared that corresponds to the alpha-subunit of $G_i$. In tissues of hypophysectomized rats, the incorporation of $^{32}$P indicative of NAD ribosylation of the inhibitory subunit was greatly increased. It is likely that in these tissues there is either more $G_i$ or that it is in a form that is more susceptible to NAD ribosylation. Although these two possibilities cannot be separated at this time, there is clearly something different about the inhibitory subunit in adipocytes after hypophysectomy. Three hours after growth hormone treatment, the change was not restored to normal, but was at least partly reversed. Similar results have been obtained in 8 or 10 experiments, and although the data are still preliminary, this is probably a very real phenomenon. The data suggest that growth hormone may affect the inhibitory subunit in a way that allows stimulatory inputs to produce greater changes in lipolysis or that sets the basal activity of adenylate cyclase at a higher level by reducing inhibitory input.

## REFERENCES

Anselmino, K. J., and F. Hoffman. 1931. Das Fettstoffwechselhormon des Hypophysenvorderlappens. I. Nachweis, Darstellung und Eifenschaften des Hormons. II. Stuffwechselwirkungen und Regulationen des Hormons. Klin. Wochenschr. 10:2380.

Armstrong, D. T., R. Steele, N. Altszuler, A. Dunn, J. S. Bishop, and R. C. DeBodo. 1961. Regulation of plasma free fatty acid turnover. Am. J. Physiol. 201:9.

Astwood, E. B. 1955. Growth hormone and corticotropin. P. 235 in The Hormones, Vol. 3, G. Pincus and K. V. Thimann (eds.). New York: Academic Press.

Birnbaum, R. S., and H. M. Goodman. 1977. Studies of the mechanism of epinephrine stimulation of lipolysis. Biochem. Biophys. Acta 476:292.

Burn, J. H., and H. W. Ling. 1929. The effect of pituitary extract and adrenalin on ketonuria and liver glycogen. J. Pharm. Pharmacol. 2:1.

Burn, J. H., and H. W. Ling. 1930. Ketonuria in rats on a fat diet (a) after injections of pituitary (anterior lobe) extract, (b) during pregnancy. J. Physiol. (London) 69:xix.

DeBodo, R. C., and N. Altszuler. 1957. The metabolic effects of growth hormone and their physiological significance. Vitamins and Hormones 15:205.

Fain, J. N. 1967. Studies on the role of RNA and protein synthesis in the lipolytic action of growth hormone in isolated fat cells. Adv. Enzyme Reg. 5:39.

Fain, J. N., and R. Saperstein. 1970. Involvement of RNA synthesis and cyclic AMP in the activation of fat cell lipolysis by growth hormone and glucocorticoids in adipose tissue. P. 20 in Adipose Tissue: Regulation and Metabolic Functions, B. Jeanrenaud and D. Hepp (eds.). New York: Academic Press.

Fain, J. N., V. P. Kovacev, and R. O. Scow. 1965. Effect of growth hormone and dexamethasone on lipolysis and metabolism in isolated fat cells of the rat. J. Biol. Chem. 240:3522.

Flower, R. J., and G. J. Blackwell. 1979. Antiinflammatory steroids induce biosynthesis of a phospholipase $A_2$ inhibitor which prevents prostaglandin generation. Nature 278:456.

Goodman, H. M. 1963. Effects of chronic growth hormone treatment on lipogenesis by rat adipose tissue. Endocrinology 72:95.

Goodman, H. M. 1968a. Effects of growth hormone on the lipolytic response of adipose tissue to theophylline. Endocrinology 82:1027.

Goodman, H. M. 1968b. Growth hormone and the metabolism of carbohydrate and lipid in adipose tissue. Ann. N.Y. Acad. Sci. 148:419.

Goodman, H. M. 1969. Endocrine control of lipolysis. P. 115 in Progress in Endocrinology. Proceedings of the Third International Congress of Endocrinology, Mexico City, C. Gual (ed.). Amsterdam: Excerpta Medica Foundation.

Goodman, H. M. 1970. Permissive effects of hormones on lipolysis. Endocrinology 86:1064.

Goodman, H. M. 1981. Separation of early and late responses of adipose tissue to growth hormone. Endocrinology 109:120.

Goodman, H. M., and G. Grichting. 1983. Growth hormone and lipolysis: A reevaluation. Endocrinology 113:1697.

Goodman, H. M., and E. Knobil. 1959. Effects of fasting and of growth hormone on plasma fatty acid concentration in normal and hypophysectomized Rhesus monkeys. Endocrinology 65:451.

Goodman, H. M., and J. Schwartz. 1974. Growth hormone and lipid metabolism. P. 211 in Handbook of Physiology: Endocrinology, Part 2, E. Knobil and W. Sawyer (eds.). Bethesda, Md.: American Physiological Society.

Goodman, H. M., E. Gorin, and T. W. Honeyman. 1986. Biochemical basis for the lipolytic activity of growth hormone. In Perspectives in Growth Hormone Research, B. Sherman and L. Underwood (eds.). New York: Marcel Dekker.

Kather, H., W. Bieger, G. Michel, K. Aktories, and K. H. Jakobs. 1985. Human fat cell lipolysis is primarily regulated by inhibitory modulators acting through distinct mechanisms. J. Clin. Invest. 76:1559.

Ketterer, B., P. J. Randle, and F. G. Young. 1957. The pituitary growth hormone and metabolic processes. Ergeb. Physiol. Biol. Chem. Expt. Pharmacol. 49:127.

Lee, M. O., and N. K. Shaffer. 1934. Anterior pituitary growth hormone and the composition of growth. J. Nutr. 7:337.

Li, C. H., M. E. Simpson, and H. M. Evans. 1949. Influence of growth and adrenocorticotropic hormones on the body composition of hypophysectomized rats. Endocrinology 44:71.

Londos, C., D. M. F. Cooper, W. Schlegel, and M. Rodbell. 1978. Adenosine analogs inhibit adipocyte adenylate cyclase by a GTP-dependent process: Basis for action of adenosine and methylxanthines on cyclic AMP production and lipolysis. Proc. Natl. Acad. Sci. USA 75:5362.

Margolis, S., and M. Vaughan. 1962. α-Glycenophosphate synthesis and breakdown in adipose tissue. J. Biol. Chem. 237:44.

Schwabe, U. R., R. Ebert, and H. G. Erbler. 1973. Adenosine release from isolated fat cells and its significance for the effects of hormones on cyclic 3′,5′-AMP levels and lipolysis. Naunyn Schmiedeberg's Arch. Pharmacol. 276:133.

Shaw, J. E., and P. W. Ramwell. 1968. Release of prostaglandin from epididymal fat pad on nervous and hormonal stimulation. J. Biol. Chem. 243:1498.

Spiegel, A. M., P. Gierschik, M. A. Levine, and R. W. Downs, Jr. 1985. Clinical implications of guanine nucleotide-binding proteins as receptor-effector couplers. N. Engl. J. Med. 312:26.

Steinberg, D. 1976. Interconvertible enzymes in adipose tissue regulated by cyclic AMP-dependent protein kinase. P. 157 in Advances in Cyclic Nucleotide Research, Vol. 7, P. Greengard, and G. A. Robinson (eds.). New York: Raven Press.

Steinberg, D., and J. K. Huttunen. 1972. The role of cyclic AMP in activation of hormone-sensitive lipase in adipose tissue. P. 47 in Advances in Cyclic Nucleotide Research, Vol. I, P. Greengard, R. Paoletti, and G. A. Robinson (eds.). New York: Raven Press.

Steinberg, D., M. Vaughan, P. Nestel, O. Strand, and S. Bergstrom. 1964. Effects of the prostaglandins on hormone-induced mobilization of free fatty acids. J. Clin. Invest. 43:1533.

Stralfors, P., P. Bjorsell, and P. Belfrage. 1984. Hormonal regulation of hormone-sensitive lipase in intact adipocytes: Identification of phosphorylated sites and effects of phosphorylation by lipolytic hormones and insulin. Proc. Natl. Acad. Sci. USA 81:3317.

Tannenbaum, G. S., J. Martin, and E. Colle. 1976. Evidence for an endogenous ultradian rhythm governing growth hormone secretion in the rat. Endocrinology 99:720.

Vane, J. R. 1971. Inhibition of prostaglandin synthesis as a mechanism of action for aspirin-like drugs. Nature (New Biol.) 231:232.

# The Use of Bioassays To Detect and Isolate Protein or Peptide Factors Regulating Muscle Growth in Meat-Producing Animals

## PEPTIDE FACTORS AFFECTING MUSCLE GROWTH

Several peptide or protein factors that have the potential to regulate muscle growth in meat-producing animals have been identified. These are discussed below.

### Somatotropin

The effect of somatotropin deficiency on muscle growth has been well established for many years. Long-term administration of somatotropin to pituitary-intact animals has been reported to increase muscling, decrease fat content, and improve feed efficiency in swine (Chung et al., 1985; Machlin, 1972); increase nitrogen retention in steers (Moseley et al., 1982) and sheep (Davis et al., 1969); increase growth rate in lambs (Wagner and Veenhuien, 1978); and improve milk production in dairy cattle (Peel et al., 1981). However, it appears unlikely that somatotropin directly affects proliferation and protein turnover in muscle cells. Although there is an increased incorporation of $^3$H-thymidine into DNA in muscle from somatotropin-treated hypophysec-

tomized rats as compared to untreated controls (Breuer, 1969), this may reflect a direct effect of somatotropin on proliferation of nonmuscle cells or an indirect effect of somatotropin on proliferation of muscle cells. It has also been reported that in in vitro incubations of rat diaphragm muscle, $10^{-8}$M somatotropin stimulates amino acid uptake (Albertsson-Wikland and Isaksson, 1976). However, recent observations that many types of cells can secrete somatomedin (Adams et al., 1984; Hill et al., 1986a) raise the possibility that responses seen in the intact diaphragm are the result of locally produced somatomedins. In fact, it is generally believed that many if not all of the effects of somatotropin on muscle growth are mediated through somatotropin-dependent plasma factors—somatomedins—produced in response to somatotropin.

In culture, muscle cells do not appear to respond to the addition of physiological levels of somatotropin. Ewton and Florini (1980) have reported that somatotropin has no detectable effect on anabolic processes in embryonic muscle cell cultures. Additionally, Allen et al. (1983) have reported that somatotropin has no direct effect on

163

the rate of actin synthesis in myotube cultures derived from rat satellite cells. These findings support the theory that the effect of somatotropin on muscle is an indirect one mediated through the somatomedins.

## Insulin-Like Growth Factors (Somatomedins)

Insulin-like growth factors are small polypeptides (approximate molecular weight of 7,500 daltons) extracted and purified from human serum. They possess insulin-like properties in vitro but do not cross-react with insulin antibodies. Multiplication stimulating activity (MSA) is the name given to a family of polypeptides isolated from media conditioned by a Buffalo rat liver (BRL) cell line (BRL 3A). To date, two classes of insulin-like growth factors (IGFs) have been characterized: IGF-I, also referred to as basic somatomedin (pH 8.2–8.4), or somatomedin-C (SM-C), and IGF-II, or neutral somatomedin. Multiplication stimulating activity appears to be the rat form of IGF-II, since the primary structure of MSA shows 93 percent identity with that of human IGF-II (Marquardt et al., 1981). At concentrations of $10^{-9}$ to $10^{-10}$M, IGFs are mitogenic for a variety of cultured cell types.

Biologically active receptors for both IGF-I/SM-C and IGF-II/MSA have been identified on the surface of cultured muscle cells (Ballard et al., 1986). IGF-I/SM-C has been shown to stimulate growth of hypophysectomized rats (Schoenle et al., 1982), proliferation of cultured myoblasts (Ballard et al., 1986), amino acid uptake in cultured myoblasts (Hill et al., 1986a), differentiation of cultured myoblasts (Ewton and Florini, 1981), and RNA synthesis and polypeptide chain initiation in an isolated muscle (Monier and Le Marchand-Brustel, 1984). IGF-II/MSA has been shown to stimulate proliferation of cultured myoblasts (Ewton and Florini, 1981; Florini and Ewton, 1981; Florini et al., 1984), amino acid transport into cultured muscle cells (Janeczko and Etlinger, 1984),

and the rate of protein synthesis in cultured myotubes (Janeczko and Etlinger, 1984). MSA has also been shown to decrease the rate of protein degradation in cultured myotubes (Janeczko and Etlinger, 1984). In addition to their well-documented presence in serum, both IGF-I/SM-C and IGF-II/MSA have been reported to be released by rat myoblasts (Hill et al., 1986b), thus raising the possibility that these peptides may be involved in autocrine or paracrine regulation of muscle growth. On the basis of this information, it appears likely that insulin-like growth factors are potent stimulators of all aspects of muscle growth and development.

## Insulin

The role of insulin in regulating general cell metabolism has been recognized for many years, but its mechanism of action is still not well understood. Similarly, its role in controlling muscle growth is not clear. Several lines of evidence suggest that insulin may have an anabolic effect on muscle tissue. Studies of a variety of animal models have demonstrated that wasting of skeletal muscle is a prominent feature of diabetes mellitus and that it is reversed by administration of insulin (Pain and Garlick, 1974). Additionally, ribosomes isolated from muscle of diabetic rats are less active in in vitro protein synthesis systems than in ribosomes from nondiabetic controls. In vitro studies with isolated muscles (Fulks et al., 1975) and the perfused rat hemicorpus (Jefferson et al., 1977) have shown that insulin increases the rate of protein synthesis and decreases the rate of protein degradation in these systems.

In cultured muscle cells as well as in fibroblasts and fibroblastic cell lines, supraphysiological concentrations of insulin ($\geq 1$ µg/ml) are required to elicit a maximum response. In muscle cell cultures, these high concentrations stimulate both proliferation and differentiation of myogenic cells

(Ewton and Florini, 1981). Insulin at high concentrations ($10^{-6}$M) is a component of synthetic media used to support growth and differentiation of myogenic cells in culture (Dollenmeier et al., 1981; Florini and Roberts, 1979). It has been proposed that the stimulation of growth of fibroblasts by insulin is mediated by insulin's weak binding to receptors for insulin-like growth factors. Affinity cross-linking studies have shown the existence of two classes of IGF receptors. Type I receptors (Massague and Czech, 1982) have a higher affinity for IGF-I than for IGF-II and a low affinity for insulin. The structure and subunit composition of type I receptors are very similar to those of the insulin receptor. Type II receptors bind IGF-II with a higher affinity than they do IGF-I and do not appear to have appreciable affinity for insulin (Massague and Czech, 1982). At high concentrations, insulin may bind to the type I receptor, and in so doing affect cell growth in a manner similar to that observed for much lower concentrations of IGF-I. This hypothesis is based on work by King et al. (1980), who showed that blockade of high-affinity insulin receptors with anti-receptor Fab fragments blocked high-affinity insulin binding but did not prevent insulin-induced stimulation of DNA synthesis in cultured fibroblasts. Furthermore, these investigators showed that anti-insulin-receptor immunoglobulin G (IgG), which triggers a number of acute insulin-like metabolic effects, does not stimulate DNA synthesis. They concluded that the growth-promoting effects of insulin on human fibroblast were due to binding of insulin to the type I receptor. Although this has not been proved in cultured muscle cells, it would seem likely that the well-documented effects of supraphysiological concentrations of insulin on proliferation and differentiation of cultured muscle cells are the result of this spillover action of insulin through IGF-I receptors.

Insulin has a wide range of effects on cell metabolism. Consequently, it is possible that physiological levels of insulin facilitate muscle cell growth by maintaining cells in a metabolic state that allows them to respond to other hormones and growth factors that stimulate cell proliferation.

## Differentiation Inhibitor

Coon's BRL cells secrete a protein that is a potent inhibitor of skeletal myoblast differentiation in vitro (Evinger-Hodges et al., 1982; Florini et al., 1984). In skeletal myoblast cultures, this protein reversibly blocks fusion, elevates creatine kinase, and increases binding of alpha-bungarotoxin. It has also been isolated from sera of embryonic origin, prompting the suggestion that it may play a role in embryonic growth of myoblasts and in satellite cell formation (Evinger-Hodges et al., 1982).

## Transferrin

Transferrin is an iron-binding glycoprotein that is present in serum (Ozawa and Kohama, 1978) and embryo extract (Ii et al., 1981). Additionally, transferrin-like molecules have been isolated from both nerve and muscle extracts (Matsuda et al., 1984). In muscle cell cultures, iron-saturated transferrin stimulates both proliferation and differentiation and is essential for maintenance of healthy myotubes. The effect of transferrin on muscle growth in culture is absolutely dependent on the presence of iron and appears to be class specific (that is, mammalian transferrins do not affect avian myoblasts, nor do avian transferrins affect mammalian myoblasts) (Shimo-Oka et al., 1986).

## Fibroblast Growth Factor

In cell cultures, fibroblast growth factor (FGF) stimulates proliferation of myogenic cells and delays their differentiation (Gospodarowicz et al., 1976; Linkhart et al., 1981). Allen et al. (1984) have proposed that FGF regulates satellite cell proliferation in skeletal muscle. However, they do not believe that serum is the source of the FGF that is affecting satellite cell proliferation. Rather, they hypothesize that FGF-like molecules are produced locally in muscle and trigger a localized response of satellite cells during muscle regeneration.

## Paracrine and Autocrine Control of Muscle Growth

Reports that various cell types secrete growth factors have sparked interest in autocrine and paracrine regulation of muscle growth. It has been reported that cultured fibroblasts secrete IGF or IGF-like molecules (Adams et al., 1984) and that fetal rat chondrocytes sequentially elaborate separate growth- and differentiation-promoting peptides during their development (Shen et al., 1985). Additionally, cultured myoblasts have been reported to synthesize and secrete IGF-I/SM-C (Hill et al., 1986a). Because all these cell types are found in muscle tissue, their ability to produce growth factors raises the possibility that muscle growth may be at least partially regulated by factors produced locally. This hypothesis is supported by reports of the purification of an FGF-like muscle growth factor present in skeletal muscle tissue (Karkami et al., 1985). The mechanism by which this factor is accumulated in skeletal muscle and the relationship of this accumulation to regulation of muscle growth and regeneration is of interest.

## BIOASSAYS FOR FACTORS INFLUENCING MUSCLE GROWTH

To develop effective strategies for controlling animal growth, a better understanding is needed of the mechanism by which known growth factors regulate proliferation, differentiation, and protein turnover in muscle cells. The potential for autocrine and paracrine regulation of muscle growth, as well as the discovery of factors such as the differentiation inhibitor, emphasize the importance of efforts to isolate currently unknown peptide factors that significantly influence the development of muscle tissue.

In addition to mitogenic growth factors, factors that inhibit the growth of cells have been reported (Harel et al., 1985; Harrington and Godman, 1980; Salmon et al., 1983). Although these factors have not been well characterized, it seems reasonable to assume that they modulate the growth-promoting effects of mitogenic serum factors such as the IGFs. In fact, both specific and nonspecific inhibitors of IGF action have been reported (Kuffer and Herington, 1984; Salmon et al., 1983). Although these inhibitors have been detected in normal sera (Kuffer and Herington, 1984), their level and activity appear to be increased by catabolic conditions in both humans and experimental animals (Salmon et al., 1983; Unterman and Phillips, 1985). Under the proper conditions, transforming growth factor-β (TGF-β) has also been shown to inhibit proliferation of certain types of cultured cells (Roberts et al., 1985). Because these inhibitory factors appear to have the potential to attenuate the action of growth-promoting factors, it is important that more is learned about their mode of action and physiological significance in meat-producing animals.

Radioimmunoassays (RIAs) cannot be used effectively to detect and characterize unknown or poorly characterized muscle growth factors. Consequently, bioassays capable of reliably detecting factors influencing muscle growth are necessary. These bioassays will augment existing RIAs by enabling us to detect and study currently unknown factors that may stimulate or inhibit muscle growth in meat-producing animals. The current lack of understanding of the mechanisms controlling muscle growth in meat animals is largely the result of difficulties encountered in devising a satisfactory bioassay system in which to study these processes. Experimental animals, isolated muscles, and muscle cell culture have been the primary systems used to study the effects of specific peptides on the growth of muscle tissue.

While experimental animals provide the most biologically complete system in which to study muscle growth, the complex interactions of their hormonal systems and large animal-to-animal variation often make it difficult to evaluate the role of any specific factor in muscle growth. Additionally, experiments with animals are expensive and labor intensive and often require several weeks or months to complete. In order to evaluate the effect of a specific factor on muscle growth, it is also necessary to measure the muscle mass of control and experimental animals. At present, this is a laborious and inaccurate procedure.

In vitro incubation of excised muscle tissue has also been used to study the effects of various peptides on muscle growth, primarily the influence of different substances on the rates of protein synthesis and degradation in skeletal muscle tissue (Fulks et al., 1975). This technique provides a more controlled experimental environment and easier measurement of protein synthesis and degradation rates than does the whole animal. However, excised muscles are generally in a catabolic state relative to protein turnover (for example, protein degradation exceeds protein synthesis) (Clark and Mitch, 1983; Fulks et al., 1975).

Muscle cell culture has been used extensively to study the effects of specific peptides on both protein turnover and muscle cell proliferation. In culture, muscle precursor cells differentiate and proliferate to form myoblasts that fuse to form multinucleated myotubes. Myotubes synthesize contractile proteins, assemble them into myofibrils, and develop the ability to contract. However, for these processes to occur, the culture media must contain blood serum or serum factors. Presumably, serum contains specific factors that are necessary for the differentiation and proliferation of muscle cells in culture. Consequently, muscle cell

culture has been used to study the effect of specific factors on proliferation, protein turnover, and differentiation in muscle cells. Although cell culture lends itself well to these kinds of studies, there is some concern about whether the findings are valid for muscle tissue in vivo. Therefore, cell culture data must ultimately be confirmed in the animal.

## EFFECT OF PORCINE GROWTH HORMONE ON BIOACTIVITY AND IGF-I CONCENTRATION IN SWINE SERUM

Although all the systems discussed in the preceding section may be useful as bioassays under the proper circumstances, my colleagues and I have focused our efforts on developing and statistically standardizing a muscle cell culture bioassay that can be used to identify factors influencing muscle growth and to determine their mode of action in meat animals. This muscle cell culture bioassay and an IGF-I radioimmunoassay have been used to measure the bioactivity and IGF-I concentration, respectively, in sera obtained from pigs before and after injection with porcine growth hormone (pGH).

Although there have been conflicting reports about the effect of exogenous growth hormone (GH) on muscle growth in pituitary-intact swine, it now appears that long-term injection of highly purified pGH increases muscling, decreases fat, and improves feed efficiency in growing pigs (Chung et al., 1985; Machlin, 1972). However, very little is known about the mechanism through which pGH affects muscle deposition in pituitary-intact swine. Although it appears likely that the GH-induced increases in the circulating level of somatomedin-C may be responsible for increased muscle deposition, little information is available on the effect of artificially increased growth hormone levels on the concentration and bioactivity of somatomedins and other growth factors whose levels might be affected by this increase. Comparison of the muscle cell culture bioassay response and the radioimmunoassayable IGF-I concentration of sera obtained from pigs before and after pGH injection should help determine whether IGF is uniquely responsible for increases in muscle growth resulting from growth hormone treatment.

## Methods

Standardized bioassays for measuring the effect of porcine serum on proliferation in cultured L6 muscle cells were done according to procedures described in detail by Kotts et al. (1987a,b). Briefly, L6 cells were plated at 600/cm$^2$ (25-cm$^2$ flasks) in Dulbecco's modified Eagle's medium (DMEM) containing 10 percent fetal calf serum. After 24 hours of attachment, the medium was removed and the cells were rinsed with 37°C DMEM without serum (SF media). Test media were applied and cells were incubated for 72 hours. The cells were removed for counting by trypsinization for 5 minutes at 37°C, and the reaction was stopped by adding ice-cold DMEM containing 10 percent fetal calf serum. Cells from each flask were quantitatively transferred to glass tubes on ice. The contents of each tube were diluted and counted in triplicate, and the counts were averaged. Triplicate flasks were assayed for each serum sample tested, and the results were expressed as the mean number of cells/cm$^2$ per flask ± standard error. The intraassay coefficient of variation was 2.6 percent (Kotts et al., 1987b). Test media consisted of DMEM containing 3 percent (volume/volume) test sera.

Porcine growth hormone was purchased from Dr. A. F. Parlow (Torrance, Calif.). The pGH used for injection was lot no. 7024-C (specific activity = 1.5 U/mg) and that used for radioimmunoassay standard was lot no. APF 6400. $^{125}$I-pGH and rabbit anti-bovine GH were supplied by Monsanto Company (St. Louis, Mo.). Crossbred bar-

rows (19 to 36 kg) from separate litters were individually penned and fed ad libitum a corn- and soybean-based diet containing 21 percent protein. Five pigs were injected with 143 μg of pGH/kg of body weight per day for 3 days.

Catheters were inserted into both jugular veins, and after a 2-day recovery period, 12-ml blood samples were removed from the catheters at 6-hour intervals (6 a.m., noon, 6 p.m., and midnight) throughout the duration of the study. Injections of pGH were given at 2 p.m. on days 4 through 6. On days 1 through 3 and 7 through 9, all pigs received sham injections containing sterile saline. Injection and postinjection blood samples were collected on days 4 through 9. The blood was allowed to clot, and serum was prepared for use in the muscle cell culture bioassays and radioimmunoassays.

Solutions of pGH for injection were prepared by dissolving the pGH in 44 mM NaHCO$_3$, pH 11.5, and then immediately lowering the pH to 9.5 by addition of 1 N HCl. Solutions were prepared on the day of the first injections and filtered through a 0.22-μm filter. Protein content of the filtered solution was determined by the microbiuret method.

The basic electrophoresis system used for analytical sodium dodecyl sulfate (SDS) polyacrylamide slab gels was that of Laemmli (1970) and consisted of a 3.5 percent acrylamide stacking gel and a 12 percent separating gel.

Radioimmunoassays were done on the individual 6-hour serum samples obtained from each pig during the study. Radioimmunoassay kits from Micromedic Systems (Horsham, Pa.) were used to quantify the levels of insulin and cortisol in the sera. The insulin kit was a homologous RIA for porcine insulin and used rabbit anti-porcine insulin antisera. The cortisol kit used rabbit anti-cortisol sera.

A heterologous radioimmunoassay for porcine growth hormone was used to quantify levels of pGH in the sera. This radioimmunoassay used pGH (pituitary; lot AFP 6400) as a standard, $^{125}$I-pGH as a trace, and rabbit anti-bovine growth hormone antisera. The sensitivity of the assay at 95 percent binding was 5 ng/ml. Serial dilution of porcine serum at 100, 150, 200, and 250 μl yielded a curve that was parallel to the pGH standard curve. Recovery of standard in the presence of 200 μl of serum was 98.6 percent. The intraassay variability was 2.95 percent, and the interassay variability was 9.8 percent. All samples compared to each other in this work were assayed in the same experiment to avoid interassay variation.

Somatomedin-C levels in serum were quantified with a kit from the Nicholls Institute (San Juan Capistrano, Calif.). Sera were treated in 1 M glycine–glycine HCl buffer (pH 3.5) for 24 hours at 37°C prior to assay. All sera were measured against a human serum SM-C standard (1 U = 36 ng of purified SM-C). The trace was $^{125}$I-human SM-C; rabbit anti-human somatomedin-C antisera were used. The intraassay variability was 5.4 percent, and the interassay variability was 9.2 percent. When acidified swine serum was assayed in the presence of $^{125}$I-human SM-C standard, 100 percent recovery was achieved. A titration of various dilutions (1:4 to 1:20) of swine sera resulted in curves parallel to those obtained with purified SM-C.

To verify that the observed increases in mitogenic activity resulted from the pGH injections and were not random daily variations in serum activity, the data obtained from the bioassay were subjected to analysis of variance. A randomized block design was used, with blocks representing pigs. To test for differences owing to pGH injection, the bioassay results from the preinjection days (1 through 3) were compared to those during (days 4 through 6) and after (days 7 through 9) injection by using the single degree of freedom contrasts on treatments.

## Results and Discussion

SDS-polyacrylamide gel electrophoresis of the pGH preparation used in this study showed a major band at 21.9 kilodaltons (kd) and a minor band at 20 kd, along with several minor bands between 15 and 9 kd. The molecular weights of the 21.9- and 20-kd bands correspond to those reported for human growth hormone (Chambach et al., 1973). The peptides banding between 9 and 15 kd may be proteolytic fragments of pGH, or they may be impurities in the preparation. Whatever their origin, any single one of these peptides represents an extremely minor contaminant in the pGH preparation.

To determine whether the pGH preparation contained contaminants that affected muscle cell proliferation, it was added at various concentrations to media containing 2.5 percent (volume/volume) control swine serum (CSS). Radioimmunoassay of the CSS showed that it contained 5.56 ng of pGH/ml and 2.18 U of SM-C/ml. Consequently, the contribution of the CSS to the final pGH or SM-C level in the bioassay was 6 × $10^{-12}$ M pGH and 2.58 × $10^{-10}$ M SM-C (based on a molecular weight of 7.6 kd and 36.1 ng of human SM-C/U and a molecular weight of 22 kd for pGH). The proliferation rate of cultured muscle cells was not significantly affected by pGH concentrations below $10^{-8}$ M, but $10^{-8}$ M pGH or higher resulted in a slight, though significant, increase in cell numbers (10 to 12 percent above control levels). The inability of pGH to stimulate proliferation of cultured muscle cells is in agreement with results obtained by others using primary myogenic cultures or L6 myogenic cells (Ewton and Florini, 1980; Gospodarowicz et al., 1976).

The slight stimulation of proliferation observed at higher pGH concentrations ($\geq 10^{-8}$ M) is consistent with the stimulation of alpha-aminoisobutyric acid uptake in 8-day-old cultures of L6 myotubes exposed to $10^{-7}$

M bovine GH (Ewton and Florini, 1980). It is possible that impurities in the GH preparation or biologically active fragments of the GH molecule (Liberti and Miller, 1978) are responsible for these increases in mitogenic activity observed at supraphysiological concentrations of GH.

In contrast to the lack of response observed when pGH was added directly to muscle cells, sera from four out of five pigs injected with pGH exhibited increased mitogenic activity. Analysis of variance on the bioassay data from all five pigs showed that the treatment effects were highly significant ($P < 0.005$). The single degree of freedom contrasts on treatment revealed that the mitogenic activity of sera obtained during and after the pGH injections was significantly higher ($P < 0.005$) than preinjection levels. Additionally, all pigs receiving pGH showed increases in SM-C levels in their sera during and after the injections.

The pGH concentration in the 24-hour pooled serum samples from the pigs on pGH injection days (days 4 through 6) was approximately 100 ng/ml, and these pools were diluted 29-fold for use in the proliferation bioassay. Thus, the maximum concentration of pGH in the bioassay media was $10^{-10}$ M. Since $10^{-10}$ M pGH had no effect on proliferation when added directly to the muscle cell cultures, the increases in bioassayable mitogenic activity of serum pools obtained during and after pGH injection were not a direct result of the increased level of pGH in the culture media.

Serum pGH levels were increased approximately 30-fold by 4 hours after each pGH injection and declined to preinjection levels by approximately 16 hours after each injection. Increases in serum SM-C levels were observed 6 to 12 hours after the increase in serum pGH concentration (10 to 16 hours after each pGH injection). The magnitude of the SM-C response was different for each pig, even though all pigs received the same dose of pGH and attained similar blood levels of pGH 4 hours after

injection. SM-C increases ranged from 1.7 to 4 times the preinjection levels. In all the pigs, the second and third injections resulted in higher concentrations of serum SM-C than the first injection. In two cases, SM-C concentrations appeared to increase in a stepwise manner with each successive injection of pGH. A similar stepwise increase in SM-C production upon successive injections of human growth hormone into hypopituitary patients was reported by Copeland et al. (1980). Serum SM-C levels remained high for 2 to 6 days after the last pGH injection.

Insulin and cortisol levels in the sera did not change during the treatment period and ranged from 3.8 to 10.6 µU/ml and 2.0 to 6.9 µg/dl, respectively.

It is well established that GH stimulates the production of somatomedins (IGFs) by the liver and possibly by other tissues as well. Administration of IGF-I/SM-C to hypophysectomized rats has been reported to restore growth to a level equivalent to that seen with GH replacement (Schoenle et al., 1982). Additionally, IGF-I/SM-C and IGF-II/MSA stimulate the proliferation of myogenic cells in culture (Ballard et al., 1986; Ewton and Florini, 1981; Florini et al., 1984; Hill et al., 1986a). Consequently, it appears likely that the increased levels of IGF-I/SM-C observed in sera obtained from pigs during and after pGH injection play a role in the increased mitogenic activity of these sera. Nonetheless, there were several instances when changes in serum IGF-I/SM-C levels did not appear to be directly related to changes in serum mitogenic activity in the bioassay. For example, sera from pig 90 showed a significant increase in SM-C concentration during and after pGH injection (2.5 U/ml preinjection to 6.5 U/ml postinjection); however, no corresponding increase in serum mitogenic activity was detectable. In contrast, sera from pig 85 exhibited a similar change in serum SM-C concentration during and after pGH injection (2 U/ml preinjection to 7 U/ml postinjection), and this corresponded to a significant increase in mitogenic activity. In addition, sera from pig 87 exhibited a relatively large increase in SM-C concentration (3.5 U/ml preinjection to 10 to 13 U/ml postinjection) but showed only a modest increase in mitogenic activity. Conversely, sera from pig 7, which exhibited relatively little increase in SM-C concentration (2 U/ml preinjection to 4 to 5.5 U/ml postinjection), showed a relatively large increase in mitogenic activity (24 percent) over the injection period.

These results suggest that factors in addition to radioimmunoassayable IGF-I/SM-C may contribute to the alterations in mitogenic activity observed in sera during and after pGH injection. There are several factors that could be involved in the mitogenic response, either by directly affecting muscle cell proliferation or by modulating the bioactivity of IGF-I. For example, IGF-II has been reported to increase fourfold in the sera of GH-deficient humans after GH administration (Schalch et al., 1982). Additionally, inhibitors of IGF-stimulated synthesis of DNA and/or sulfate incorporation in costal cartilage have been reported in sera from starved, diabetic, or hypophysectomized rats (Kuffer and Herington, 1984; Salmon et al., 1983; Unterman and Phillips, 1985), and a specific inhibitor of IGF has been isolated and partially purified from normal sera (Kuffer and Herington, 1984). Somatomedin-binding proteins ranging in molecular weight from 40 to 70 kd have also been reported to bind and inactivate IGF (Hossenlopp et al., 1986; Martin and Baxter, 1985; Romanus et al., 1986). In addition, a protein that inhibits differentiation of myogenic cells has been identified in fetal calf serum and in media obtained from BRL cells in culture (Evinger-Hodges et al., 1982; Florini et al., 1984). It is possible that these factors or other, as yet unidentified, factors are affecting the mitogenic activity of sera in the muscle cell culture bioassay used in this study.

Results of this study demonstrate the importance of developing bioassays for muscle growth. Used in conjunction with radioimmunoassays, bioassays can help elucidate the mode of action of known growth factors such as somatotropin. They also provide a valuable tool for use in identifying unknown growth factors that affect muscle growth in meat animals. Identification of these factors and clarification of their mode of action is crucial to an eventual understanding of the biological control of muscle growth.

## REFERENCES

Adams, S. O., M. Kapadia, B. Mills, and W. H. Daughaday. 1984. Release of insulin-like growth factors and binding protein activity into serum-free medium of cultured human fibroblasts. Endocrinology 115:520.

Albertsson-Wikland, K., and O. Isaksson. 1976. Development of responsiveness of young normal rats to growth hormone. Metabolism 25:747.

Allen, R., K. C. Masak, P. K. McAllister, and R. A. Merkel. 1983. Effects of growth hormone, testosterone and serum concentration on actin synthesis in cultured satellite cells. J. Anim. Sci. 56:833.

Allen, R. E., M. V. Dodson, and L. S. Luiten. 1984. Regulation of skeletal muscle satellite cell proliferation by bovine pituitary fibroblast growth factor. Exp. Cell Res. 152:154.

Ballard, F. J., L. C. Read, G. L. Francis, C. J. Bagley, and J. C. Wallace. 1986. Binding properties and biological potencies of insulin-like growth factors in L6 myoblasts. Biochem. J. 233:223.

Breuer, C. B. 1969. Stimulation of DNA synthesis in cartilage of hypophysectomized rats by native and modified placental lactogen and anabolic hormones. Endocrinology 85:989.

Chambach, A., R. A. Yadley, M. Ben-David, and D. Rodbard. 1973. Characterization of human growth hormone by electrophoresis and isoelectric focusing in polyacrylamide gel. Endocrinology 93:848.

Chung, C. S., T. D. Etherton, and J. P. Wiggins. 1985. Stimulation of swine growth by porcine growth hormone. J. Anim. Sci. 60:118.

Clark, A. S., and W. E. Mitch. 1983. Comparison of protein synthesis and degradation in incubated and perfused muscle. Biochem. J. 212:649.

Copeland, K. C., L. E. Underwood, and J. J. Van Wyk. 1980. Induction of immunoreactive somatomedin-C in human serum by growth hormone: Dose response relationships and effects on chromatographic profiles. J. Clin. Endocrinol. Metab. 50:690.

Davis, S. L., U. S. Garrigus, and F. C. Hinds. 1969. Metabolic effects of growth hormone and diethylstilbestrol in lambs. II. Effects of daily ovine growth hormone injections in plasma metabolites and nitrogen-retention in fed lambs. J. Anim. Sci. 30:236.

Dollenmeier, P., D. C. Turner, and H. M. Eppenberger. 1981. Proliferation of chick skeletal muscle cells cultured in a chemically defined medium. Exp. Cell Res. 135:47.

Evinger-Hodges, M. J., D. Ewton, Z. S. C. Seifert, and J. R. Florini. 1982. Inhibition of myoblast differentiation *in vitro* by a protein isolated from liver cell medium. J. Cell Biol. 93:395.

Ewton, D. Z., and J. R. Florini. 1980. Relative effects of the somatomedins, MSA and growth hormone on myoblasts and myotubes in culture. Endocrinology 106:577.

Ewton, D. Z., and J. R. Florini. 1981. Effects of the somatomedins and insulin on myoblast differentiation *in vitro*. Dev. Biol. 86:31.

Florini, J. R., and D. Z. Ewton. 1981. Insulin acts as a somatomedin analog in stimulating myoblast growth in serum-free medium. In Vitro 17:763.

Florini, J. R., and S. B. Roberts. 1979. A serum-free medium for the growth of muscle cells in culture. In Vitro 15:983.

Florini, J. R., D. Z. Ewton, M. J. Evinger-Hodges, S. L. Fallen, R. L. Lau, J. F. Ragan, and B. M. Vertel. 1984. Stimulation and inhibition of myoblast differentiation by hormones. In Vitro 20:942.

Fulks, R. M., J. B. Li, and A. L. Goldberg. 1975. Effects of insulin, glucose and amino acids on protein turnover in rat diaphragm. J. Biol. Chem. 250:290.

Gospodarowicz, D., J. Weseman, J. S. Moran, and J. Lindstrom. 1976. Effect of fibroblast growth factor on the division and fusion of bovine myoblasts. J. Cell Biol. 70:395.

Harel, L., C. Blat, and G. Chatelain. 1985. Regulation of cell proliferation inhibitory and stimulatory factors diffused by 3T3 cultured cells. J. Cell. Physiol. 123:139.

Harrington, W. N., and G. C. Godman. 1980. A selective inhibitor of cell proliferation from normal serum. Proc. Natl. Acad. Sci. USA 77:423.

Hill, D. J., C. J. Crace, S. P. Nissley, D. Morrell, A. T. Holder, and R. D. G. Milner. 1986a. Fetal rat myoblasts release both rat somatomedin-C (SM-C)/insulin-like growth factor I (IGF I) and multiplication-stimulating activity *in vitro*: Partial characterization and biological activity of myoblast-derived SM-C/IGF I. Endocrinology 117:2061.

Hill, D. J., C. J. Crace, A. J. Strain, and R. D. G. Milner. 1986b. Regulation of amino acid uptake and deoxyribonucleic acid synthesis in isolated human fetal fibroblasts and myoblasts: Effect of human placental lactogen, somatomedin-C, multiplication stimulating activity, and insulin. J. Clin. Endocrinol. Metab. 62:753.

Hossenlopp, P., D. Seurin, B. Segoria-Quinson, S. Hardouin, and M. Binoux. 1986. Analysis of serum insulin-like growth factor binding proteins using Western blotting: Use of the method for titration of the binding proteins and competitive binding studies. Anal. Biochem. 154:138.

Ii, I., I. Kimura, T. Hasegawa, and E. Ozawa. 1981. Transferrin is an essential component of chick embryo extract for avian myogenic cell growth in vitro. Proc. Jpn. Acad. 57:211.

Janeczko, R. A., and J. D. Etlinger. 1984. Inhibition of intracellular proteolysis in muscle cultures by multiplication-stimulating activity. Comparison of effects of multiplication-stimulating activity and insulin on proteolysis, protein synthesis, amino acid uptake, and sugar transport. J. Biol. Chem. 259:6292.

Jefferson, L. S., J. B. Li, and S. R. Rannels. 1977. Regulation by insulin of amino acid release and protein turnover in perfused rat hemicorpus. Proc. Natl. Acad. Sci. USA 69:816.

Karkami, E., D. Spector, and R. C. Strohman. 1985. Myogenic growth factor present in skeletal muscle is purified by heparin-affinity chromatography. Proc. Natl. Acad. Sci. USA 82:8044.

King, G. L., C. R. Kahn, M. M. Rechler, and S. P. Nissley. 1980. Direct demonstration of separate receptors for growth and metabolic activities of insulin and multiplication-stimulating activity (an insulin-like growth factor) using antibodies to the insulin receptor. J. Clin. Invest. 66:130.

Kotts, C. E., M. E. White, C. E. Allen, and W. R. Dayton. 1987a. Stimulation of in vitro muscle cell proliferation by sera from swine injected with porcine growth hormone. J. Anim. Sci. 64:623.

Kotts, C. E., M. E. White, F. Martin, C. E. Allen, and W. R. Dayton. 1987b. A statistically standardized bioassay for measuring the proliferation rate of myogenic cells in culture. J. Anim. Sci. 64:615.

Kuffer, A. D., and A. C. Herington. 1984. Partial purification of a specific inhibitor of the insulin-like growth factors by reversed-phase high-performance liquid chromatography. J. Chromatogr. 336:87.

Laemmli, U. K. 1970. Cleavage of structural proteins during the assembly of the head of bacteriophage T4. Nature 227:680.

Liberti, J. P., and M. S. Miller. 1978. Somatomedin-like effects of biologically active bovine growth hormone fragments. Endocrinology 103:680.

Linkhart, T. A., C. H. Clegg, and S. D. Hauschka. 1981. Myogenic differentiation in permanent clonal mouse myoblast cell lines: Regulation by macromolecular growth factors in the culture medium. Dev. Biol. 86:19.

Machlin, L. J. 1972. Effect of porcine growth hormone on growth and carcass composition of the pig. J. Anim. Sci. 35:794.

Marquardt, H., G. J. Todaro, L. E. Henderson, and S. Oroszlan. 1981. Purification and primary structure of a polypeptide with multiplication-stimulating activity from rat liver cell cultures. J. Biol. Chem. 256:6859.

Martin, J. L., and R. C. Baxter. 1985. Antibody against acid-stable insulin-like growth factor binding protein detects 150,000 mol wt growth hormone-dependent complex in human plasma. J. Clin. Endocrinol. Metab. 61:799.

Massague, J., and M. P. Czech. 1982. The subunit structures of two distinct receptors for insulin-like growth factors I and II and their relationship to the insulin receptor. J. Biol. Chem. 257:5038.

Matsuda, R., D. Spector, and R. C. Strohman. 1984. There is selective accumulation of a growth factor in chicken skeletal muscle. I. Transferrin accumulation in adult anterior latissimus dorsi. Dev. Biol. 103:267.

Monier, S., and Y. Le Marchand-Brustel. 1984. Effects of insulin and IGF-I on RNA synthesis in isolated soleus muscle. Mol. Cell. Endocrinol. 37:109.

Moseley, W. M., L. F. Krabill, and R. F. Olsen. 1982. Effect of bovine growth hormone administered in various patterns on nitrogen metabolism in the Holstein steer. J. Anim. Sci. 55:1062.

Ozawa, E., and K. Kohama. 1978. Partial purification of a factor promoting chicken myoblast multiplication in vitro. Proc. Jpn. Acad. 49:852.

Pain, V. M., and P. J. Garlick. 1974. Effect of streptozotocin diabetes and insulin treatment on the rate of protein synthesis in tissues of the rat in vivo. J. Biol. Chem. 249:4510.

Peel, C. J., D. E. Bauman, R. C. Gorewit, and C. J. Sniffen. 1981. Effect of exogenous growth hormone on lactational performance in high yielding dairy cows. J. Nutr. 111:1662.

Roberts, A. M., M. A. Anzano, L. M. Wakefield, N. S. Roche, D. F. Stern, and M. B. Sporn. 1985. Type beta transforming growth factor: A bifunctional regulator of cellular growth. Proc. Natl. Acad. Sci. USA 82:119.

Romanus, J. A., J. E. Terrell, Y. W.-H. Yang, S. P. Nissley, and M. M. Rechler. 1986. Insulin-like growth factor carrier proteins in neonatal and adult rat serum are immunologically different: Demonstration using a new radioimmunoassay for the carrier protein from BRL-3A rat liver cells. Endocrinology 118:1743.

Salmon, W. D., L. A. Holladay, and V. J. Burkhalter. 1983. Partial characterization of somatomedin inhibitors in starved rat serum. Endocrinology 112:360.

Schalch, D. S., S. E. Tollefsen, G. J. Klingensmith, R. W. Gotlin, and M. J. Diehl. 1982. Effects of growth hormone administration on serum somatomedins, somatomedin carrier proteins and growth rates in children with growth hormone deficiency. J. Clin. Endocrinol. Metab. 55:49.

Schoenle, E., J. Zapf, R. E. Humbel, and E. R. Froesch. 1982. Insulin-like growth factor I stimulates growth in hypophysectomized rats. Nature 296:252.

Shen, V., L. Rifas, G. Kohler, and W. Peck. 1985. Fetal rat chondrocytes sequentially elaborate separate growth- and differentiation-promoting peptides during their development in vitro. Endocrinology 116:920.

Shimo-Oka, T., Y. Hagiwara, and E. Ozawa. 1986. Class specificity of transferrin as a muscle trophic factor. J. Cell. Physiol. 126:341.

Unterman, T. G., and L. S. Phillips. 1985. Glucocorticoid effects on somatomedins and somatomedin inhibitors. J. Clin. Endocrinol. Metab. 61:618.

Wagner, J. F., and E. L. Veenhuien. 1978. Growth performance, carcass deposition and plasma hormone levels in wether lambs when treated with growth hormone and thyroprotein. J. Anim. Sci. 46(Suppl. 1):397.

# Effects of Beta-Adrenergic Agonists on Growth and Carcass Characteristics of Animals

LARRY A. MUIR

Until recently, few mechanisms were known through which a drug could promote the growth performance or improve the carcass characteristics of livestock and poultry (Muir, 1985). Antimicrobial agents, such as antibiotics and antibacterials, improve growth performance of livestock and poultry by killing or inhibiting the growth of microorganisms (Muir et al., 1977). Estrogenic agents improve growth performance and carcass characteristics of cattle and sheep, but the specific mechanism is not well understood (Burroughs et al., 1954; Dinusson et al., 1950; Muir et al., 1983). Progestational agents improve the growth performance of cyclic heifers by inhibiting estrus and therefore its adverse affects, such as hyperactivity and reduced feed consumption (Davis, 1969). Androgenic agents improve growth performance and carcass characteristics of cattle and swine, especially females, supposedly through a direct, receptor-mediated action on skeletal muscle cells (Heitzman, 1980). In addition, exogenous growth hormone administration reportedly improves growth performance and carcass characteristics of livestock (Machlin, 1972; Wagner and Veenhuizen, 1978).

Now a new mechanism has been found through which the growth performance and carcass characteristics of all poultry and livestock species are dramatically improved (Baker et al., 1984; Beermann et al., 1986; Dalrymple et al., 1984; Moser et al., 1986; Muir et al., 1985; Ricks et al., 1984). This mechanism involves the activation by beta-adrenergic agonists (beta-agonists) of specific beta-adrenoceptors on the surface of adipocytes and skeletal muscle cells. This paper describes what is known about beta-agonists and the mechanisms through which they work.

## WHAT ARE BETA-AGONISTS?

Beta-agonists are structural analogs of the catecholamines epinephrine and norepinephrine. Epinephrine and norepinephrine are very similar in structure, and both bind to four different cell surface receptors called adrenoceptors (specifically, the $alpha_1$, $alpha_2$, $beta_1$, and $beta_2$ receptors). Of special interest are the effects of beta-agonists on adipose and muscle tissues. The adipose tissue of most species contains beta-receptors that, when activated, stimulate lipolysis. Most muscle tissue contains primarily beta$_1$ or beta$_2$ receptors, which, when activated, cause a specific muscular function. Skeletal muscle is known to have beta$_2$ receptors, but their response function is not well understood.

The structures of the beta-agonists that will be discussed in this paper—isoproterenol, clenbuterol, cimaterol, L-640,033, and BRL35135—are shown in Figure 1. Isoproterenol is a very potent beta$_1$/beta$_2$ agonist that is not orally active but is very effective in vitro. Clenbuterol and cimaterol (American Cyanamid) and L-640,033 (Merck) are orally active beta-agonists that have been shown to stimulate animal growth and change carcass characteristics (Dalrymple et al., 1984; Muir et al., 1985; Ricks et al., 1984). BRL35135 (Beecham) is an orally active

beta-agonist that has been shown to stimulate lipolysis (Arch et al., 1983, 1984).

## EFFECTS OF BETA-AGONISTS ON GROWTH PERFORMANCE AND CARCASS CHARACTERISTICS

Numerous growth trials have been conducted with different beta-agonists at varying dose levels in poultry, swine, sheep, and, to a lesser extent, cattle (Baker et al., 1984; Beermann et al., 1986; Dalrymple et al., 1984; Moser et al., 1986; Muir et al., 1985; Ricks et al., 1984). The results of these trials are summarized in Tables 1 and 2. In general, beta-agonists work best when used during the finisher period, regardless of species. Optimum responses are obtained when these drugs are administered right to

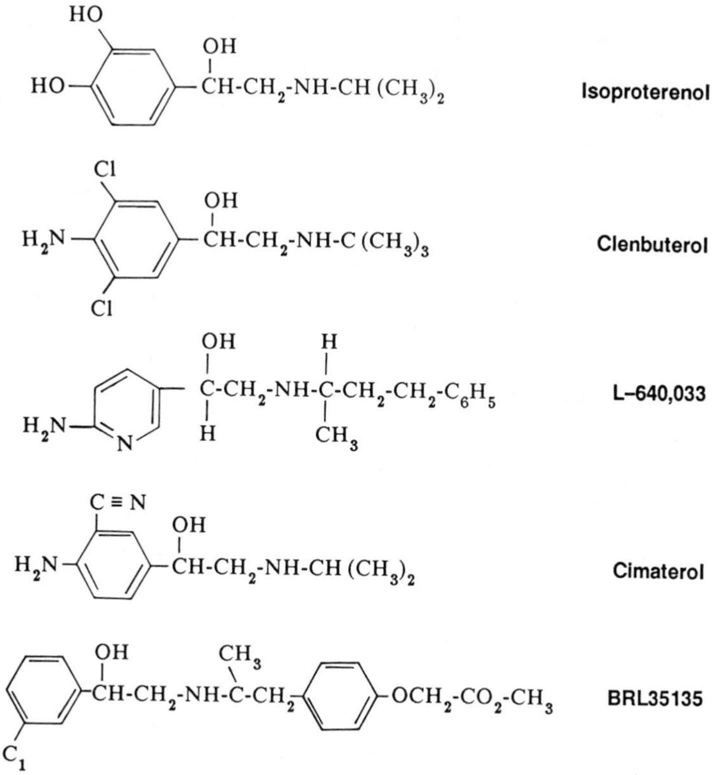

**FIGURE 1** Structures of the beta-adrenergic agonists isoproterenol, clenbuterol, L-640,033, cimaterol, and BRL35135.

TABLE 1    Profile of a Beta-Adrenergic Agonist Product for Livestock Growth
Promotion—Growth Performance

| Characteristic | Poultry | Ruminant | Swine |
|---|---|---|---|
| Dietary use level (ppm) | 0.2–2 | 1–10[a] | 0.2–4 |
| Growth rate (% increase) | 4 | 0–20[b] | 0–6 |
| Feed conversion (% improvement) | 5 | 0–20[b] | 0–6 |

[a]Sheep and cattle data.
[b]Sheep data only; cattle data not available.

SOURCE: Based on studies by Muir et al. (1985), Ricks et al. (1984), Baker et al. (1984), Beermann et al. (1986), Moser et al. (1986), and Dalrymple et al. (1984) using different beta-agonists.

the time of marketing. How close to marketing time that beta-agonists will actually be used will depend on the withdrawal time for each drug; actual withdrawal times have not yet been established.

In poultry, the dietary use levels for beta-agonists range from 0.2 to 2 ppm in the feed. When given during the final 2 to 4 weeks of the 7-week period before slaughter, improvements in growth rate and feed conversion of 4 and 5 percent, respectively, are usually obtained with broilers. Also, total carcass protein is increased approximately 6 percent, while total carcass fat is reduced. Abdominal fat is reduced, but the reduction is less than expected. In addition, the effect of beta-agonists on abdominal fat appears to differ between sexes, with males showing little or no reduction and females a reduction of 5 to 20 percent. As a result of these changes, carcass yield of broilers is usually increased by approximately 1 percent.

In ruminants, the dietary use levels for beta-agonists range from 1 to 10 ppm in the feed. In sheep, feeding of 1 to 2 ppm for the last 3 to 6 weeks of the finishing period appears to be most effective. In most sheep growth trials, responses in growth rate and feed conversion of 20 percent are obtained, although occasionally no response is observed. In terms of carcass composition, sheep respond with a 10 percent increase in total carcass protein and a 15 to 30 percent increase in the loineye area. Total carcass fat is reduced 20 to 30 percent, with even larger decreases in back fat and abdominal fat.

Data on the effects of beta-agonists in cattle are extremely limited but do show changes in carcass composition that are similar to those observed for sheep.

Swine appear to be more sensitive to beta-agonists than other species, with 0.2 to 4 ppm in the feed appearing to yield optimum results. Unlike other species, swine

TABLE 2    Profile of a Beta-Adrenergic Agonist Product for Livestock Growth
Promotion—Carcass Characteristics

| Characteristic | Poultry | Ruminant[a] | Swine |
|---|---|---|---|
| Carcass protein (% increase) | 6 | 10 | 4–8 |
| Loineye area (% increase) | — | 15–20 | 9–15 |
| Carcass fat (% decrease) | 4–8 | 20–30 | 10–16 |
| Back fat (% decrease) | — | 20–50 | 10–17 |
| Abdominal fat (% decrease) | 2–8 | 20–45 | — |

[a]Sheep and cattle data.

SOURCE: Based on studies by Muir et al. (1985), Ricks et al. (1984), Baker et al. (1984), Beermann et al. (1986), Moser et al. (1986), and Dalrymple et al. (1984) using different beta-agonists.

have failed in most reported trials to respond with improved growth rate or feed conversion. The studies in which improved growth performance was observed have used short-duration treatment (4 weeks or less). Swine do show very consistent improvement in carcass characteristics when medicated with beta-agonists. Total carcass protein is increased 4 to 8 percent, and loineye area muscle protein is increased 9 to 15 percent. Total carcass fat and back fat are reduced 10 to 17 percent.

In addition to food animal species, beta-agonists are also very effective in laboratory animals. For example, clenbuterol has been shown to improve the growth performance and shift the carcass composition of young, rapidly growing male rats (Table 3; Rickes et al., 1985). Apparently, a dose of 10 ppm in the feed produces the maximum response: a 9 percent improvement in weight gain, a 10 percent improvement in feed conversion, a 9 percent increase in total carcass protein, and a 20 percent reduction in total carcass fat. These responses to beta-agonists in the rat are very similar to those observed in food-producing animals. Thus, the rat appears to be an excellent model for studying beta-agonists as growth promoters.

Beta-agonists have been examined for their effects on milk production by dairy cows. Cows producing 17 to 18 kg of milk per day were medicated with the beta-agonists formoterol, zinterol, or Z1170. The beta-agonists were fed at 20 mg per head per day for 10 days. Milk production on days 5 to 10 of treatment was not different from that of controls or from milk production before or 5 days after treatment. In addition, the composition of the milk was not altered. These data suggest that beta-agonists, unlike growth hormone, apparently are not able to stimulate milk production, even though both beta-agonists and growth hormone appear to function through a repartitioning of nutrients.

## EFFECTS OF BETA-AGONISTS ON LIPID METABOLISM

Free fatty acid (FFA) synthesis is the conversion of glucose, acetate, or both to free fatty acids. Lipogenesis is the sum of FFA synthesis and the esterification of FFAs to triglycerides (TGs). Lipolysis is the breakdown of TGs to FFAs and glycerol. The rate of glycerol production can be used to estimate lipolysis because the glycerol produced during lipolysis cannot be reused for FFA esterification since adipocytes lack the necessary enzyme for phosphorylation of glycerol (phosphokinase). A scheme for the regulation of lipolysis by beta-agonists through specific adrenoceptors is shown in Figure 2. The activation of the beta-receptor on the outer surface of the adipocyte plasma membrane activates the chain of events that eventually leads to the breakdown of stored triglycerides to FFAs and glycerol.

Many beta-agonists effectively reduce lipid accumulation in adipose tissue. The mechanisms through which they act were studied at Merck in an in vitro system (Duquette and Muir, 1984). Adipose tissue was taken from an animal source, for example, rat epididymal or perirenal fat, using the procedure of Rodbell (1964). Adipocytes were incubated with treatment for 2 hours at

TABLE 3 Effects of a Beta-Adrenergic Agonist, Clenbuterol, on Growth Performance and Carcass Composition of the Rat (percent change over control)

| Characteristic | Clenbuterol, ppm in diet | | |
| --- | --- | --- | --- |
| | 2 | 10 | 50 |
| Weight gain (g/day) | 4.8* | 9.6* | 8.5* |
| Feed intake (g/day) | 0.4 | −3.4 | 1.7 |
| Feed conversion (g feed/g gain) | −3.6 | −10.7* | −7.2* |
| Carcass protein (g/carcass) | 5.1* | 8.5** | 9.2** |
| Carcass fat (g/carcass) | −8.5* | −19.9** | −23.3** |

*$P < 0.05$ compared with control.
**$P < 0.01$ compared with control.

SOURCE: Ricks et al. (1985).

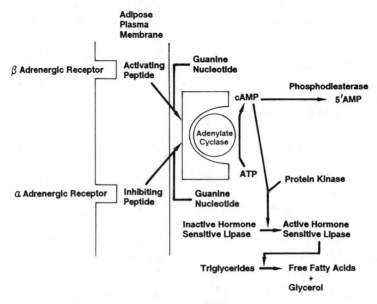

**FIGURE 2**   Scheme for the regulation of lipolysis by beta-agonists through specific adrenoceptors. Source: Adapted from J. A. Garcia-Sarnz and J. N. Fain. 1982. Regulation of adipose tissue metabolism by catecholamines: Roles of alpha₁, alpha₂, and beta-adrenoceptors. Trends Pharmacol. Sci. 3:201.

37°C. Lipolysis was estimated by measuring glycerol production. Glycerol was measured by a fluorometric modification of the enzymatic method of Wieland (1974). Lipogenesis was estimated by measuring the incorporation of [14]C-acetate into fatty acids from TGs.

Isoproterenol is very effective for stimulating lipolysis (glycerol release) in rat adipose tissue in vitro. At a concentration of 0.001 μM, isoproterenol had no effect on the basal rate of glycerol release; maximum stimulation occurred at 1 μM. The half-maximal effect dose was 0.017 μM. The idea that beta-agonists stimulate lipolysis through a specific beta-receptor is supported by the observation that the stimulation of lipolysis by isoproterenol can be blocked by beta-antagonists, such as propranolol or betaxolol.

Isoproterenol was also studied for its effects on lipogenesis ([14]C-acetate incorporation into FFAs in TGs) in rat adipose

tissue in vitro (Duquette and Muir, 1985). Insulin was used in this study to increase lipogenesis and to simulate in vivo conditions. Isoproterenol at concentrations of 0.01, 0.05, and 0.25 μM reduced [14]C-acetate incorporation into TGs in a dose-related manner. In addition, when the TGs were hydrolyzed and the resulting FFAs and glycerol were tested for [14]C activity, the results showed that the effect of isoproterenol was primarily to reduce the incorporation of [14]C-acetate into FFAs with only minor effects on glycerol. These observations support the validity of this test system for estimating lipogenesis.

These in vitro test systems for lipolysis and lipogenesis were used to compare the activities of four different beta-agonists. Isoproterenol, clenbuterol, L-640,033, and BRL35135 were dose-titrated in rat adipose tissue to study their effects on lipolysis and lipogenesis (Duquette and Muir, 1985). All four inhibited lipogenesis and stimulated lipolysis. The intrinsic activity of all beta-agonists was similar for both actions. This means that the maximum effects of the beta-agonists, independent of dose, were of similar magnitude for each effect. Three of the four beta-agonists were 5 to 10 times more potent as inhibitors of lipogenesis than as stimulators of lipolysis; BRL35135 was equally potent for both. A comparison of the potencies of these drugs for inhibition of lipogenesis, as measured by 50 percent effective concentration, were isoproterenol > BRL35135 > L-640,033 > clenbuterol. Similar comparisons for stimulation of lipolysis were BRL35135 > isoproterenol > L-640,033 > clenbuterol. These observations suggest that in the animal a drug's efficacy for reducing body lipids may be even more dependent on that drug's activity for blocking lipogenesis than for stimulating lipolysis. They also indicate that there is considerable variation between beta-agonists in their potencies for blocking lipogenesis and stimulating lipolysis.

The ability of adipocytes from different animal species to initiate lipolysis in response to similar concentrations of isoproterenol was investigated by Muir et al. (1985). Adipocytes from sheep, pigs, and rats all responded with increases of 380 to 2,300 percent over their controls. Adipocytes from chickens failed to respond.

Because chicken adipocytes failed to respond to isoproterenol, a more detailed study was conducted. The beta-agonists isoproterenol, clenbuterol, and L-640,033 and the positive control glucagon were all tested at concentrations of 0.01, 0.05, 0.25, 1.25, and 6.25 $\mu$M for effects on lipolysis in isolated chicken adipocytes (Muir et al., 1985). As expected, the chicken adipocytes responded to glucagon with increased lipolysis. However, none of the three beta-agonists stimulated lipolysis at any of the concentrations tested.

Since the chicken, unlike the other species studied, synthesizes FFAs in the liver, the effects of beta-agonists on lipogenesis

in isolated chicken hepatocytes were investigated. Isoproterenol, clenbuterol, and L-640,033 and the positive control glucagon were tested on chicken hepatocytes in a design identical to the one described for chicken adipocytes (Muir et al., 1985). As expected, glucagon caused a dose-related inhibition in $^{14}$C-acetate incorporation into FFAs in TGs (that is, inhibition of lipogenesis). All three beta-agonists also caused a dose-related inhibition of lipogenesis. Thus, beta-agonists block body fat accumulation in chickens by inhibiting lipogenesis in the liver, but they are not able to stimulate lipolysis in adipose tissue.

In summary, beta-agonists have been shown to stimulate lipolysis and inhibit lipogenesis in the adipose tissue of the rat (Muir et al., 1985). In adipose tissue from sheep and swine, beta-agonists can stimulate lipolysis, but no data are available regarding their effects on lipogenesis in these species. Beta-agonists are ineffective in chicken adipocytes. However, they inhibit lipogenesis in chicken hepatocytes, the primary site for fatty acid synthesis in poultry.

## EFFECTS OF BETA-AGONISTS ON SKELETAL MUSCLE PROTEIN METABOLISM

Skeletal muscle cells have beta-receptors, and beta-agonists increase skeletal muscle protein in animals. Thus, beta-agonists might exert a direct effect on skeletal muscle cells, or their effect could be indirect through changes in plasma hormone concentrations or nutrient partitioning. Herbert et al. (1986) measured the effects of clenbuterol on urinary nitrogen excretion by sheep by infusing clenbuterol together with feedstuffs directly into the abomasum. Within 6 hours after the initiation of infusion, nitrogen excretion dropped about 25 percent and remained depressed over the entire 7-day test. These results suggest that clenbuterol caused an immediate improvement in nitrogen retention.

Muscle protein accumulation is the net balance of protein synthesis minus protein degradation. A drug like clenbuterol that dramatically increases muscle protein accumulation might be expected to act by altering the rate of muscle protein synthesis, degradation, or both. This was examined by Reeds et al. (1986), who fed clenbuterol at 0 or 2 ppm in the diet to young male rats. The rates of protein synthesis in two skeletal muscles—the gastrocnemius and soleus— were estimated by the method of Garlick et al. (1980). Rats were injected with a large dose of labeled phenylalanine and killed 10 minutes later. The rate of protein synthesis was estimated from the amount of labeled phenylalanine in the muscle protein and from the specific activity of the free phenylalanine. Protein deposition was calculated from the slope of the line of the log of the protein content versus time. Protein content was estimated from body weight. The rate of protein degradation was estimated from the differences between rates of synthesis and deposition. The effects of clenbuterol on muscle protein mass and rates of protein synthesis and degradation were determined on days 4, 11, and 21 of treatment.

After only 4 days of clenbuterol treatment, the protein masses of the gastrocnemius and soleus muscles were increased 17.7 and 50.6 percent, respectively, over the controls. These larger muscle protein masses were maintained throughout the 21-day test period. In both the gastrocnemius and soleus muscles, the rate of protein degradation was decreased on day 4 by 55 percent, with no change in the rate of protein synthesis. By day 11, this decrease in the rate of protein degradation relative to the controls was still evident, but the magnitude of the decrease was slightly less (39 and 25 percent for the gastrocnemius and soleus muscles, respectively). The rates of protein synthesis were still the same as for the controls. At day 21, the rates of protein degradation were still reduced (20 and 30 percent, respectively), but the rates

of protein synthesis had decreased 20 percent relative to the controls.

These observations suggest that clenbuterol increases skeletal muscle protein in the rat by reducing the rate of muscle protein degradation. Apparently, after muscle protein mass is increased by a certain amount, the rate of protein synthesis is reduced. At this point, the rate of muscle protein accumulation is reduced to normal, but the extra muscle protein mass is maintained.

## SEPARATION OF LIPID AND PROTEIN EFFECTS OF BETA-AGONISTS

The information presented thus far demonstrates that beta-agonists reduce the content of lipids in the carcass, increase the accumulation of skeletal muscle protein, and improve the growth rate and feed conversion of the animal. To understand the mode of action of beta-agonists, studies were undertaken to determine whether the growth and feed conversion responses were associated with the effects of the beta-agonists on lipid metabolism, protein metabolism, or both.

L-640,033 is an excellent growth-promoting beta-agonist. BRL35135 is a potent inhibitor of lipogenesis and a potent stimulator of lipolysis, but it does not appear to affect muscle protein metabolism. Both beta-agonists were evaluated in similar rat growth trials. In each trial, 110 young male rats (10 per treatment and 20 controls) were fed the beta-agonist at 0, 0.25, 1.0, 2.5, 5.0, 10, 15, 25, or 50 ppm for 2 weeks. Clenbuterol at 10 ppm was used as a positive control. Rate of gain, feed intake, and feed conversion were determined. In addition, the weights of the gastrocnemius muscle and epididymal fat pads were measured to assess the effects of the drugs on skeletal muscle protein and carcass fat.

L-640,033 increased rate of gain in a dose-related manner (Rickes et al., 1985). Feed consumption was increased only at the two highest doses (25 and 50 ppm). Feed conversion was improved 4 to 6 percent, independent of dose. Also, L-640,033 increased gastrocnemius muscle weight and decreased epididymal fat pad weight, both in dose-related manners (Rickes et al., 1985). Both responses were similar to those observed with clenbuterol at 10 ppm.

BRL35135 had no effect on either rate of gain or feed conversion at any of the doses tested. Clenbuterol, the positive control, increased rate of gain and improved feed conversion. As expected, BRL35135 reduced epididymal fat pad weight in a dose-related manner, with the maximum effect at 5 ppm. The reduction in epididymal fat pad weight with BRL35135 was significantly greater than that with clenbuterol. BRL35135 did not increase gastrocnemius muscle weight, while clenbuterol increased it 17 percent. Thus, BRL35135 reduced carcass lipids in the rat without increasing skeletal muscle protein or improving rate of gain or feed conversion.

These observations suggest that improvements in growth rate and feed conversion obtained with beta-agonists are associated with the effects of the drugs on skeletal muscle protein metabolism and not with their effects on lipid metabolism. Thus, while the ability of a beta-agonist to reduce carcass fat is an important benefit, this activity does not appear to be related to any growth-promoting activity.

### EFFECTS OF BETA-AGONISTS ON PLASMA HORMONES

The effect of beta-agonists on plasma hormone levels is an important consideration when assessing the possible modes of action of these drugs in promoting growth. Thus, a study was carried out in which 50 young male rats (10 per treatment and 20 controls) were fed clenbuterol at 10 ppm, BRL35135 at 15 ppm, or L-640,033 at 15 ppm for 2 weeks (L. A. Muir, unpublished data). At necropsy, gastrocnemius muscle

and epididymal fat pad weights were measured to assess the effects of the beta-agonists on skeletal muscle protein and carcass lipids. In addition, blood samples were obtained and assayed for plasma growth hormone, insulin, somatomedin-C (SM-C), and glucose.

All three beta-agonists produced the expected changes in gastrocnemius muscle and epididymal fat pad weights. Clenbuterol and L-640,033 increased gastrocnemius muscle weight and decreased epididymal fat pad weights. BRL35135 decreased epididymal fat pad weight, but did not alter gastrocnemius muscle weight. Plasma insulin levels were decreased approximately 30 percent by clenbuterol and L-640,033, but were not decreased by BRL35135. Similar effects were observed for SM-C. Plasma growth hormone was decreased by all three drugs, especially BRL35135, but the responses were so variable that none of these growth hormone reductions was statistically significant. Clenbuterol decreased plasma glucose, while the other beta-agonists had no effect on glucose.

Beermann et al. (1985) reported that cimaterol fed to lambs for 12 weeks reduced plasma insulin and elevated plasma $T_4$ (thyroid hormone thyroxine) but did not alter plasma levels of $T_3$ (thyroid hormone triiodothyronine), cortisol, or prolactin.

### SUMMARY

Beta-adrenergic agonists are analogs of the catecholamines epinephrine and norepinephrine. They appear to work through specific beta-adrenoceptors on the surface of adipocytes and skeletal muscle cells. Beta-adrenergic agonists that are known to promote growth, such as clenbuterol, cimaterol, and L-640,033, improve the growth rate and feed conversion of sheep and poultry. Effects on swine are more variable, while definitive data on cattle are not yet available. These drugs have also been shown to decrease total carcass fat and to increase total carcass protein in all four animal species. Many beta-adrenergic agonists reduce carcass lipids by stimulating lipolysis and blocking lipogenesis in adipose tissue. The exception occurs in poultry, where these drugs inhibit lipogenesis in the liver but do not stimulate lipolysis in adipose tissue. Less is known about the effects of beta-adrenergic agonists on protein metabolism in skeletal muscle. However, recent studies suggest that some of these drugs increase skeletal muscle protein accretion by reducing the rate of protein degradation without altering the rate of protein synthesis. Studies in rats comparing the growth-promoting and carcass-altering effects of two beta-adrenergic agonists, L-640,033 and BRL35135, indicate that improvements in growth rate and feed conversion with beta-adrenergic agonists are associated with improved protein accretion rather than altered lipid metabolism. Finally, growth-promoting beta-adrenergic agonists were found to reduce plasma levels of insulin and somatomedin-C in the rat but did not elevate plasma growth hormone levels. These observations support the concept that growth-promoting beta-adrenergic agonists work directly through skeletal muscle cell receptors and not indirectly through the elevation of plasma growth hormone or insulin concentrations. In addition, beta-adrenergic agonists that reduce carcass lipids appear to work directly through beta-adrenoceptors on the surface of adipocytes in livestock and hepatocytes in poultry.

## ACKNOWLEDGMENT

The author wishes to acknowledge the work of Paul Duquette, Eric Rickes, and Sandra Wien, who contributed to numerous aspects of the beta-agonist research at Merck, and Dr. Y. T. Yang, whose ideas and research findings supported our beta-agonists research program.

## REFERENCES

Arch, J. R. S., M. A. D. Phil, and A. T. Ainsworth. 1983. Thermogenic and antiobesity activity of a novel beta-adrenoceptor agonist (BRL26830A) in mice and rats. Am. J. Clin. Nutr. 38:549.

Arch, J. R. S., A. T. Ainsworth, M. A. Cawthorne, V. Piercy, M. V. Sennitt, V. E. Thody, C. Wilson, and S. Wilson. 1984. Atypical beta-adrenoceptor on brown adipocytes as target for anti-obesity drugs. Nature 309:163.

Baker, P. K., R. H. Dalrymple, D. L. Ingle, and C. A. Ricks. 1984. Use of a beta-adrenergic agonist to alter muscle and fat deposition in lambs. J. Anim. Sci. 59:1256.

Beermann, D. H., W. R. Butler, D. E. Hogue, R. H. Dalrymple, and C. A. Ricks. 1985. Plasma metabolic hormone, glucose, and free fatty acid concentrations in lambs fed the repartitioning agent, cimaterol (CL 263,780). J. Anim. Sci. 61(Suppl. 1):254 (Abstr.).

Beermann, D. H., D. E. Hogue, V. K. Fishell, R. H. Dalrymple, and C. A. Ricks. 1986. Effects of cimaterol and fishmeal on performance, carcass characteristics and skeletal muscle growth in lambs. J. Anim. Sci. 62:370.

Burroughs, W., C. C. Culbertson, J. Kastelic, E. Cheng, and W. H. Hale. 1954. The effects of trace amounts of diethylstilbesterol in rations of fattening steers. Science 120:66.

Dalrymple, R. H., P. K. Baker, P. E. Gingher, D. L. Ingle, J. M. Pensack, and C. A. Ricks. 1984. A repartitioning agent to improve performance and carcass composition of broilers. Poultry Sci. 63:2376.

Davis, L. W. 1969. MGA—A new concept in heifer feeding. Pp. 72–82 in Proceedings of the 24th Kansas Formula Feed Conference, Manhattan: Kansas State University of Agricultural and Applied Sciences.

Dinusson, W. E., F. N. Andrews, and W. M. Beeson. 1950. The effects of stilbesterol, testosterone, thyroid alteration and spaying on the growth and fattening of beef heifers. J. Anim. Sci. 9:321.

Duquette, P. F., and L. A. Muir. 1984. Effects of ovine growth hormone and other anterior pituitary hormones on lipolyis of rat and ovine adipose tissue in vitro. J. Anim. Sci. 58:1191.

Duquette, P. F., and L. A. Muir. 1985. Effect of the beta-adrenergic agonists isoproterenol, clenbuterol, L-640,033 and BRL35135 on lipolysis and lipogenesis in rat adipose tissue in vitro. J. Anim. Sci. 61(Suppl. 1):265 (Abstr.).

Garcia-Sarnz, J. A., and J. N. Fain. 1982. Regulation of adipose tissue metabolism by catecholamines: Roles of alpha$_1$, alpha$_2$ and beta-adrenoceptors. Trends Pharmacol. Sci. 3:201.

Garlick, P. S., M. A. McNurlan, and V. R. Preedy. 1980. A rapid and convenient technique for measuring the rate of protein synthesis in tissues by injection of "3H" phenylalanine. Biochem. J. 192:719.

Heitzman, R. J. 1980. Manipulation of protein metabolism, with special reference to anabolic agent. Pp. 193–203 in Protein Deposition in Animals, P. J. Buttery and D. B. Lindsay, eds. Boston: Butterworth.

Herbert, F., F. D. DeB. Hovell, and P. J. Reeds. 1986. Some preliminary observations on the immediate effects of clenbuterol on heart rate, body temperature and nitrogen retention in lambs wholly nourished by intragastric infusion. Br. J. Nutr. 56:483 (Abstr.).

Machlin, L. J. 1972. Effect of porcine growth hormone on growth and carcass composition of the pig. J. Anim. Sci. 35:794.

Moser, R. L., R. H. Dalrymple, S. G. Cornelius, J. E. Pettigrew, and C. E. Allen. 1986. Effect of cimaterol (CL 263,780) as a repartitioning agent in the diet for finishing pigs. J. Anim. Sci. 62:21.

Muir, L. A. 1985. Mode of action of exogenous substances on animal growth—an overview. J. Anim. Sci. 61(Suppl. 2):154.

Muir, L. A., M. W. Stutz, and G. E. Smith. 1977. Feed additives. Pp. 27–37 in Livestock Feeds and Feeding, D. C. Church, ed. Corvallis, Oreg.: O&B Books.

Muir, L. A., S. Wien, P. F. Duquette, E. L. Rickes, and E. H. Cordes. 1983. Effects of exogenous growth hormone and diethylstilbesterol on growth and carcass composition of growing lambs. J. Anim. Sci. 56:1315.

Muir, L. A., S. Wien, P. F. Duquette, and G. Olson. 1985. Effect of the beta-adrenergic agonist L-640,033 on lipid metabolism, growth and carcass characteristics of female broiler chickens. J. Anim. Sci. 61(Suppl. 1):263 (Abstr.).

Reeds, P. J., S. M. Hay, P. M. Dorwood, and R. M. Palmer. 1986. Stimulation of muscle growth by clenbuterol: Lack of effect on muscle protein biosynthesis. Br. J. Nutr. 56:249.

Rickes, E. L., L. A. Muir, and P. F. Duquette. 1985. Effect of the beta-adrenergic agonist L-640,033 on growth and carcass composition of growing male rats. J. Anim. Sci. 61(Suppl. 1):264 (Abstr.).

Ricks, C. A., R. H. Dalrymple, P. K. Baker, and D. L. Ingle. 1984. Use of beta-agonist to alter fat and muscle deposition in steers. J. Anim. Sci. 59:1247.

Rodbell, M. 1964. Metabolism of isolated fat cells. I. Effects of hormone on glucose metabolism and lipolysis. J. Biol. Chem. 239:375.

Wagner, J. F., and E. L. Veenhuizen. 1978. Growth performance, carcass deposition and plasma hormone levels in wether lambs when treated with growth hormone and thyroprotein. J. Anim. Sci. 47(Suppl. 1):397.

Wieland, O. 1974. Glycerol UV-method. Pp. 1404–1409 in Methods of Enzymatic Analysis, H. U. Bergmeyer, ed. New York: Academic Press.

# Anabolic Effects of Porcine Somatotropin on Pig Growth

TERRY D. ETHERTON

Animal agriculture must develop ways to enhance the growth performance of animals raised for meat production in order to provide consumers with a product that is leaner and, therefore, more nutritious. Because leaner meat products will be sought by consumers concerned about the relation between the consumption of saturated fatty acids and the incidence of coronary heart disease, strategies to increase growth rate and improve feed efficiency (ratio of feed consumed to body weight gained) will economically benefit producers. The central question is, what research options are available now and in the foreseeable future that may provide effective ways to manipulate meat animal growth performance?

This paper focuses on the concept that an elevation of blood concentrations of growth hormone (GH, or somatotropin) in meat animals markedly increases growth rate, improves feed efficiency, and dramatically increases muscle mass while decreasing adipose tissue (fat) mass (Chung et al., 1985; Etherton et al., 1986a, 1986b, 1987; Machlin, 1972). Table 1 shows the extent to which growth hormone can affect the growth performance of pigs. The stimulatory effects of GH on growth performance have created great interest in developing a GH-based product for practical use in animal agriculture. In fact, it is likely that such a product will be available for use within the next 2 to 3 years. The mechanisms by which GH works are discussed in the following section, since a better understanding of them may lead to ways to improve the effectiveness of GH or of alternative strategies for enhancing growth performance.

Growth hormone is a protein that is synthesized in the anterior pituitary gland of mammals. It plays a central role in stimulating normal growth and is both anabolic and catabolic in that it stimulates growth rate and muscle accretion and concurrently decreases adipose tissue growth (Etherton et al., 1986b, 1987). The positive effects of GH on growth rate are indirect, being mediated largely by the GH-dependent insulin-like growth factor I (IGF-I, or somatomedin-C) (Etherton and Kensinger, 1984). The effects of GH on adipose tissue growth and metabolism are direct, not being mediated by IGF-I (Walton and Etherton, 1986; Walton et al., 1986, 1987a).

Observations by Etherton and coworkers

TABLE 1  Effects of Porcine Growth Hormone on Growth Performance (in percent)

| Performance Factor | Dosage of Porcine Growth Hormone[a] (µg/kg body wt) | | |
|---|---|---|---|
| | 35 | 70 | 140 |
| Carcass lipid | −29 | −32 | −68 |
| Muscle | +21 | +26 | +24 |
| Feed/gain | −12 | −21 | −24 |

[a] Dose of porcine GH given daily per kilogram of body weight for 77 days by intramuscular injection. Values are percentage response versus that for control pigs. For example, carcass lipid decreased 68 percent, muscle mass increased 24 percent, and the amount of feed consumed per unit body weight gain decreased 24 percent in pigs given 140 µg/kg body wt.

SOURCE: Adapted from T. Etherton, C. Evock, C. Chung, P. Walton, M. Sillence, K. Magri, and R. Ivy. 1986. Stimulation of pig growth performance by long-term treatment with pituitary porcine growth hormone (pGH) and a recombinant pGH. J. Anim. Sci. 63(Suppl. 1):219.

that GH enhances growth performance suggest that any strategy that increases the blood levels of GH should be a viable approach for manipulating growth performance. However, the extent to which GH must be elevated and for how long is still not clear. Since administration of exogenous GH effectively stimulates growth performance, it is reasonable to ask whether an increase in the secretion of endogenous GH can lead to similar anabolic effects. Implicit in this question is that tools are available that allow GH secretion to be modulated.

In 1982, a hypothalamic peptide that stimulates GH release was purified from tumors of patients with acromegaly (Guillemin et al., 1982; Rivier et al., 1982). Subsequently, the growth hormone releasing factor (GRF) from porcine and bovine hypothalami was purified and sequenced (Bohlen et al., 1983; Esch et al., 1983). GRF is a potent, specific stimulant of GH release in pigs and cattle (Etherton et al., 1986b; Moseley et al., 1984). Aside from studies done in our laboratory (Etherton et al., 1986b), there are few published data on the effects of long-term administration of GRF on growth performance of meat animals. Our studies have shown positive effects; however, the magnitude has been less than that observed for GH-treated pigs (Etherton et al., 1986b). Because so little is known about the optimal dose and temporal profile of GRF administration, it is premature to conclude that GRF is less effective than GH treatment. Nonetheless, it has been established that chronic GRF treatment does not result in pituitary refractoriness to the stimulatory effects of GRF. This indicates that the capacity of the pituitary to respond to GRF is not diminished over time, thereby suggesting that GRF treatment is a viable candidate for promoting growth. Furthermore, GRF analogs have been synthesized that are considerably more potent than the 44-amino-acid peptide synthesized in the hypothalamus and that therefore may be more effective in promoting growth than the naturally occurring peptide.

The counter-regulatory peptide to GRF is somatostatin, which inhibits GH release. The paper by Schelling and Byers in this volume discusses neutralization of somatostatin as a possible means to enhance growth performance. It is likely that concurrent stimulation of GRF and inhibition of somatostatin would enhance growth performance more than either approach alone.

The elevation of blood GH by exogenous GH treatment leads to a cascade of biological events that account for the increase in growth performance. One such event is an increase in the level of somatomedin (IGF-I) in the blood. Given that many of the somatogenic effects of GH appear to be mediated by IGF-I, it is reasonable to speculate that administration of exogenous IGF-I may be a feasible way to enhance growth performance. But because sufficient quantities of recombinant IGF-I are scarce, this hypothesis has not yet been tested in meat animals.

At least two points must be considered regarding IGF-I treatment as a potential growth promoter. First, it is transported by a specific carrier protein (Martin and Baxter, 1986; Zapf et al., 1975) that also affects bioavailability of the hormone to the target tissue. For example, free (unbound) IGF-I is an insulin mimic in bovine and porcine adipose tissue in terms of stimulating lipid metabolism (Etherton and Evock, 1986; Walton et al., 1987a), but addition of the carrier protein blocks these effects in rat and pig adipose tissue (Walton et al., 1987b). Because the circulating carrier protein is normally relatively saturated with IGF-I in serum from pigs (P. Walton and T. Etherton, unpublished data), exogenously administered IGF-I would be mostly free in the blood and act as an insulin mimic, resulting in hypoglycemia. Guler et al. (1986) have demonstrated this in mini-pigs treated with a bolus dose of IGF-I. More recent studies with pigs in our laboratory with recombinant human IGF-I have confirmed this (R. Gopinath and T. Etherton, unpublished data). However, the effects of IGF-I on growth performance in meat animals when the dose is below that which causes hypoglycemia and is given in a sustained manner still must be determined. A central question that arises is whether chronic treatment of animals with IGF-I stimulates expression of the gene that encodes for the carrier protein. If not, then exogenous treatment of meat animals with IGF-I may not be an effective approach to growth manipulation since hypoglycemia would ensue. Also, when pigs are treated with GH, the increase in circulating IGF-I concentration is associated with a concurrent increase in carrier protein (P. Walton and T. Etherton, unpublished data).

The second point to consider in IGF-I treatment pertains to the effects of GH on adipose tissue metabolism. In cultured porcine and bovine adipose tissue, GH antagonizes insulin action (Etherton and Evock, 1986; Walton et al., 1986). In vivo, treatment of pigs with GH decreases the rate of synthesis of fatty acids and markedly blunts the sensitivity and responsiveness of adipocytes to insulin and free IGF-I (Walton et al., 1987a). Therefore, it seems unlikely that IGF-I treatment will decrease adipose tissue growth when the effects of the free hormone are stimulatory in the tissue and, hence, anabolic. It has been routinely found that in pigs treated with GH (Etherton et al., 1986b, 1987), adipose tissue growth is decreased rather than increased. Thus, the marked increase in IGF-I concentration in pigs treated with GH is not associated with an increase in adipose tissue growth. This suggests that the inhibition of the insulin-like effects of free IGF-I by the binding protein observed in vitro in pig adipose tissue also occurs in vivo (P. Walton and T. Etherton, unpublished data). And because the sensitivity of pig adipocytes to free IGF-I is blunted by GH in vivo, it appears that even if there were an increase in free IGF-I in blood or tissue, the adipocytes would be less responsive to the insulin-like effects of free IGF-I.

The unique characteristic of GH that appears to account for the remarkable improvement in feed efficiency of GH-treated animals is that it decreases adipose tissue growth. In the pig, this is associated with a decrease in the rate of fatty acid synthesis. This adaptation by the adipocytes results in a redirection of the nutrients from adipose tissue to other target tissues (such as muscle). This change in nutrient utilization not only accounts for the decrease in adipose tissue growth but also offers a possible explanation for how muscle growth is increased. In all our studies, we have consistently noted that blood urea nitrogen (BUN) is decreased in a GH-dependent manner. This indicates that hepatic amino acid oxidation is decreased, which, in turn, infers that delivery of amino acids from peripheral tissues (such as muscle) is decreased. The glucose carbon normally destined for deposition in adipose tissue may spare amino acids from being oxidized in muscle, thereby providing more amino acids for protein synthesis. Also, in tissue culture, IGF-I inhibits myofibrillar protein degradation and increases the rate of protein synthesis (Ewton and Florini, 1986). Collectively, these observations illustrate the remarkable coordination of nutrient partitioning that occurs among the various tissues in an animal. It is only now that we are beginning to appreciate the extent to which nutrient partitioning can be manipulated.

For some time endocrinologists have recognized that circulating protein hormones play a role in regulating the number and affinity of their respective receptors in the target cell. For example, treatment of rats with insulin has been shown to result in a decrease (down regulation) of insulin binding. Thus, a point of regulation occurs when the target cell recognizes the hormone. It may well be that differences exist among meat animals and that this contributes to the variations seen in growth performance. We thought that chronic treatment of pigs with GH might induce down regulation of GH binding and result in a decrease in tissue sensitivity. To assess this we measured GH binding to membranes prepared from livers from pigs treated with different doses of GH for 35 days. In contrast to our original speculation, GH treatment increased binding (Chung and Etherton, 1986), suggesting that tissue sensitivity to GH increases after treatment. If this is indeed the case, then future research must focus on the mechanisms that regulate GH receptor number, since this information may lead to alternative strategies for increasing growth performance. In particular, it will be important to increase our understanding of how the GH receptor produces signals that alter cell function so markedly and how this differs among the different target tissues (for example, muscle, liver, fat).

## PROSPECTS FOR INCREASING GROWTH PERFORMANCE

Growth hormone clearly increases meat animal growth performance, but before a GH-based product is developed for application in animal agriculture, two questions must be answered. First, will recombinant DNA technology enable sufficient quantities of the protein to be produced at a cost that will not limit product development? Little concrete information has been published on this topic; however, it is our belief that this is no longer a problem. Second, and more important, how will GH be administered at the farm level? Daily injections are impractical for large-scale production. Thus, a delivery system must be developed where GH is administered in a vehicle that provides for controlled delivery of the protein over a sustained period of time (e.g., 30 days). At present, this is the limiting step in the development of a GH-based product, although intense research in the area is ongoing.

It is possible that alternative means can be developed for enhancing growth performance, but it has been questioned whether there is really any need for them "after" GH. We contend that there is indeed such need. For one thing, strategies may be developed that improve the effectiveness of GH or that are synergistic to GH. In fact, there are data from studies that indicate that such approaches are possible. It has been found that blocking adrenal function significantly enhances responsiveness to GH in rats treated chronically with GH and trilostane (Sillence et al., 1987). Trilostane is a specific inhibitor of glucocorticoid hormone synthesis. It remains to be established whether trilostane also enhances GH potency in pigs.

Several conceptual approaches to manipulating growth performance have been presented, and it is likely that one or more will be developed into a product that dramatically affects animal agriculture. It is also reasonable to assume that other strategies will evolve as our understanding of the biological mechanisms that regulate growth and nutrient partitioning increases. For instance, certain monoclonal antibodies to GH, when complexed to the hormones, increase its bioactivity in mice (Holder et al., 1985).

An exciting era is evolving in animal agriculture. We now have available the means to alter growth performance in a way that is beneficial to both the producer and the consumer.

It should be emphasized that attempts to manipulate meat animal growth performance are not under way solely to produce larger animals that grow more rapidly but, rather, to enhance the efficiency of growth performance. Thus, it is remarkable that GH has its greatest effects on feed efficiency and carcass composition. In terms of the former, it is reasonable to conclude that the savings in feed costs could be on the order of $1 billion to $3 billion a year in the United States alone. This, along with the dramatic beneficial changes observed in carcass composition, sufficiently illustrates the need for this technology and its benefit to animal agriculture and society.

## REFERENCES

Bohlen, P., F. Esch, P. Brazeau, N. Ling, and R. Guillemin. 1983. Isolation and characterization of the porcine hypothalamic growth releasing factor. Biochem. Biophys. Res. Commun. 116:726.

Chung, C. S., and T. Etherton. 1986. Characterization of porcine growth hormone (pGH) binding to porcine liver microsomes: Chronic administration of pGH induces pGH binding. Endocrinology 119:780.

Chung, C. S., T. Etherton, and J. Wiggins. 1985. Stimulation of swine growth by porcine growth hormone. J. Anim. Sci. 60:118.

Esch, F., P. Bohlen, N. Ling, P. Brazeau, and R. Guillemin. 1983. Isolation and characterization of the bovine hypothalamic growth hormone releasing factor. Biochem. Biophys. Res. Commun. 117:772.

Etherton, T., and C. Evock. 1986. Stimulation of lipogenesis in bovine adipose tissue by insulin and insulin-like growth factor. J. Anim. Sci. 62:357.

Etherton, T., and R. Kensinger. 1984. Endocrine regulation of fetal and postnatal meat animal growth. J. Anim. Sci. 59:511.

Etherton, T., C. Evock, C. Chung, P. Walton, M. Sillence, K. Magri, and R. Ivy. 1986a. Stimulation of pig growth performance by long-term treatment with pituitary porcine growth hormone (pGH) and a recombinant pGH. J. Anim. Sci. 63(Suppl. 1):219.

Etherton, T., J. Wiggins, C. Chung, C. Evock, J. Rebhun, and P. Walton. 1986b. Stimulation of pig growth performance by porcine growth hormone and growth hormone-releasing factor. J. Anim. Sci. 63:1389.

Etherton, T., J. Wiggins, C. Evock, C. Chung, J. Rebhun, P. Walton, and N. Steele. 1987. Stimulation of pig growth performance by porcine growth hormone: Determination of the dose-response relationship. J. Anim. Sci. 64:433.

Ewton, D., and J. Florini. 1986. Binding to and actions of somatomedins on myoblasts and myotubes: Demonstration of actions mediated by the type I receptor. Paper presented at the 68th annual meeting of The Endocrine Society. P. 167. Bethesda, Md.: The Endocrine Society.

Guillemin, R., P. Brazeau, P. Bohlen, F. Esch, N. Ling, and W. Wehrenbert. 1982. Growth hormone-releasing factor from a human pancreatic tumor that caused acromegaly. Science 218:585.

Guler, H., P. Zenobi, J. Zapf, E. Scheiwiller, J. Merryweather, C. Scandella, W. Marki, and E. Froesch. 1986. IGF-I and II and recombinant human (RH) IGF-I are hypoglycemic in the rat, mini-pig, and men. Paper presented at the 68th annual meeting of The Endocrine Society. P. 129. Bethesda, Md.: The Endocrine Society.

Holder, A., R. Aston, M. Preece, and J. Ivanyi. 1985. Monoclonal antibody-mediated enhancement of growth hormone activity in vivo. J. Endocrinol. 107:R9.

Machlin, L. 1972. Effect of porcine growth hormone on growth and carcass composition of the pig. J. Anim. Sci. 35:794.

Martin, J., and R. Baxter. 1986. Insulin-like growth factor-binding protein from plasma: Purification and characterization. J. Biol. Chem. 261:8754.

Moseley, W., L. Krabill, A. Friedman, and R. Olsen. 1984. Growth hormone response of steers injected with synthetic human pancreatic growth hormone-releasing factor. J. Anim. Sci. 58:430.

Rivier, J., J. Spiess, M. Thorner, and W. Vale. 1982. Characterization of a growth hormone-releasing factor from a human pancreatic islet tumor. Nature 300:276.

Sillence, M. N., T. D. Etherton, and K. A. Magri. 1987. Growth response of normal female rats to porcine growth hormone is improved by trilostane. Paper presented at the 69th Annual Meeting of The Endocrine Society. Bethesda, Md.: The Endocrine Society.

Walton, P., and T. Etherton. 1986. Stimulation of lipogenesis by insulin in swine adipose tissue: Antagonism by porcine growth hormone. J. Anim. Sci. 62:1584.

Walton, P., T. Etherton, and C. Evock. 1986. Antagonism of insulin action in cultured pig adipose tissue by pituitary and recombinant porcine growth hormone: Potentiation by hydrocortisone. Endocrinology 118:2577.

Walton, P., T. Etherton, and C. Chung. 1987a. Exogenous pituitary and recombinant porcine growth hormones induce insulin and insulin-like growth factor I resistance in pig adipose tissue. Dom. Anim. Endocrinol. 4:183.

Walton, P. E., R. Gopinath, B. D. Burleigh, and T. D. Etherton. 1987b. An acid-stable subunit of porcine serum IGF binding protein specifically blocks biological action of IGF-I on adipose tissue. J. Anim. Sci. 65(Suppl. 1):274.

Zapf, J., M. Waldvogel, and E. Groesch. 1975. Binding of nonsuppressible insulin-like activity to human serum. Evidence for a carrier protein. Arch. Biochem. Biophys. 1687:638.

# Immunization of Beef Cattle Against Somatostatin

G. T. SCHELLING and F. M. BYERS

The roles and interactions of somatostatin, growth hormone releasing factor, somatotropin, and somatomedin are of great biological interest and appear to offer considerable potential for the modification of growth and production in food-producing animals. It is now clear that single hormones do not function independently to regulate growth. Rather, a number of events or cascading effects come into play to generate animal growth responses.

Somatotropin (ST) has been recognized as an important growth regulating factor for some time. Li (1973) demonstrated its anabolic nature relative to protein synthesis, and Raben (1973) demonstrated its catabolic nature through its ability to stimulate lipolysis. Daughaday et al. (1972) indicated that somatomedin (SM) was a factor induced by plasma ST, and Thorner et al. (1982) isolated several growth hormone releasing factor (GRF) peptides that induced ST release. The liver release of SM may require insulin (Schalch et al., 1979), and thyroxine may be required at the tissue level for SM to be effective (Froesch et al., 1976). The relationships among these agents became clearer when Vale et al. (1976) demonstrated that somatostatin (SS) inhibited ST release (Figure 1). It is also recognized that SS inhibits thyrotropin (Vale et al., 1976); insulin and glucagon (Mortimer et al., 1974); and gastrin, gastric inhibitory peptide, pepsin secretion, motilin, and vasoactive intestinal polypeptide (C. N. Bloom et al., 1974; S. R. Bloom et al., 1974). The current general state of knowledge indicates the potential to stimulate growth by exogenously providing additional GRF, ST, or SM. This paper explores the potential for achieving stimulated growth by immunologically alleviating the inhibitory effects of SS. Antibody binding of SS would reduce available SS and therefore shift the balance of control toward GRF, which presumably would result in greater ST production (Figure 2). The other inhibitory roles of SS cannot be neglected, however, since these influences could benefit the animal through enhanced metabolism or improved nutrient uptake and utilization.

## METHODS AND RESULTS

### Passive Immunization Against Somatostatin

Immunological approaches to generate antibodies for binding biologically active

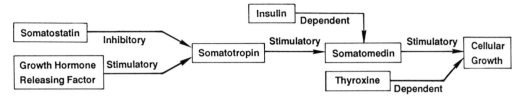

FIGURE 1 General hormonal relationships leading to increased growth.

molecules have been used as an analytical laboratory technique for some time. Subsequent studies extended passive immunization to animal studies. Arimura et al. (1975) generated SS-specific antiserum to study the effect of inhibiting SS on serum ST concentrations. The passive immunization of rats resulted in increased ST levels (Ferland et al., 1976), and rats injected with SS antiserum had a surge in plasma ST that continued for a 6-hour sampling period (Tannenbaum et al., 1978). Arimura and Fishback (1981) administered SS antiserum to rats daily for 3 days and found that the

mean serum ST of the treated rats was 76 ng/ml, while that of the control rats was 16.8 ng/ml.

Lawrence et al. (1985) conducted long-term passive immunization studies with rats to study ST concentrations and animal responses. After SS antiserum was produced in goats, rats were prepared with indwelling jugular vein catheters to facilitate the daily SS antiserum administration for 21 days. During this time, serum ST levels and performance criteria were measured weekly. An ST response was evident and peaked by day 10, when the immunized animals showed

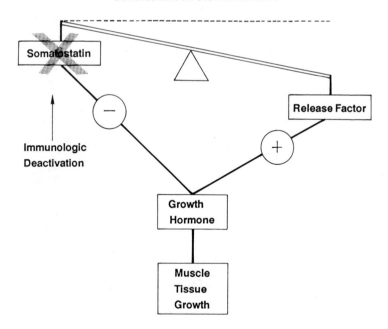

FIGURE 2 Imbalance created by deactivation of somatostatin.

an ST level of 184.9 ng/ml as compared with 7.6 ng/ml for the controls. However, the ST response diminished with time, and the levels in the test rats were similar to those in the controls by day 20. Table 1 indicates the weekly gains of the animals. There was a significant ($P < 0.05$) gain response during the first week, but the response gradually diminished over the next 2 weeks. This loss of response with time may have been due to secondary immunological responses, since whole serum was administered to the rats as the source of antibodies.

### Active Immunization Against Somatostatin

#### Hormonal Responses

Active immunity techniques appear to provide the best approach for taking advantage of the potential to immunize against SS. They involve establishing immunity to SS in the target animal by immunizing it with SS conjugated to an appropriate immunostimulating molecule (Figure 3). The animal should falsely recognize SS as a foreign molecule and begin the active production of antibodies that would bind the SS produced by the animal, thereby reducing available SS.

**TABLE 1** Average Weekly Gain of Rats Passively Immunized Against Somatostatin (in grams)

| Treatment | Week 1 | Week 2 | Week 3 |
|-----------|--------|--------|--------|
| Control   | 6.0    | 6.8    | 5.5    |
| Immunized | 7.4[a] | 6.8    | 5.7    |

[a]Different from the control ($P < 0.05$).

SOURCE: M. E. Lawrence, G. T. Schelling, T. W. Welsh, F. M. Byers, and L. W. Greene. 1985. Effect of passive immunization against somatostatin on plasma growth hormone and performance of growing rats. J. Anim. Sci. 61(Suppl. 1):47.

To study hormonal responses, Varner et al. (1980) actively immunized lambs against SS with an egg albumin-conjugated SS. The episodic nature of ST was thoroughly studied by taking frequent blood samples. Mean baseline and overall mean ST concentrations were significantly greater in the treated lambs (Table 2). The frequency of ST peaks was not influenced by the treatment, and peak amplitude was not statistically different because of high variation.

A number of other studies have not indicated a statistically significant ST response to active immunization in sheep (Chaplin et al., 1984; Galbraith et al., 1985; Spencer and Williamson, 1981). Similar studies with growing cattle (Lawrence et al., 1986)

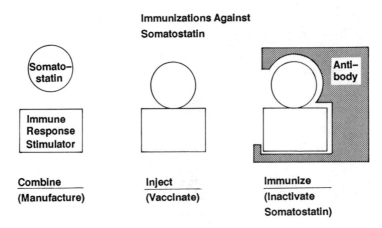

**Immunizations Against Somatostatin**

**FIGURE 3** Generation of antigen and subsequent somatostatin antibody production.

TABLE 2   Somatotropin Response to Active Immunization of
Lambs Against Somatostatin

| Variable | Control | Immunized | P |
|---|---|---|---|
| Baseline | 4.0 | 6.8 | <0.05 |
| Amplitude (ng/ml) | 10.0 | 18.1 | NS[a] |
| Overall mean (ng/ml) | 4.2 | 7.1 | <0.05 |
| Frequency (spikes/12 hours) | 1.7 | 2.0 | NS |

[a]NS = not significant.

SOURCE: M. A. Varner, S. L. Davis, and J. J. Reeves. 1980. Temporal
concentrations of growth hormone, thyrotropin, insulin and glucagon in sheep
immunized against somatostatin. Endocrinology 106:1027.

weighing 250 or 350 kg not only showed no
positive ST response, but trends were toward lower ST levels with active immunization. Although some studies have indicated the ability of metabolically challenged
immunized sheep to yield a greater ST
response (Spencer et al., 1983b; Varner et
al., 1980), GRF challenge studies with actively immunized growing beef cattle (D.
C. Kenison, G. T. Schelling, F. M. Byers,
and L. W. Greene, unpublished data) resulted in only slightly higher ST responses.

While ST level and challenge studies do
not provide convincing evidence of consistent ST responses to active immunization,
subtle ST changes of biological importance
should not be ruled out, since thorough
studies of the measurement of ST turnover
have not yet been reported. Increased ST
turnover rate in actively immunized animals
could be responsible for the inconsistent
responses in the other ST parameters reported. A general ST response is supported
by reports of consistent SM responses in
sheep actively immunized against SS (Spencer and Williamson, 1981; Spencer et al.,
1983b). An SM response would presumably
be mediated through ST.

### Growth Responses

Spencer and Williamson (1981) were the
first to show that lambs actively immunized
against somatostatin gained weight more
rapidly than lambs not actively immunized.

Lambs immunized at 3 weeks of age and at
regular intervals thereafter with SS conjugated to human serum globulin gained weight
faster than their twin counterparts injected
with human serum globulin alone. This
finding was in contrast to the earlier results
of Varner et al. (1980). The lack of a growth
response in the work of Varner et al. (1980)
was probably due to the nearly mature sheep
used in that study. The experiment was
designed to specifically investigate hormonal responses, and young, rapidly growing animals were not used. Recent work by
Spencer et al. (1983b), which is more detailed in nature, resulted in similar positive
gain responses with growing lambs immunized against SS.

Chaplin et al. (1984) immunized lambs at
3 weeks of age and every 11 days thereafter
for 103 days. The treated lambs gained
weight 16.6 percent faster than the control
animals. Other lamb studies by Bass et al.
(1983), Spencer et al. (1985), and Spencer
and Hallett (1985) have confirmed a rate of
gain response with immunization against
SS.

Lawrence et al. (1986) conducted immunization studies with 26 young, rapidly
growing, Charolais crossbred steers weighing 147 kg. Each treated steer was injected
with protein-conjugated SS every 2 weeks
during a 154-day study, and each control
steer was injected with the conjugated protein alone. Blood samples, taken every 2
weeks, indicated the development of a sig-

nificant SS antibody titer in each treated steer. A response in gain was observed after 56 days and was maintained ($P < 0.001$) throughout the 154-day study (Table 3). The treated cattle gained weight 17.6 percent faster than did the control cattle over the 154-day study. There was a positive correlation ($P < 0.001$) between SS antibody titer and average daily gain of the immunized steers.

Other work also indicates a gain response in beef cattle. G. T. Schelling, F. M. Byers, and L. W. Greene (unpublished data) studied 28 crossbred beef steers on ryegrass pasture. Fourteen were immunized against SS at the beginning of a 105-day trial and then twice during the trial. The control steers received placebo injections at the same time intervals. Table 4 shows that the treated cattle gained 115 kg compared with 103 kg for the control cattle, for an 11.6 percent gain response ($P < 0.05$) during the study. Another study, with a limited number of young dairy calves (Vicini et al., 1986), indicated that immunized calves gained more weight.

The efficiency of feed utilization is of utmost importance from the production standpoint. The feed efficiency associated with rate of gain was studied in some of the previously cited gain research. Spencer et al. (1983a) fed early-weaned lambs until slaughter to study feed efficiency. Beginning

at 3 weeks of age, the animals were immunized at regular intervals and showed a 14 percent improvement in feed efficiency. The lambs also gained weight faster, and there was a 20 percent reduction in time to reach slaughter weight. Other lamb studies indicated feed efficiency improvements of 11 percent (Spencer and Hallett, 1985) and 27 percent (Spencer, 1986).

In the beef cattle study of Lawrence et al. (1986), steers were fed a completely mixed feed that met or exceeded the nutrient requirements established by the National Research Council. The control and treated feed efficiencies (ratio of feed/gain) were 6.11 and 5.42, respectively, for a 12.7 percent improvement ($P < 0.01$) for the immunized steers (Table 3).

## Composition of Growth

A limited amount of data has been reported on the composition of growth in immunized animals. Spencer et al. (1983a) reported that lambs immunized against SS had an increased stature, as measured by shoulder height. This was subsequently confirmed by the observation of elongated bones during postmortem carcass dissection. Work by Spencer (1986) has demonstrated the increase in carcass weight and soft tissue that would be expected from lambs that gained weight faster and were heavier. The

TABLE 3   Effect of Active Immunization Against Somatostatin in Growing Cattle

| Variable | Control | Immunized |
| --- | --- | --- |
| Initial body weight (kg) | 147 | 147 |
| Final body weight (kg) | 329 | 361 |
| Average daily gain (kg) | 1.19 | 1.40[a] |
| Average daily gain response (%) | — | 17.6 |
| Feed efficiency (feed/gain) | 6.11 | 5.42[a] |
| Feed efficiency response (%) | — | 12.7 |

[a]Different from control ($P < 0.001$).

SOURCE:   M. E. Lawrence, G. T. Schelling, F. M. Byers, and L. W. Greene. 1986. Improvement of growth and feed efficiency in cattle by active immunization against somatostatin. J. Anim. Sci. 63(Suppl. 1):215.

TABLE 4   Effect of Active Immunization Against Somatostatin in Growing Cattle on Pasture

| Variable | Control | Immunized |
|---|---|---|
| Initial body weight (kg) | 235 | 235 |
| Final body weight (kg) | 338 | 350[a] |
| Gain (kg) | 103 | 115[a] |
| Average daily gain (kg) | 0.98 | 1.09[a] |
| Average daily gain response (%) | — | 11.6 |

[a]Different from control ($P < 0.05$).

SOURCE:   G. T. Schelling, F. M. Byers, and L. W. Greene (unpublished data).

work indicated no significant difference in the proportion of muscle (54 versus 53 percent) or fat (29 versus 31 percent) in control and treated lambs, even though the treated lamb carcasses were heavier (14.4 versus 17.1 kg). This suggests that treated animals would be leaner at a weight equal to that of the controls. There is a limited amount of research (Spencer and Hallett, 1985) with lambs slaughtered at the same weight to support the concept of leaner carcasses.

## Somatostatin Effects at the Gastrointestinal Tract

The role of SS at the level of the gastrointestinal tract (GIT) was recognized early. S. R. Bloom et al. (1974) reported effects of SS on motilin levels and gastric emptying. Boden et al. (1976) reported effects on duodenal motility. Other studies (Reichlin, 1987) have reported the influences of SS at the GIT level. Recent work by Gyr et al. (1986) has suggested that circulating plasma SS is a regulator of pancreatic function. Thus, control at the GIT level is probably more than just an effect of locally produced SS, and therefore, circulating antibodies could play an important role there.

Several studies have indicated an effect of SS on the rate of passage through the GIT of sheep. Faichney and Barry (1984) reported that the administration of SS in-

creased rate of passage. Subsequent work (Fadlalla et al., 1985) indicated an effect of passive immunization on the rate of passage. The intravenous administration of antibodies to SS resulted in an increase in the GIT retention time of chromic oxide, a GIT marker. Further elucidation of the net digestion and absorption effects of SS modification is not available at this time.

## Somatostatin Effects on Other Hormones

Evidence is emerging to indicate that immunization against SS may result in a fairly consistent increase in SM (Spencer, 1985). The general positive relationships among GH, SM, and growth are becoming more clearly formulated (Etherton and Kensinger, 1984). Thus, the concept of a growth response resulting from immunization against SS must also consider SM. The work of Plotsky and Vale (1985), which suggests a direct SS relationship with GRF release, must also be considered in evaluating all factors influencing growth. While the inhibitory relationships of SS to insulin and glucagon (Mortimer et al., 1974) and to thyrotropin (Vale et al., 1976) are clear, the importance of these relationships in the stimulation of growth by immunization is less evident. These possible associations make an understanding of the biology of the situation even more difficult.

## CONCLUSIONS

The original simple concept of immunizing against SS to reduce its general availability and thereby allow for increased ST release has turned into something very complex. It now appears that the relationships between SS and ST, other hormones, and GIT agents must also be considered. While direct ST involvement should by no means be ruled out as a mechanism of action at this time, it is clear that the striking serum ST concentration increases suggested by earlier rat studies do not occur in the active immunization of ruminants. It must be kept in mind that subtle ST responses, such as turnover, are difficult to detect and could very well be causing important biological influences. Considerable work will be required to elucidate the mechanisms of action. It is likely that significant progress will be made in this area in the near future because of current interest and the availability of resource materials to study growth regulation.

The immunization approach exhibits excellent potential, but its development will be challenging. The inherent complexity of the immunological response and our superficial understanding of hormonal relationships will present a formidable task. However, the application of "natural" biology to enable the animal to produce its own growth regulators in an appropriate pattern has an element of safety that should be readily accepted by the wary consumer. This approach could be an important new way to promote growth not only in beef cattle but in other species as well.

## REFERENCES

Arimura, A., and J. B. Fishback. 1981. Somatostatin: Regulation of secretion. Neuroendocrinology 33:246.

Arimura, A., H. Sato, D. Coy, and A. Schally. 1975. Radioimmunoassay for growth hormone release inhibiting hormone. Proc. Soc. Exp. Biol. Med. 148:784.

Bass, J. J., P. D. Gluckman, R. J. Fairclough, A. J. Peterson, and S. R. Davis. 1983. Effect of immunization against somatostatin and feed quality on growth controlling hormones and body composition. Proc. End. Soc. Australia 26(Suppl. 2):30.

Bloom, C. N., D. H. Coy, and A. V. Schally. 1974. Inhibition of gastrin and gastric-acid secretion by growth hormone release inhibiting hormone. Lancet 2:1106.

Bloom, S. R., D. N. Ralphs, G. M. Besser, R. Hall, D. H. Coy, A. J. Kastin, and A. V. Schally. 1974. Effect of somatostatin on motilin levels and gastric emptying. Gut 16:834.

Boden, G., H. Jacoby, and A. Staus. 1976. Somatostatin interacts with basal and carbachol stimulated antral and duodenal motility. Gastroenterology 70:961.

Chaplin, R. K., D. E. Kerr, and B. Laarveld. 1984. Somatostatin immunization and growth in lambs. Can. J. Anim. Sci. 64(Suppl.):312.

Daughaday, W. H., K. Hall, M. S. Raben, W. D. Salmon, Jr., J. L. Van den Brande, and J. J. Van Wyk. 1972. Somatomedin: Proposed designation for sulphation factor. Nature 235:107.

Etherton, T. D., and R. S. Kensinger. 1984. Endocrine regulation of fetal and postnatal meat animal growth. J. Anim. Sci. 59:511.

Fadlalla, A. M., G. S. G. Spencer, and D. Lister. 1985. The effect of passive immunization against somatostatin on marker retention time in lambs. J. Anim. Sci. 61:234.

Faichney, G. J., and T. N. Barry. 1984. Intravenous somatostatin infusion affects gastro-intestinal tract function in sheep. Can. J. Anim. Sci. 64(Suppl.):93.

Ferland, I., F. Labrie, M. Jobin, A. Arimura, and A. V. Schally. 1976. Physiological role of somatostatin in the control of growth hormone and thyrotropin secretion. Biochem. Biophys. Res. Commun. 68:149.

Froesch, E. R., J. Zapf, T. K. Audhya, E. Benporath, B. J. Segen, and K. B. Gibson. 1976. Non-suppressible insulin-like activity and thyroid hormones: Major pituitary-dependent sulphation factors for chick embryo cartilage. Proc. Natl. Acad. Sci. USA 73:2904.

Galbraith, H., S. Wigzell, J. R. Scaife, and G. D. Henderson. 1985. Growth and metabolic response of rapidly growing male castrate lambs to immunization against somatostatin. Anim. Prod. 40:523.

Gyr, K., C. Beglinger, E. Kohler, and U. Keller. 1986. Circulating somatostatin (S-14) inhibits both endo- and exocrine pancreatic function in man. International Conference on Somatostatin. P. 78, Abstract No. II-43. Serono Symposia, Washington, D.C.

Lawrence, M. E., G. T. Schelling, T. W. Welsh, F. M. Byers, and L. W. Greene. 1985. Effect of passive immunization against somatostatin on plasma growth hormone and performance of growing rats. J. Anim. Sci. 61(Suppl. 1):47.

Lawrence, M. E., G. T. Schelling, F. M. Byers, and L. W. Greene. 1986. Improvement of growth and feed efficiency in cattle by active immunization against somatostatin. J. Anim. Sci. 63(Suppl. 1):215.

Li, C. H. 1973. Growth hormone: Purification and biochemical characterization. P. 257 in Methods in Investigative and Diagnostic Endocrinology, S. A. Benson and R. S. Yalow, eds. Amsterdam: North-Holland.

Mortimer, C. H., D. Carr, T. Lind, S. R. Bloom, C. N. Mallinson, A. V. Schally, W. M. G. Tunbridge, L. Yeomans, D. H. Coy, A. Kastin, G. M. Besser, and R. Hall. 1974. Effects of growth hormone release inhibiting hormone on circulating glucagon, insulin and growth hormone in normal, diabetic, acromegaly and hypopituitary patients. Lancet 1:697.

Plotsky, P. M., and W. Vale. 1985. Patterns of growth hormone-releasing factor and somatostatin secretion into the hypophysial-portal circulation of the rat. Science 230:461.

Raben, M. S. 1973. Physiology: Hormonal effects. P. 257 in Methods in Investigative and Diagnostic Endocrinology, S. A. Benson and R. S. Yalow, eds. Amsterdam: North-Holland.

Reichlin, S., ed. 1987. Somatostatin, basic and clinical studies. Pp. 221–290. New York: Plenum Press.

Schalch, D. S., U. E. Heinrich, B. Draznin, C. J. Johnson, and L. L. Miller. 1979. Role of liver in regulating somatomedin activity: Hormonal effect on the synthesis and release of insulin-like growth factor and its carrier protein by the isolated perfused rat liver. Endocrinology 104:1143.

Spencer, G. S. G. 1985. Hormonal systems regulating growth. A review. Livestock Prod. Sci. 12:31.

Spencer, G. S. G. 1986. Immuno-neutralization of somatostatin and its effects on animal production. Dom. Anim. Endocrinol. 3:55.

Spencer, G. S. G., and K. G. Hallett. 1985. Immunization against somatostatin in a commercial breed of sheep and its effect on growth and efficiency. Anim. Prod. 40:523.

Spencer, G. S. G., and E. D. Williamson. 1981. Increased growth in lambs following auto-immunization against somatostatin. Anim. Prod. 32:376.

Spencer, G. S. G., G. J. Garssen, and P. L. Bergstrom. 1983a. A novel approach to growth promotion using auto-immunization against somatostatin. II. Effects on appetite, carcass composition and food utilization in lambs. Livestock Prod. Sci. 10:409.

Spencer, G. S. G., G. J. Garssen, and I. C. Hart. 1983b. A novel approach to growth promotion using auto-immunization against somatostatin. I. Effects on growth and hormone levels in lambs. Livestock Prod. Sci. 10:25.

Spencer, G. S. G., K. G. Hallett, and A. M. Fadlalla. 1985. A novel approach to growth promotion using auto-immunization against somatostatin. III. Effects in a commercial breed of sheep. Livestock Prod. Sci. 13:43.

Tannenbaum, G. S., J. Epelbaum, E. Colle, P. Brazeau, and J. B. Martin. 1978. Dissociation of effects of somatostatin antiserum on growth hormone and insulin secretion. Metabolism 27:1263.

Thorner, M. D., R. L. Perryman, M. J. Cronin, M. Draznin, A. Johanson, A. D. Rogol, J. Jane, L. Rudolf, E. Horvath, K. Kovacs, and W. Vale. 1982. Acromegaly with somatotroph hyperplasia: Successful treatment by restriction of a pancreatic tumor secreting a GH-releasing factor. Clin. Res. 30:555.

Vale, W., P. Brazeau, C. Rivier, M. Brown, B. Boss, J. Rivier, R. Burgus, N. Ling, and R. Guillemin. 1976. Somatostatin. Rec. Prog. Hormone Res. 31:365.

Varner, M. A., S. L. Davis, and J. J. Reeves. 1980. Temporal concentrations of growth hormone, thyrotropin, insulin and glucagon in sheep immunized against somatostatin. Endocrinology 106:1027.

Vicini, J. L., J. H. Clark, W. L. Hurley, and J. M. Bahr. 1986. Effect of immunization against somatostatin on growth of young dairy calves. J. Anim. Sci. 63(Suppl. 1):242.

# Lactation Biology and Methods of Increasing Efficiency

RONALD C. GOREWIT

Breakthroughs in biotechnology have made it possible to manipulate physiological mechanisms controlling the growth and development of organ systems, as well as processes such as milk secretion that are of economic importance. Recombinant derived bovine growth hormone (bSTH) has a dramatic effect on increasing milk production and mammary growth in dairy cattle. This paper briefly summarizes the biology of lactation, using the dairy cow as a model. It then reviews a number of experiments in which the dramatic influence of bSTH on milk secretion and mammary gland development has been shown and alternative methods for increasing the efficiency of mammary gland function have been examined.

## MAMMARY ANATOMY

The cow has four mammary glands grouped into a structure called an udder, which is located in the inguinal region of the cow's body. Milk is secreted by alveolar epithelial cells, which are grouped into small clusters called lobules. Lobules are surrounded by connective tissue capsules (Schmidt, 1971;

Turner, 1939, 1952), often referred to as stroma. Groups of lobules form larger structures called lobes and are considered to be the parenchymal elements. The entire mammary gland is composed of lobules and lobes. The lobules are drained by small ducts. The smaller ducts or capillary milk ducts are lined with a single layer of epithelial cells and are capable of secretion. The ducts get progressively larger until they reach a cistern, which is connected to a teat by which milk is released upon suckling or machine milking (Schmidt, 1971; Turner, 1939, 1952).

A group of cells called basket cells or myoepithelial cells surround each alveolus (Schmidt, 1971; Pitelka and Hamamoto, 1983). The neurohypophysial hormone oxytocin causes the myoepithelial cells to contract, forcing newly synthesized milk into the lumen of the alveoli. Most milk present between milkings is in the epithelial cells and alveolar lumen.

At six months of fetal age, the calf has mammary glands consisting of a small teat with a meatus, a teat cistern, a gland cistern, and a primitive duct system. Very little further development takes place before birth.

A small amount of growth in secretory tissue occurs from birth to puberty, most of which is due to deposition of adipose tissue. With each recurring estrous cycle after puberty, some further mammary gland development takes place (Sinha and Tucker, 1969). Estrogen produced during each estrous cycle is primarily responsible for ductal growth and progesterone for development of the secretory tissue. When pregnancy occurs, a marked increase in mammary gland growth takes place (Hammond, 1927). Most of the ductal growth occurs during the first part of pregnancy, and the lobulo-alveolar system takes form during the middle and later parts of pregnancy. A wave of mitosis occurs shortly before or after parturition (Paape and Tucker, 1969; Tucker and Reece, 1963a,b,d). A slight amount of growth may occur until the peak of lactation, and some evidence indicates that growth may continue throughout certain stages of lactation (Trauig, 1967). At some point during lactation, however, cells are destroyed or eliminated and involution (regression) of the gland begins.

Much is being learned about the hormonal requirements for mammary growth as more precise tools for quantifying growth are developed. Nuclear magnetic resonance (NMR) imaging and computerized tomography (CT scan) technology will help pinpoint hormonal requirements for mammary gland growth at various physiological stages of the animal's development.

Experimental results to date indicate that estrogen, progesterone, prolactin, and somatotropin are required for mammary gland development in the intact animal (Forsyth, 1983). The placenta may also influence mammary gland development during pregnancy. Hormones with mammogenic, lactogenic, and luteotrophic stimulating properties have been found in a variety of animal placentas. These proteins are the placental lactogens, which have been characterized biochemically in numerous animals including cattle (Forsyth, 1983). Insulin and the adrenal corticoids appear to be more directly involved in maintaining a normal metabolic state in hypophysectomized animals, but they have direct effects on mammary gland proliferation in in vitro systems (Forsyth, 1983; Tucker, 1974). Epithelial cells must divide in organ culture (this process is under the control of insulin) and proliferate in the presence of cortisol in order to synthesize casein in response to prolactin (Anderson, 1974; Lockwood et al., 1967; Rivera and Bern, 1961).

## INITIATION OF LACTATION (LACTOGENESIS)

Colostrum or first milk accumulates in the epithelial cells before parturition (Mepham, 1983; Schmidt, 1971). It is concentrated with antibodies and passively immunizes the young to a variety of antigenic factors. In the rat, lactose does not appear in milk until parturition. The initiation of lactation, called lactogenesis, is characterized by increases in the RNA/DNA ratio, the number of ribosomes, the endoplasmic reticulum, and the number of mitochondria per cell. Histological changes are primarily associated with changes due to milk accumulation within the lumen of the alveolus. The anterior pituitary produces hormones essential for lactogenesis. Prolactin causes localized initiation of milk secretion when injected into the rabbit mammary gland (Forsyth, 1983; Schmidt, 1971; Tucker, 1974), but corticoids are required for lactogenesis in most animals (Forsyth, 1983; Tucker, 1974).

Insulin and cortisol are the minimal hormone requirements for maintaining viable mammary gland tissue explants in vitro (Forsyth, 1983). As mentioned previously, the cells must first divide in order to synthesize casein. For prolactin and human placental lactogen to stimulate casein synthesis, cell division must take place in the presence of insulin and cortisol (Forsyth, 1983).

The hormonal control of lactogenesis is not completely defined. Most theories center on either a rise in the blood levels of prolactin and adrenal glucocorticoids at the time of parturition or a drop in progesterone or glucocorticoid binding globulin (transcortin) (Forsyth, 1983; Schwalm and Tucker, 1978; Tucker, 1974). Transcortin is proposed to bind the adrenal corticoids, thus inhibiting their biological activity (Tucker, 1974). Several years ago, it was shown that progesterone inhibited the synthesis of alphalactalbumin, a protein essential in forming lactose synthetase. Lactose synthetase is postulated to be a rate-limiting enzyme for lactose biosynthesis. It is thought that estrogen levels increase before parturition, which stimulates prolactin secretion. At this time, prostaglandin $F_2a$ causes regression of the corpus luteum, which normally maintains pregnancy (Forsyth, 1983; Schwalm and Tucker, 1978; Tucker, 1974). Progesterone concentrations fall, leading to the unmasking of glucocorticoid receptors. Estrogen continues to increase, thereby increasing prolactin concentrations (Forsyth, 1983; Schwalm and Tucker, 1978; Tucker, 1974). Prolactin may up-regulate its own receptors, and the biosynthetic processes (lactose and casein production) involved in milk synthesis are activated (Forsyth, 1983; Schwalm and Tucker, 1978; Tucker, 1974).

## CONTROL OF PROLACTIN PRODUCTION

Prolactin secretion, release by the pituitary gland, or both are under control of the hypothalamus (Schmidt, 1971; Tucker, 1974). The hypothalamus produces a chemical compound called prolactin inhibiting factor (PIF) that normally inhibits prolactin secretion or release from the pituitary. Compounds such as reserpine, epinephrine, and other biogenic amines and acetylcholine decrease PIF and therefore increase blood concentrations of prolactin. Thyrotropin releasing hormone, estradiol, triiodothyronine ($T_3$), and tetraiodothyronine ($T_4$) stimulate prolactin release (Forsyth, 1983; Schmidt, 1971; Tucker, 1974). Stress, milking or suckling, high temperatures, and light will also influence prolactin secretion (Forsyth, 1983; Tucker, 1974, 1985a).

## MAINTENANCE OF LACTATION (GALACTOPOIESIS)

Galactopoiesis is dependent on removal of milk and a suckling or milking stimulus in all animals. Milk synthesis will not continue if the product is not effectively removed. Prolactin is released at milking along with adrenocorticotrophic hormone (ACTH) and oxytocin. Complete restoration of milk production in hypophysectomized goats has been obtained with injection of prolactin, bSTH, $T_3$, insulin, and corticosteroids (Cowie, 1969).

Much work has been done on the feeding and injection of hormones to intact animals, especially ruminants. Anterior pituitary extracts have been found to increase milk secretion in dairy cows, primarily because of the bSTH content of the extracts (Forsyth, 1983; Schmidt, 1971; Tucker, 1985a). Several workers have shown that bSTH isolated from the pituitary increases milk production in cows (Tucker, 1985a). Recombinant-derived bSTH has been shown to increase milk production in short- and long-term experiments with no deleterious effects. These experiments are discussed later.

Pituitary prolactin is not galactopoietic in dairy cattle (Plaut et al., 1985). Large doses of ACTH or adrenal corticoids inhibit lactation in the rat and ruminant (Tucker, 1985a).

Feeding of thyroprotein, $T_4$, or $T_3$ increases milk production in lactating cows (Meites, 1961; Thomas and Moore, 1953; Thomas et al., 1957). Thyroprotein feeding increases milk production for 2 to 4 months and also results in a transitory increase in butter fat percentage. It appears that feeding thyroprotein causes an increased need for nutrients; a loss of body weight; and an increase in heart rate, respiration rate, and body temperature (Meites, 1961). Several workers have shown that long-term treatment increases milk production in early lactation (Schmidt, 1971). However, there is a rapid decline in production in later lactation, resulting in overall lower production than is normal for the cow. No detrimental health effects have been seen with prolonged thyroprotein treatment, provided the nutritional needs of the animal are always considered.

## MILK EJECTION

Removal of milk from the mammary gland is dependent on a functional milk ejection reflex. This is a neurohormonal-dependent process. The ejection of milk results from a nervous stimulus that an animal associates with milking or suckling activity, such as manual massage of the udder teats, suckling, or sight and smell of the calf (Tucker, 1985a). The milking machine itself can also stimulate the reflex (Gorewit et al., 1983). The neural stimulus reaches the central nervous system and causes the posterior lobe to release oxytocin (Tucker, 1985a). Oxytocin reaches the mammary gland and myoepithelial cells, and contraction of these cells forces milk from the alveoli into the duct system. Milk then flows freely into the larger ducts and cisterns. Adrenalin inhibits milk ejection primarily by reducing blood flow to the gland so that sufficient concentrations of oxytocin cannot reach the receptors on the myoepithelial cells (Gorewit and Aromando, 1985).

The posterior pituitary hormones are produced in the hypothalamus and travel to the posterior pituitary where they are stored until release (Tucker, 1985a). The paraventricular nuclei are particularly involved with oxytocin production. However, the supraoptic nuclei can also release oxytocin.

Oxytocin is a peptide containing eight amino acids. It has a molecular weight of about 1,000 daltons. Vasopressin is a similar molecule and has some oxytocic properties, but oxytocin appears to have five to six times more activity in causing milk ejection than does vasopressin. Also, considerably more oxytocin than vasopressin is released during milk ejection (Schmidt, 1971; Tucker, 1985a).

A very significant advancement in lactation research was made when a nonextraction radioimmunoassay for measuring oxytocin was developed at Cornell University (Gorewit, 1979). This allowed researchers to define more precisely the physiology of milk ejection. Milking or suckling of the cow causes a marked increase in blood oxytocin concentrations (Gorewit, 1979; Gorewit and Aromando, 1985; Gorewit et al., 1983; Wachs et al., 1984a,b). The level of oxytocin drops to resting concentrations within 20 minutes of release. The synthesis, metabolic clearance rate, and half-life of oxytocin have been determined for the cow and change during the lactational cycle (Wachs et al., 1984a,b).

Oxytocin exerts a vasoactive influence on the bovine mammary gland (Gorewit et al., 1988). During the normal milking process, there is a 30 to 50 percent increase in mammary blood flow, which is primarily caused by oxytocin release (Gorewit et al., in press). This increased blood flow may have a rejuvenating effect on the metabolically active cells or aid in the expulsion of milk via pressure differentials between the myoepithelial cells and the capillaries surrounding them.

Myoepithelial cells contain specific receptors for oxytocin and are under direct hormonal control (Forsyth, 1983; Soloff and Swartz, 1973; Zhao and Gorewit, 1986, 1987). The motor innervation of the mammary gland per se plays no part in normal milk ejection. Myoepithelial cells have been isolated and grown in primary cell culture (Gorewit and McOsker, 1983) on both plastic and collagen matrices, but they appear to remain more differentiated on collagen (Gorewit and Rizzo, 1986).

## MAMMARY INVOLUTION

Regression or involution of the mammary gland takes place after the peak of lactation and after cessation of milking or suckling (Lenfers, 1907; Schmidt, 1971). The involutionary process is more drastically affected by cessation of milk removal than it is after peak lactation (Schmidt, 1971; Schmidt et al., 1962). Involution is thought to be due to decreases in cell numbers, the decline in rate of milk synthesis of remaining cells, or both.

There are characteristic changes in mammary histology during the involutionary process, including decreases in the size of the alveoli, the number of alveoli per lobule, the total number of alveoli and lobular volume, and the number of cells per alveolus (Schmidt, 1971). Complete lobules disintegrate in parts of the mammary gland during advanced involution, and by the end of involution, the gland resembles that of the virginal state. However, the essential lobular structure of the gland is still recognizable (Schmidt, 1971).

Mammary gland engorgement occurs after cessation of milking or suckling and causes irreversible changes in the cytoplasm of the secretory epithelial cells (Schmidt, 1971). The changes are thought to be due to interference with the blood supply to the mammary epithelium. Alveoli eventually rupture and secretion moves into the intercellular spaces. Phagocytes then begin to enzymatically break down milk components. Changes similar to those that occur normally during lactation are believed to take place during involution, but the entire process is not so abrupt.

Biochemical changes also occur in the mammary gland during involution. There is a tremendous decrease in the secretory activity of the cell (Schmidt, 1971; Tucker and Reece, 1963b). A decrease in the respiratory quotient, a decrease in oxygen consumption, and an accumulation of lactic acid in the tissue take place. Oxidative phosphorylation within the mitochondria is uncoupled within 12 to 24 hours after the young have been removed (Schmidt, 1971; Schmidt et al., 1962).

The suckling stimulus plays an important role in galactopoiesis, since it has been shown that involution is retarded by the suckling of ligated mammary glands (Schmidt, 1971). Suckling stimuli also maintain the nucleic acid content of the lactating mammary gland (Thatcher and Tucker, 1966; Tucker, 1964; Tucker and Reece, 1963c). The suckling stimulus without milk removal, however, neither prevents a decrease in cell loss nor maintains the protein synthetic activity of the cells (Schmidt, 1971). Prolactin injections also retard involution (Hooker and Williams, 1941; Schmidt, 1971; Williams, 1945).

Oxytocin injections retard involution in the rat after cessation of milking (Schmidt, 1971). This may be because of periodic milk ejection caused by oxytocin, which releases milk from the alveoli into the ducts and stromal tissue where it can be absorbed, thereby allowing further milk synthesis to occur. Prolactin will not maintain the full biochemical integrity of the cell unless the secretory products are removed (Schmidt, 1971).

## MILK SECRETION RATE

Milk secretion rate is important in the dairy industry. It influences the required frequency for milking of cows and the acceptable intervals between milkings. In part, milk secretion rate depends on the pressure that accumulates within the mammary gland. When milk accumulates within the mammary gland for a long enough period of time, pressure is built up to a sufficient level to inhibit secretion and milk is resorbed by the blood (Schmidt, 1971). A marked increase in pressure occurs after 1 hour of milking. Residual milk or complementary milk moves from the alveoli into the teat and gland cisterns. Thereafter, a gradual increase in the pressure occurs owing to the movement of milk from the alveoli to the teat and gland cisterns. The rate of milk secretion is linear for about 10 to 12 hours after the last milking, after which it decreases slightly. It continues to decrease until it finally reaches zero about 35 hours after the last milking (Schmidt, 1971; Tucker et al., 1961).

Part of the early increase in intramammary pressure is due to residual milk that is left in the udder after normal milking. The amount of residual milk can be as great as 15 to 30 percent (Gorewit and Sagi, 1984; Gorewit et al., 1983; Schmidt, 1971). This percentage is higher in low-producing cows than high-producing cows (Schmidt, 1971).

Increasing the time interval between milkings can increase milk production. Decreasing the milking interval from 2 to 1 will lower milk production in cows by as much as 40 percent (Schmidt, 1971).

## FACTORS AFFECTING THE YIELD AND COMPOSITION OF MILK

Milk fat, lactose, and proteins are synthesized in the cells from precursors absorbed from blood (Davies et al., 1983; Schmidt, 1971). These components are released in the milk by apocrine, merocrine, or holocrine secretion (Tucker, 1974). Water, minerals, and vitamin components of milk enter the lumen of the alveolus primarily through diffusion (Mather and Keennan, 1983; Schmidt, 1971), although some may be bound to other compounds.

Mammary gland blood flow rate is highly correlated to milk production. In fact, about 500 volumes of blood flow through the cow's udder for each volume of milk produced (Mepham, 1983; Schmidt, 1971). The ratio of blood flow to milk yield is higher in lower milk producing goats and in animals in late lactation.

Many physiological and environmental factors can influence milk secretion. For cows, factors related to increases in milk yield are increased body weight, advancing age, increased plane of nutrition, fall and winter calving, moderate or cool environmental temperatures, and good body condition at calving. Factors that tend to decrease milk yield are advancing lactation, advanced stage of gestation, short dry period, spring and summer calving, high environmental temperatures and humidity, diseases that affect the udder or feed intake of the cow, and a decreased plane of nutrition (Schmidt, 1971).

During a normal lactation of the dairy cow, the milk yield starts out at a high level, peaks 3 to 6 weeks after calving, and then gradually declines toward the end of lactation. The milk fat and protein percentages are inversely related to the milk yield (Davies et al., 1983; Mepham, 1983; Schmidt, 1971). The percentage composition starts out at a moderate level, decreases to a low level during peak lactation, and then gradually increases toward the end of lactation (Mepham, 1983; Schmidt, 1971; Tucker and Reece, 1963c).

Certain changes in the cow's diet adversely influence milk fat percentage. Most of these are related to a high-concentrate, low-roughage diet that contains a low amount of fiber. The reason for milk fat depression is unclear. The depressed milk fat percentage is accompanied by a change in rumen fermentation. There is a decrease in rumen acetate production, an increase in rumen propionate production, and a decrease in rumen pH. Feeding sodium or potassium bicarbonate, magnesium bicarbonate, magnesium oxide, and calcium hydroxide partly prevents the milk fat depression caused by restricted roughage intake (Davies et al., 1983; Schmidt, 1971).

## BIOCHEMISTRY OF MILK SECRETION

The mammary gland secretory epithelial cells break down substrates to provide energy for synthetic processes within the mammary gland. From these substrates, the gland synthesizes milk components such as fat, lactose, and protein. The cells regulate milk composition by controlling amounts of constituents such as water, vitamins, and minerals that are not synthesized in the mammary gland.

The major blood precursors for milk synthesis are glucose, acetate, beta-hydroxybutyrate, triglyceride fatty acids, and amino acids (Kuhn, 1983; Smith et al., 1983). The two major energy sources are glucose and acetate. Other compounds are absorbed and used by the mammary gland, but they do not contribute significantly to the quantitative aspects of milk composition, even though their qualitative aspects are extremely important.

Compounds that are broken down by oxidation in mitochondria are used for energy in milk synthesis. Approximately 90 percent of the adenosine triphosphate (ATP) is formed via the electron transport system. The terminal phosphate group of ATP is transferred to a specific acceptor molecule. The acceptor molecule has its energy content raised to a level at which it can participate in the energy-requiring processes within the cell, such as the synthesis of triglycerides, lactose, and proteins. The liberated adenosine diphosphate (ADP) molecule can be reused for the generation of ATP (Smith et al., 1983).

Energy in the mammary epithelial cell is generated by one of three pathways (Smith et al., 1983). The Embden-Meyerhof glycolytic pathway degrades glucose and other hexose molecules into two lactic acids with the generation of ATP at the substrate level of phosphorylation. The pyruvate produced can enter the citric acid cycle. The citric acid cycle is the final common pathway for mammary metabolism. It can also utilize acetyl coenzyme A (acetyl-CoA) from fatty acid metabolism and carbon skeletons from amino acid metabolism. A third pathway operating in the mammary gland is the pentose phosphate shunt. Its primary function in the mammary cell is to provide hydrogen ions for reductive stages of fatty acid synthesis. Breakdown products of the pentose phosphate shunt are also involved in nucleic acid synthesis. The pentose phosphate shunt is the major pathway for glucose oxidation in the epithelial cell. A sudden increase in enzyme activity occurs during parturition in the rat but has not been described for the cow.

## Milk Protein Synthesis

There are a number of proteins that are specific to milk. Among the major ones are casein, alpha-lactalbumin, and beta-lactoglobulin. Most of the milk proteins are synthesized within the mammary gland. Gamma-casein, blood serum albumin, and the immune globulins are absorbed as preformed proteins from the blood (Mercier and Gaye, 1983).

Most of the protein synthesized by the epithelial cells is synthesized from amino acids that are absorbed from the bloodstream. This has been determined by measuring arteriovenous differences across the mammary gland and relating uptake by the mammary gland to the composition of amino acids in milk protein (Mercier and Gaye, 1983). Radioisotopes have been used to follow the pathways of incorporation of labeled elements of amino acids into the proteins in the milk. The peptides in blood plasma provide less than 10 percent of the amino acids in milk protein (Mercier and Gaye, 1983). Plasma proteins may provide a small portion of the essential amino acids of milk protein synthesized in the mammary gland. However, less than 10 percent of these proteins come from plasma proteins. The essential amino acids are absorbed from the bloodstream, and most of the nonessential amino acids are also absorbed from blood. The mammary gland is capable of producing nonessential amino acids from other amino acids (Mercier and Gaye, 1983). For example, ornithine can be converted to proline by the secretory epithelial cell.

Carbohydrates and volatile fatty acids can act as substrates for nonessential amino acids.

The protein synthetic reaction mechanisms appear to be comparable to those found in most other protein-synthesizing cells.

## Milk Fat Synthesis

Fat is the most variable component of milk. Both the percentage composition of fat and the fatty acid composition of triglycerides within and among species vary. Most milk fat is made up of triglycerides. Glucose, acetate and beta-hydroxybutyrate, triglycerides of the chylomicra, and low-density lipoproteins from blood serve as major precursors for milk lipids (Dils, 1983). The beta-hydroxybutyrate is also used for fatty acid synthesis (Dils, 1983). The ruminant mammary gland cannot effectively utilize acetyl-CoA formed from glucose in the mitochondria.

The short-chain fatty acids from $C_4$ to $C_{14}$ and some palmitic acid are synthesized within the mammary gland from acetate derived as absorbed acetate in the ruminant or from glucose in the nonruminant (Dils, 1983). About 30 percent of palmitic acid is derived from acetate, and the remainder comes from triglycerides of blood. Stearic and oleic acids come primarily from plasma triglycerides. Stearic acid is absorbed in greater quantities from blood than is oleic acid, yet oleic acid is the most prevalent $C_{18}$ fatty acid in milk. Stearate can be converted to oleic acid by the bovine, caprine, and swine mammary glands. Oleic acid cannot be saturated to form stearate.

Free glycerol from the bloodstream provides less than 10 percent of the glycerol portion of milk triglycerides. Most glycerol comes from glycerol-3-phosphate from glycolysis and the remainder from lipoprotein glycerides (Dils, 1983).

The malonyl-CoA pathway appears to be the predominant route of fatty acid synthesis. Two pathways for esterification of fatty acids may be present in the mammary gland: the phosphatidic acid pathway, which is the most common, and formation of 1,2-diglyceride from acylation of 2-monoglyceride (Dils, 1983).

## Lactose, Minerals, and Vitamins

The major sugar of milk is lactose. Lactose is a disaccharide made up of a glucose and a galactose molecule. The primary precursor of lactose is glucose (Davies et al., 1983; Kuhn, 1983; Smith et al., 1983). The glucose molecule is phosphorylated to form glucose-6-phosphate, which is then converted into glucose-1-phosphate. The glucose-1-phosphate, in the presence of uridine triphosphate, forms uridine diphosphate (UDP) glucose, which is converted to UDP galactose. The UDP galactose is united with free glucose to form lactose with the liberation of UDP. The last step is catalyzed by the enzyme lactose synthetase. This is a unique enzyme that is composed of two subunits: the common galactosyl transferase and the milk protein alpha-lactalbumin.

The major mineral constituents of milk are calcium, phosphorus, potassium, chlorine, sodium, and magnesium. Potassium, chlorine, and sodium are in soluble form. Phosphates, citrates, and casein bind various minerals such as calcium and sodium. The buffering capacity of milk is due to citrates, phosphates, and bicarbonates, along with the proteins in the milk. Serum calcium is in equilibrium with bone calcium, making it difficult to increase the calcium content of the milk by increasing the calcium content of the feed. Inorganic phosphate of blood serum is the precursor of milk phosphates.

There is considerable evidence that healthy cows have constant amounts of lactose, potassium, sodium, and chlorine in their milk (Schmidt, 1971). The exact amount appears characteristic for each cow. There is a close inverse relationship between lactose content of milk and the molar sum of sodium and potassium contents, as well as between lactose and potassium contents of milk. Water moves into the milk with casein to maintain osmotic equilibrium with the blood. Consequently, secretion of lactose, potassium, sodium, and chlorine controls the milk volume (Peaker, 1983). Milk contains trace amounts of some other minerals and can take up large amounts of iodine when excessive amounts are fed.

Vitamins are absorbed by the mammary gland from the bloodstream. Generally, the vitamin content of milk can be increased by increasing the vitamin content of blood supplying the mammary gland. The ruminant animal depends on feed supply and exposure to sunlight for its fat-soluble vitamins A, D, and E. Beta-carotene is converted to vitamin A in the intestinal mucosa of the ruminant. Vitamin D in the milk of cows comes from activation of ergosterol in feed or from the animal's exposure to sunlight. This activates 7-dehydrocholesterol in the skin of the animal. Milk contains vitamins E and K.

The B vitamins are synthesized by microflora in the rumen. Consequently, changes in the B vitamin contents of the diet do not change the contents in milk except for riboflavin. The ascorbic acid (vitamin C) content of cow milk cannot be changed by dietary content, since it is synthesized in the ruminant's body.

## EFFECTS OF HORMONES ON MILK SECRETION AND MAMMARY DEVELOPMENT

### Milk Secretion

Asimov and Krouze (1937) injected dairy cows with anterior pituitary extracts and found significant increases in milk production. British workers established that growth hormone was the active hormone responsible for these increases (Young, 1947). Almost a decade later, Brumby and Hancock (1955) reported results of treating lactating cows for 12 weeks with pituitary growth hormone. Twin cows received daily injections of somatotropin and produced approximately 50 percent more milk than their twin mates. Their live weights were unchanged.

Machlin (1973) studied the effect of growth hormone on milk production and feed utilization in dairy cows. Growth hormone injections increased milk production and appeared to increase feed efficiency. More recently, researchers at Cornell University and the National Institute for Research in Dairying demonstrated that growth hormone increased significantly both milk production and feed utilization in high-producing, genetically superior cows (Hart et al., 1985; Peel et al., 1981).

Bauman et al. (1982) were the first research group to administer recombinant methionyl bovine growth hormone to high-producing dairy cows. The recombinant growth hormone was as effective as pituitary-derived growth hormone in enhancing milk production. It is now possible to apply this breakthrough in biotechnology to widespread use on commercial dairy farms.

Since 1981, several studies have compared the effectiveness of natural pituitary growth hormone versus recombinant growth hormone in increasing milk production and feed utilization as well as the effectiveness of various routes and methods of hormone administration.

In high-yielding Holstein cows, milk production has been consistently increased from 2 to 5 kg/day in early, mid, and late lactation by administration of bSTH (Bauman et al., 1982; Hart et al., 1985; Peel et al., 1981, 1982, 1983; Richard et al., 1985). Additional nutrients in the form of glucose and casein (Peel et al., 1982) or lipids (Lough et al., 1984) have had no additive effect compared to bSTH treatment alone. There is a curvilinear relationship between milk production and dose of growth hormone (Eppard et al., 1985). However, the pattern in which somatotropin is administered does not appear to affect the increases in milk production observed (Fronk et al., 1983).

In most short-term trials, feed intake did not increase upon administration of bSTH, despite significant increases in milk production. To date, no changes in digestibility or the efficiency with which energy is used for maintenance of milk synthesis during growth hormone administration have been observed.

Long-term studies have been done with both natural pituitary growth hormone and recombinant derived hormone (Bauman et al., 1985; Brumby and Hancock, 1955; Fronk et al., 1983; Machlin, 1973). Production increases were very similar in studies carried out by Brumby and Hancock (1955) and Machlin (1973) for 12 and 10 weeks, respectively, using pituitary-derived somatotropin.

Studies by Bauman et al. (1985) were carried out for 27 weeks. High-yielding Holstein cows received treatments of 0 (control), 13.5, 27.0, and 40.5 mg/day of recombinant-derived bovine growth hormone or 27.0 mg/day of pituitary-derived growth hormone. They showed increases in milk production ranging from 16 to 41 percent over the control production. Injections were carried out for 188 days commencing around day 84 of lactation. There were no significant differences in live weight gains even though feed intake increased. Feed intake gradually increased to support the higher milk production. Cows treated with natural anterior pituitary growth hormone responded with substantial increases in milk production.

Peel et al. (1985) treated five sets of monozygotic twins in which the animals' sole diet was ryegrass and clover pasture. They were treated with natural pituitary-derived bSTH. Like the trials carried out at Cornell, milk production increased and so did feed intake to support the increased production. The improved milk production seen in the two long-term studies was related to the greater efficiency with which

feed was utilized for milk secretion (kg of milk/kg of feed). This was primarily related to dilution of feed costs for maintenance at the higher production levels.

## Effects of Somatotropin on Mammary Growth

Somatotropin has been shown to be essential for pubertal mammary development (Forsyth, 1983; Tucker, 1985a). The lack of available growth hormone necessary to carry out studies on large animals, such as cattle, has made it difficult to study the hormone's effects on enhancing normal rates of mammary growth at puberty in these animals. Recently, Sejrsen et al. (1986) have examined the effects of daily administration of exogenous somatotropin on mammary development in dairy heifers. Nine pairs of identical twins were used. One twin received a daily subcutaneous injection of somatotropin (20 IU) and the other received excipient. Treatments commenced at 8.0 months of age (179 kg live weight) and continued for 15.6 weeks. At that time, heifers were slaughtered and mammary development was evaluated. Somatotropin resulted in an increase in mammary parenchyma and decreases in extraparenchymal tissue and weight of the mammary glands. Increases in parenchyma were 56 percent as determined by computer assisted x-ray tomography and 18 percent as determined by dissection. Chemical composition (39 percent water, 7 percent protein, and 54 percent fat) and histological and cytological appearance of the mammary gland parenchyma were not affected by the treatment. Treatment with exogenous somatotropin around puberty enhanced the growth rate of mammary parenchymal tissue. This increase in tissue might well lead to increased future milk production in these animals.

It is likely that somatotropin does not directly stimulate milk secretion and mammary growth. Receptors for bSTH have not been found in mammary tissue from dairy cows. Moreover, the infusion of bSTH directly into the mammary artery has not stimulated milk production in sheep. Somatotropin is thought to activate the production of somatomedins or insulin-like growth factors (IGFs). The role of somatomedins is well documented for growth but not for lactation.

Davis et al. (1984) and Peel et al. (1985) have shown that somatotropin administration increases IGF. IGF-I and IGF-II receptors have been reported in bovine and porcine mammary tissue (Gregor and Burleigh, 1985; Peel and Bauman, 1987). There is no doubt that growth factors play a pivotal role in mammary gland function and development.

## GENETICALLY SUPERIOR COWS AND bSTH-TREATED COWS

There are many similarities between genetically superior cows and cows treated with growth hormone (Peel and Bauman, 1987). Both consume more feed and preferentially partition nutrients to the mammary gland for milk synthesis. Somatotropin treatment does not change the digestibility of feed maintenance requirements of animals or the efficiency with which milk is synthesized. The gross feed efficiency is improved, however. This is because maintenance represents a smaller proportion of consumed nutrients in both the genetically superior cow and the cow that has higher milk yields during bSTH treatment.

In genetically superior cows, there is a greater use of body reserves in early lactation. In bSTH-treated cows, increased mobilization of nutrient reserves to support increased milk yields in the first weeks of hormone treatment occurs. Genetically superior cows are thought to contain large quantities of secretory tissue, even though the synthetic activity per secretory cell is not known.

Improved management is necessary to optimize reproductive performance in genetically superior cows. In cows receiving somatotropin, it is not known what effect the increased milk production will have on reproductive performance. It is likely that there will be no difficulty in well-managed herds.

## ALTERNATE METHODS FOR INCREASING THE EFFICIENCY OF LACTATION

### Optimizing Milk Removal

For copious milk secretion to continue, the milk must be effectively extracted from the udder. Oxytocin is the principal hormonal factor responsible for milk ejection. Under normal conditions, 15 to 30 percent of the milk produced by the udder can be left in the udder after milking. Moreover, there appears to be a negative feedback system wherein the milk remaining in the udder can influence further secretion rates. If milk ejection can be optimized to reduce this residual milk, then milk yields can be increased significantly.

### Growth Factors and Other Biological Compounds

Animals can be made to produce milk more efficiently by treatment with specific agents such as somatomedins, neurotransmitters, or specific growth factors. Monoclonal antibodies directed toward key enzymes controlling milk secretion could be utilized. Once the mechanisms underlying autocrine regulation of growth are determined, the chemical factors can be isolated, identified, and produced by genetic engineering. Genes for specific growth factors can also be incorporated into appropriate somatic cells of animals. These cells in turn can be transplanted back into the animal's body after their genetic code has been altered to produce the desired growth factor.

## Hormone Receptors

One of the key steps in the action of a hormone is the binding of that hormone to its receptor within or on the cell. Increases in animal efficiency may come about in the future if the amplification steps to subsequent hormonal binding of the ligand with its receptor can be regulated. Methods that will increase the affinities of the ligand for its receptor so that the desired physiological response will take place can be developed. Alternatively, undesired or negative control mechanisms brought about by interactions of hormones or growth factors with their receptors can be modulated.

## Controlling Involution

The mammary gland undergoes a natural period of regression or involution. During this time, either the rate of milk synthesis diminishes or the cells begin to age and die. The mechanisms of senescence in the mammary gland must be examined so that lactation can be extended indefinitely, thereby increasing the efficiency of milk secretion.

## Controlling the Environment

Cows are very sensitive to environmental stresses such as heat and humidity. Fortunately, great progress has been made in improving the management practices of farms in areas where heat and humidity are a problem. Hormones critical for the control of lactation are sensitive to temperature, humidity, and photoperiod (Tucker, 1985b). Development of methods to optimize the environmental conditions to promote secretion of galactopoietic factors would certainly lead to increased animal efficiency.

## Genetic Selection

Dairy scientists conducting research in animal breeding have made great progress in improving lactational efficiency. How-ever, it takes a long time for improvements to be realized through the genetic selection process, and scientists are constantly searching for physiological factors that can be correlated immediately to the animal's future ability to produce milk. Several workers have shown that serum concentrations of growth hormone are associated with milk production (Barnes et al., 1985; Flux et al., 1984; Hart et al., 1978). Substances like bSTH that can be directly correlated with milk production could be used effectively for the genetic selection of animals.

## SUMMARY

The mammary gland is a very complex organ system typically classified as an exocrine or duct gland. It is an "accessory organ" to the reproductive system and is specialized in both structure and function.

Most of the major development of the gland occurs after the start of pregnancy. Blood hormones during pregnancy play a major role in controlling the extent of mammary gland development. Lactogenesis is also under the influence of hormones. The mammary gland, therefore, provides a tissue system in which the action of a hormone can be isolated and the precise role of the hormone inducing the synthesis process can be studied.

Milk secretion is controlled by several factors. The total amount of milk produced and its composition can be altered by changes in the hormonal, environmental, and nutritional status of the animal. Growth hormone and thyroactive compounds are galactopoietic. However, for milk secretion to continue, the secretory products must be effectively removed. This requires a functional milk ejection reflex. Milk removal requires neural stimulation through suckling or milking procedures. The nerve stimulus induces the release of the hormone oxytocin, which causes the myoepithelial cells surrounding the milk-producing alveoli to contract, thus forcing the milk from the alveoli into the ducts. If milk is not evacuated, milk synthesis decreases and eventually stops with the complete involution of the secretory tissue. Thus, milk secretion requires the interplay of hormonal, nutritional, and neurohormonal processes in addition to evacuation of the milk by suckling or milking.

A very unique aspect of the mammary gland is that a gradual drop in the level of milk production occurs after the peak level of secretion. This happens regardless of the nutritional regime of the animal or the intensity of the suckling stimulus. This is a normal process similar to senescence or aging and leads to the complete cessation of secretion. Normal secretion can only resume after another pregnancy, after which the secretory tissue has developed in the udder.

With the recent breakthroughs in molecular biology, it is now possible to increase mammary growth and the efficiency of milk production in dairy animals. Bovine somatotropin increases mammary growth in prepubertal calves. This increase in growth could lead to greater milk production per individual animal during lactation. Increases in milk production of up to 40 percent have been demonstrated with exogenous administration of bSTH. Cows adjust their nutrient intake upward to support this increase.

Additional ways of increasing the efficiency of lactation could be achieved by treating animals with specific agents such as somatomedins, antibodies, or specific growth factors. Once the mechanisms underlying autocrine regulation of growth are determined, the chemical factors involved can be isolated, identified, and produced by genetic engineering. Genes for these substances can also be incorporated directly into the host's cells. Numbers of hormonal receptor sites and amplification steps subsequent to binding may be manipulated to alter the efficiency of milk production. Milk secretion will be optimized further after it

is more thoroughly understood how to increase the efficacy of milk ejection. Increased milk production can be achieved per animal by developing methods that retard mammary involution, thereby lengthening the period of lactation.

Environmental factors can adversely influence milk production. When those factors that optimize milk secretion are controlled, the efficiency of lactation is increased. If strong correlations between blood hormone concentrations and total milk production can be made, there is a potential for selecting animals for high milk production.

The milk of the dairy cow is a very important economic commodity because of its nutritional nature and the products that are produced from it and its by-products. With the increasing size of the world population and the decreasing numbers of dairy farms, it is imperative that we seek ways to increase animal production by increasing the animal's own efficiencies.

## REFERENCES

Anderson, R. R. 1974. Endocrinological control. P. 97 in Lactation: A Comprehensive Treatise, Vol. 4, B. L. Larson, ed. New York: Academic Press.

Asimov, G. J., and N. K. Krouze. 1937. The lactogenic preparations from the anterior pituitary and the increase of milk yield in cows. J. Dairy Sci. 20:289.

Barnes, M. A., G. W. Kazmer, R. M. Akers, and R. E. Pearson. 1985. Influence of selection for milk yield on endogenous hormones and metabolites in Holstein heifers and cows. J. Anim. Sci. 60:271.

Bauman, D. E., M. J. DeGeeter, C. J. Peel, G. M. Lanza, R. C. Gorewit, and R. W. Hammond. 1982. Effects of recombinantly derived bovine growth hormone (bGH) on lactational performance of high yielding dairy cows. J. Dairy Sci. 65(Suppl. 1):121 (Abstr.).

Bauman, D. E., P. J. Eppard, M. J. DeGeeter, and G. M. Lanza. 1985. Responses of high-producing dairy cows to long-term treatment with pituitary somatotropin and recombinant somatotropin. J. Dairy Sci. 68:1352.

Brumby, P. J., and J. Hancock. 1955. The galactopoietic role of growth hormone in dairy cattle. N.Z. J. Sci. Technol. 36A:417.

Cowie, A. T. 1969. General hormonal factors involved in lactogenesis. P. 157 in Lactogenesis: The Initiation of Milk Secretion at Parturition, M. Reynolds and S. I. Folley, eds. Philadelphia: University of Pennsylvania Press.

Davies, D. T., C. Holt, and W. W. Christie. 1983. The composition of milk. In Biochemistry of Lactation, T. B. Mepham, ed. Amsterdam: Elsevier.

Davis, S. R., P. D. Gluckman, and I. C. Hart. 1984. Effects of growth hormone and thyroxine treatment of lactating cows on milk production and plasma concentrations of IGF-I and IGF-II. Proc. Endocrinol. Soc. Aust. 27(Suppl. 1):16 (Abstr.).

Dils, R. R. 1983. Milk fat synthesis. P. 142 in Biochemistry of Lactation, T. B. Mepham, ed. Amsterdam: Elsevier.

Eppard, P. J., D. E. Bauman, and S. N. McCutcheon. 1985. Effect of dose of bovine growth hormone on lactation of dairy cows. J. Dairy Sci. 68:1109.

Flux, D. S., D. D. S. McKenzie, and G. F. Wilson. 1984. Plasma metabolite and hormone concentrations in Friesian cows of differing genetic merit measured at two feeding levels. Anim. Prod. 38:377.

Forsyth, I. A. 1983. The endocrinology of lactation. P. 309 in Biochemistry of Lactation, T. B. Mepham, ed. Amsterdam: Elsevier.

Fronk, T. J., C. J. Peel, D. E. Bauman, and R. C. Gorewit. 1983. Comparison of different patterns of exogenous growth hormone administration on milk production in Holstein cows. J. Anim. Sci. 57:699.

Gorewit, R. C. 1979. Method for determining oxytocin concentration in unextracted sera, characterization in lactating cattle. Proc. Soc. Exp. Biol. Med. 160:80.

Gorewit, R. C., and M. C. Aromando. 1985. Mechanisms involved in the adrenalin-induced blockade of milk ejection in dairy cattle. Proc. Soc. Exp. Biol. Med. 180:340.

Gorewit, R. C., and J. McOsker. 1983. Isolation, separation and pure culture of mammary secretory and myoepithelial cells from lactating cows. J. Dairy Sci. 66(Suppl. 1):106 (Abstr.).

Gorewit, R. C., and N. Rizzo. 1986. Ultrastructural features of mammary gland myoepithelial cells cultured on plastic and mammary gland collagen substrates. J. Dairy Sci. 69(Suppl. 1):204 (Abstr.).

Gorewit, R. C., and R. Sagi. 1984. Effects of exogenous oxytocin on production and milking variables of cows. J. Dairy Sci. 67:2050.

Gorewit, R. C., R. Sagi, E. A. Wachs, and W. G. Merrill. 1983. Current concepts on the role of oxytocin in milk ejection. J. Dairy Sci. 66:2236.

Gorewit, R. C., M. C. Aromando, and D. G. Bristol. In press. Measuring mammary gland blood flow using a transit-time ultrasonic flow probe. J. Appl. Physiol.

Gregor, P., and B. D. Burleigh. 1985. Presence of high affinity somatomedin/insulin-like growth factor receptors in porcine mammary gland. Endocrinology 116(Suppl. 1):223 (Abstr.).

Hammond, J. 1927. The Physiology of Reproduction in the Cow. London: Cambridge University Press.

Hart, I. C., J. A. Bines, S. V. Morant, and J. L. Ridley. 1978. Endocrine control of the levels of hormones (prolactin, growth hormone, thyroxine and insulin) and metabolites in the plasma of high- and low-yielding cattle at various stages of lactation. J. Endocrinol. 77:333.

Hart, I. C., J. A. Bines, S. James, and S. V. Morant. 1985. The effect of injecting or infusing low doses of bovine growth hormone on milk yield, milk composition and the quantity of hormone in the milk serum of cows. Anim. Prod. 40:243.

Hooker, C. W., and W. F. Williams. 1941. Retardation of mammary involution in mice by injection of lactogenic hormone. Endocrinology 28:42.

Kuhn, N. J. 1983. The biosynthesis of lactose. P. 159 in Biochemistry of Lactation, T. B. Mepham, ed. Amsterdam: Elsevier.

Lenfers, P. 1907. Zur Histolgie der Milchdruse des Rindes. Z. Fleisch- Milchhygiene 17:340.

Lockwood, D. H., F. E. Stockdale, and Y. J. Topper. 1967. Hormone-dependent differentiation of mammary gland: Sequence of action of hormones in relation to cell cycle. Science 156:945.

Lough, D. S., L. D. Muller, R. S. Kensinger, T. F. Sweeney, L. C. Griel, and T. D. Etherton. 1984. Effect of dietary fat and exogenous growth hormone on the performance of early lactation Holstein cows. J. Dairy Sci. 67(Suppl. 1):115 (Abstr.).

Machlin, L. J. 1973. Effect of growth hormone on milk production and feed utilization in dairy cows. J. Dairy Sci. 56:575.

Mather, I. H., and T. W. Keennan. 1983. Function of endomembranes and the cell surface in the secretion of organic milk constituents. P. 231 in Biochemistry of Lactation, T. B. Mepham, ed. Amsterdam: Elsevier.

Meites, J. 1961. Farm animals: Hormonal induction of lactation and galactopoiesis. Ch. 8 in Milk: The Mammary Gland and Its Secretion, Vol. 1, S. K. Kon and A. T. Cowie, eds. New York: Academic Press.

Mepham, T. B. 1983. Physiological aspects of lactation. P. 13 in Biochemistry of Lactation, T. B. Mepham, ed. Amsterdam: Elsevier.

Mercier, J. C., and P. Gaye. 1983. Milk protein synthesis. P. 177 in Biochemistry of Lactation, T. B. Mepham, ed. Amsterdam: Elsevier.

Paape, M. J., and H. A. Tucker. 1969. Influence of length of dry period on subsequent lactation in the rat. J. Dairy Sci. 52:518.

Peaker, M. 1983. Secretion of ions and water. P. 292 in Biochemistry of Lactation, T. B. Mepham, ed. Amsterdam: Elsevier.

Peel, C. J., and D. E. Bauman. 1987. Somatotropin and lactation. J. Dairy Sci. 70:474.

Peel, C. J., D. E. Bauman, R. C. Gorewit, and C. J. Sniffen. 1981. Effect of exogenous growth hormone on lactational performance in high-yielding dairy cows. J. Nutr. 111:1662.

Peel, C. J., T. J. Fronk, D. E. Bauman, and R. C. Gorewit. 1983. Effect of exogenous growth hormone in early and late lactation on lactational performance in dairy cows. J. Dairy Sci. 66:776.

Peel, C. J., T. J. Fronk, D. E. Bauman, and R. C. Gorewit. 1982. Lactational response to exogenous growth hormone and abomasal infusion of a glucose-sodium caseinate mixture in high-yielding dairy cows. J. Nutr. 112:1770.

Peel, C. J., L. D. Sandles, K. J. Quelch, and A. C. Herington. 1985. The effects of long term administration of bovine growth hormone on the lactational performance of identical twin dairy cows. Anim. Prod. 41:135.

Pitelka, D. R., and S. T. Hamamoto. 1983. Ultrastructure of the mammary secretory cell. P. 249 in Biochemistry of Lactation, T. B. Mepham, ed. Amsterdam: Elsevier.

Plaut, K., D. E. Bauman, and N. Agergaard. 1985. Effects of exogenous prolactin on lactational performance of dairy cows. J. Dairy Sci. 68(Suppl. 1):169 (Abstr.).

Richard, A. L., S. N. McCutcheon, and D. E. Bauman. 1985. Responses of dairy cows to exogenous bovine growth hormone administered during early lactation. J. Dairy Sci. 68:2385.

Rivera, E. M., and H. A. Bern. 1961. Influence of insulin on maintenance and secretory stimulation of mouse mammary tissues by hormones in organ-culture. Endocrinology 69:340.

Schmidt, G. H. 1971. Biology of Lactation. San Francisco: W. H. Freeman.

Schmidt, G. H., R. T. Chatterton, and W. Hansel. 1962. Histological changes during involution of the mammary gland of ovariectomized and intact lactating goats. J. Dairy Sci. 45:1380.

Schwalm, J. W., and H. A. Tucker. 1978. Glucocorticoids in mammary secretions and blood serum during reproduction and lactation and distributions of glucocorticoids, progesterone and estrogens in fractions of milk. J. Dairy Sci. 61:550.

Sejrsen, K., J. Foldager, M. T. Sorensen, R. M. Akers, and D. E. Bauman. 1986. Effect of exogenous bovine somatotropin on pubertal development in heifers. J. Dairy Sci. 69:1528.

Sinha, Y. N., and H. A. Tucker. 1969. Mammary development and pituitary prolactin level of heifers from birth through puberty and during the estrous cycle. J. Dairy Sci. 52:507.

Smith, G. H., B. Crabtree, and R. A. Smith. 1983. Energy metabolism in the mammary gland. P. 121 in Biochemistry of Lactation, T. B. Mepham, ed. Amsterdam: Elsevier.

Soloff, M. S., and T. L. Swartz. 1973. Characterization of a proposed oxytocin receptor in rat mammary gland. J. Biol. Chem. 248:6471.

Thatcher, W. W., and H. A. Tucker. 1966. Effects of intense nursing stimulation on lactation. J. Anim. Sci. 25:932 (Abstr.).

Thomas, J. W., and L. A. Moore. 1953. Thyroprotein feeding to dairy cows during successive lactations. Dairy Sci. 36:657.

Thomas, J. W., D. V. Kopland, E. A. Keyes, and L. A. Moore. 1957. A study of the short-term use of iodinated casein for milk production. J. Dairy Sci. 40:128.

Trauig, H. H. 1967. Cell proliferation in the mammary gland during late pregnancy and lactation. Anat. Rec. 157:189.

Tucker, H. A. 1964. Influence of number of suckling young on nucleic acid content of lactating rat mammary gland. Proc. Soc. Exp. Biol. Med. 116:218.

Tucker, H. A. 1974. General endocrinological control of lactation. P. 277 in Lactation: A Comprehensive Treatise, Vol. 4, B. L. Larson, ed. New York: Academic Press.

Tucker, H. A. 1985a. Endocrine and neural control of the mammary gland. P. 39 in Lactogenesis: The Initiation of Milk Secretion at Parturition, M. Reynolds and S. I. Folley, eds. Philadelphia: University of Pennsylvania Press.

Tucker, H. A. 1985b. P. 211 in Recent Advances in Animal Nutrition, W. Haresign and D. J. A. Cole, eds. Storeham, Mass.: Butterworth.

Tucker, H. A., and R. P. Reece. 1963a. Nucleic acid content of mammary glands of pregnant rats. Proc. Soc. Exp. Biol. Med. 112:370.

Tucker, H. A., and R. P. Reece. 1963b. Nucleic acid content of mammary glands of lactating rats. Proc. Soc. Exp. Biol. Med. 112:409.

Tucker, H. A., and R. P. Reece. 1963c. Nucleic acid content of mammary glands of rats lactating 41 and 61 days. Proc. Soc. Exp. Biol. Med. 112:688.

Tucker, H. A., and R. P. Reece. 1963d. Nucleic acid content of rat mammary glands during post-lactational involution. Proc. Soc. Exp. Biol. Med. 112:1002.

Tucker, H. A., R. P. Reece, and R. E. Mather. 1961. Udder capacity estimates as affected by rate of milk secretion and intramammary pressure. J. Dairy Sci. 44:1725.

Turner, C. W. 1939. The Comparative Anatomy of the Mammary Gland. Columbia, Mo.: University of Missouri Press.

Turner, C. W. 1952. The Mammary Gland, Vol. 1, The Anatomy of the Udder of Cattle and Domestic Animals. Columbia, Mo.: Lucas.

Wachs, E. A., R. C. Gorewit, and W. B. Currie. 1984a. Half-life, clearance, and production rate for oxytocin in cattle during lactation and mammary involution. I. Dom. Anim. Endocrinol. 1:121.

Wachs, E. A., R. C. Gorewit, and W. B. Currie. 1984b. Oxytocin concentrations of cattle in response to milking stimuli through lactation and involution. II. Dom. Anim. Endocrinol. 1:141.

Williams, W. L. 1945. The effect of lactogenic hormone on post parturient unsuckled mammary glands of the mouse. Anat. Rec. 93:171.

Young, F. G. 1947. Experimental stimulation (galactopoiesis) of lactation. Br. Med. Bull. 5:155.

Zhao, X., and R. C. Gorewit. 1986. Characterization of oxytocin receptors in mammary tissue from lactating and nonlactating cows. J. Dairy Sci. 69(Suppl. 1):165 (Abstr.).

Zhao, X., and R. C. Gorewit. 1987. Oxytocin receptors in bovine mammary tissue. J. Recept. Res. 7:729–741.

# Factors Affecting the Composition of Milk from Dairy Cows

J. G. LINN

Milk composition is economically important to milk producers and processors and nutritionally important to consumers. It has been known for years that variations in milk composition occur; however, the composition of milk marketed nationally has been rather constant over the last 15 years, averaging 3.6 percent fat, 3.2 percent protein, and 4.7 percent lactose (Young et al., 1986). This is probably partly because of the prominence of the Holstein breed and the pricing of milk based on fat concentration. The introduction of milk pricing on a component basis and the perception by consumers that animal fats are unhealthy have created new interest in how milk components can be altered to accommodate these emerging markets. The paper starts with a brief overview of the biosynthesis of milk components since changes in these reflect changes in the mammary gland synthesis or secretion of the component. Factors affecting milk composition such as breed, genetic variation within breed, health, environment, management practices, and diet are then reviewed.

## LIPIDS

### Biosynthesis

The synthesis of milk fat has been recently reviewed (Dils, 1983, 1986; Larson, 1985; Rook and Thomas, 1980). The following discussion highlights relevant stages of biosynthesis where fat composition can be altered.

The predominant fat in milk is triacylglycerol, which contains fatty acids of short- ($C_4$–$C_{10}$), intermediate- ($C_{12}$–$C_{16}$), or long-chain ($C_{18}$) length. The short-chain acids are synthesized within the mammary gland from acetate and beta-hydroxybutyrate; long-chain acids are almost exclusively derived from blood plasma fatty acids of dietary origin; and intermediate-chain acids arise from both sources. In broad terms, about 50 percent of the fatty acids in milk are synthesized in the mammary gland and the other 50 percent are derived directly from blood.

Fatty acids are synthesized in the mammary gland via the malonyl coenzyme A (malonyl-CoA) pathway. Blood beta-hydroxybutyrate is primarily used for the first four carbons initiating fatty acid synthesis. Chain length occurs two carbons at a time, with acetate being the major carbon donor. Once formed, fatty acyl-CoAs may combine with glycerol or diacylglycerol or monoacylglycerol to form triacylglycerol. Placement of the fatty acids on the glycerol molecule is not random. Short-chain fatty acids are essentially in the 3 position, and $C_{18}$ acids are on either the 1 or 3 position.

Triacylglycerols are synthesized in the endoplasmic reticulum. As they are formed, they are rapidly incorporated into lipid-covered droplets. The droplets then migrate toward the apical membrane of the secretory cell, where they become encapsulated by the membrane, pinched off, and released into the lumen.

## Factors Affecting Milk Fat Content

### Breed/Genetics

Between and within breeds, fat varies the most and lactose the least (Woodford et al., 1986). Gaunt (1980) reported cattle in the United States tend to have the lowest percentage of milk fat. This may be partly because of environmental factors, but some genetic variation within a breed in different countries must exist.

The repeatability from one lactation to another for the percentage of constituents in milk is quite high, an average of 0.67 (Gaunt, 1980). Repeatability of milk fat percentage for Holsteins is 0.76. Other breeds appear to have a similar repeatability.

Jerseys have the highest heritability for milk fat percentage (0.71), with other breeds ranging from 0.51 to 0.57. The small variation between ratios of one milk constituent to another, particularly fat to protein, suggests little hope for drastic changes in milk yield and milk composition (Gaunt, 1973; Wilcox, 1978). Heritabilities of solids-not-fat (SNF) to fat and protein to fat ratios are highest for Ayrshire followed by Jersey,

Guernsey, Brown Swiss, and Holstein. Differences in heritabilities of breeds other than Holstein may be overestimated because of a small sample population.

Genetic correlations between milk composition percentages are high and positive, averaging 0.74. However, milk yield and composition percentages are negatively correlated, $-0.3$ for milk yield and fat percentage (Gaunt, 1980). Thus, it is very difficult to improve milk yield and milk percentage composition simultaneously.

Selection in Holstein cattle for the single trait of milk fat percentage would decrease milk yield by 287 pounds but increase fat percentage by 0.19 percent per generation. Selection for milk yield only increases milk yield by 607 pounds and decreases fat percentage by 0.036 percent. Selection for milk fat yield is the most effective method for increasing fat percentage ($+0.058$ percent) and milk yield ($+443$ pounds) (Gaunt, 1980).

### Environment/Management

A decrease in milk fat percentage of 0.2 percent over five lactations has been reported by Rogers and Stewart (1982). Fat yields would be expected to increase, since the increase in milk yields with age more than offsets the drop in fat percentage.

Milk fat percentages vary with stage of lactation. The highest percentages are usually found in colostrum, followed by a decline during the first 2 months of lactation, then a slow increase as lactation progresses. Davies et al. (1983) reported distinct changes in the fatty acid content of milk over the lactation cycle. During the first half, the proportions of short- and intermediate-chain fatty acids increase, and the proportion of long-chain fatty acids decreases. No further changes occur during the last half of lactation. Some of these changes are influenced by environment, diet, and rates of fatty acid synthesis in the mammary gland.

Seasonal variations in milk fat percentages are well recognized, with summer months averaging 0.4 percentage units less than winter months (Jenness, 1985). The higher environmental temperatures during the summer also affect milk fatty acid composition. Milk fat in the summer tends to be lower in palmitic acid relative to stearic and octadecanoic acids than milk fat from the same cows during the winter (Christie, 1979). Some of the changes in milk fat percentage and composition with temperature change can be related to changes in blood plasma lipids, but these observations are also confounded by dietary changes. Milam et al. (1986) observed no change in milk fat percentage when heat-stressed cows were given water at 10 or 28°C.

The fat percentage of milk increases continuously during the milking process, with the lowest fat milk drawn first and the highest fat milk drawn last. The increase in fat percentage throughout the milking process is due to the clustering of fat globules trapped in the alveoli (Jenness, 1985). Thus, if cows are not milked out completely, fat percentage will be lower than normal, but, at the next milking, fat content will be higher than normal. Furthermore, when milking intervals are unequal, the highest fat percentage is obtained after the shortest interval (Wheelock, 1980). Milk fatty acid composition is not affected by milking interval or time of day milking (Christie, 1979). The effect of milking three versus two times a day on milk fat percentage has varied, with some researchers reporting no change (Amos et al., 1985; DePeters et al., 1985; Gisi et al., 1986) and others reporting decreases (Allen et al., 1986; Gisi et al., 1986).

### Health/Physiology

Mastitis (inflammation of the udder) generally causes a decline in milk fat percentage and a change in milk fat composition (Kitchen, 1981; Needs and Anderson, 1984; Schultz, 1977). The decrease in fat percentage, however, is less (about 10 percent) than that observed for lactose or casein (about 15 percent). Reported changes in milk fat composition from mastitis have varied. There is general agreement on increases in amounts of free fatty acids and short-chain fatty acids, but both increases (Needs and Anderson, 1984) and decreases (Kitchen, 1981; Schultz, 1977) in phospholipid and long-chain fatty acids have been reported.

The effects of hormones on milk fat percentage are not well known (Bauman and Elliot, 1983; Tucker, 1985). It has been demonstrated that adrenaline and noradrenaline increase lipolytic activity in adipose tissue, but their effect on milk fat is unknown. Administration of exogenous growth hormone has resulted both in no change (Bauman et al., 1985; Peel et al., 1985) and in changes (Eppard et al., 1985) in milk fat percentage and composition. At low doses (5 and 10 IU/day), growth hormone lowered fat percentage with no change in fat composition, but at high doses (50 and 100 IU/day), milk fat percentage was increased and milk fat contained more endogenous fatty acids (Eppard et al., 1985). Growth hormone affected both synthesis of fatty acids in the mammary gland and uptake of preformed fatty acids from the blood, depending on dose level and energy balance of the cow. Sutton (1980) reported that the use of thyroprotein, 1,3-butanediol, and glucocorticoids have generally not increased milk fat percentage.

### Nutrition

Diets for today's high-producing dairy cows are typically higher in energy from readily fermentable carbohydrates than fats. Feeding of these diets often causes a condition known as low-milk-fat syndrome. Characteristics of low-milk-fat syndrome are a reduction in milk fat percentage (as much as 60 percent) and changes in milk fat composition (an increase in $C_{18}$ polyunsaturated and monounsaturated acids and decreases in $C_{16:0}$ and $C_{18:0}$ fatty acids) (Banks et al., 1983; Christie, 1979). Causes of low-milk-fat syndrome probably involve both an alteration in rumen fermentation and availability of endogenous fatty acid sources (Christie, 1979). Feeding of readily fermentable carbohydrates depresses fiber digestion and pH in the rumen and thus decreases acetic and butyric acid production and increases propionic acid production. Increased propionic acid concentrations in the rumen lead to increased lactic acid and glucose production, which, in turn, stimulates insulin production, reducing free fatty acid release from adipose tissue. Thus, the main precursors of milk fat (acetic and butyric acids derived from rumen fermentation, long-chain fatty acids of dietary origin, and acetic acid and long-chain fatty acids from endogenous sources) can be affected by diet through changes in rumen fermentation or addition of fats for direct absorption and inclusion into milk fat.

*Rumen fermentation.*   Milk fat percentage is related positively to rumen molar percentages of acetic and butyric acids and negatively to that of propionic acid. Davis (1978) reported that rumen molar percentage of propionate must be above 25 before a highly significant negative relationship between milk fat percentage and propionate exists. Sutton (1980) estimated that 60 percent of the variations observed in milk fat percentage can be accounted for by changes in the molar proportion of propionate in the rumen.

A positive relationship exists between the molar ratio of acetate to propionate and milk fat percentage. A linear increase in milk fat percentage occurs as the ratio of acetate to propionate increases up to 2.2 (Davis, 1978). Above a ratio of 2.2 there is little change in milk fat percentage. Thus, diets that increase propionate production have the greatest effect on milk fat percentage.

Numerous dietary factors affect rumen fermentation (Sutton, 1980). Those most commonly associated with changes in the acetate to propionate ratio are forage to concentrate ratio, type of carbohydrate in the diet, physical form of the diet, processing of ingredients, additives, and the frequency and method of offering feed. The following discussion summarizes the influence of these factors on rumen fermentation, acetate to propionate ratio, and change in milk fat percentage.

The general effect of decreasing the forage to concentrate ratio on rumen fermentation is to decrease pH, increase propionic acid production, and reduce fiber digestion. Thus, as forage declines, milk fat percentage falls proportionately; however, milk fat yields may increase (Sutton, 1980). The critical forage to concentrate ratio appears to be about 40:60, beyond which additional concentrate drastically lowers milk fat percentage (Coppock, 1985; Sutton, 1985). However, Sutton (1980) reported that the actual level of forage needed in a diet to maintain normal milk fat percentage may be affected by total feed intake. At high levels of intake, more forage is needed than at low-intake levels to maintain the same milk fat percentage. Recent work by Shaver et al. (1986) has shown similar results, with milk fat percentages being higher in milk from cows fed a 60:40 forage to grain diet at 2.93 percent of body weight than at 3.75 percent of body weight. Declines in milk fat percentage with high-grain feeding are accompanied by a change in milk fatty acid composition from saturated fatty acids to more unsaturated acids, especially those containing 16 carbons or less (Banks et al., 1983; Sutton, 1980).

The type of forage and its effect on milk fat percentage are influenced by forage particle size, maturity, and fiber content of the forage. It has been known for a while that finely ground forages reduce milk fat percentage. Finely ground forages apparently result in higher levels of propionate being produced during rumen fermentation than forages of adequate particle size (Sutton, 1980). Recent work by Woodford et al.

(1986) has shown that a mean forage particle length of 0.64 cm or more is needed to keep rumen molar percentage of propionate below 25 and milk fat above 3.6 percent. Mertens (1985) recommended a minimum of 28 percent neutral detergent fiber and about 18 percent acid detergent fiber in diets to maximize milk production and fat percentage. The daily amount of neutral detergent fiber needed was estimated to be 1.2 percent of body weight.

Stage of forage maturity is an important factor in the supply of adequate fiber in the diet. More immature alfalfa hay was required in the diet to obtain maximum production of 4 percent fat-corrected milk than when mid- or late-bloom alfalfa hay was fed (Kawas et al., 1983). Recent work (Hansen et al., 1984) has shown that an interaction between forage species and concentrate level in the diet affects milk fat percentage. Bromegrass supported a higher milk fat percentage at higher concentrate feeding than did alfalfa. No difference between the two forage sources was observed at lower concentrate levels.

Carbohydrate source can influence rumen fermentation and consequently milk fat percentage. Sutton (1985) reported that the lower ruminal degradability of corn compared with that of barley would result in the production of milk with a higher fat percentage. Recent work (DePeters and Taylor, 1985) has confirmed that barley-based concentrates tend to depress fiber digestibility, resulting in lower ruminal acetate to propionate ratios and lower milk fat percentages than those with corn-based concentrates. The higher digestion of barley in the rumen produces more propionate and results in less starch being presented to the lower digestive tract for conversion to glucose than with corn. However, the increased production of propionate in the rumen from barley appeared to stimulate milk yield more than glucose derived directly from corn in the lower digestive tract. The mechanism(s) by which these two differences in

nutrient supply affect milk fat is not well known. Processing of grains such as grinding, rolling, heating, steam flaking, and pelleting increases digestion of the starch in the rumen and produces effects similar to those reported above for barley (Sutton, 1980).

Increasing butyric acid production in the rumen should also help to maintain or increase milk fat percentages. Sutton (1980) suggested that beet pulp is a promoter of butyric acid production in the rumen. Other carbohydrates such as whey (Casper and Schingoethe, 1986; Schingoethe, 1976), sucrose, and lactose (Sutton, 1980) have been evaluated as sources of soluble carbohydrate to prevent milk fat depression.

The pattern of feeding, often referred to as feeding strategy, was found to have little if any benefit in terms of increasing milk fat percentage under normal conditions (Linn and Otterby, 1984). However, under feeding regimes where fat-depressing conditions are likely, increasing the frequency of offering concentrates to six or more times per day appears to stabilize the rumen environment (Bragg et al., 1986) and increase milk fat percentage (Sutton, 1980, 1985).

The mixing of all feed ingredients before feeding does not affect milk fat yield or percentage any differently than if the ingredients were fed separately (Holter et al., 1977; Marshall and Voigt, 1975; Owen, 1981).

Thomas and Chamberlain (1984) summarized the effects of infusion of specific nutrients into cows on changes in milk constituents. Intraruminal infusions of acetic acid consistently increase milk yield, lactose yield, and milk fat yield, whereas infusions of propionate reduce milk fat yield. Glucose infusions, either intraabomasal or intravenous, increase milk yield and decrease milk constituent percentages. Infusions of protein or amino acids (Schwab et al., 1976) have had variable or no effect on milk fat percentage.

The effects of dietary protein on milk fat

percentage are variable but generally small when diets within normally accepted ranges of nutrients have been fed (Sutton, 1980; Thomas and Chamberlain, 1984). Changes in fat percentage result from changes in milk yield rather than from a direct effect of dietary protein source or amount. Insufficient amounts of rumen-degradable protein may lower milk fat percentage because of a lack of ruminal ammonia for optimal microbial digestion of fiber and other feedstuffs.

Additives such as buffers and methionine hydroxy analog have been used to promote increases in milk fat percentage. Cows in early lactation fed high-concentrate diets were shown to benefit from the inclusion of the methionine hydroxy analog in their rations (Lundquist et al., 1983). Feeding of 25 grams of methionine hydroxy analog daily during the first 120 days of lactation increased milk fat 0.35 percentage units.

Buffers are compounds used to raise rumen pH through the neutralization of volatile fatty acids. However, other modes of action have been indicated for the group of compounds commonly alluded to as buffers (sodium bicarbonate, potassium bicarbonate, limestone, magnesium oxide, and bentonite) (Chalupa and Schneider, 1985). In general, the bicarbonates have been effective in maintaining or increasing milk fat percentages of cows fed high-grain diets, especially when corn silage was the main forage source (Chalupa and Schneider, 1985; Davis, 1978; Sutton, 1980). Magnesium oxide has also been shown to help prevent milk fat percentage depression; however, it appears that the mechanism of action is through transfer of lipid into the mammary gland from blood rather than through a change in rumen fermentation (Chalupa and Schneider, 1985).

*Added fats.* Dietary fats can alter milk fat composition in a number of ways (Christie, 1979). One route is for fatty acids to be unaltered during digestion and absorption and therefore appear in milk fat directly. Another route is for the rumen microorganisms to hydrogenate the fatty acid, which can then appear in milk fat in this form or be further modified by desaturation before appearing in milk fat. Dietary fatty acids can appear in milk fat in the same form in which they were fed or be completely changed to another form before entering milk. In addition, the amount of particular fatty acids in the diet can alter lipid metabolism in the animal through mammary gland uptake problems or enzyme inhibitions. Dietary long-chain fatty acids can affect rumen fermentation and thus alter the amount of volatile fatty acids (acetic, propionic, and butyric acids) available for fat synthesis in the mammary gland.

The use of fats and oils in the diets of dairy cows has received considerable attention (Fogerty and Johnson, 1980; Linn, 1983; Palmquist and Jenkins, 1980; Storry, 1980; Storry and Brumby, 1980). Numerous lipid sources, from natural to manufactured, have been evaluated. Their effects on milk yield and composition depend on type of fat, characteristics of the diet into which they are incorporated, rate and form fed, and method of feeding. Only a brief summary of changes in milk fat percentage and composition is reported here.

The changes in milk fat percentage and composition observed with the use of fat in diets of dairy cows are a reflection of the change in output of different fatty acids from the mammary gland; short- and medium-chain fatty acids ($C_4$ to $C_{14}$) are synthesized in the mammary gland, the $C_{18}$ fatty acids come from the diet, and the $C_{16}$ fatty acids come from both synthesis and dietary sources. Although dietary fats and oils may alter milk fat composition, the output of total milk fat depends on the balance of increased dietary transfer and decreased synthesis. However, there is probably a minimum content of short-chain fatty acids necessary to maintain melting points at body temperatures (Christie, 1979).

Both protected and unprotected fats and oils have been fed to dairy cows. Some of the unprotected fat or oil sources reported in the literature are tallow, yellow grease, vegetable oils, blends of animal-vegetable fats, and whole oilseeds (soybeans, sunflowers, cottonseed, and rapeseed). The common protected fat sources, so called because they are unavailable in the rumen and therefore do not alter rumen fermentation, fed are tallow and vegetable oils. Common methods of protection are formaldehyde-protein coating (Storry and Brumby, 1980) and formation of insoluble calcium salts of the fat (Jenkins and Palmquist, 1984).

In general, the addition of unprotected fat to dairy diets results in variable effects on milk yield and milk fat composition. The addition of fats, oils, or long-chain fatty acids depresses the synthesis of $C_4$ to $C_{16}$ fatty acids in the mammary gland. This most likely results from an alteration in rumen fermentation rather than an inhibition of mammary gland acetyl-CoA carboxylase activity (Banks et al., 1983; Storry, 1980; Thomas, 1980). The effect on rumen fermentation is most pronounced with unsaturated fatty acid feeding. Long-chain fatty acid sources (more than 20 carbons) such as fish oils and Seterculia seed fats have a specific inhibitory action on the uptake of preformed fatty acids by the mammary gland. The changes in milk fat composition that occur with fat feeding are predominantly in the triglyceride fraction, with very little change occurring in the phospholipid and fat membrane fractions (Storry, 1980).

Protected polyunsaturated fatty acids appear to be the most promising for consistently increasing milk fat percentage and altering milk fat composition. Protected oilseeds or oils rich in linoleic acid (sunflower, corn, and soybean) produce large, rapid increases in the linoleic acid content of milk fat when fed. The increases in linoleic acid content are generally associated with declines in myristic, palmitic, and oleic acids. Transfer of linoleic acid from protected

supplements to milk is reported to be between 20 and 40 percent (Christie, 1979; Fogerty and Johnson, 1980).

Feeding of protected saturated fats, the most common source being tallow, generally invokes the same response in increase of milk fat percentage as feeding of protected polyunsaturated fats. However, protected hydrogenated soybean oil has decreased the milk fat percentage (Banks et al., 1983). Protected tallow increases the amounts of $C_4$, $C_{16:1}$, $C_{18:0}$, and $C_{18:1}$ fatty acids found in milk fat (Christie, 1979). Similar results were reported for unprotected tallow.

## PROTEIN

The total (crude) protein content of milk is determined by analyzing milk for nitrogen and multiplying by a factor of 6.38. The total protein percentage of milk is generally considered to be about 3.5, of which 94 to 95 percent is in the form of true protein (Davies et al., 1983; Jenness, 1985). Casein accounts for approximately 80 percent of the true protein, and milk serum or whey proteins account for about 20 percent. Urea is the largest single nonprotein nitrogen (NPN) component, accounting for approximately 50 percent of the total NPN (Wolfschoon-Pombo and Klostermeyer, 1981).

Milk proteins fall into several families of polypeptide chains, for which a systematic nomenclature system has been defined (Eigel et al., 1984). Casein proteins are characterized by ester-bound phosphate, high proline contents, and few or no cysteine residues and are precipitable from milk at pH 4.6 and 20°C. The main casein types in milk are alpha-, beta-, gamma-, and kappa-caseins. Whey proteins are distinguished from casein by remaining in solution upon precipitation of casein proteins. The major whey proteins are beta-lactoglobulin and alpha-lactalbumin. Serum albumin, immunoglobulins, proteose peptones, lactoferrin, and transferrin represent a smaller proportion of the whey protein fraction (Davies et al., 1983; Jenness, 1985; Kuzdzal-Savoie et al., 1980).

## Biosynthesis

The synthesis of milk proteins has been extensively reviewed (Larson, 1979, 1985; Mercier and Gaye, 1983). In general, protein synthesis in mammary alveolar cells is similar to other protein synthesis systems in which DNA controls protein synthesis. Messenger RNA carries the encoded DNA message from the nucleus to the ribosomes located in the rough endoplasmic reticulum (RER) and cytoplasm. Ribosomes are composed of ribosomal RNA and several proteins combined into a ribonucleoprotein complex, which, in conjunction with transfer RNA, combines amino acids into peptide chains. As the polypeptide chains are elongated to form proteins, they pass out of the RER, through the lumen, and into the region of the Golgi apparatus where they accumulate and polymerize into different milk protein molecules. Casein must be phosphorylated, bound with calcium, and stabilized by calcium phosphate linkages and other ionic bonds before being released from the vesicles. The presence of alpha-lactalbumin in the region of the Golgi apparatus promotes synthesis of lactose. The secretory vesicles containing essentially nonfat milk constituents leave the cell by moving to the apical surface and fusing with the plasma membrane and discharging the vesicular contents into the cell lumen.

Most of the proteins present in milk are synthesized in the mammary gland, although some immunoglobulins and albumins are transferred from the blood (Larson, 1979). Blood leukocytes can also cross mammary barriers either by passing between secretory cells or by pushing secretory cells directly into the lumen. Urea diffuses freely across mammary cells, so there is a high correlation between blood plasma and milk urea concentrations (Thomas, 1980).

The synthesis of milk protein requires that both essential and nonessential amino acids be supplied to the mammary gland (Clark et al., 1978; Mepham, 1982). Uptake of free amino acids from the blood by the mammary gland can occur via several transport systems (Baumrucker, 1985). Mepham (1982) has classified essential and nonessential amino acids into three groups according to uptake by the mammary gland. Group I essential amino acids (methionine, histidine, phenylalanine, tyrosine, and tryptophan) are taken up in amounts just sufficient to meet milk protein synthesis needs. Group II essential amino acids (valine, leucine, isoleucine, arginine, lysine, and threonine) are taken up in excess. However, some data (Thomas, 1983) suggest that lysine and possibly leucine, isoleucine, and threonine should also be included in group I. Group III is the nonessential amino acids. The amounts taken up vary with animal, time, and availability. In addition to free amino acid uptake from blood, there is evidence that red blood cells and the recycling of amino acids also contribute to the cellular amino acid pool (Baumrucker, 1985). Breakdown of red blood cell glutathionine can make a significant contribution to the amount of cysteine, glycine, and glutamic acid available in the cell. Recycling of casein proteins is reported to account for at least 7 percent of the protein synthetic capacity in the mammary gland.

## Factors Affecting Milk Protein Content

### Breed/Genetics

Breeds differ in total milk protein percentage and type of milk protein produced. Jersey and Guernsey cattle have the highest percentages of total protein, casein, and whey. Variability of the major protein fractions within breeds has also been reported (Rolleri et al., 1956), with Holstein milk containing less of the major caseins and more gamma-casein than milk from other breeds. Genetic variants have been demonstrated for the milk protein groups, and breed differences have been found for the frequency of occurrence of these variants (Gaunt, 1980).

Genetic selection would increase the percentage of protein in milk 0.075 percentage units but decrease milk yield 231 pounds. Joint selection for milk yield, protein, and fat is recommended if the desired result is increased yield of protein and fat (Gaunt, 1980; Van Vleck, 1978; Wilcox, 1978). Gaunt (1980) estimated that it would take about 11 generations for milk protein percentages to equal milk fat percentages if protein yield with no change in fat percentage were used as the selection criterion.

### Environment/Management

Age has a significant effect on milk protein percentage and composition in cows (Jenness, 1985; Ng-Kwai-Hang et al., 1982; Rogers and Stewart, 1982). Milk protein percentage declines in cows older than 3 years, with a 0.4 percentage unit drop being reported over five lactations (Rogers and Stewart, 1982). This decline appears to be primarily in the casein fraction; however, changes in whey protein fractions have also been reported (Kroeker et al., 1985). Suggested reasons for the change are deterioration of udder tissue, selective culling for high production, and increased incidences of mastitis. The increase in immunoglobulins with advancing age reported by Kroeker et al. (1985) supports the latter suggestion.

Stage of lactation has a considerable influence on milk protein concentration (Davies et al., 1983; Ng-Kwai-Hang et al., 1982, 1985; Rogers and Stewart, 1982). At the beginning of lactation, colostrum is exceptionally rich in protein containing large quantities of immunoglobulins and about twice the levels of casein, beta-lactoglobulin, and alpha-lactalbumin found in mid-lactation milk. Total protein amounts fall rapidly during the first few days of transition from colostrum to normal milk and reach a minimum about 5 to 10 weeks into lactation, corresponding inversely to maximum milk yield. Thereafter, the amount of protein tends either to increase gradually as lactation progresses or to rise sharply when the cow becomes pregnant.

Milk protein percentage (Ng-Kwai-Hang et al., 1982) and yield (Keown et al., 1986) are higher during fall and winter than spring and summer. However, stage of lactation and feeding practices confound these observations as cows on spring pasture have elevated milk protein concentrations (Rogers and Stewart, 1982). Whey proteins have been found to have no definite seasonal variations (Kroeker et al., 1985). High environmental temperatures, above 29°C, have been suggested to depress milk protein percentage, but cows offered cold water (10°C) during heat stress do not show increased milk protein concentrations over cows offered 28°C water (Milam et al., 1986).

Variations in milking procedure or frequency have a minor effect, if any, on milk protein percentage. Milk protein or SNF percentages do not change during the milking process (Jenness, 1985). Extended milking intervals do not change milk protein or SNF percentages until intervals exceed 16 hours (Rogers and Stewart, 1982). Increasing milking frequency from twice to three times daily for more than 15,000 Holstein cows did not change the percentage of SNF (Gisi et al., 1986). Similar results were reported by Amos et al. (1985) and DePeters et al. (1985).

### Health/Physiology

Mastitis has very little effect on total milk protein percentage; however, it drastically alters the composition of milk protein (Kitchen, 1981; Schultz, 1977). The general effect of mastitis is to impair milk synthesis and loosen the connections between cells, thereby increasing permeability of blood constituents (Jenness, 1985; Wheelock, 1980). Milk proteins synthesized in the mammary gland (caseins, beta-lactoglobulin, and alpha-lactalbumin) decrease (Kitchen, 1981; Schultz, 1977), whereas blood serum proteins (whey proteins) increase (Kitchen, 1981;

Kroeker et al., 1985; Poutrel et al., 1983; Schultz, 1977). Grappin et al. (1981) reported a whey protein to total protein ratio increase of 2.08 percent and a casein to total protein ratio decrease of 1.85 percent for every 1 log unit increase in somatic cell count. The same change in somatic cell count was reported by Ng-Kwai-Hang et al. (1982) to decrease the ratio of casein to total protein by 2.79 percent.

The hormone requirement for milk synthesis and secretion is prolactin, adrenocorticotrophic hormone, and estrogens and the relative absence of progesterone. Of particular importance to milk protein synthesis is prolactin (Tucker, 1985). Current studies (Bauman et al., 1985; Peel et al., 1985) on administration of exogenous growth hormone have generally shown increases in milk yield without significant changes in composition. However, Eppard et al. (1985) observed a slight decrease in milk protein percentage and an increase in alpha-lactalbumin as a percentage of total milk protein with increasing dosage levels (0 to 100 IU/day) of bovine growth hormone.

### Nutrition

Dietary crude protein affects milk yield and consequently milk protein yield more than milk protein percentage (Emery, 1978; Kaufman, 1980; Thomas, 1980, 1983). A small effect of dietary crude protein concentration on milk protein percentage was reported by Emery (1978): a 0.02 percentage unit increase in milk protein with every 1 percentage unit increase in dietary crude protein between 9 and 17 percent. More recently, Cragle et al. (1986) reported an increase of 0.1273 Mcal in milk protein energy content per 1 Mcal gross energy increase in feed protein. Neither of these studies, however, considered source of dietary crude protein or change in milk protein composition. Thus, the increases in milk protein observed may have been in milk NPN and not true milk protein. Elevated milk protein concentrations from cows fed diets high in rumen-degradable protein or NPN most likely will be from increased milk urea or NPN levels (Oltner et al., 1985; Thomas, 1980). On the other hand, diets low in rumen-degradable protein or balanced for optimal microbial protein synthesis should increase supplies of amino acids available to the mammary gland for protein synthesis, and thus, more true milk protein should be produced (Kaufman, 1980; Oldham, 1984; Thomas, 1980). However, the proportions between true milk proteins (caseins, beta-lactoglobulin, and alpha-lactalbumin) do not appear to change with increases or decreases in milk protein synthesis (Thomas, 1983).

In experiments where protein (usually casein) has been abomasally infused to increase amino acid supplies to the tissue, increases in milk protein percentage along with milk yield have been reported (Clark, 1975; Clark et al., 1977). Abomasal infusions of amino acid mixtures also increased milk protein percentage, with methionine and lysine accounting for more than 68 percent of the observed increase (Schwab et al., 1976). Based on these responses, it could be concluded that increasing the intestinal supply of amino acids through increased rumen protein synthesis or low rumen-degradable protein sources would increase milk protein percentage and probably milk yield. However, on a practical feeding basis, milk protein responses to dietary proteins with different rumen degradabilities have been quite variable but generally of no effect. A number of studies (Crawford and Hoover, 1984; Crooker et al., 1983; Forester et al., 1983; Henderson et al., 1985; Holter et al., 1985; Kung and Huber, 1983; Lundquist et al., 1986) reported no increases in milk protein when protected proteins were fed. Madsen's (1982) study, however, reported significant increases. Again, none of the studies cited determined milk protein composition except that of Lundquist et al. (1986), which showed no change in milk

NPN content within equal dietary crude protein percentages due to feeding formaldehyde-treated soybean meal compared with feeding an untreated soybean meal.

Kaufman (1980) summarized the effects of dietary protein supply on milk protein concentration. Insufficient amounts of dietary protein will reduce milk protein concentrations, but the reduction is minimized when low rumen-degradable protein supplements are fed. Increasing dietary crude protein supply has little effect on milk protein percentage.

The amount of energy consumed, density of energy in the diet, and the source of energy in the diet all influence milk protein percentage and yield. Cragle et al. (1986) compared 59 percent versus 49 percent concentrate feeding and found that cows fed rations containing 59 percent concentrate produced an average of 11 percent more milk, 13 percent more protein, 3 percent more fat, and 11 percent more lactose than cows fed 49 percent concentrate rations. Of the increase in milk protein, 85 percent was attributed to increased yield and only 15 percent to increased percentage in the milk. Emery (1978) reported that milk protein percentage increases 0.015 percent for each Mcal of additional net energy fed from 9 to 40 Mcal/day and that the increased protein percentage was usually accompanied by an increased milk yield. Mild energy malnutrition has been reported to slightly reduce milk protein percentage; however, under severe energy malnutrition, milk protein percentage is unaltered but yields decrease drastically (Thomas, 1980, 1983).

Rogers and Stewart (1982) reviewed the effects of various forage sources in the diet on milk composition. Cows grazing early spring pastures were reported to have increased milk protein percentages. However, the confounding of energy, protein, and condition of the cow in most forage studies where milk composition is reported prohibits the drawing of definite conclusions.

Thomas (1980, 1983) discussed the notion that increasing propionic acid in the rumen through increased concentrate feeding or reduced forage particle size affects milk protein percentage. To summarize, there is a strong positive correlation between rumen production of propionic acid and milk protein; however, the exact mechanism is unknown. One suggestion is that propionate increases glutamic acid availability to the mammary gland and, through its role in amino acid transamination, enhances synthesis of nonessential amino acids. A second hypothesis is that propionate through insulin could enhance plasma concentrations of glutamine and alanine. Propionate could also enhance glutamate output from the liver by increasing its synthesis or reducing usage in gluconeogenesis.

Intake of energy can also be increased through inclusion of fats or oils in the diet. Feeding protected lipids, vegetable fats, or vegetable oils to lactating cows depressed milk protein percentage, whereas animal fats had no effect or minimal effect on milk protein percentages (Linn, 1983; Palmquist and Jenkins, 1980). Dunkley et al. (1977) indicated that the depressing effect was on the casein fraction. Although the exact depressing mechanism is unknown, it may be through altered glucose metabolism (Palmquist and Jenkins, 1980), changes in rumen metabolism (Jenkins and Palmquist, 1984), or both. Thus, the source of increased dietary energy (carbohydrate versus lipid) fed to lactating cows has a significant effect on milk protein percentage changes.

## CARBOHYDRATES

The predominant carbohydrate in milk is the disaccharide lactose. It is composed of one molecule of glucose and one molecule of galactose joined in a 1-4 carbon linkage as beta-galactoside. The principal biological function of lactose in milk is the regulation of water content and, thus, the regulation of osmotic content (Davies et al., 1983; Jenness, 1985). Because of this function, lactose is the most constant constituent in milk, averaging 4.6 percent.

Carbohydrates other than lactose that are found in milk are monosaccharides, sugar phosphates, nucleotide sugars, free neutral and acid oligosaccharides, and glycosyl groups of peptides and proteins (Jenness, 1985). Free glucose and galactose and the sugar alcohol myo-inositol are also present in milk. However, the amounts of these carbohydrate fractions are minor compared with that of lactose.

## Biosynthesis

Glucose is the primary substrate for lactose synthesis, with 85 percent of the carbon secreted in lactose derived from blood glucose (Thomas and Chamberlain, 1984). Lactose synthesis is initiated in the Golgi apparatus and continues in the vesicles with an influx of water and ionic constituents that causes the vesicles to swell as they pass toward the cell surface. Glucose and uridine diphosphate (UDP)-galactose, derived from glucose, combine to form lactose under the action of the enzyme lactose synthetase. The milk protein beta-lactalbumin must be present for glucose and UDP-galactose to combine. Thus, beta-lactalbumin appears to be a prime regulator of lactose synthesis (Kuhn, 1983; Larson, 1985). Entry of water into the vesicle is linked with lactose synthesis to maintain osmotic equilibrium with surrounding fluids. Thus, the rate of lactose synthesis regulates water secretion and consequently milk yield.

## MINERALS

### Factors Affecting Milk Mineral Content

The mineral content of milk is derived from minerals found in circulating body fluids. The factors influencing mineral content of milk are discussed below.

### Breed/Genetics

Cerbulis and Farrel (1976) reported the ash, calcium, phosphorus, and magnesium contents of milk from different breeds of dairy cattle. The average ash content varied from 0.74 percent for Holsteins to 0.83 percent for Jerseys. The highest calcium and phosphorus contents in milk were reported for Jerseys.

### Environment/Management

It is well documented that the mineral composition of colostrum is higher than that of milk. Calcium, phosphorus, potassium, and chloride concentrations follow the same lactation curves as fat and protein—that is, high in colostrum, lowest at peak milk yield, and then gradually increasing as lactation progresses (Iyengar, 1982; Jenness, 1985). Milk inorganic phosphorus levels were shown to be higher in first lactation cows than in multiparous cows, and milk phosphate levels were lowest during the summer (Forar et al., 1982).

### Health/Physiology

Mastitis increases the percentages of sodium and chloride in milk and decreases the percentage of potassium (Kitchen, 1981; Peaker and Faulkner, 1983; Schultz, 1977). Bacterial infection of the udder results in damage to the ductal and secretory epithelium and increases the permeability of blood capillaries. Thus, sodium and chloride, which are higher in blood, pour into the lumen of the alveolus, and in order to maintain osmolarity, potassium is decreased proportionally. Fernando et al. (1985) reported the decline in lactose and potassium and increase in sodium and chloride in mastitic milk was most prominent in strippings of milk after milking.

The percentages of calcium and phosphorus in milk decline with mastitis infections (Kitchen, 1981; Schultz, 1977). Most likely this reflects lower casein levels, since both ions are complexed with casein micelles. Contradictory evidence exists regarding the effect of mastitic infections on levels of magnesium. Trace elements may increase slightly in mastitic milk (Tallamy and Randolph, 1970).

Administration of exogenous growth hormone has relatively little effect on the percentages of minerals in milk, but yields of minerals increased with increasing milk production (Eppard et al., 1985).

### Nutrition

Normal dietary regimes have little influence on the mineral composition of milk, especially the macromineral constituents. Forar et al. (1982) fed two levels of phosphorus (0.31 and 0.54 percent) and two levels of calcium (1.0 and 1.8 percent) in four diets to lactating cows and found no differences in milk inorganic phosphorus percentages. Diets depressing milk fat percentage have been shown to lower the percentage of citrate and soluble calcium in milk (Davies et al., 1983). Changes in milk phosphorus and calcium percentages would not be expected, since very few of these ions are in the free form in milk. Dietary factors affecting citrate and casein contents of milk would be expected to correspond with small changes in calcium, since calcium is complexed and secreted with these substances.

Fettman et al. (1984) observed decreases in milk chloride percentage when cows were fed chloride-deficient rations during early lactation. Milk potassium percentage declined along with chloride levels, reflecting altered mineral metabolism in chloride-deficient cows. A recent report (Schneider et al., 1986) evaluating dietary sodium and potassium effects on heat-stressed cows found no change in milk potassium percentages based on quantity of potassium fed or source of sodium fed. However, cows offered shade had higher milk potassium percentages than cows given no shade. Percentages of sodium in milk were lowered significantly by feeding cows sodium bicarbonate and only slightly by feeding salt or high levels of potassium, as compared with results for control cows. The lower milk sodium percentages corresponded with lower plasma sodium levels in cows fed sodium bicarbonate.

Milk iodine levels have been shown to increase with increased feeding of iodine. Franke et al. (1983) observed progressive increases in milk iodine concentrations during lactation when as little as 4 ppm of organic iodine were added to the diet. Larson et al. (1983) found cow age, season of calving, milk production, and health status to have no effect on the concentration of iodine in milk.

Iyengar (1982) reported that iodine, manganese, molybdenum, selenium, zinc, and cobalt concentrations in milk could be altered by dietary means. However, very limited research has been directed toward this end. Most of the changes that have been observed are the result of marked dietary changes. The effects of slightly underfeeding or overfeeding a required dietary mineral or the effects of mineral interactions on the mineral composition of milk are not well known.

## OTHER MILK SOLUBLES

There are many other components in milk in addition to those already discussed. They can be categorized as either natural or contaminant. They appear in milk both from leakage during the normal secretory process and by actual secretion. Whatever the mode of entry, their concentrations can vary considerably, but their significance and purpose remain largely unknown.

The natural compounds that have been detected in milk are gases, alcohol, aldehydes, ketones, carboxylic acid, sulfur-containing compounds, nucleotide material, hormones, phosphate esters, glucose, acetate, and citrate. Many of these are products of intermediary metabolism of the mammary gland (Davies et al., 1983; Jenness, 1985; Peaker and Faulkner, 1983). The reasons for changes in the concentrations of these compounds in milk are unknown.

An exception to the above is the compound citrate. The concentration of citrate in milk is modifiable and is important from a milk-processing standpoint. Alteration of citrate concentrations changes the amount of free calcium in the soluble phase of milk, which, in turn, affects the precipitation of milk proteins. Milk citrate concentrations are highly correlated with fat percentage, and therefore diets that lower milk fat percentage also decrease the citrate content of milk (Faulkner and Peaker, 1982). Stage of lactation and season of the year also affect milk citrate levels. It appears that the source of milk citrate is from synthesis within secretory cells and that secretion into milk is similar to that of lactose and casein (Faulkner and Peaker, 1982).

The other category of components—contaminants—includes compounds that are not normally found in milk but that enter accidentally or by design. Included here are chemicals, pesticides, herbicides, fungicides, heavy metals, and drugs. These items are mentioned as a reminder that milk can contain compounds other than those of nutritional importance to humans and that maintaining a nutritious, wholesome milk supply is of utmost importance.

## MANIPULATING MILK CONSTITUENTS—SUMMARY AND CONCLUSIONS

Variations in milk composition arise from differences in relative rates of synthesis and secretion of milk components by the mammary gland. The processes involved for lactose, protein, and fat synthesis and secretion are independent but regulated through nutrient or substrate availability and hormonal control of nutrient utilization. Thus, genetics, which mediates hormonal

effects, and diet, which regulates nutrient availability, are the major factors affecting milk composition.

The most variable milk constituent is fat. Considerable variation exists between and within dairy cattle breeds. Genetic selection for fat percentage can change fat content of milk but will also affect other constituents since there is a high correlation between the percentage of components in milk. Genetic selection for fat content would alter the quantity of fat produced but not the composition of the fat. The best hope for altering composition is through diet. Changes in fat percentage and composition can be accomplished by altering the diet to produce changes in fermentation patterns or the composition of fat absorbed from the digestive tract. Diets that increase the proportion of propionate in the rumen depress milk fat percentage, but changes in fat composition are minimal, including slight increases in $C_{18}$ polyunsaturated fatty acids and slight decreases in $C_{16:0}$ and $C_{18:0}$ fatty acids. Inclusion of fats in the diet, particularly rumen-protected fats, is the most effective way to alter milk fat composition. Significant increases in long-chain fatty acids can be achieved by including fat containing these acids in the diet. However, the amount and composition of fats in the diet need to be controlled to avoid impairment of digestion of other dietary constituents in the rumen. Unsaturated fatty acids are hydrogenated extensively in the rumen.

Milk protein percentage and composition can be manipulated through genetic selection. Variations in the casein, beta-lactoglobulin, and alpha-lactalbumin fractions are known to exist. Heritability estimates of protein percentage range from 0.3 to 0.7. Increasing milk protein percentage through genetic selection is feasible; however, increasing milk protein yield through selection is more desirable. The percentage of true proteins in milk cannot be manipulated through feeding. Total protein percentage in milk can be lowered by including fats in the diet or raised in relation to milk fat percentage by feeding high-concentrate diets. Dietary protein percentage has a minimal effect on milk protein percentage when it is within practical feeding ranges.

Levels of other nutritional components of milk—lactose, vitamins, and minerals—are rather constant and not subject to large changes through genetic or nutritional manipulation.

The manipulation of milk components through changes in dairy management practices, breeding, feeding, health, environment, and general management appears to be rather limited. Milk fat percentage and composition can be changed through feeding, whereas milk protein percentage is best changed through genetics. Any changes will be slow in coming and minor compared to those achieved through processing and manufacturing. The goal of milk producers should be to modify composition as much as possible to meet market demand but to emphasize maximum yield of components in high-quality, wholesome milk.

## REFERENCES

Allen, D. B., E. J. DePeters, and R. C. Laben. 1986. Three times a day milking: Effects on milk production, reproductive efficiency and udder health. J. Dairy Sci. 69:1441.

Amos, H. E., T. Kiser, and M. Loewenstein. 1985. Influence of milking frequency on reproductive and productive efficiencies of cows. J. Dairy Sci. 68:732.

Banks, W., J. L. Clapperton, and W. Steele. 1983. Dietary manipulation of the content and fatty acid composition of milk fat. Proc. Nutr. Soc. 42:399.

Bauman, D. E., and J. M. Elliot. 1983. Control of nutrient partitioning in lactating ruminants. Ch. 14 in Biochemistry of Lactation, T. B. Mepham, ed. Amsterdam: Elsevier.

Bauman, D. E., P. J. Eppard, M. J. DeGeeter, and G. M. Lanza. 1985. Responses of high-producing dairy cows to long term treatment with pituitary somatotropin and recombinant somatotropin. J. Dairy Sci. 68:1352.

Baumrucker, C. R. 1985. Amino acid transport systems in bovine mammary tissue. J. Dairy Sci. 68:2436.

Bragg, D. St. A., M. R. Murphy, and C. L. Davis. 1986. Effect of source of carbohydrate and frequency of feeding on rumen parameters in dairy steers. J. Dairy Sci. 69:392.

Casper, D. P., and D. J. Schingoethe. 1986. Evaluation of urea and dried whey in diets of cows during early lactation. J. Dairy Sci. 69:1346.

Cerbulis, J., and H. M. Farrell, Jr. 1976. Composition of the milk of dairy cattle. II. Ash, calcium, magnesium and phosphorus. J. Dairy Sci. 59:589.

Chalupa, W., and P. L. Schneider. 1985. Buffers for dairy cattle. 20th Annual Proceedings of the 1985 Pacific Northwest Animal Nutrition Conference, sponsored by the Pacific Northwest Feed Manufacturers. October 1985, Boise, Idaho.

Christie, W. W. 1979. The effects of diet and other factors on the lipid composition of ruminant tissues and milk. Prog. Lipid Res. 17:245.

Clark, J. H. 1975. Lactational responses to post-ruminal administration of proteins and amino acids. J. Dairy Sci. 58:1178.

Clark, J. H., H. R. Spires, R. G. Derrig, and M. R. Bennik. 1977. Milk production, nitrogen utilization and glucose synthesis in lactating cows infused post-ruminally with sodium caseinate and glucose. J. Nutr. 107:631.

Clark, J. H., H. R. Spires, and C. L. Davis. 1978. Uptake and metabolism of nitrogenous compounds by the lactating mammary gland. Fed. Proc. 37:1233.

Coppock, C. E. 1985. Energy nutrition and metabolism of the lactating cow. J. Dairy Sci. 68:3403.

Cragle, R. G., M. R. Murphy, S. W. Williams, and J. H. Clark. 1986. Effects of altering milk production and composition by feeding on multiple component milk pricing system. J. Dairy Sci. 69:282.

Crawford, R. J., Jr., and W. H. Hoover. 1984. Effects of particle size and formaldehyde treatment of soybean meal on milk production and composition for dairy cows. J. Dairy Sci. 67:1945.

Crooker, B. A., J. H. Clark, and R. D. Shanks. 1983. Effects of formaldehyde treated soybean meal on milk yield, milk composition and nutrient digestibility in the dairy cow. J. Dairy Sci. 66:492.

Davies, D. T., C. Holt, and W. W. Christie. 1983. The composition of milk. Ch. 5 in Biochemistry of Lactation, T. B. Mepham, ed. Amsterdam: Elsevier.

Davis, C. L. 1978. The use of buffers in the rations of lactating dairy cows. In Proceedings of the Regulation of Acid-Base Balance, sponsored by the University of Arizona and Church and Dwight Co., Inc., W. H. Hale and P. Meinhardt, eds. Tuscon: University of Arizona.

DePeters, E. J., and S. J. Taylor. 1985. Effects of feeding corn or barley on composition of milk and diet digestibility. J. Dairy Sci. 68:2027.

DePeters, E. J., N. E. Smith, and J. Acedo-Rico. 1985. Three or two times daily milking of older cows and first lactation cows for entire lactations. J. Dairy Sci. 68:123.

Dils, R. R. 1983. Milk fat synthesis. Ch. 5 in Biochemistry of Lactation, T. B. Mepham, ed. Amsterdam: Elsevier.

Dils, R. R. 1986. Comparative aspects of milk fat synthesis. J. Dairy Sci. 69:904.

Dunkley, W. L., N. E. Smith, and A. A. Franke. 1977. Effects of feeding protected tallow on composition of milk and milk fat. J. Dairy Sci. 60:1863.

Eigel, W. N., J. E. Butler, C. A. Ernstrom, H. M. Farrell, Jr., V. R. Harwalker, R. Jenness, and R. McL. Whitney. 1984. Nomenclature of proteins of cow's milk: Fifth revision. J. Dairy Sci. 67:1599.

Emery, R. S. 1978. Feeding for increased milk protein. J. Dairy Sci. 61:825.

Eppard, P. J., D. E. Bauman, J. Bitman, D. L. Wood, R. M. Akers, and W. A. House. 1985. Effect of dose of bovine growth hormone on milk composition: Alpha-lactalbumin, fatty acids, and mineral elements. J. Dairy Sci. 68:3047.

Faulkner, A., and M. Peaker. 1982. Secretion of citrate into milk. J. Dairy Res. 49:159.

Fernando, R. S., S. L. Spahr, and E. H. Jaster. 1985. Comparison of electrical conductivity of milk with other indirect methods for detection of subclinical mastitis. J. Dairy Sci. 68:449.

Fettman, M. J., L. E. Chase, J. Bentinck-Smith, C. E. Coppock, and S. A. Zinn. 1984. Nutritional chloride deficiency in early lactation Holstein cows. J. Dairy Sci. 67:2321.

Fogerty, A. C., and A. R. Johnson. 1980. Influence of nutritional factors on the yield and content of milk fat: Protected polyunsaturated fat in the diet. Int. Dairy Fed. Bull. Doc. 125:96.

Forar, F. L., R. L. Kincaid, R. L. Preston, and J. K. Hillers. 1982. Variation of inorganic phosphate in blood plasma and milk lactating cows. J. Dairy Sci. 65:760.

Forester, R. J., D. G. Grieve, J. G. Buchanan-Smith, and G. K. MacLeod. 1983. Effect of dietary protein degradability on cows in early lactation. J. Dairy Sci. 66:1653.

Franke, A. A., J. C. Bruhn, and R. B. Osland. 1983. Factors affecting iodine concentration of milk of individual cows. J. Dairy Sci. 66:997.

Gaunt, S. N. 1973. Genetic and environmental changes in milk consumption. J. Dairy Sci. 56:270.

Gaunt, S. N. 1980. Genetic variation in the yields and contents of milk constituents. Int. Dairy Fed. Bull. Doc. 125:73.

Gisi, D. D., E. J. DePeters, and C. L. Pelissier. 1986. Three times daily milking of cows in California dairy herds. J. Dairy Sci. 69:863.

Grappin, R., V. S. Packard, and R. E. Ginn. 1981. Variability and interrelationship of various herd milk components. J. Food Prot. 44:69.

Hansen, W. P., D. E. Otterby, J. D. Donker, R. G. Lundquist, and J. G. Linn. 1984. Influence of grain concentrations, forage type, and methionine hydroxy analog on lactational performance of dairy cattle. J. Dairy Sci. 67(Suppl. 1):99 (Abstr.).

Henderson, S. J., H. E. Amos, and J. J. Evans. 1985. Influence of dietary crude protein concentration and degradability on milk production, composition, and ruminal protein metabolism. J. Dairy Sci. 68:2227.

Holter, J. B., W. E. Urban, Jr., H. H. Hayes, and H. A. Davis. 1977. Utilization of diet components fed blended or separately to lactating cows. J. Dairy Sci. 60:1288.

Holter, J. B., W. E. Hylton, and C. K. Bozak. 1985. Varying protein content and nitrogen solubility for pluriparous, lactating Holstein cows: Lactation performance and profitability. J. Dairy Sci. 68:1984.

Iyengar, G. V. 1982. Elemental Composition of Human and Animal Milk: A Review. International Atomic Energy Agency Technical Document 269. Vienna: International Atomic Energy Agency.

Jenkins, T. C., and D. L. Palmquist. 1984. Effect of fatty acids of calcium soaps on rumen and total nutrient digestibility of dairy rations. J. Dairy Sci. 67:978.

Jenness, R. 1985. Biochemical and nutritional aspects of milk and colostrum. Ch. 5 in Lactation, B. L. Larson, ed. Ames: Iowa State University Press.

Kaufman, W. 1980. Protein degradation and synthesis within the reticulorumen in relation to milk protein synthesis. Intl. Dairy Fed. Bull. Doc. 125:152.

Kawas, J. R., N. A. Jorgensen, A. R. Hardie, and J. L. Danelon. 1983. Change in feeding value of alfalfa hay with stage of maturity and concentrate level. J. Dairy Sci. 66:181 (Abstr.).

Keown, J. F., R. W. Everett, N. B. Empet, and L. H. Wadell. 1986. Lactation curves. J. Dairy Sci. 69:769.

Kitchen, B. J. 1981. Bovine mastitis: Milk compositional changes and related diagnostic tests. J. Dairy Res. 48:167.

Kroeker, E. M., K. F. Ng-Kwai-Hang, J. F. Hayes, and J. E. Moxley. 1985. Effect of beta-lactoglobulin variant and environmental factors on variation in the detailed composition of bovine milk serum proteins. J. Dairy Sci. 68:1637.

Kuhn, N. J. 1983. The biosynthesis of lactose. Ch. 6 in Biochemistry of Lactation, T. B. Mepham, ed. Amsterdam: Elsevier.

Kung, L., Jr., and J. T. Huber. 1983. Performance of high producing cows in early lactation fed protein of varying amounts, sources, and degradability. J. Dairy Sci. 66:227.

Kuzdzal-Savoie, S., W. Manson, and J. H. Moore. 1980. The constituents of cow's milk. Int. Dairy Fed. Bull. Doc. 125:4–13.

Larson, B. L. 1979. Biosynthesis and secretion of milk protein: A review. J. Dairy Res. 46:161

Larson, B. L. 1985. Biosynthesis and cellular secretion of milk. Ch. 4 in Lactation, B. L. Larson, ed. Ames: Iowa State University Press.

Larson, L. L., S. E. Wallen, F. G. Owen, and S. R. Lowry. 1983. Relation of age, season, production and health indices to iodine and beta-carotene concentrations in cow's milk. J. Dairy Sci. 66:2257.

Linn, J. G. 1983. The addition of fats to diets of lactating dairy cows: A review. In Proceedings of a Feed Fat Seminar, sponsored by Central Bi-Products. Redwood Falls, Minn.

Linn, J. G., and D. E. Otterby. 1984. Feeding strategies in dairy nutrition. Pp. 13–22 in Proceedings of the 45th Minnesota Nutrition Conference. St. Paul, Minn.: University of Minnesota Press.

Lundquist, R. L., J. G. Linn, and D. E. Otterby. 1983. Influence of dietary energy and protein on yield and composition of milk from cows fed methionine hydroxy analog. J. Dairy Sci. 66:475

Lundquist, R. L., D. E. Otterby, and J. G. Linn. 1986. Influence of formaldehyde-treated soybean meal on milk production. J. Dairy Sci. 69:1337.

Madsen, J. 1982. The effect of formaldehyde-treated protein and urea on milk yield and composition in dairy cows. Acta Agric. Scand. 32:389.

Marshall, S. P., and A. R. Voigt. 1975. Complete rations for dairy cattle. I. Methods of preparation and roughage-to-concentrate ratios of blended rations with corn silage. J. Dairy Sci. 58:891.

Mepham, T. B. 1982. Amino acid utilization by lactating mammary gland. J. Dairy Sci. 65:287.

Mercier, J.-C., and P. Gaye. 1983. Milk protein synthesis. Ch. 7 in Biochemistry of Lactation, T. B. Mepham, ed. Amsterdam: Elsevier.

Mertens, D. R. 1985. Effect of fiber on feed quality for dairy cows. Pp. 209–224 in Proceedings of the 46th Minnesota Nutrition Conference. St. Paul, Minn.: University of Minnesota Press.

Milam, K. Z., C. E. Coppock, J. W. West, J. K. Lanham, D. H. Nave, J. M. Labore, R. A. Stermer, and C. F. Brasington. 1986. Effects of drinking water temperature on production responses in lactating Holstein cows in summer. J. Dairy Sci. 69:1013.

Needs, E. C., and M. Anderson. 1984. Lipid composition of milk from cows with experimentally induced mastitis. J. Dairy Res. 51:239.

Ng-Kwai-Hang, K. F., J. F. Hayes, J. E. Moxley, and H. G. Monardes. 1982. Environmental influences on protein content and composition of bovine milk. J. Dairy Sci. 65:1993.

Ng-Kwai-Hang, K. F., J. F. Hayes, J. E. Moxley, and H. G. Monardes. 1985. Percentages of protein and nonprotein nitrogen with varying fat and somatic cells in bovine milk. J. Dairy Sci. 68:1257.

Oldham, J. D. 1984. Amino acid metabolism in ruminants. Pp. 137–151 in Proceedings of the Cornell Nutrition Conference, sponsored by Cornell University and American Feed Manufacturers Association. Ithaca, N.Y.: Cornell University.

Oltner, R., M. Emanuelson, and H. Wiktorsson. 1985. Urea concentrations in milk in relation to milk yield, live weight, lactation number and amount and composition of feed given to dairy cows. Livestock Prod. Sci. 12:47.

Owen, J. B. 1981. Complete-diet feeding of dairy cows. In Recent Development in Ruminant Nutrition, W. Haresign and D. J. A. Cole, eds. London: Butterworth.

Palmquist, D. L., and T. C. Jenkins. 1980. Fat in lactation rations: Review. J. Dairy Sci. 63:1

Peaker, M., and A. Faulkner. 1983. Soluble milk constituents. Proc. Nutr. Soc. 42:419.

Peel, C. J., L. D. Sandles, K. J. Quelch, and A. C. Herington. 1985. The effects of long-term administration of bovine growth hormone on the lactational performance of identical-twin dairy cows. Anim. Prod. 41:135.

Poutrel, B., J. P. Caffin, and P. Rainard. 1983. Physiological and pathological factors influencing bovine serum albumin content in milk. J. Dairy Sci. 66:535.

Rogers, G. L., and J. A. Stewart. 1982. The effects of some nutritional and nonnutritional factors on milk protein concentration and yield. Aust. J. Dairy Technol. 37:26.

Rolleri, G. D., B. L. Larson, and R. W. Touchberry. 1956. Protein production in the bovine. Breed and individual variations in the specific protein constituents of milk. J. Dairy Sci. 39:1683.

Rook, J. A. F., and P. C. Thomas. 1980. Principles involved in manipulating the yields and concentrations of constituents in milk. Int. Dairy Fed. Bull. Doc. 125:66.

Schingoethe, D. J. 1976. Whey utilization in animal feeding: A summary and evaluation. J. Dairy Sci. 59:556.

Schneider, P. L., D. K. Beede, and C. J. Wilcox. 1986. Responses of lactating cows to dietary sodium source and quantity and potassium quantity during heat stress. J. Dairy Sci. 69:99

Schultz, L. H. 1977. Somatic cell in milk—physiological aspects and relationship to amount and composition of milk. J. Food Prot. 40:125.

Schwab, C. G., L. D. Satter, and A. B. Clay. 1976. Response of lactating cows to abomasal infusions of amino acids. J. Dairy Sci. 59:1254.

Shaver, R. D., A. J. Nytes, L. D. Satter, and N. A. Jorgensen. 1986. Influence of amount of feed intake and forage physical form on digestion and passage of prebloom alfalfa hay in dairy cows. J. Dairy Sci. 69:1545.

Storry, J. E. 1980. Influence of nutritional factors on the yield and content of milk: Nonprotected fat in the diet. Int. Dairy Fed. Bull. Doc. 125:88.

Storry, J. E., and P. E. Brumby. 1980. Influence of nutritional factors on yield and content of milk: Protected nonpolyunsaturated fat in the diet. Int. Dairy Fed. Bull. Doc. 125:105.

Sutton, J.D. 1980. Influence of nutritional factors on the yield and content of milk fat: Dietary components other than fat. Int. Dairy Fed. Bull. Doc. 125:126.

Sutton J. D. 1985. Digestion and absorption of energy substrates in the lactating cow. J. Dairy Sci. 68:3376.

Tallamy, P. T., and H. E. Randolph. 1970. Influence of mastitis on properties of milk. V. Total and free concentrations of major minerals in skim milk. J. Dairy Sci. 53:1386.

Thomas, P. C. 1980. Influence of nutrition on the yield and content of protein in milk: Dietary protein and energy supply. Int. Dairy Fed. Bull. Doc. 125:142.

Thomas, P. C. 1983. Milk protein. Proc. Nutr. Soc. 42:407.

Thomas, P. C., and D. G. Chamberlain. 1984. Manipulation of milk composition to meet market needs. Ch. 14 in Recent Advances in Animal Nutrition, W. Haresign and D. J. A. Cole, eds. London: Butterworth.

Tucker, H. A. 1985. Endocrine and neural control of the mammary gland. Ch. 2 in Lactation, B. L. Larson, ed. Ames: Iowa State University Press.

Van Vleck, L. D. 1978. Breeding for increased milk protein. J. Dairy Sci. 61:815.

Wheelock, J. V. 1980. Influence of physiological factors on the yields and contents of milk constituents. Int. Dairy Fed. Bull. Doc. 125:83.

Wilcox, C. J. 1978. Genetic considerations of economic importance: Milk yield, composition and quality. Ch. 2 in Large Dairy Herd Management, C. J. Wilcox, H. H. Van Horn, B. Harris, Jr., H. H. Head, S. P. Marshall, W. W. Thatcher, D. W. Webb, and J. M. Wing, eds. Gainesville: University Presses of Florida.

Wolfschoon-Pombo, A., and H. Klostermeyer. 1981. The NPN-fraction of cow milk. I. Amount and composition. Milchwissenschaft 36:598.

Woodford, J. A., N. A. Jorgensen, and G. P. Barrington. 1986. Impact of dietary fiber and physical form on performance of lactating dairy cows. J. Dairy Sci. 69:1035.

Young, C. W., J. K. Hillers, and A. E. Freeman. 1986. Production, consumption, and pricing of milk and its components. J. Dairy Sci. 69:272.

# Methodologies for Measuring Body Composition in Humans

HWAI-PING SHENG

*"Nothing is measured with greater error than the human body."*
Beneke, 1878

Studies of the composition of the human body are relatively new in human biology. Although interest in the effects of malnutrition on body tissues, morbidity, and mortality dates back to the time of Hippocrates, the primary research interest in body composition began in the 1940s. Since that time, many procedures and techniques have been developed to assess indirectly the various components of the body. These techniques have been discussed and evaluated at a number of symposia and in review articles (Brozek, 1963, 1965; Brozek and Henschel, 1961; Garrow, 1982; Lohman, 1984; National Academy of Sciences, 1968; Siri, 1961).

This paper briefly reviews the indirect methods that are currently available to measure adipose tissue (fat) in the body. These procedures are directed either to whole-body measurement or to specific sites and regions, in which case they extrapolate data to whole-body fat content using previously determined relationships. Methods range from the simple to the complex; most make use of constants and assumptions derived from either the guinea pig data of Pace and Rathbun (1945) or cadaver analyses, which form the basis for the "reference man" (Brozek et al., 1963). Most indirect methods were validated against another indirect method; few studies were validated by direct cadaver analysis (Knight et al., 1986) or carcass analysis of an animal (Lewis et al., 1986; Sheng and Huggins, 1979).

The terms *lean body mass* (LBM) and *fat-free mass* (FFM) are used interchangeably and sometimes cause confusion among investigators. Body mass can be considered as the sum of adipose tissue and LBM or, alternatively, of ether-extractable fat and FFM. The terms would be synonymous if adipose tissue were composed of pure fat instead of approximately 80 to 85 percent fat, 2 percent protein, and 13 to 18 percent water. Thus, the distinction between LBM and FFM is not critical in a fairly lean individual, but it is important in an obese individual in whom the contribution of the nonfat component to the adipose tissue can be large. The terms fat and FFM will be used in this paper.

## WHOLE-BODY MEASUREMENTS

### Fat-Soluble Gases

Because most anesthetic gases are rare inert gases (for example, cyclopropane, xe-

242

none, and krypton) and are highly soluble in fat but not in water, it is theoretically possible to use the dilution principle to calculate total body fat by measuring the absorption of these gases. Measurements of fat by this technique have been reported by several investigators who used either the absorption phase (Lesser and Zak, 1963) or both the absorption and desorption phases of the gas (Mettau et al., 1977) to calculate body fat. Results for small animals agreed with those obtained by carcass analysis; results for humans were in the range of published data for fat (Mettau et al., 1977). The disadvantages of this method include the necessity of a closed respiratory system and the length of time required to attain equilibrium conditions, both of which inconvenience the subject. Attempts to reduce the duration of the experiment by extrapolation of the early phase of measurements have been relatively unsuccessful.

## Body Compartmentalization into Two Components

Most indirect methods compartmentalize the body in numerous ways, depending on the purpose of the study and the requirements of the investigators. In its simplest form, body mass can be considered to consist of two phases: fat and FFM. In the research setting, body fat content is often determined by deriving FFM from a set of measurements and then calculating body fat content as part of the body mass not accounted for by FFM. The concept of a fat-free body was originally suggested in 1915 by Dubois and Benedict, who proposed that the FFM was metabolically important and had a constant chemical composition. Research on FFM was accelerated markedly during the 1940s by Behnke et al. (1942), who attempted to measure the amount of "primary energy-exchanging mass" of tissues in the body, which they called the LBM. The LBM or FFM has been estimated by several methods, all of which, as summarized by Wedg-

wood (1963), assume that LBM has a constant density, LBM has a constant proportion of water, bone is a constant proportion of LBM, and cell water is a constant proportion of cell mass. It is also frequently assumed that LBM has a constant percentage of potassium.

### Determination of Fat by Densitometry

Densitometric determination of body fat is considered by many investigators as the "reference method" or the "standard" against which other indirect methods are compared. Equations have also been developed to predict body fat from anthropometric measurements using fat data obtained by densitometry. The estimation of body fat from densitometry was pioneered by Behnke et al. (1942), who reasoned that if the densities of the two body components (fat and LBM) were known and if the density of the whole body could be measured, then the proportional masses of fat and LBM could be calculated. Although the concept of densitometry is theoretically sound, an accurate measurement of body density and, for the two-compartment approach, the known densities for body fat and FFM are required.

Theoretically, body density can be measured with an accuracy of $\pm 0.001$ to $\pm 0.025$ g/ml (Siri, 1961), but in practice this is difficult to achieve. Body density is calculated using an Archimedean principle:

Body density = Body mass/body volume.

Many different methods have been developed to measure body volume, but as yet, none appears to yield a satisfactory level of accuracy.

The original, and still most widely used, physical method to measure body volume uses either underwater weighing (Gnaedinger et al., 1963) or water displacement (Garn and Nolan, 1963). This measurement can be made with a relatively simple apparatus, but it suffers from two practical problems: (1) subject cooperation is required because whole body submersion is essential, and (2) residual volumes of air in the lungs and the gut have to be measured separately. Although the residual volume of air in the lungs can be measured easily, no adequate method is available for measuring air in the gut.

Photogrammetry has been suggested as a tool for the measurement of body volume (Pierson, 1963), but thus far has not proved successful because photomapping requires complicated mathematics and highly skilled personnel. An additional drawback in this method is the inclusion of the residual volumes of air in the lungs and gut.

Diethelm et al. (1977) and Garrow et al. (1979) have reported the successful use of a combination of water displacement (to measure a partially submerged body) and air displacement (to measure the nonsubmerged head region). Certain technical difficulties, such as volume of air in the gut and thermodynamic problems with the air-displacement method, have yet to be resolved. Body volume measured by air displacement is theoretically simple but technically difficult. In theory, the volume of air displaced by an infant placed in a rigid chamber can be measured by either the helium dilution method or by measuring the pressure difference as described by Boyle's law (Faulkner, 1963; Fomon et al., 1963; Gnaedinger et al., 1963; Lim, 1963; Taylor et al., 1985). If the chamber volume is 30 liters and if a piston changes the volume by 0.3 liters, a 2-liter premature infant would only change the incremental pressure over that of the empty chamber by 0.76 cm of water (or 0.073 percent). To measure such small pressure changes accurately is difficult, since a change of temperature from 36 to 37°C at a constant volume and an ambient pressure of 760 mm Hg would cause a pressure rise of 3.34 cm of water. This technical difficulty can be resolved by the development of a differential dynamic system where identical volume changes in two identical chambers are induced by two yoked pistons (Taylor et al., 1985). Any differential pressure, as measured by a manometer between the two chambers, would be due entirely to the difference in air volume between the chambers. This system would require a resolution of the differential pressure of 1 percent (instead of 0.073 percent) for a 1 percent change in body volume (Taylor et al., 1985). Body volume measurements obtained by this system are generally reasonable, although widely divergent values are produced occasionally, probably because of pressure fluctuations from respiratory movement and temperature changes (Taylor et al., 1985). When the technical difficulties are resolved, this method may be particularly suited for infants, because corrections for residual volumes of air in the lungs and gut are not necessary.

The acoustic plethysmograph is another method being explored to measure body volume (Deskins et al., 1985). It makes use of the Helmholtz principle that resonant frequency is inversely proportional to the volume of the resonating chamber; that is, the volume of an object placed inside the resonating chambers can be calculated from the difference in resonant frequencies. The acoustic plethysmograph can be constructed and operated relatively inexpensively and can be easily used to measure body volume in infants. Its disadvantages include a lack of ability to measure the residual volume of air in the lungs and gut.

Even with the assurance that body density can be measured with great "precision" for a given individual, and perhaps with great "accuracy," the application of the densitometric approach to measure FFM and fat is not without error. The values of 0.9 for the density of body fat and 1.10 or 1.095 for the density of mixed tissues of the FFM are used in the calculations (Brozek et al., 1963). Although the density of body fat varies at different body sites and from consumption of different diets, the variations reported are less than 2 percent (Pearson et al., 1968). Therefore, their contribution to the error in the estimation of fat is small. However, there is an increasing realization that it is invalid to assume the chemical constancy of FFM (Wedgwood, 1963); thus, the value of 1.095 for the density of FFM (derived from cadaver analysis) must be used cautiously. The greatest change in the chemical composition of FFM occurs during the growth of the infant, resulting in an increase of FFM density from 1.064 in infants (Fomon et al., 1982) to 1.095 for the reference man (Brozek et al., 1963). The extent of error in fat estimation can be calculated for an infant: Fat content was estimated as 11 percent of body weight when a density value of 1.064 was used for FFM and 23 percent when 1.095 was used. Thus, reported percentages of body fat must be viewed with caution. As Brozek et al. (1963) concluded after a detailed review of the method, "It appears that no universally valid formulas for densitometric estimation of the fat content can be offered."

## Determination of FFM by Hydrometry

A value for body fat may be derived simply from the total body water (TBW) measurement based on the assumption that FFM has a constant water content of 73.2 percent:

$$FFM = TBW/0.732.$$

Measurement of TBW is theoretically simple, requiring the estimation of dilution spaces of small-molecular-weight substances or tracer doses of isotopically labeled water (Schoeller et al., 1980; Sheng and Huggins, 1979). However, increasing evidence suggests that tritiated water overestimates TBW to varying degrees in animals in various nutritional and physiological states, especially in rapidly growing young animals (McManus et al., 1969; Sheng and Huggins, 1979). The degree of overestimation of TBW would affect the degree by which body fat was underestimated.

Use of a "constant" for the hydration of FFM has been questioned. In the derivation of this constant from eviscerated guinea pigs and several other species of animals, Pace and Rathbun (1945) recognized that the constant—73.2 percent—can be applied only to adult animals, a provision that has occasionally been overlooked. Even in adult animals, fatter animals tend to have a higher FFM water content. Moulton (1923) recognized in 1923 that relative water content was reduced during early growth in a number of animal species. The animal reaches chemical maturity only when its relative water content stabilizes, and the age at which stabilization occurs depends on the species. This concept has been challenged by various investigators and lately by Shields et al. (1983), who could find no evidence of a constant chemical composition in the fat-free body portion of pigs. The pigs in the growth study reached a body weight of 150 kg. Consequently, care must be exercised when the value 73.2 percent is applied in the young; otherwise, underestimation of the fat will result.

## Determination of Fat from Potassium

FFM can be estimated from potassium (K) by the following equation:

$$FFM = Total\ body\ K/68.1.$$

In this equation, FFM is assumed to have a constant proportion of K throughout life: 68.1 mmol/kg of FFM, a value derived from cadaver analysis (Kirton and Pearson, 1963). This assumption, however, does not apply in all circumstances; evidence has shown that infants have a lower concentration of K (Forbes and Hursh, 1963) and that adult K concentrations may differ between populations and ethnic groups (Meneely et al., 1963).

Total body K has been measured with the dilution of $^{42}K$, a radioisotope of K (Corsa et al., 1950). Alternatively, body K can be estimated by measuring the naturally occurring radioisotope $^{40}K$ which constitutes approximately 0.012 percent of the natural K in humans (Forbes, 1962). The high-energy gamma ray emitted from $^{40}K$ can be measured with highly sensitive, but expensive, whole-body counters. Proper calibration of this system has permitted quantification of the K concentration in the human body from which FFM, and hence fat, can be estimated.

### Total Body Electrical Conductivity and Impedance

Total body electrical conductivity (TOBEC) and bioelectrical impedance analysis (BIA) have recently been used to assess adiposity (Cochran et al., 1986; Harrison and Van Itallie, 1982; Lukaski et al., 1985; Segal et al., 1985). These methods are discussed in greater detail in the paper by Boileau in this volume. Briefly, these two techniques use the basic principle that lean tissue conducts an electrical current better than fat tissue. Values for FFM obtained by these techniques compare favorably with those obtained by other indirect methods, such as anthropometry, densitometry, hydrometry, and total body K (Cochran et al., 1986; Harrison and Van Itallie, 1982; Lukaski et al., 1985; Segal et al., 1985), and with direct carcass analysis of animals (Fiorotto et al., 1987). However, as discussed by Cohn (1985), data that validate these techniques are incomplete and additional studies are needed.

### Multicompartmentalization of the Body

The above methods to estimate body fat from FFM assume that the chemical composition of FFM is constant, an assumption that undoubtedly introduces an error whose boundaries are not well defined. In contrast, the recent development of more sophisticated and complex techniques for the elemental analysis of the body allows a more accurate estimate of body fat without such an assumption. This multicompartmental approach (Anderson, 1963; Cohn et al., 1984, 1985) was first used by Moore et al. (1963), who objected to using FFM as a reference standard because it contained a significant amount of extracellular tissues, primarily skeleton and extracellular fluid. Moore suggested that the term "body cell mass" (BCM), which is a more homogeneous mass responsible for basal metabolism, replace the term FFM. The calculation of BCM is based on the assumptions that nearly all K is in the cells, the ratio of K to nitrogen (N) is constant (3 mmol of K/g of N), and N is a constant proportion of BCM. Thus, BCM can be calculated from measured K multiplied by a coefficient factor of 8.33. The three-compartment approach, as conceived by Moore and colleagues, divides the body mass into fat, BCM, and extracellular tissue (ECT) compartments.

The concept of BCM only recently received the attention it deserves. The development of total body neutron activation analysis allows the estimation of extracellular tissues—the solid phase estimated from body calcium (Ca) and the aqueous phase from body chlorine (Cl). Body cell mass can be estimated from body K by measuring $^{40}K$ (Cohn et al., 1984, 1985). Body fat then can be calculated after estimation of the BCM and ECT compartments (Cohn et al., 1984, 1985). This approach, although theoretically superior to the two-compartment approach, also uses assumptions derived from cadaver analysis—that is, a constant proportion of body Ca in the extracellular solids, a constant ratio of K/N, and a constant proportion of N in the BCM. Body Ca can be measured accurately by a well-calibrated neutron activation system; a relatively small error is introduced into the final estimation of fat by assuming a constant proportion of body Ca in extracellular solids. The potential error resulting from the use of the K/N ratio of 3 mmol/g may be substantial (Sheng and Huggins, 1973).

Expansion of the three-compartment approach to the four-compartment approach reduces the body into its four elemental phases: fat, water, protein, and minerals. An accurate estimate of fat is possible if water (measured by dilution technique), protein (calculated from body nitrogen measured by prompt gamma neutron activation analysis), and body minerals (calculated from body Ca measured by delayed neutron activation analysis) are accurately measured (Cohn et al., 1984, 1985). The only assumption made is that Ca is a constant proportion of body minerals. Any error introduced into the body fat estimation by this assumption is small because of the small proportion of minerals in the whole body (4 percent). The predominant disadvantages of neutron activation analysis are its complexity, cost, and the radiation exposure, however minimal, to growing infants and adults of childbearing age.

The densitometric method has been applied recently to the pediatric population using the four-compartment approach in which total body water was measured with a tracer, and the mineral content and the densities of fat, water, protein, and minerals were obtained from relevant literature (Sheng et al., 1984). The use of literature values for mineral content and the various densities to estimate fat appeared to introduce only a small error. Body volume was measured using either the pressure-differential method (Dell et al., 1987; Taylor et al., 1985) or the acoustic plethysmograph (Deskins et al., 1985).

As discussed earlier, the overestimation of TBW by tritium, particularly in the infant, may introduce error to the four-compartment approach of estimating fat. Recently, Lewis et al. (1986) reported that TBW in the infant baboon can be measured accurately by nuclear magnetic resonance (NMR). NMR's potential for the analysis of body composition appears promising; also with NMR imaging, regional distribution of body fat can be analyzed (Fuller et al., 1985). Further developments of this technique may result in the measurement of total body fat without the use of assumptions as in the compartmental approaches.

## REGIONAL FAT MEASUREMENT

Progress has been made in the development of methods to measure composition at various regions of the body. Body fat is calculated from these measurements using equations that establish a relationship between these measurements and body fat estimated by another indirect method. Such methods, which will not be discussed in detail, range from simple anthropometric measures used primarily for population studies to sophisticated computerized methods in a research setting. For all these methods, validation has been primarily with another indirect method; that is, the values obtained were compared with reported body fat values in the literature or compared against values obtained by other indirect methods performed on the same individual. The least expensive and most frequently used method uses calipers to measure skinfold thicknesses at specific sites. Other methods include soft-tissue radiography (Garn, 1957) and ultrasonography (Borkan et al., 1982), both of which use expensive and nonportable instruments. More recently, infrared interactance has been proposed as a rapid, safe, and noninvasive method to measure subcutaneous fat in both research and field settings (Conway et al., 1984). Numerous studies have attempted to validate the extrapolation of subcutaneous fat thickness measured at a number of sites on the body to total body fat and to establish subcutaneous fat thickness as a "standard" for the assessment of total body fat (Durnin and Rahaman, 1967). Although the thickness of subcutaneous fat is roughly proportional to the total weight of body fat, body fat calculated by this method may be inaccurate and misleading because of the variation among population norms. Equations are being developed to overcome this difficulty; specific formulas for body fat estimation are suggested for specific population groups (Lohman, 1981).

Interest in adapting complex diagnostic tools to estimate body fat is increasing. Images depicting fat and muscle of body regions can be obtained with computerized axial tomography (Borkan et al., 1983; Heymsfield and Noel, 1981; Sjostrom et al., 1986), dual-photon absorptiometry (Gotfredsen et al., 1986; Mazess et al., 1984), and nuclear magnetic resonance (Fuller et al., 1985). Sophisticated software allows total body fat to be computed from a series of cross-sectional fat areas along the length of the body. Although all these techniques show great potential in the estimation of body fat, they are expensive and relatively unavailable for routine measurements. Furthermore, a degree of radiation exposure is involved with both computerized axial tomography and dual-photon absorptiometry methods.

## SUMMARY

Many indirect methods of varying degrees of complexity are available for estimation of body fat. Most of the methods have been validated for predictability and precision using other indirect methods. The reference method most commonly used is that based on densitometry to estimate body fat from a two-compartment approach (Sheng et al., 1984). The accuracy of most of these methods has been validated only in a few instances by direct carcass analysis. The final choice of an indirect method ultimately depends on its cost, the objective of the experiment, and the physical conditions under which it is to be used.

## ACKNOWLEDGMENTS

This work is a publication of the U.S. Department of Agriculture/Agricultural Research Service Children's Nutrition Research Center, Department of Pediatrics, Baylor College of Medicine and Texas Children's Hospital, Houston, Texas. This project has been partially funded by the U.S. Department of Agriculture, Agricultural Research Service, under Cooperative Agreement 58-7MN1-6-100.

## REFERENCES

Anderson, E. C. 1963. Three-component body composition on analysis based upon potassium and water determinations. Ann. N.Y. Acad. Sci. 110:189–212.

Behnke, A. R., B. G. Feen, and W. C. Welham. 1942. The specific gravity of healthy men: Body weight and volume as an index to obesity. J. Am. Med. Assoc. 118:495–498.

Borkan, G. A., D. E. Hults, J. Cardarelli, and B. A. Burrows. 1982. Comparison of ultrasound and skinfold measurements in assessment of subcutaneous and total fatness. Am. J. Phys. Anthropol. 58:307–313.

Borkan, G. A., D. E. Hults, S. G. Gerzof, B. A. Burrows, and A. H. Robbins. 1983. Relationships between computed tomography tissue areas, thicknesses and total body composition. Ann. Human Biol. 10:537–546.

Brozek, J. 1963. Body composition, Parts I and II. Ann. N.Y. Acad. Sci. 110:1–1018.

Brozek, J., ed. 1965. Human Body Composition: Approaches and Applications. New York: Pergamon.

Brozek, J., and A. Henschel, eds. 1961. Techniques for Measuring Body Composition. Washington, D.C.: National Academy of Sciences.

Brozek, J., F. Grande, J. T. Anderson, and A. Keys. 1963. Densitometric analysis of body composition: Revision of some quantitative assumptions. Ann. N.Y. Acad. Sci. 110:113–140.

Cochran, W. J., W. J. Klish, W. W. Wong, and P. D. Klein. 1986. Total body electrical conductivity used to determine body composition in infants. Pediatr. Res. 20:561–564.

Cohn, S. H. 1985. How valid are bioelectric impedance measurements in body composition studies? Am. J. Clin. Nutr. 44:306–308.

Cohn, S. H., A. N. Vaswani, S. Yasumura, K. Yuen, and K. J. Ellis. 1984. Improved models for determination of body fat by in vivo neutron activation. Am. J. Clin. Nutr. 40:255–259.

Cohn, S. H., A. N. Vaswani, S. Yasumura, K. Yuen, and K. J. Ellis. 1985. Assessment of cellular mass and lean body mass by noninvasive nuclear techniques. J. Lab. Clin. Med. 105:305–311.

Conway, J. M., K. H. Norris, and C. E. Bodwell. 1984. A new approach for the estimation of body composition: Infrared interactance. Am. J. Clin. Nutr. 40:1123–1130.

Corsa, J., Jr., J. M. Olney, Jr., R. W. Steenburg, M.

R. Ball, and F. D. Moore. 1950. The measurement of exchangeable potassium in many by isotope dilution. J. Clin. Invest. 29:1280–1295.

Dell, R., Y. Aksoy, S. Kashyap, M. Forsythe, R. Ramakrishnan, C. Zucker, and W. C. Heird. 1987. Relationship between density and body weight in prematurely born infants receiving different diets. Pp. 91–97 in In Vivo Body Composition Studies, K. J. Ellis, S. Yasamura, and W. D. Morgan, eds. London: The Institute of Physical Medicine.

Deskins, W. G., D. Winter, H.-P. Sheng, and C. Garza. 1985. Use of a resonating cavity to measure body volume. J. Acoust. Soc. Am. 77:756–758.

Diethelm, R., J. S. Garrow, and S. F. Stalley. 1977. An apparatus for measuring the density of obese subjects. J. Physiol. 267:14P.

Durnin, J. V. G. A., and M. M. Rahaman. 1967. The assessment of the amount of fat in the human body from measurements of skinfold thickness. Br. J. Nutr. 21:681–689.

Faulkner, F. 1963. An air displacement method for measuring body volume in babies: A preliminary communication. Ann. N.Y. Acad. Sci. 110:75–79.

Fiorotto, M. L., W. J. Cochran, R. C. Funk, H.-P. Sheng, and W. J. Klish. 1987. Total body electrical conductivity measurements: Effects of body composition and geometry. Am. J. Physiol. 252:R794–R800.

Fomon, S. J., R. L. Jensen, and G. M. Owen. 1963. Determination of body volume of infants by a method of helium displacement. Ann. N.Y. Acad. Sci. 110:80–90.

Fomon, S. J., F. Haschke, E. E. Ziegler, and S. E. Nelson. 1982. Body composition of reference children from birth to age 10 years. Am. J. Clin. Nutr. 35:1169–1175.

Forbes, G. B. 1962. Methods for determining composition of the human body. Pediatrics 29:477–494.

Forbes, G. B., and J. B. Hursh. 1963. Age and sex trends in lean body mass calculated from $K^{40}$ measurements: With a note on the theoretical basis for the procedure. Ann. N.Y. Acad. Sci. 110:255–263.

Fuller, M. F., M. A. Foster, and J. M. S. Hutchison. 1985. Estimation of body fat by nuclear magnetic resonance imaging. Proc. Nutr. Soc. 44:108A.

Garn, S. M. 1957. Roentgenogrammetric determinations of body compositions. Human Biol. 29:337–353.

Garn, S. M., and P. Nolan, Jr. 1963. A tank to measure body volume by water displacement (BOVOTA). Ann. N.Y. Acad. Sci. 110:91–95.

Garrow, J. S. 1982. New approaches to body composition. Am. J. Clin. Nutr. 35:1152–1158.

Garrow, J. S., S. Stalley, R. Diethelm, P. H. Pittet, R. Hesp, and D. A. Halliday. 1979. A new method for measuring the body density of obese adults. Br. J. Nutr. 42:173–183.

Gnaedinger, R. H., E. P. Reineke, A. M. Pearson, W. D. Van Huss, J. A. Wessel, and H. J. Montoye. 1963. Determination of body density by air displacement, helium dilution, and underwater weighing. Ann. N.Y. Acad. Sci. 110:96–108.

Gotfredsen, A., J. Jensen, J. Borg, and C. Christiansen. 1986. Measurement of lean body mass and total body fat using dual photon absorptiometry. Metabolism 35:38–93.

Harrison, G. G., and T. B. Van Itallie. 1982. Estimation of body composition: A new approach based on electromagnetic principles. Am. J. Clin. Nutr. 35:1176–1179.

Heymsfield, S. B., and R. A. Noel. 1981. Radiographic analysis of body composition by computerized axial tomography. Pp. 161–172 in Nutrition and Cancer: Etiology and Treatment, G. R. Newell and N. M. Ellison, eds. New York: Raven.

Kirton, A. H., and A. M. Pearson. 1963. Relationships between potassium content and body composition. Ann. N.Y. Acad. Sci. 110:221–228.

Knight, G. S., A. H. Beddoe, S. J. Streat, and G. L. Hill. 1986. Body composition of two human cadavers by neutron activation and chemical analysis. Am. J. Physiol. 250:E179–E185.

Lesser, G. T., and G. Zak. 1963. Measurement of total body fat in man by the simultaneous absorption of two inert gases. Ann. N.Y. Acad. Sci. 110:40–54.

Lewis, D. S., W. L. Rollwitz, H. A. Bertrand, and E. J. Masoro. 1986. Use of NMR for measurement of total body water and estimation of body fat. J. Appl. Physiol. 60:836–840.

Lim, T. P. 1963. Critical evaluation of the pneumatic method for determining body volume: Its history and technique. Ann. N.Y. Acad. Sci. 110:72–74.

Lohman, T. G. 1981. Skinfolds and body density and their relation to body fatness: A review. Human Biol. 53:181–225.

Lohman, T. G. 1984. Research in progress in validation of laboratory methods of assessing body composition. Med. Sci. Sports Exerc. 16:596–603.

Lukaski, H. C., P. E. Johnson, W. W. Bolonchuk, and G. I. Lykken. 1985. Assessment of fat-free mass using bioelectrical impedance measurements of the human body. Am. J. Clin. Nutr. 41:810–817.

Mazess, R. B., W. W. Peppler, and M. Gibbons. 1984. Total body composition by dual-photon ($^{153}Gd$) absorptiometry. Am. J. Clin. Nutr. 40:834–839.

McManus, W. R., R. K. Prichard, C. Baker, and M. V. Petruchenia. 1969. Estimation of water content by tritium dilution of animals subjected to rapid live-weight changes. J. Agric. Sci. Cambridge 72:31–40.

Meneely, G. R., R. M. Heyssel, C. O. T. Ball, R. L. Weiland, A. R. Lorimer, C. Constantinides, and E. U. Meneely. 1963. Analysis of factors affecting body composition determined from potassium content in 915 normal subjects. Ann. N.Y. Acad. Sci. 110:271–281.

Mettau, J. W., H. J. Degenhart, and H. K. A. Visser. 1977. Measurement of total body fat in newborns and infants by absorption and desorption of nonradioactive xenon. Pediatr. Res. 11:1097–1101.

Moore, F. D., K. H. Olesen, J. D. McMurrey, H. V. Parker, M. R. Ball, and C. M. Boyden. 1963. The Body Cell Mass and Its Supporting Environment. Philadelphia: W. B. Saunders.

Moulton, C. R. 1923. Age and chemical development in mammals. J. Biol. Chem. 57:79–97.

National Academy of Sciences. 1968. Body Composition in Animals and Man. Washington, D.C.: National Academy of Sciences.

Pace, N., and E. N. Rathbun. 1945. Studies on body composition, III. Water and chemically contained nitrogen content in relation to fat content. J. Biol. Chem. 158:685–691.

Pearson, A. M., R. W. Purchas, and E. P. Reineke. 1968. Theory and potential usefulness of body density as a predictor of body composition. Pp. 153–169 in Body Composition in Animals and Man. Washington, D.C.: National Academy of Sciences.

Pierson, W. R. 1963. A photogrammetric technique for the estimation of surface area and volume. Ann. N.Y. Acad. Sci. 110:109–122.

Schoeller, D. A., E. van Santen, D. W. Peterson, W. Dietz, J. Jaspan, and P. D. Klein. 1980. Total body water measurement in humans with $^{18}O$ and $^{2}H$ labeled water. Am. J. Clin. Nutr. 33:2686–2693.

Segal, K. R., B. Gutin, E. Presta, J. Wang, and T. B. Van Itallie. 1985. Estimation of human body composition by electrical impedance methods: A comparative study. J. Appl. Physiol. 58:1565–1571.

Sheng, H.-P., and R. A. Huggins. 1973. Body cell mass and lean body mass in the growing beagle. Proc. Soc. Exp. Biol. Med. 142:175–180.

Sheng, H.-P., and R. A. Huggins. 1979. A review of body composition studies with emphasis on total body water and fat. Am. J. Clin. Nutr. 32:630–647.

Sheng, H.-P., W. G. Deskins, D. Winter, and C. Garza. 1984. Estimation of total body fat and protein by densitometry. Pediatr. Res. 18:212A.

Shields, R. G., Jr., D. C. Mahan, and P. L. Graham. 1983. Changes in swine body composition from birth to 145 KG. J. Anim. Sci. 57:43–54.

Siri, W. E. 1961. Body composition from fluid spaces and density: Analysis of methods. Pp. 223–244 in Techniques for Measuring Body Composition, J. Brozek and A. Henschel, eds. Washington, D.C.: National Academy of Sciences.

Sjostrom, L., H. Kvist, A. Cederblad, and U. Tylen. 1986. Determination of total adipose tissue and body fat in women by computed tomography, $^{40}K$, and tritium. Am. J. Physiol. 250:E736–E745.

Taylor, A., Y. Aksoy, J. W. Scopest, G. du Mont, and B. A. Taylor. 1985. Development of an air displacement method for whole body volume measurement of infants. J. Biomed. Eng. 7:9–17.

Wedgwood, R. J. 1963. Inconstancy of the lean body mass. Ann. N.Y. Acad. Sci. 110:141–152.

# Utilization of Total Body Electrical Conductivity in Determining Body Composition

R. A. BOILEAU

Assessment of body composition is an important part of evaluating nutritional status, health, and physical fitness. In general, body composition analysis uses concepts and measurement techniques that permit partitioning of body weight into two or more components. The simplest conceptual model partitions body weight into a fat weight component and a fat-free or lean body weight component. These are of particular interest in relation to human nutrition and health, since obesity is a major health problem in Western societies, both among children (Coates et al., 1982; Ylitalo, 1981) and adults (Buskirk, 1971; McArdle et al., 1981). Furthermore, body composition analysis has many applications for the animal scientist, including nondestructive monitoring of meat production.

Measurement of human body composition has been a somewhat perplexing problem because of the necessity to use noninvasive techniques and the lack of a substantial data base characterizing the chemical composition of the body for validation purposes. Hence, the status of our understanding of human body composition has developed from use of indirect measurement techniques, the conceptual framework of which is based on the chemical analysis of only a few cadavers. The reference techniques judged to be most accurate, precise, and conceptually sound include densitometry, hydrometry, and body potassium ($^{40}K$) spectroscopy. The methodology of these techniques has been reviewed in a number of reports (Behnke and Wilmore, 1974; Boileau and Lohman, 1977; Boileau et al., 1985; Keys and Brozek, 1953; Lohman et al., 1984a).

Other techniques, considered to be less precise but applicable in large population studies, involve skinfold thickness and other anthropometric measurements. More recent technologies have spawned development of several new techniques including total body neutron activation analysis (Cohn et al., 1974), computerized axial tomography (Borkan and Hults, 1983), nuclear magnetic resonance imaging (Lohman, 1984), whole-body impedance (Nyboer, 1972), and total body electrical conductivity analysis (Harrison and Van Itallie, 1982). The focus of this report is on total body electrical conductivity (TOBEC) as a technique for body composition analysis.

## BACKGROUND AND MEASUREMENT PRINCIPLE

Electrical conductivity analysis is a method of compositional analysis that uses an instrument (U.S. Patent 3,735,247, 1973)—called electronic meat measuring equipment (EMME)—to measure the fat and lean content of live swine (model SA-1). EMME SA-1 was later modified for measurement of packaged meat and in vivo measurements of humans (EMME/TOBEC HA-1). Data presented in the literature are primarily based on the EMME/TOBEC HA-1, which is the prototype of the new TOBEC HA-2.

Application of the electrical conductivity method to the two-component body composition model is based on the concept that the fat-free body (FFB) component conducts electrical current more readily than the fat component. This is due to the higher water and electrolyte content found in the tissues and extracellular water making up the FFB. Electrical conductivity of various biological materials indicates that constituents associated with the FFB (for example, muscle, liver, and blood) have conductivity values of about 4 mmho-cm versus conductivity values for fat of about 0.3 mmho-cm in the 2.5- to 5.0-MHz range, an FFB/fat ratio of about 13 (Geddes and Baker, 1968; Pethig, 1979). Van Itallie et al. (1985) have suggested that the FFB/fat conductivity ratio may be as high as 20 to 1.

Current flow induced in a biological system is a function of conductive and dielectric properties. The conductive properties are related to the intra- and extracellular ionic content, and the dielectric effect is associated primarily with capacitance related to cell membranes. Impedance to current flow in the system results in an irreversible loss of energy as heat. This energy loss is related to the conductive mass. The dielectric or capacitance properties of current flow in a biological system must also be considered; these represent the reactive part of impedance in which energy transfer is reversible due to temporary storage of electrical energy. Capacitance is partly determined by the geometry of the conductor, which may produce an effect whereby capacitance increases as cross-sectional area, length, or both increase. While theoretically both electrical properties define the flow of current in a conductive mass, the conductive properties appear to exert a more dominant effect in estimating FFB mass. A detailed treatment of the electrical properties of biological tissues can be found in Pethig (1979).

There are two basic bioelectrical techniques used to measure whole-body conductivity for body composition assessment: (1) direct injection of current and (2) non-contact total body electrical conductivity (TOBEC). This discussion focuses on TOBEC. In this technique current applied to a coil induces an electromagnetic field in which the body is statically situated (HA-1) or scanned (HA-2). The conducting mass (subject) passing through the electromagnetic field of the coil absorbs heat energy, thereby perturbing the electrical field of the coil. The loss of energy detected in the coil is an index of the conductive mass of the body. The power dissipated in the subject at any one time is less than 1 $\mu$W/cm$^2$—less than 1/100th of the standard set by the American National Standards Institute for human exposure. The oscillating current frequency applied to the coil is an important aspect of the measurement, since the degree of separation in the conductivities of FFB and fat has been shown to be frequency dependent (Pethig, 1979). The first TOBEC model (HA-1) used 5-MHz oscillating coil current and required a 0.5-second measurement on the statically situated subject (Harrison and Van Itallie, 1982). The new TOBEC instrument (HA-2) is a scanning device in which the subject moves on a motor-driven sled through a 2.5-MHz coil electromagnetic field at a constant rate. It requires about 40 seconds for one measurement, during which conductivity is measured at 64 equidistant intervals. The change in coil energy as the body moves through the length of the coil is detected as change in conductance and capacitance relative to an empty coil. The measured conductance and capacitance of the conductor (subject) is reflected in a phase angle/distance curve. The area under the curve is an index of total body conductivity. The phase angle/distance curve generated from the HA-2 model is transformed by a Fourier series analysis, which partitions components of the average phase curve into discrete terms of phase (PC) and amplitude (AM) coefficients. Van Itallie et al. (1985) have reported a high correlation ($r = 0.98$) between the phase average readings of HA-1 and HA-2 in 40 men and women.

## MEASUREMENT PRECISION AND VALIDITY OF TOBEC

Most available information on the reliability and validity of TOBEC analysis has been reported on the SA-1 or HA-1 instrument. Measurement precision was reported for two studies on animals. Domermuth et al. (1976), using the SA-1 model, measured 12 pigs 14 times a day for 2 days and found an average coefficient of variation (CV) among the animals of 4 percent. Bracco et al. (1983) evaluated measurement reliability on 30 lightly anesthetized rats using a DMe 100 Ground Meat Fat Tester and reported an average intraday reliability coefficient of 0.99 for three consecutive trials.

High reliability coefficients have also been reported on humans measured with the HA-1 instrument. Presta et al. (1983) measured 32 subjects 10 times consecutively over a period of 3 minutes with a reported intraclass correlation of 0.99 among the trials. Segal et al. (1985), using the same reliability assessment method on 75 subjects, also reported an intraclass correlation of 0.99 and found the CV to be less than 2 percent for each subject. Using the HA-2 instrument, Van Loan and Mayclin (1987) meas-

ured 14 subjects five times a day for 5 days. No significant differences were found either within subjects or between test days. Precision of the HA-2 measurement has also been evaluated in 12 subjects, measured five consecutive times a day for 3 consecutive days, with the University of Illinois HA-2 instrument. No significant variability was detected for the within-day trials or the between-day trials for either the HA-2 readings or body density. The relative errors were lower for the HA-2 readings than for body density. With the exception of one subject who had one within-day CV of 3.6 percent, all individual daily CVs were less than 2 percent. On the other hand, 17 of 36 CVs exceeded 2 percent for the body density measurement. Therefore, the measurement precision of TOBEC appears to be excellent relative to that of other techniques for the assessment of body composition. This can be partly attributed to minimal requirements for subject learning and participation in the measurement process.

Validation of the TOBEC method has been studied in both animals and humans. In animal studies, two approaches have been used: (1) comparison of TOBEC values to [40]K total, body water, and FFB components derived from carcass analysis, and (2) FFB derived from densitometry, total body water, and/or [40]K spectroscopy. In humans, validation studies have compared TOBEC-derived FFB values with FFB derived from several indirect reference methods.

Domermuth et al. (1976) were the first to report the relationship between TOBEC and other body composition methods including total potassium ([40]K) and carcass analysis in pigs. Two experiments were conducted, one with 42 pigs and the other with 35 pigs, in which the animals were fasted for 16 to 18 hours to obtain a shrunk body weight before being measured by TOBEC and [40]K. The animals were then killed and their carcasses analyzed for specific gravity and fat, water, and protein content. The linear correlations between the live animal TOBEC readings and $^{40}$K measurements were 0.75 and 0.81 for experiments 1 and 2, respectively. The correlations of carcass analysis-derived total body water weight and protein weight to the TOBEC reading in experiment 1 were higher ($r$ = 0.87 and 0.83, respectively) than for the respective live animal $^{40}$K data ($r$ = 0.78 and 0.69). The same trend was observed in experiment 2, but because of the homogeneity of this sample, the coefficients were somewhat depressed.

Bracco et al. (1983) observed a high association between TOBEC values in 30 live rats and FFB estimated by densitometry ($r$ = 0.97; the standard error of estimate [SEE] was 13.6 g) and by chemical analysis of the carcass ($r$ = 0.97; SEE = 14.2 g). High linear correlations were also observed between TOBEC and total protein ($r$ = 0.95) and total body water ($r$ = 0.98). Klish et al. (1984) reported a correlation of 0.99 between the natural log of the TOBEC (Infant Model, HI-1) reading determined on live rabbits (mean weight = 2.8 kg) and the FFB chemically determined from carcass analysis. Similarly, Cochran et al. (1985), using five infant miniature pigs (weight range, 2.3 to 4.7 kg) found a high linear correlation ($r$ = 0.99) between the natural log of the TOBEC (HI-1) signal and total body water measured by desiccation. The data on animals indicate a strong relationship between TOBEC and FFB estimated directly by chemical and carcass analyses as well as indirectly by various reference methods.

The basic approach to both calibration and validation of TOBEC in the human has been to investigate the association of the TOBEC reading to FFB and fat estimated by one or more of the reference body composition methods. Four of the five studies reported used the HA-1 or HI-1 instruments, and all but one studied adult samples (age range, 18 to 63 years). In the infant study, Cochran et al. (1986) measured subjects (aged 2 days to 9.7 months) and re-

ported the relationships between the TO-BEC (HI-1 model) reading and total body water (deuterium dilution). FFB was estimated from total body water (TBW) and the sum of the triceps and subscapular skinfolds. A high correlation ($r$ = 0.96) was obtained for the observed TOBEC reading and FFB was estimated from TBW (using 0.82 as the fraction of water in FFB), with a somewhat lower correlation ($r$ = 0.82) found for TO-BEC and the sum of skinfolds. The adult HA-1 data, all of which have been reported by the Columbia University St. Luke's-Roosevelt Hospital group, indicate a strong relationship between TOBEC and the various reference methods. On this basis, it is possible to calibrate the TOBEC number with FFB estimated from body density or another method. While the high correlations reported for the HA-1 device and FFB derived from the reference methods are impressive, it is noteworthy that the SEE represents CVs of 7.3 percent (Presta et al., 1983) and 5.9 percent (Segal et al., 1985). When sex was considered as a categorical variable, the correlations increased (0.95 to 0.97) and the SEE was reduced (3.4 to 2.5 kg) (Segal et al., 1985). The error associated with estimating fat content derived from body density ($D_B$) for the various indirect methods is lowest for the TOBEC method (SEE = 3.5 percent fat) (Van Itallie et al., 1985).

At present, five TOBEC HA-2 instruments are in use for pilot testing. In one study (Van Loan and Mayclin, 1987), FFB from $D_B$ and also $D_B$ and TBW were predicted from a series of TOBEC variables (Fourier coefficients) in a group of young adult males and females (aged 18 to 35 years). High multiple $r$ values (0.98) were obtained from regression analysis, with the SEE ranging from 1.4 to 1.7 kg. The remarkably low FFB SEE observed from the $D_B$ and $D_B$-TBW methods of 2.6 and 3.2 percent, respectively, may in part be sample specific, but also may indicate that the HA-2 predicts FFB better than the HA-1, where the best prediction of FFB was 5.9 percent (Segal et al., 1985).

## UNIVERSITY OF ILLINOIS TOBEC STUDIES

The TOBEC HA-2 was recently evaluated in relation to densitometry and body potassium to assess the relationship of TOBEC to independent measures of body composition. A diverse sample of 190 children and adults were classified by the following levels of maturation: (1) prepubescent and pubescent children (aged 8 to 12 years), (2) postpubescent youths (aged 13 to 18 years), (3) young adults (aged 19 to 34.9 years), and (4) mature adults (aged 35 years and older). Classification was deemed important, since evidence suggests that the composition of the FFB is unstable during growth, development, and aging (Boileau et al., 1985).

Each subject was measured densitometrically and with the TOBEC HA-2. Body density was measured weighing the subject underwater; pulmonary residual volume was measured at the time of weighing (Boileau et al., 1984). Fat and FFB expressed both in absolute and relative terms were estimated from density (Siri, 1961). The TOBEC technique was described above. From a TOBEC scan, several orders of phase angle coefficients (PC-I, PC-II, PC-III, and PC-AVE) and amplitude coefficients (AM-1, AM-II, AM-III, and AM-AVE) were generated by Fourier series analysis. Each subject underwent at least three TOBEC scans. In addition to the $D_B$ and TOBEC measurements, 44 subjects were measured for body potassium and 126 for bone mineral content. Body potassium was measured by $^{40}K$ spectroscopy in a $\pi$ liquid scintillation counter (Boileau et al., 1973). Bone mineral was measured by single-photon absorptiometry (Lohman et al., 1984b). The bone mineral content was used to estimate the percentage of mineral FFB, which in turn was used to calculate a mineral-free FFB (MF-FFB) that could be related to TOBEC variables (Boileau et al., 1985).

The results of this analysis suggest an excellent empirical relationship between TOBEC and FFB estimated by either the $D_B$ or $^{40}K$ methods. Correlations of the phase angle coefficients (PC) with FFB $D_B$ reflecting conductivity appear to be slightly higher than the amplitude (AM) coefficients reflecting capacitance. Regression analysis was then conducted to predict FFB $D_B$ using linear combinations of the individual TOBEC variables and the conductivity indexes (for example, PC-I$^{1/2} \times Ht$, AM-III$^{1/2} \times Ht$) with the best prediction equations for each selected on the basis of the highest $r^2$ and the lowest SEE. Overall, the SEEs for predicting $FFB_{D_B}$ from the conductivity indexes were slightly lower than were those from a combination of individual TOBEC variables, except in the postpubescent group.

The next step in the analysis was to evaluate the applicability of the prediction equations across maturation levels. Since the densitometric method assumes that the FFB is stable and chemically mature, and since this assumption may not be valid in growing children, youths, and aging adults, the equation for young adults was used to predict FFB from TOBEC in the other three groups.* Analysis indicates that while the slopes of the regression of actual ($FFB_{D_B}$) and predicted ($FFB_{TOBEC}$) were somewhat similar to the line of identity (1.0), the intercepts varied considerably and were significantly different from zero. Furthermore, significant mean differences between actual and predicted FFB were observed for the prepubescent/pubescent and mature adult groups, but not for the postpubescent group. This suggests that specific equations may need to be considered, at least for the youngest and oldest groups. The lack of precise estimation of FFB from TOBEC analysis in these groups may partly be due to assumptions implicit in the $D_B$ method

---

* This equation is:
$$FFB_{TOBEC} = 1.545 + 0.28 \, (\text{PC-II}^{1/2} \times Ht)$$
$$- 0.010 (\text{PC-III}^{1/2} \times Ht).$$

that may not be valid. The Siri (1961) equation used to compute percent fat and FFB from $D_B$ assumes an FFB density of 1.100 g/cm³. However, this assumption appears to be invalid in children and older adults, since changes in water and mineral content of the FFB have been shown to lower the FFB density (Layman and Boileau, 1986). Thus, part of the variability associated with the predictors of FFB from the equation for the young adult group may be related to biological error in the FFB estimated densitometrically in the other three groups.

To further study the relationship between $FFB_{D_B}$ and $FFB_{TOBEC}$, $FFB_{D_B}$ was expressed as MF-FFB. The MF-FFB was calculated by subtracting the estimated bone mineral weight, measured by photon absorptiometry, from the $FFB_{D_B}$. Since bone mineral contains little water and electrolytes, its conductivity is relatively low compared with other components of the FFB; therefore, theoretically the MF-FFB better represents the conductive component of the FFB. Although the SEE is reduced from 2.60 to 2.41 kg, the CV is similar for $FFB_{D_B}$ (6.1) and $MF\text{-}FFB_{D_B}$ (6.0), suggesting that a correction for bone mineral content does relatively little to reduce the error in predicting the actual FFB.

Body potassium was also found to be highly related to TOBEC ($r = 0.99$). The best predictors of body potassium were PC-$I^{1/2} \times Ht$ and PC-$II^{1/2} \times Ht$, yielding an SEE of 6.6 g (CV = 5.7 percent). These independent variables represent the conductance function of the TOBEC measurement. Potassium is associated primarily with the mineral-free FFB, since only a negligible amount of potassium is found in either fat or bone. Therefore, a high correlation between body potassium and TOBEC further supports the validity of the TOBEC method.

Total body electrical conductivity analysis appears to be a promising method for assessing body composition on both theoretical and empirical grounds. The association demonstrated between TOBEC and FFB determined by both densitometry and $^{40}K$ spectroscopy statistically confirms the theoretical basis of the method. The reported error in estimating FFB from TOBEC, ranging from 2.6 percent in a homogeneous group (Van Loan and Mayclin, 1987) to 5.0 percent in a heterogeneous group of children, youth, and adults (University of Illinois study), indicates that the method can be applied to a variety of subjects with good prediction precision. This study further suggests that population-specific calibration equations may improve the precision of estimating body composition. Although the ability of the TOBEC method to detect changes in body composition during weight reduction appears excellent (M. Van Loan, personal communication, 1986), further validation is needed in terms of the technique's capacity for detecting change in FFB, body water, and body potassium as a consequence of dietary, physical training, and dehydration treatments.

## REFERENCES

Behnke, A. R., and J. H. Wilmore. 1974. Evaluation and Regulation of Body Build and Composition. Englewood Cliffs, N.J.: Prentice-Hall.

Boileau, R. A., and T. G. Lohman. 1977. The measurement of human physique and its effect on physical performance. Orthopedic Clin. N. Am. 8:563–581.

Boileau, A., B. H. Massey, and J. E. Misner. 1973. Body composition changes in adult men during selected weight training and jogging programs. Res. Q. 44:158–168.

Boileau, R. A., T. G. Lohman, M. H. Slaughter, T. E. Ball, S. B. Going, and M. K. Hendrix. 1984. Hydration of the fat-free body in children during maturation. Human Biol. 56:651–666.

Boileau, R. A., T. G. Lohman, and M. H. Slaughter. 1985. Exercise and body composition of children and youth. Scan. J. Sports Sci. 7:17–27.

Borkan, G. A., and D. E. Hults. 1983. Change in body fat content and distribution with aging. Am. J. Phys. Anthropol. 60:175.

Bracco, E. F., M. U. Yang, K. Segal, S. A. Hashim, and T. B. Van Itallie. 1983. A new method for estimation of body composition in the live rat. Proc. Soc. Exp. Biol. 174:143–146.

Buskirk, E. R. 1971. Obesity. Pp. 229–242 in Physiological Basis of Rehabilitation Medicine, J. A. Downey and R. C. Darling, eds. Philadelphia: W. B. Saunders.

Coates, T., J. Killen, and L. Slinkard. 1982. Parent participation in a treatment program for overweight adolescents. Int. J. Eating Disorders 1:37–48.

Cochran, W. J., W. J. Klish, W. W. Wong, M. L. Fiorott, P. D. Klein, and B. L. Nichols. 1985. The use of total body impedance to determine body composition in infants. Pediatr. Res. 4:216 (Abstr.).

Cochran, W. J., W. J. Klish, W. W. Wong, and P. D. Klein. 1986. Total body electrical conductivity used to determine body composition in infants. Pediatr. Res. 20:561–686.

Cohn, S. H., K. J. Ellis, and S. Wallach. 1974. In vivo neutron activation analysis: Clinical potential in body composition studies. Am. J. Med. 57:683–686.

Domermuth, W., T. L. Veum, M. A. Alexander, H. B. Hedrick, J. Clark, and D. Eklund. 1976. Prediction of lean body composition of live market weight swine by indirect methods. J. Anim. Sci. 43:966–976.

Geddes, L. A., and L. E. Baker. 1968. P. 155 in Principles of Applied Biomedical Instrumentation. New York: John Wiley & Sons.

Harrison, G. G., and T. B. Van Itallie. 1982. Estimation of body composition: A new approach based on electromagnetic principles. Am. J. Clin. Nutr. 35:1176–1179.

Keys, A., and J. Brozek. 1953. Body fat in adult man. Physiol. Rev. 33:245–325.

Klish, W. J., G. B. Forbes, A. Gordon, and W. J. Cochran. 1984. New method for the estimation of lean body mass in infants (EMME instrument): Validation in nonhuman models. J. Pediatr. Gastroenterol. Nutr. 3:199–204.

Layman, D. K., and R. A. Boileau. 1986. Aerobic exercise and body composition. Pp. 125–141 in Nutrition and Aerobic Exercise, D. K. Layman, ed. Washington, D.C.: American Chemical Society.

Lohman, T. G. 1984. Research progress in validation of laboratory methods of assessing body composition. Med. Sci. Sports Exercise 16:596–603.

Lohman, T. G., R. A. Boileau, and M. H. Slaughter. 1984a. Body composition in children and youth. Pp. 29–59 in Advances in Pediatric Sports Sciences, R. A. Boileau, ed. Champaign, Ill.: Human Kinetics Publishers.

Lohman, T. G., M. H. Slaughter, R. A. Boileau, J. Bunt, and L. Lussier. 1984b. Bone mineral measurements and their relation to body density in children, youth and adults. Human Biol. 56:667–697.

McArdle, W. D., F. I. Katch, and V. L. Katch. 1981. Exercise Physiology: Energy, Nutrition and Performance. Philadelphia: Lea & Febiger.

Nyboer, J. 1972. Workable volume and flow concepts of bio-segments by electrical impedance plethysmography. T-I-T J. Life Sci. 2:1–13.

Pethig, R. 1979. Pp. 207–243 in Dielectric and Electronic Properties of Biological Materials. New York: John Wiley & Sons.

Presta, E., K. R. Segal, B. Gutin, G. G. Harrison, and T. B. Van Itallie. 1983. Comparison in man of total body electrical conductivity and lean body mass derived from body density: Validation of a new body composition method. Metabolism 32:524–527.

Segal, K. R., B. Gutin, E. Presta, J. Wang, and T. B. Van Itallie. 1985. Estimation of human body composition by electrical impedance methods: A comparative study. J. Appl. Physiol. 58:1565–1571.

Siri, W. E. 1961. Body composition from fluid spaces and density: Analysis of methods. Pp. 223–244 in Techniques for Measuring Body Composition, J. Brozek and A. Henschel, eds. Washington, D.C.: National Academy of Sciences.

U.S. Patent 3,735,247. May 22, 1973. Method and Apparatus for Measuring Fat Content in Animal Tissue Either In Vivo or in Slaughtered and Prepared Form, W. H. Harker (inventor). The EMME Company, Assiguee. Washington, D.C.: U.S. Patent Office.

Van Itallie, G. G., K. Segal, M. U. Yang, and R. C. Funk. 1985. Clinical assessment of body fat content in adults: Potential role of electrical impedance methods. Pp. 5–8 in Body Composition Assessment in Youth and Adults: Report of the Sixth Ross Conference on Medical Research, A. Roche, ed. Columbus, Ohio: Ross Laboratories.

Van Loan, M., and P. Mayclin. 1987. A new TOBEC instrument and procedure for the assessment of body composition: Use of Fourier coefficients to predict lean body mass and total body water. Am. J. Clin. Nutr. 45:131–137.

Ylitalo, V. 1981. Treatment of obese school children. Acta Paediatr. Scand. (Suppl. 290):1–108.

# Live Animal and Carcass Composition Measurement

DAVID G. TOPEL and ROBERT KAUFFMAN

Animals of all species vary considerably in composition (Reid et al., 1968) as a result of their stage of growth, nutritional history, and genetic base. This is of concern to livestock producers, the meat industry, and consumers because the economic value of a meat-producing animal depends greatly on its composition. During the last 15 to 20 years, the meat industry has made dramatic progress in reducing the fat content of domestic animals in response to consumer demand for more lean meat and the economic pressure to produce animals more efficiently. Nevertheless, the average pork carcass and U.S. Department of Agriculture Choice beef carcass are still about 30 to 35 percent fat (Topel, 1986).

The proportion of muscle in an animal's body varies from less than 35 percent to nearly 50 percent of the body weight (Webster, 1986). In addition to stage of growth, nutrition, and genetics, several other factors contribute to variation in body composition, such as contents of the alimentary canal, pregnancy, and presence of abnormalities. All these traits collectively complicate the accurate measurement of body composition. Nevertheless, it is important to seek meth-

ods that will reliably approximate body composition because of its contribution to the total worth of meat-producing animals. Therefore, this paper identifies the various techniques that have been used to estimate body composition, as well as new techniques that have potential for future application.

## LINEAR MEASUREMENTS OF LIVE ANIMALS

Some years ago, some livestock evaluators believed that measurements of the length, width, height, and circumference of live animals could be used to predict various carcass characteristics including composition (Busch et al., 1969; Cook et al., 1951; Green et al., 1969; Kidwell, 1955). They used tape measures, centrex curves, and several types of rather elaborate calipers that were designed to make almost any linear measurement imaginable on the non-symmetrical surfaces of live animals. Reference points were usually confined to anatomically defined locations of the skeleton. Animals (primarily cattle) were led onto a flat surface and constrained in a neck stanchion. If the animal was not gentle, it was nearly impossible to palpate the body to locate the skeletal reference points, let alone make the measurements. From the numerous dimensions measured, the evaluator could very accurately reconstruct the topography of the animal's body; however, most if not all of the data were of limited value in determining compositional patterns. Many of the measurements were obviously related to weights of carcass wholesale cuts, but not to percent fat or muscle. This approach may have provided some insight into the variations in frame and skeletal size and their relationship to live weight, breed, and stage of maturity; but it was not useful in predicting the muscle, fat, and bone content of animals.

## LINEAR MEASUREMENTS OF THE CARCASS

A simple, inexpensive ruler to measure fat thickness and length and width of the longissimus dorsi muscle has been used by animal scientists for many years. Palsson (1939) evaluated lamb carcasses, Hirzel (1939) measured beef carcasses, and McMeekan (1941) reported strong relationships between linear measurements of back fat thickness and carcass fat percentage. These workers also reported good estimates of carcass muscle when carcass length was combined with the depth and length of the longissimus dorsi. From these early studies have come more than 200 papers relating linear measurements of body fat thickness and longissimus dorsi area to the muscle, fat, and bone percentage of the carcass as well as to its chemical fat, protein, and water content (see, for example, Berg and Butterfield, 1976; Breidenstein et al., 1968; Brozek, 1961; Cross, 1982; Doornenbal, 1968; Kauffman, 1971; Kempster, 1986; Zobrisky, 1963). The relationships of back fat thickness and size of the longissimus dorsi are considered to be good, but not excellent, predictors of body composition.

## THE BACK FAT PROBE

The back fat probe was first described scientifically by Hazel and Kline (1952) and has been used often to determine quantitatively the actual thickness of subcutaneous fat on live animals. It has been used more extensively on pigs than on cattle and sheep because a greater proportion of the pig's fat is deposited subcutaneously and there is greater variation in the measurement obtained when comparing lean and fat pigs. With cattle there is the problem of hide thickness, and with sheep there are minimal variations of fat depth.

To measure the actual fat depth, a small incision is made in the skin with a scalpel and a narrow metal ruler is forced through the fat layers, or a ruler containing a needle point is forced directly through the skin and fat layers. (Since the nerve and vascular supplies in the skin and subcutaneous fat are minimal, pain and bleeding are not much of a problem.) The measuring device must penetrate the false lean or aponeurosis (sheet of fascial connective tissue separating the outer and middle layers of subcutaneous fat) and continue until there is a second resistance due to the epimysial connective tissue covering the muscle (usually the longissimus dorsi when probing the thoracic and lumbar portions of the back). The depth should be visually verified and recorded after slipping a flat object over the ruler, firmly sliding it to the skin surface (avoiding undue pressure), and then removing the ruler, needle, or both.

Once the fat depth is known, it can be used in a previously developed regression equation with other variables such as live weight and muscling score to estimate composition. Fat depth alone usually accounts for most of the variation in composition, but live weight and degree of muscling should improve the accuracy of the measurement (Fahey et al., 1977).

The major advantages of this method are that it affords a reasonably accurate prediction of composition, it is relatively easy to standardize, it makes a rapid measurement, and it is inexpensive. On the other hand, it requires that the animal be restrained, and it is too slow if large numbers of animals are involved. For cattle, a restraining chute is needed, and for lambs, the variations in fat depth may be so small that the method might not be sophisticated enough to yield an accurate measurement.

## REFLECTANCE PROBE

The reflectance probe was developed by researchers at the Danish Meat Research Institute for use on pork carcasses. It is widely used in Europe, but not in the United States. The instrument measures reflectance of the muscle and fat components when inserted into the loin section of the pork carcass. Desmoulin (1984) summarized its value for estimating fat and muscle thickness. Fat content was estimated with greater accuracy than lean content when weight was not included in the prediction equation ($r^2 = 0.82$). The combination of weight and carcass length with the reflectance probe measurement correlates well ($r^2 = 0.77$) with muscle percent.

The cost of the equipment is relatively high but not excessive if it is used on a daily basis for grading pork carcasses in large slaughter plants. It is simple to use, and readings can be obtained in less than a minute. The optical probe is used on cold carcasses only, since these yield the largest differences in light reflection between muscle and fat tissue. The reflection probe can also indicate the meat quality characteristics of the carcass (Barton, 1983).

## LIVE WEIGHT

The development of growth curves from the animal's live weight provides a practical and simple method for estimating body composition if the genetic history for body composition is known. As animals grow,

their carcass composition changes and the proportion of fat increases at the expense of muscle and bone (Rouse et al., 1970). When comparing animals of similar type grown in the same environment, live weight will normally show a high positive correlation with the percentage of fat in the carcass and, because of the close relationship between muscle and bone, a high negative correlation with the proportion of muscle in the carcass (Busch et al., 1969).

Even in mixed-breed populations with animals obtained from different production systems, there is often a strong association between weight and fatness, although the degree of correlation is more variable. Used sensibly, live weight can be a guide to carcass composition. It can be made more effective when a sample of cattle, swine, or sheep representative of the population or production group is slaughtered to establish the relationship between weight and composition (Cianzio et al., 1982; Hammack and Shrode, 1986).

The relationship between live weight and fatness is such that it will be influenced by the way animals are fed, the environment in which they are grown, and any subclinical disease that may alter their growth rate. Live weight and its relationship to composition are also dependent on the contents of the digestive tract, which can vary from 10 to 20 percent of live weight depending on diet. Any relationship developed to predict fatness from live weight in one set of circumstances is therefore unlikely to apply with acceptable accuracy in other circumstances. For these reasons, it is difficult to establish guidelines that can apply to the general population of domestic animals. The farmer or livestock feeder should, however, be monitoring the performance, weight, and carcass traits of the animals used for his or her production system (Kempster, 1982). If a farmer has these records, live weight can be used to predict composition.

Live weight of cattle, swine, and sheep is still the major and, in many markets, the only factor used in deciding when animals will be sold for slaughter. Therefore, livestock breeders and farmers must select for cattle, swine, and sheep that have the genetic traits for low fat and high muscle percentage at live weights that will provide conveniently sized cuts of meat for the consumer and meet the standards established by the packing industry to operate economically.

## VISUAL ASSESSMENT AND SUBJECTIVE EVALUATION

Visual assessment and subjective evaluation methods are the most commonly used techniques to estimate body muscle and fat characteristics in meat-producing animals. A major problem with visual evaluation is distinguishing between muscling and fatness. Visual assessments of muscling are therefore likely to be more effective as indicators of muscle deposition within a narrow range of fatness and particularly when fat levels are low.

Gregory et al. (1962, 1964) and Wilson et al. (1964) reported on the extent to which carcass traits can be predicted from live characteristics in beef cattle. Their studies included the use of subjective techniques of appraisal in selecting breeding stock from relatively homogeneous populations under similar feeding regimes. They concluded that subjective live scores can account for only 20 to 40 percent of the variation in carcass traits and are of moderate value in ranking individual animals for selection from a breeding population.

Lewis et al. (1969) identified the variation in carcass cutability and grade characteristics that could be accounted for by visual appraisal. After live estimates were statistically compared with carcass measurements, the coefficients of determination of either a weight-adjusted or a weight-unadjusted basis indicated that trained personnel could account for more than half of the variation in carcass traits and that their estimates account for, on the average, over twice the variation accounted for by untrained personnel. Three-fourths of the variation in fat thickness could be detected by experienced evaluators.

## ULTRASONICS

Recent developments in ultrasonics have led to new interest in the use of ultrasonic techniques for estimating body composition in meat-producing animals (Recio et al., 1986).

Ultrasonics is based on the principle of high-frequency sound signals passing through tissues, but that when an interface between two tissues is encountered, some sound is reflected back. A pulse generator sends electrical pulses that are converted into sound signals in the transmitter. These signals are then passed through the tissues until they are reflected at an interface. The reflected signals are picked up by the receiver and can be amplified and shown in a visual form by an oscilloscope. Variations in the time taken for the reflected signals to return to the transmitter-receiver are used to measure variations in the distances of the boundaries between tissues. These concepts are outlined by Miles (1978).

The "A" mode ultrasonic machines display echo amplitude against time which is shown on the screen as peaks superimposed on a time baseline. The distance between the peaks represents the thickness of the tissues being measured. For "B" mode machines, the signals are shown on a cathode ray tube as a series of bright spots. The thickness of the tissues is represented by the distance between successive bright spots. Generally, these machines have a single transducer that moves across the body of the animal on a track. As the transducer moves, a picture is built up either on polaroid film or on a cathode ray screen. An example is the Scanogram machine.

Real-time machines produce a practically instantaneous picture by rapid electronic switching from element to element. The principle involved is similar to that already described except that movements of the tissues can be seen because of the continuous nature of the picture. The Danscanner is an example. The interpretation of results for "B" mode machines and real-time scanning usually requires the tracing of depths and areas from pictures. This can now be done by using planimeters linked to microprocessors or computers (Alliston, 1983).

Of all the nondestructive evaluation techniques used to evaluate the body composition of living animals, the new ultrasonic techniques appear to have the greatest potential for practical application at this time. A large cooperative research study between scientists in Denmark and the United Kingdom on ultrasonic methods was reported by Andersen et al. (1982).

The application of ultrasonics to the measurement of carcass traits of meat-producing animals was first reported in the United States by Stouffer et al. (1959). Since then, ultrasonic techniques have improved considerably, and Andersen et al. (1982) provide an excellent comparative report on five ultrasonic machines: the Scanogram, the Danscanner, the Philips, the Ohio, and the Bruel and Kjaer. A summary follows.

Ultrasonic scanning predicts body composition with a degree of accuracy similar to that of the corresponding cut surface measurements on the carcass. The ultrasound prediction was somewhat better than would be expected from the relationship between ultrasonic measurements and the corresponding cut surface measurements such as fat thickness over the loin.

When the five ultrasonic units were evaluated, the Bruel and Kjaer scanner was less accurate than the other four. No clear differences were detected for the other four units between the machine-operator combinations in terms of predicting body composition traits. Although the Philips and Ohio machines were only able to scan a section of the longissimus dorsi muscle and its overlying subcutaneous fat, they provided an acceptable description of the carcass composition traits. Among the operators, however, there was a preference for the Danscanner and Scanogram, which are specially constructed for use with farm animals. Because the four ultrasonic machines had similar technical capabilities, other factors to consider include capital investment, ease of use, operating costs, and quality of service.

A review of the recent literature (Miller et al., 1986; Recio et al., 1986) indicates that real-time ultrasound measurements obtained by very experienced operators can accurately predict carcass composition traits. The real-time ultrasound live measures of longissimus dorsi area, 12th rib, and shoulder fat thickness were significantly correlated ($P < 0.05$) to the comparable carcass measurements ($r^2 = 0.98$, 0.88, and 0.79, respectively). For predicting percentage of carcass fat, the 9th-10th-11th rib fat percentage (coefficient of determination [CD] = 85.4), the U.S. Department of Agriculture (USDA) yield grade (CD = 74.0), the real-time ultrasound, the 12th rib fat thickness (CD = 55.8), and the carcass specific gravity (CD = 48.8) were all significantly correlated ($P < 0.05$). Adjusted fat thickness was the single most useful carcass measurement for predicting percentage of carcass fat (CD = 69.3).

## VIDEO IMAGE ANALYSIS

Video image analysis (VIA) has been studied as a replacement for or supplement to the subjective visual assessment of grading carcasses. The concept is based on the use of a video camera to obtain a video image (a numerical array of gray values) through an analog/digital converter. The values can then be manipulated by computer. In practice, the application of VIA to carcass grading is not simple. Some of the potential difficulties are as follows:

1. Development of image analysis procedures with optimal correlation to carcass anatomy and carcass composition;

2. Technical problems associated with daily use of electronic equipment in the harsh slaughterhouse environment;

3. Standardization of the video inspection process (relative position of the object, background contrast, lighting); and

4. Development of software with the ability to handle carcasses with large variations in size.

In the United Kingdom, the VIA principle is now commercially used to measure visible lean in fabricated beef. In Sweden, a version of the VIA system called Electronic Scanning Planimetry has been developed and evaluated for prediction of carcass composition in pigs.

In 1978, the U.S. Department of Agriculture, in cooperation with the National Aeronautics and Space Administration and the Jet Propulsion Laboratory, began a project to develop an instrument for objective evaluation of carcass quality and yield grade. Video image analysis was identified as having the greatest potential. The best combination of VIA-measured traits for predicting kilograms of lean was total lean area at the 12th rib, rib weight (kilograms), total fat area at the 12th-13th rib, and fat thickness (centimeters). This equation had a CD of 93.6. The results of the study clearly indicate that strong potential exists for VIA as a yield-grading device.

Wassenberg et al. (1986) reported that VIA is as reliable as an expert three-member committee using USDA traits to evaluate the percent beef carcass yield of primal lean. In addition, it might be less subject to human error. It also shows potential for use as a predictor of total production weight yields which could facilitate the sale of boxed beef products. This method could be used in the U.S. commercial beef industry in the near future.

## WHOLE-BODY $^{40}$K COUNTING

Estimating the body composition of a living subject by whole-body $^{40}$K counting is feasible because of the direct relation of potassium to lean body mass and its indirect relation to fat. Potassium is the only single element found in body tissue in significant amounts that has any predictive value of body composition. It is found mostly in the intracellular space, and thus, total body potassium is indicative of total body cell mass. Potassium is not found in fat in any significant amount, and therefore, if potassium is present in the fat-free tissue as a constant percentage, then a value for total body potassium can be converted to a weight of lean body mass (Ward, 1968).

Approximately 0.012 percent of all naturally occurring potassium is made up of the radioactive isotope $^{40}$K. The rest is composed of the stable isotopes $^{39}$K and $^{41}$K. Because $^{40}$K emits gamma radiation at 1.46 MeV, the intensity of 1.46-MeV gamma emission from the body can be used to estimate total potassium content. From these values, total body protein and lean mass can be estimated, assuming that the mass of protein or muscle versus potassium is constant (Schmidt et al., 1974).

Lohman et al. (1968) reported that the standard error for the estimation of the total mass of potassium in beef carcass was 3.4 percent and that the corresponding figure for carcass lean mass was 4.2 percent. Breidenstein et al. (1968) used 103 steers representing four breed types and slaughtered at four different weights to compare several alternative methods of determining carcass lean muscle mass (CLMM). Fifty-four steers were subjected to whole-body counting after consuming a low-counting diet for a week. Constants for breed type were included in all regressions except those using whole-body potassium and physical measurements of the live animal. The dependent variable was weight or percentage of CLMM. Results were similar to those obtained by other scientists working in the $^{40}$K area.

The inclusion of either live weight or carcass weight in a regression model results in an appreciable decrease in the coefficient of variation. Fat thicknesses measured at one-half and three-fourths of the medial to lateral axis of the longissimus dorsi were useful criteria, but little or no reduction in the coefficient of variation resulted from including fat thickness measured at one-fourth of the medial to lateral axis. Inclusion of the longissimus dorsi area generally reduced the coefficient of variation. Carcass specific gravity was a useful indicator of CLMM, and the coefficient of variation was further reduced by including carcass weight and fat thickness. Measurement of trimmed hindquarter was no better than other more easily acquired measures. Whole-body $^{40}K$ counting resulted in the lowest coefficient of variation of any regression model except the model including standard trimmed lean, which had a coefficient of variation of only 1.4 percent (which was not reduced by including fat thicknesses).

The $^{40}K$ method has proved useful in research projects where the research center has a $^{40}K$ Whole Body Counter, which only a few agricultural experiment stations in the United States have. Furthermore, facilities must be specially shielded from background radiation because of the low levels of $^{40}K$ being measured. Uncertainties in the measurement of total-body potassium arise from various sources including random error due to counting statistics, instability of the counting apparatus, and variation in sensitivity due to differences in body geometry and position of the animal. These factors restrict the use of $^{40}K$ in the commercial industry. The topic of $^{40}K$ estimation of body composition was reviewed in detail in *Body Composition in Animals and Man* in 1968 by the National Academy of Sciences (see Reid et al., 1968; Breidenstein et al., 1968; Lohman et al., 1968; Ward, 1968).

## BODY DENSITY

Discovery of the principle of density is credited to Archimedes, around 200 B.C. The Archimedean principle is based on the fact that a body displaces a volume equal to its own. Density is expressed in relation to the density of a reference standard, usually water at 20°C. In the case of gas, however, the standard is generally air.

The rationale for estimating fatness or muscling from density is based on the assumption that the body can be considered a two-component system, with the components being of different but constant densities (Keys and Brozek, 1953). If this is the case and the densities of the components are known, the proportions of the two components can be estimated from the density of the whole body. The two components in meat-producing animals are usually considered to be the fatty tissue and the fat-free body. There is considerable evidence that the fat-free body is fairly constant in composition in mature animals (Elsley et al., 1964; Messinger and Steele, 1949; Morales et al., 1945; Murray, 1922). The water content in the fat-free body is not constant in young, growing animals, however; and therefore, the density measurements are not likely to be as accurate for predicting composition (Pearson et al., 1968). The commonly reported density value for lean is 1.10; for fat it is 0.90.

The major problem in determining density is the measurement of volume. Although this would appear to be a simple procedure, it is not, especially in live animals. Even water displacement, which is the simplest method, has numerous pitfalls. Air displacement procedures, such as helium dilution, are even more complicated.

Timon and Bichard (1965) reported an inverse relationship between fat and carcass specific gravity in lambs. The correlation coefficients ranged from $-0.56$ to $-0.88$. Working with 83 lambs, they found that carcass specific gravity accounted for 86.1 and 78.1 percent of the respective variances in carcass fat and muscle percentages.

Kraybill et al. (1951) determined the specific gravity of the beef carcass and the empty body (without blood, hide, and lungs) of 30 beef animals. The correlation coefficient between carcass and empty-body specific gravities was 0.98. Empty-body specific gravity was correlated ($-0.95$) with the percentage of carcass fat. Zinn et al. (1966) and Albin et al. (1967) found that the crude protein content of beef cattle estimated from carcass specific gravity using the relationship of Kraybill et al. (1951) is higher than values obtained by actual laboratory analysis. The accuracy of specific gravity for estimating body composition traits varies from average to good. At the 1986 meeting of the American Society of Animal Science, Miller et al. (1986) reported an average relationship (CD = 48.8) for specific gravity in predicting carcass fat.

The variation in predicting carcass composition in pork carcasses is similar to that for cattle and sheep. Garrett (1968) provided a summary of the variation.

Density techniques are slow and have no commercial use, but the specific gravity technique is still used to a limited degree in the research field.

## ELECTRONIC MEAT-MEASURING EQUIPMENT

The electronic meat-measuring equipment (EMME) principle works on eddy currents being induced in the animal by an alternating magnetic field produced by a current passing through a coil surrounding the animal. The eddy currents generate a magnetic field that can be picked up by a change of impedance in the coil. The concept is based on the method that the conductivity of muscle is much higher than that of fat.

Domermuth et al. (1976) investigated the predictive value of EMME for body composition of pigs and found that EMME values in combination with fasted weight could predict carcass protein ($r^2 = 0.78$) and lean cuts ($r^2 = 0.80$).

Fredeen et al. (1979) found correlations of $-0.79$ between EMME values and the percentage of total fat and 0.79 and 0.40 for percentage of muscle for 130 and 228 pigs, respectively. The results obtained with the EMME method in general were too variable to be acceptable.

Each EMME machine has to be calibrated and a formula established for the specific machine. Temperature and humidity can influence the results. At present, the EMME machine is not used to estimate body composition of swine on a commercial basis. Some units have been used to estimate the fat content of boneless meat packaged in boxes for interstate shipment.

## ANYL-RAY

The Anyl-ray technique is based on x-ray attenuation as an index of tissue fatness. It is used on a regular basis by the commercial meat industry in the United States to determine the fat content in ground meat used for meat processing. The method is fast, requires a small sample (2 to 3 kg), and has a high degree of accuracy.

## TISSUE SAWDUST TECHNIQUE

Vance et al. (1970) reported a correlation ($P < 0.01$) between the chemical components of beef carcass sides and the meat sawdust from sawing through the frozen round, loin, rib, and chuck at 2.54-cm intervals. This technique was further evaluated by Williams et al. (1974), who evaluated 20 bull carcasses averaging 282 kg. Correlations between the chemical composition of the carcass and the tissue sawdust were 0.82, 0.94, 0.64, and 0.68 for moisture, fat, protein, and ash, respectively. Also, 12 carcass sides from six Holstein calves averaging 138 kg were used to evaluate storage methods (chilling versus freezing of the carcass) and two types of sawdust (cross-section every 2.54 cm versus retail cut) for estimating carcass composition. Chilled carcasses yielded only 23 percent as much sawdust as frozen carcasses. The reliability of the sawdust procedure for predicting carcass composition was greatest from frozen carcasses sawed every 2.54 cm, followed by the meat sawdust from cutting frozen carcasses into retail cuts. Chemical composition of meat sawdust can provide a good estimate of the chemical composition of cattle when samples are collected from frozen carcasses. The method is simple but time-consuming. Slight devaluation of the carcass occurs. This method has value as a research tool, but is not feasible for commercial application (Williams et al., 1974).

### DILUTION TECHNIQUES

The dilution technique involves the introduction of a known amount of tracer, which will become uniformly distributed throughout a compartment in the animal body (Cuthbertson, 1975; Odwongo et al., 1985). A sample of the compartment is then taken and the concentration of the tracer measured. A tracer should not be toxic, must be metabolized, should be easily measurable, and must diffuse homogeneously into all the volume to be measured (Robelin, 1982). Some of the different tracers used in animals include antipyrine and $N$-acetyl-1,4-aminoantipyrine, urea, tritiated water (TOH), and deuterium oxide ($D_2O$). Deuterium oxide and urea appear to be the most suitable tracers because they are more accurate and not radioactive. Results from research with antipyrine generally demonstrate that antipyrine dilution is too variable to give good estimation of total body water (Panaretto and Till, 1963).

### UREA DILUTION

Urea dilution has been used to estimate body composition in cattle (Bartle et al., 1983; Kock and Preston, 1979; Meissner et al., 1980; Preston and Kock, 1973) and in lambs (Bartle et al., 1985). Because urea is inexpensive and the technical requirements of plasma urea N analysis are minimal, the urea dilution technique could be used for both research and industrial purposes where measurement of body composition during growth is necessary. The correlation between urea space and fatness ranged from 0.71 to 0.82. The technique works best with heavy cattle having a relatively large degree of fatness, compared to lighter cattle with a small degree of fatness. Rule et al. (1986) reported that some equations developed for urea dilution estimates of body water overestimated empty body water in 6-month-old steers by 7.59 percent, but that for 12- and 18-month-old steers the calculated and percentage empty body water did not differ ($P > 0.05$).

Bartle and Preston (1986) further evaluated the amount of urea diffusing from the blood into the rumen and urine of cattle after urea infusion and found that urea did not diffuse into the reticulo-ruminal water. They indicated that the urea dilution method overestimates empty body water by the urine volume produced in the 12-minute collection period.

To ensure more accurate data, it is suggested that before using any prediction equation to calculate body composition by dilution techniques, the equation should be tested with a subsample of cattle from the population for which its use is intended (Rule et al., 1986).

Cuthbertson (1975) and Robelin (1982) examined the problems associated with the estimation of body water in ruminants caused by the variation in the water content of the alimentary tract. Robelin used $D_2O$ to study 340 beef cattle for whole-body composition and found that the weight of water and protein was fairly closely related to fat-free mass. He reported that for a single beef animal, an accuracy of 13 percent for lipid and 7 percent for protein deposition is obtained for a total body weight gain of 300 kg.

Foot and Greenhalgh (1970) used the $D_2O$ procedure to estimate body fat content in sheep. The values they obtained differed from those obtained by analysis of the slaughtered animals by 0.8 to 1.7 kg in seven ewes containing 5.2 to 21.4 kg of fat. The standard deviation was ±1.2 percentage units.

The $D_2O$ dilution method has no commercial application and is used on a limited basis as a research tool to estimate body composition. It is relatively simple for scientists to use but too complex for industrial application. It is a good way to estimate total body water but is limited in its level of accuracy for total body fat.

Application of a kinetic technique to solve an anatomic problem with no documentation of the congruity of the kinetic and anatomic models is clearly limited. Simulation analysis indicates that the kinetic model is very insensitive to changes in anatomic pool sizes, but very sensitive to changes in exchange rates of water among pools (R. W. Russell and R. B. Reed, personal communication, 1986).

## COMPUTERIZED TOMOGRAPHY

The Nobel Prize was awarded to A. M. Cormack and G. N. Houndsfield for the development of the computerized tomography (CT) technique. The concept is based on presentation of anatomic areas of the body by computed synthesis of an image from x-ray transmission data obtained in many different directions through the plane under consideration (Cormack, 1980; Houndsfield, 1980). An x-ray tube rotates around an object, and the computer reconstructs from a series of pictures a slide through the object. By this technique, the density (CT number) of different body tissues at different distances from the x-ray tube can be calculated.

One of the first applications of this technique for estimating composition of meat-producing animals was reported by Skjervold (1982) from the Agricultural University of Norway. Their study of 23 pigs indicated that it was possible to obtain a good predic-

tion of the body composition on the basis of the relative CT distribution from one tomographic plane. Skjervold also reported the CT numbers of different body tissues. Lung tissue had values of −200 to −100; fat tissue, −100 to 0; muscle tissue, +30 to +100; and bone, +400 to +500.

Allen and Vangen (1984) used computerized tomography to estimate the body composition of 207 pigs ranging in weight from 59 to 120 kg. The values they obtained are similar to those reported by Skjervold (1982).

European researchers have been active in evaluating CT for use in estimating body composition of meat-producing animals, but only limited research is being done in the United States. Researchers at the Meat and Animal Science Department of the University of Wisconsin are cooperating with medical college faculty and are currently collecting data from pigs.

The main drawbacks to computerized tomography are expense, the time required to obtain an estimate, and the necessity to anesthetize the animal before scanning. Even with these limitations, however, improved techniques are expected that will make computerized tomography acceptable for scanning animals for genetic selection of breeding stock. This method therefore has great potential for future use in the livestock industry.

## NUCLEAR MAGNETIC RESONANCE IMAGING

The nuclear magnetic resonance (NMR) method for estimating body composition is based on a strong static magnetic field and pulsed radio waves that induce resonance of protons in the measured body. The signals emitted are a reaction of the body to the high-frequency disturbance. Therefore, they are a product of the matter itself, with intensities depending on the proton spin densities and molecular structures. The NMR signal does not continue indefinitely. Environmental influences cause the individual flipped magnetic moments to get out of phase and return to the orientation they had before the radio frequency pulse was applied. The time required to reestablish original conditions has been defined as spin-lattice relaxation time T1 and spin-spin relaxation time T2. Procedures to determine T1 are known as inversion recovery, and for T2 as spin-echo methods. Both systems produce a data matrix of the size 128–128 or 256–256 that contains in x-ray CT the normalized Houndsfield units ranging from −1,000 (air) to more than 1,400 (compact bone). There are several ways to produce images. On a device with seven colors, the total data space in a matrix is subdivided into seven regions, with each region representing a different color. Fat, muscle, bone, and connective tissue are always presented if the total data space is mapped onto seven colors (Groeneveld et al., 1984).

Fuller et al. (1984) used the Aberdeen NMR imaging machine to evaluate pigs for body composition. Only three pigs were evaluated. Images were obtained at nine sites along the body, three each of the shoulder, midback, and rump. Good images reportedly were obtained of the muscle, fat, and bone portions of the sites scanned.

Nuclear magnetic resonance imaging has great potential, but very limited data are available on its usefulness for predicting body composition traits of meat-producing animals. The equipment is very expensive, and the method is very complex; its future will depend on the amount of resources available for its development as an agricultural tool.

## NEAR-INFRARED REFLECTANCE

Near-infrared reflectance (NIR) is widely used to predict the composition of various plant materials and may have potential application for estimating carcass composition. Mitchell et al. (1986) used 20 pigs for each weight group of 30, 60, and 90 kg to evaluate the NIR method. Readings were taken at specific sites on the ham, shoulder, and side of the pig. Carcass composition was determined by analysis of the soft tissue dissected from the eviscerated carcass for lipid, protein, and water content. Multiterm regression correlations were generated for carcass fat as a percentage of live body weight. For the carcass, percent fat correlated best with NIR readings taken on the ham. The measurements taken from the carcass accounted for about 50 to 60 percent of the variation. The values for the live pig were lower. These relationships indicate that with refinement in instrumentation and technique, this method may be useful in predicting body composition. It is simple, and the equipment is not prohibitively expensive. More research is needed, however, before NIR can be considered for commercial use.

## SOLUBLE SHORT-LIVED RADIOACTIVE GAS TRACERS

A range of halogenated gases with a particular affinity for adipose tissue could be considered for predictors of body composition. The commonly used anesthetic halothane (2-bromo-2-chloro-1,1,1-trifluoroethane) is an example. The label can be $^{11}$C, $^{18}$F, $^{77}$Br, or $^{38}$Cl. This idea was reported by Ettinger et al. (1984), who suggested that an animal can be given labeled halogenated gases in concentrations small enough to have no noticeable anesthetic effect but large enough that the gases are taken up by the adipose tissue. The amount taken up could be measured by a conventional whole-body counter or a whole-body scanner. The hypothesis has not been tested, but a good theoretical basis exists for the concept.

## SUMMARY OF THE PRACTICABILITY/ COST-BENEFIT COMPARISON OF BODY COMPOSITION MEASURES

More than 30 techniques for estimating live animal or carcass composition were reported in this review. The cost of the equipment to measure body composition can range from 1 dollar to over 1 million dollars. Accuracy, precision, and practicality are also considerations. Many promising techniques have been rejected for commercial use, not because of costs but because of practicability.

One of the least costly techniques available for estimating fat thickness in cattle and swine is the ruler back fat probe. Its accuracy is as high as the best ultrasonic techniques and almost as high as the computerized tomography methods recently developed for meat-producing animals. The cost of a ruler probe can range from 1 to 50 dollars, but still, the device is not used extensively in the meat industry because personnel are concerned about its practicality. (This concern is not really valid; a trained person can probe an individual pig or steer in less than a minute when the animal is restrained.)

The scientific community must understand that most producers and buyers of livestock in the United States prefer the use of live weight and visual assessment methods for estimating body composition because of their practicality, low cost, and rapidity in making the measurements. This must reflect the limited interest of the U.S. livestock industry in reducing fat in meat-producing animals by objective methods. One reason for this is the small margin paid by the packing industry for trim, well-muscled animals versus fat, less muscular ones. We need an improved marketing program that will pay farmers for producing trim, muscular animals. A system of this type will encourage the use of more objective methods for the selection of breeding animals and the marketing of animals for meat production.

From the research standpoint, many techniques are available to estimate body composition, but their accuracies are not outstanding. Most can account for 60 to 80 percent of the variation in muscle, fat, or

bone of the carcass. Thus, more accurate methods are needed for researchers working in the body composition field. Based on recent literature, it may be possible to improve accuracy with such new methods as computerized tomography and nuclear magnetic resonance imaging. The cost of the equipment currently prevents their widespread use, but with further research on new methods, we may, in the near future, develop the ultimate technique—one that is cost-effective, simple, and accurate.

## REFERENCES

Albin, R. C., D. W. Zinn, S. E. Curl, and G. H. Tatsch. 1967. Growth and fattening of the bovine. III. Effect of energy intake upon carcass composition. J. Anim. Sci. 26:209.

Allen, P., and O. Vangen. 1984. x-ray tomography of pigs—some preliminary results. P. 52. in In Vivo Measurements of Body Composition in Meat Animals, D. Lister, ed. London and New York: Elsevier Applied Science Publications.

Alliston, J. C. 1983. Evaluation of carcass quality in live animals. P. 79 in Sheep Production, W. Haresign, ed. Boston: Butterworth.

Andersen, B. B., H. Busk, J. P. Chadwick, A. Cuthertson, G. A. J. Fursey, D. W. Jones, P. Lewin, C. A. Miles, and M. G. Owen. 1982. CEC supported ultrasonic trial in U.K. and Denmark. Pp. 13–41 in In Vivo Estimation of Body Composition in Beef, CEC Workshop Report, B. B. Andersen, ed. Copenhagen: National Institute of Animal Sciences.

Bartle, S. J., and R. L. Preston. 1986. Plasma, rumen and urine pools in urea dilution determination of body composition in cattle. J. Anim. Sci. 63:77.

Bartle, S. J., J. R. Males, and R. L. Preston. 1983. Evaluation of urea dilution as an estimator of body composition in mature cows. J. Anim. Sci. 56:410.

Bartle, S. J., R. L. Preston, M. A. McCann, and F. B. Craddock. 1985. Evaluation of urea dilution as an estimator of body composition in finishing lambs. J. Anim. Sci. 61(Suppl. 1):265.

Barton, P. 1983. Quality traits of pork carcasses. P. 15 in Annual Report of the Danish Meat Research Institute. Copenhagen: Danish Meat Research Institute.

Berg, R. T., and R. M. Butterfield. 1976. New Concepts of Cattle Growth. New York: John Wiley & Sons.

Breidenstein, B. C., T. G. Lohman, and H. W. Norton. 1968. Comparison of potassium-40 method with other methods of determining carcass lean muscle mass in steers. P. 393 in Body Composition in Animals and Man. Washington, D.C.: National Academy of Sciences.

Brozek, J. 1961. Body measurements including skinfold thickness as indicators of body composition. P. 3 in Techniques for Measuring Body Composition. Washington, D.C.: National Academy of Sciences.

Busch, D. A., C. A. Dinkel, and J. A. Minyard. 1969. Body measurements, subjective scores and estimates of certain carcass traits as predictors of edible portion in beef cattle. J. Anim. Sci. 29:557.

Cianzio, D. S., D. G. Topel, G. B. Whitehurst, D. C. Beitz, and H. L. Self. 1982. Adipose tissue growth in cattle representing two frame sizes: Distribution among depots. J. Anim. Sci. 55:305.

Cook, A. C., M. L. Kohli, and W. M. Dawson. 1951. Relationship of five body measurements to slaughter grade, carcass grade and dressing percentage in milking Shorthorn steers. J. Anim. Sci. 10:386.

Cormack, A. M. 1980. A presentation of anatomical information by computed synthesis of an image from x-ray transmission data obtained in many different directions through the plan under consideration. Nobel Lecture. J. Computer Assisted Tomography 4:658.

Cross, H. R. 1982. In vivo and in vitro measurements of composition. Proc. Recip. Meat Conf. 35:1.

Cuthbertson, A. 1975. Carcass quality. P. 147 in Meat, D. J. A. Cole and R. A. Lawrie, eds. London: Butterworth.

Desmoulin, B. 1984. Pig carcass evaluation by linear measurement and the fat-o-meater (reflectance probe). P. 167 in In Vivo Measurements of Body Composition in Meat Animals, D. Lister, ed. London and New York: Elsevier Applied Science Publications.

Domermuth, W., T. L. Veum, M. A. Alexander, H. B. Hedrick, J. Clark, and D. Eklund. 1976. Prediction of mean body composition of live market weight swine by indirect methods. J. Anim. Sci. 43:966.

Doornenbal, H. 1968. Relationship to body composition of subcutaneous backfat, blood volume, and total red-cell mass. Pp. 218–230 in Body Composition in Animals and Man. Washington, D.C.: National Academy of Sciences.

Elsley, F. W. H., I. McDonald, and V. R. Fowler. 1964. The effect of plane of nutrition on the carcass of pigs and lambs when variations in fat content are excluded. Anim. Prod. 6:141.

Ettinger, K. V., M. A. Foster, and U. J. Miola. 1984. Future developments in the in vivo measurements of body composition of pigs. P. 207 in In Vivo Measurements of Body Composition in Meat Animals, D. Lister, ed. London and New York: Elsevier Applied Science Publications.

Fahey, T. J., D. M. Schaefer, R. G. Kauffman, R. J. Epley, P. F. Gould, J. R. Romans, G. C. Smith, and D. G. Topel. 1977. A comparison of practical methods to estimate pork carcass composition. J. Anim. Sci. 44:8.

Foot, J. Z., and J. F. D. Greenhalgh. 1970. The use of deuterium oxide space to determine the amount of body fat in pregnant blackface ewes. Br. J. Nutr. 24:815.

Fredeen, H. T., A. H. Martin, and A. P. Sather. 1979. Evaluation of an electronic technique for measuring lean content of the live pig. J. Anim. Sci. 48:536.

Fuller, M. F., M. A. Foster, and J. M. S. Hutchison. 1984. Nuclear magnetic resonance imaging of pigs. P. 123 in In Vivo Measurements of Body Composition in Meat Animals, D. Lister, ed. London and New York: Elsevier Applied Science Publications.

Garrett, W. N. 1968. Expenses in the use of body density as an estimator of body composition of animals. P. 170 in Body Composition in Animals and Man. Washington, D.C.: National Academy of Sciences.

Green, W. W., W. R. Stevens, and M. B. Gauch. 1969. Use of body measurements to predict the weights of wholesale cuts of beef carcasses: Wholesale round of 900 pound steers. Pp. 1–18 in Agricultural Experiment Station Bulletin A-165. College Park: University of Maryland.

Gregory, K. E., L. A. Swiger, V. H. Arthaud, R. B. Warren, D. K. Hallet, and R. M. Koch. 1962. Relationships among certain live and carcass characteristics of beef cattle. J. Anim. Sci. 21:720.

Gregory, K. E., L. A. Swiger, B. C. Breidenstein, V. H. Arthaud, R. B. Warren, and R. M. Koch. 1964. Subjective live appraisal of beef carcass traits. J. Anim. Sci. 23:1176.

Groeneveld, E., E. Kollweitt, M. Henning, and A. Pfau. 1984. Evaluation of body composition of live animals by x-ray and nuclear magnetic resonance computed tomography. P. 52 in In Vivo Measurements of Body Composition in Meat Animals, D. Lister, ed. London and New York: Elsevier Applied Science Publications.

Hammack, S. P., and R. R. Shrode. 1986. Calfhood weights, body measurements and measures of fatness vs. criteria of overall size and shape for predicting yearling performance in beef cattle. J. Anim. Sci. 63:447.

Hazel, L. N., and E. A. Kline. 1952. Mechanical measurement of fatness and carcass value of live hogs. J. Anim. Sci. 11:313.

Hirzel, R. 1939. Factors affecting quality in mutton and beef with special reference to the proportions of muscle, fat and bone. Onderstepoort J. Vet. Sci. 12:379.

Houndsfield, G. M. 1980. Computer medical imaging. Nobel Lecture. J. Computer Assisted Tomography 4:665.

Kauffman, R. G. 1971. Variation in gross composition of meat animals. Proc. Recip. Meat Conf. 24:292.

Kempster, A. J. 1982. Management and selection of cattle for slaughter. Pp. 127–133 in In Vivo Estimation of Body Composition in Beef, CEC Workshop Report, B. B. Andersen, ed. Copenhagen: National Institute of Animal Sciences.

Kempster, A. J. 1986. Correlations between indirect and direct measurements of body composition. Proc. Nutr. Soc. 45:55.

Keys, A., and J. Brozek. 1953. Body fat in adult man. Physiol. Rev. 33:245.

Kidwell, J. F. 1955. A study of the relationship between body composition and carcass quality in fat calves. J. Anim. Sci. 14:233.

Kock, S. W., and R. L. Preston. 1979. Estimation of bovine carcass composition by urea dilution technique. J. Anim. Sci. 48:319.

Kraybill, H. F., H. L. Bitter, and O. G. Hankins. 1951. Body composition of cattle. II. Determination of fat and water content from measurement of body specific gravity. J. Appl. Physiol. 4:575.

Lewis, T. R., G. G. Suess, and R. G. Kauffman. 1969. Estimation of carcass traits by visual appraisal of market livestock. J. Anim. Sci. 28:601.

Lohman, T. G., W. J. Coffman, A. R. Twardock, B. C. Breidenstein, and H. W. Norton. 1968. Factors affecting potassium-40 measurement in the whole body and body components. P. 291 in Body Composition in Animals and Man. Washington, D.C.: National Academy of Sciences.

McMeekan, C. P. 1941. Growth and development in the pig with special references to carcass quality characteristics. J. Agric. Sci. 31:1.

Meissner, H. H., J. H. van Staden, and E. Pretorius. 1980. In vivo estimation of body composition in cattle with tritium and urea dilution. I. Accuracy of prediction equations for the whole body. South African J. Anim. Sci. 10:165.

Messinger, W. J., and J. M. Steele. 1949. Relationship of body specific gravity to body fat and water content. Proc. Soc. Exp. Biol. Med. 70:316.

Miles, C. A. 1978. A note on recent advances in ultrasonic scanning of animals. P. W133 in Proceedings of the 24th European Meat Research Workers Conference. Kulmbach, West Germany: European Meat Research Workers.

Miller, M. F., H. R. Cross, G. C. Smith, J. F. Baker, F. M. Byers, and H. A. Recio. 1986. Evaluation of live and carcass techniques for predicting beef carcass composition. J. Anim. Sci. 63(Suppl. 1):234 (Abstr.).

Mitchell, A. D., K. H. Norris, H. H. Klueter, N. C. Steele, and M. B. Soloman. 1986. Estimation of live body and carcass composition of pigs by near-infrared reflectance. J. Anim. Sci. 63(Suppl. 1):234 (Abstr.).

Morales, M. F., E. N. Rathbun, R. E. Smith, and N. Pace. 1945. Studies on body composition. II. Theoretical consideration regarding the major body tissue components with suggestions for application to men. J. Biol. Chem. 158:677.

Murray, J. A. 1922. The chemical composition of animal bodies. J. Agric. Sci. 12:103.

Odwongo, W. O., H. R. Conrad, A. E. Staubus, and J. H. Harrison. 1985. Measurement of body water kinetics with deuterium oxide in lactating dairy cows. J. Dairy Sci. 68:1155.

Palsson, H. 1939. Meat quality in sheep with special reference to Scottish breeds and crosses. J. Agric. Sci. 29:544.

Panaretto, B. A., and A. R. Till. 1963. Body composition in vivo. II. The composition of mature goats and its relationship to antipyrine, tritiated water and N-acetyl-4-amine antipyrine spaces. Aust. J. Agric. Res. 14:926.

Pearson, A. M., R. W. Purchas, and E. P. Reineke. 1968. Theory and potential usefulness of body density as a predictor of body composition. P. 153 in Body Composition in Animals and Man. Washington, D.C.: National Academy of Sciences.

Preston, R. L., and S. W. Kock. 1973. In vivo prediction of body composition in cattle from urea space measurements. Proc. Soc. Exp. Biol. Med. 143:1057.

Recio, H. A., J. W. Savell, H. R. Cross, and J. M. Harris. 1986. Use of real-time ultrasound for predicting beef cutability. J. Anim. Sci. 63(Suppl. 1):260 (Abstr.).

Reid, J. T., A. Bensadaum, L. S. Bull, J. H. Burton, P. A. Gleeson, I. K. Han, Y. D. Joo, D. G. Johnson, W. R. McManus, O. L. Paladines, J. W. Straud, H. F. Tyrrell, B. D. H. Van Nickerk, and G. W. Wellington. 1968. Some peculiarities in the body composition of animals. P. 19 in Body Composition in Animals and Man. Washington, D.C.: National Academy of Sciences.

Robelin, J. 1982. Measurement of body water in cattle by dilution technique. P. 107 in In Vivo Estimation of Body Composition in Beef, CEC Workshop Report, B. B. Andersen, ed. Copenhagen: National Institute of Animal Sciences.

Rouse, G. H., D. G. Topel, R. L. Vetter, R. E. Rust, and T. W. Wickersham. 1970. Carcass composition of lambs at different stages of development. J. Anim. Sci. 31:846.

Rule, D. C., R. N. Arnold, E. J. Hentges, and D. C. Beitz. 1986. Evaluation of urea dilution as a technique for estimating body composition in beef steers in vivo: Validation of published equations and comparison with chemical composition. J. Anim. Sci. 63:1935.

Schmidt, M. K., J. L. Clark, T. L. Veum, and G. E. Krause. 1974. Prediction of composition of crossbred swine from birth to 136 kg live weight via the liquid scintillation whole body counter. J. Anim. Sci. 39:855.

Skjervold, H. 1982. Estimation of body composition in live animals by the use of computerized tomography. P. 148 in In Vivo Estimates of Body Composition in Beef, CEC Workshop Report, B. B. Andersen, ed. Copenhagen: National Institute of Animal Sciences.

Stouffer, J. R., M. V. Vallentine, and G. H. Wellington. 1959. Ultrasonic measurements of fat thickness and loin eye area on live cattle and hogs. J. Anim. Sci. 18:1483.

Timon, V. M., and M. Bichard. 1965. Quantitative estimates of lamb carcass composition. Anim. Prod. 7:183.

Topel, D. G. 1986. Future meat animal composition: Industry adaptation of new technologies. J. Anim. Sci. 63:633.

Vance, R. D., H. W. Ockerman, V. R. Cahill, and R. F. Plimpton, Jr. 1970. Carcass composition as related to meat sawdust and analysis. J. Anim. Sci. 31:192 (Abstr.).

Ward, G. M. 1968. Introduction to whole-body counting. P. 263 in Body Composition in Animals and Man. Washington, D.C.: National Academy of Sciences.

Wassenberg, R. L., D. M. Allen, and K. E. Kemp. 1986. Video image analysis prediction of total kilograms and percent primal lean and fat yield in beef carcasses. J. Anim. Sci. 62:1609.

Webster, H. J. F. 1986. Factors affecting the body composition of growing and adult animals. Proc. Nutr. Soc. 45:45.

Williams, D. B., D. G. Topel, and R. L. Vetter. 1974. Evaluation of a tissue-sawdust technique for predicting beef carcass composition. J. Anim. Sci. 39:849.

Wilson, L. L., C. A. Dinkel, H. J. Turna, and J. A. Minyard. 1964. Live animal prediction of cutability and other beef carcass characteristics by several judges. J. Anim. Sci. 23:1102.

Zinn, D. W., R. C. Albin, S. E. Curl, and C. T. Gaskins. 1966. Growth and fattening of the bovine. II. Postweaning protein and gross energy composition. Proc. W. Sec. Am. Soc. Anim. Sci. 17:151.

Zobrisky, S. E. 1963. Status of methods in pork carcass evaluation. Proc. Recip. Meat Conf. 16:266.

# Altering Carcass Measurements and Composition of the Pig

V. C. SPEER

## GENETICS AND SELECTION

The pig and fat are closely linked in the mind of the consumer, much to the detriment of the pig. But in reality the amount and type of fat in a pig carcass is quite similar to that in other red meat animals. A dramatic change in carcass measurements and composition has come about with the development of the modern lean-type pig. The lean-type pig utilizes and deposits protein more efficiently than a fat-type pig, yielding a carcass with more lean tissue. This change came about through selection (genetics) during the period 1955 to 1970. In the late 1960s, the incidence of sudden pig death, or Porcine Stress Syndrome (PSS), became an acute problem among heavily muscled pigs developed through genetic improvement (Cassens et al., 1972). The improvement in muscling since 1970 has declined for the barrows submitted to the Iowa Swine Testing Station (Evans, 1986), largely because of the association of PSS with heavy muscling.

## SEX

At typical slaughter weights for pigs, the intact male (boar) yields a carcass with the least fat and most lean, followed by the female (gilt). The castrated male (barrow) yields a carcass with the most fat and least lean. During the growth phase and until male aggressiveness (ranting) develops, the boar will gain weight the most rapidly and most efficiently. There is the potential problem of strong odor or flavor in the meat from boars slaughtered at typical market weights in the United States. Carcasses from boars are readily accepted in some other countries (for example, Australia and England) but are slaughtered at light weights to reduce the possibility of boar taint in the carcass.

## WEIGHT

Beyond a live weight of about 90 kg, the rate of lean tissue deposition reaches a plateau and, in many pigs, actually declines as fat deposition increases. Furthermore, daily gain seems to decline slightly, although the daily feed requirement increases.

## NUTRITION

### Protein

Ashton et al. (1955) and Jensen et al. (1955) reported that an increase in protein levels in corn-soybean meal diets produced only minimal carcass responses in fat-type pigs. Genetically improved pigs fed similar corn-soybean meal diets 10 years later (Johnson, 1965) were more responsive to protein level: An increase in dietary protein level yielded a greater reduction in back fat depth and a greater increase in ham and loin percent. Responsiveness to protein level as related to type (fat versus lean) is evident in the U.S. Department of Agriculture's selection study, reported by Davey and Morgan (1969).

### Amino Acids

In the typical protein level study, the levels and ratios of the essential amino acids change, so it is difficult to determine whether responses are due to protein level or to one or more amino acids. In the typical corn-soybean meal diet, lysine is the first limiting amino acid as protein level is reduced. Carcass measurements improved in response to increases in lysine levels when all other diet components were held constant (Asche et al., 1985).

### Energy

Diet density (energy level) will affect carcass measurements of pigs that are fed ad libitum. Feeding pigs a diet with added fat (3,600 kcal of metabolizable energy [ME]/kg) versus a corn-soybean meal diet (3,100 kcal of ME/kg) reduced the feed requirement but increased the back fat measurement (Wagner et al., 1963).

### Calorie/Protein Ratio

Increasing the energy content of a corn-soybean meal diet by adding fat may depress daily gain, and feed efficiency may not improve as much as expected. Carcass measurements are also adversely affected. To counteract these adverse performance and carcass criteria, the diet can be formulated to contain a constant calorie/protein ratio. Daily gain and feed efficiency were shown by Allee et al. (1976) to improve markedly when the protein level in the diet was adjusted proportionately to the energy level. Carcass back fat, however, increased compared with those pigs given a control diet (1.35 versus 1.22 inches). Generally, diets are formulated to constant calorie/protein ratios using metabolizable energy values for the ingredients. Because fat has a proportionately lower heat increment than normal energy sources such as grain, its energy value is underestimated. Perhaps if diets were formulated to contain constant calorie/protein ratios using net energy values for the ingredients when fat is included in the diet, the adverse effects on carcass measurements would be corrected.

### Grain Source

The two most commonly fed grain sources for pigs are corn and barley. Corn is better than barley in terms of performance criteria, but barley is superior to corn with regard to carcass measurements (Greer et al., 1965). Much, if not all, of the positive carcass response to barley is related to its lower energy composition compared with that of corn.

### RESTRICTED FEED INTAKE

Reducing the feed intake of growing-finishing pigs will improve carcass measurements (Braude, 1972; Greer et al., 1965; Speer, 1966). Restricted or controlled feeding is commonly practiced in pig production in Europe, but because daily gain is reduced it has not been adopted by U.S. producers. The improved feed efficiency reported by Braude (1972) in response to restricted feeding compared to ad libitum feeding was not evident from the studies of Speer (1966) and Greer et al. (1965).

## TEMPERATURE

At environmental temperatures higher than ideal, the pig reduces feed intake and expends energy in an attempt to stay cool. The result is an adverse effect on production criteria but an improvement in carcass measurements (Stahly and Cromwell, 1979). At lower environmental temperatures, the pig increases feed intake and once again expends energy to maintain body temperature. With respect to carcass measurements, the increased energy expenditure to maintain body temperature may counteract the effect of increased feed intake.

## HORMONES AND RELATED COMPOUNDS

### Diethylstilbestrol

Plimpton and Teague (1972) implanted diethylstilbestrol in boars weighing 70 kg and then slaughtered them at about 110 kg live weight. This procedure retained the positive carcass attributes of the young boar, while the effects of objectionable odor and flavor of boar meat were reduced.

### Diethylstilbestrol and Methyltestosterone

A combination of diethylstilbestrol (2.2 mg/kg of diet) and methyltestosterone (2.2 mg/kg of diet) added to the feed improved the feed efficiency and carcass measurements of growing-finishing pigs (Baker et al., 1967). This product was never approved by the Food and Drug Administration for use in the United States, but it was approved and marketed in Great Britain.

### Epinephrine and Epinephrine-Like Stimulators

Cunningham et al. (1963) used epinephrine to increase fat mobilization, lipolysis, and nitrogen deposition in the pig. Results were encouraging, but the required daily injection was a distinct disadvantage. In subsequent studies, Cunningham and Friend (1964) and Cunningham (1968) added nicotine or caffeine to the feed in an attempt to stimulate epinephrine-like responses. Both compounds seemed to improve carcass measurements of growing-finishing pigs. Similarly, the action of the beta-adrenergic agonists clenbuterol and cimaterol (Jones et al., 1985; Moser et al., 1984) improved carcass measurements in growing-finishing pigs. The beta-adrenergic agonists are orally active, making them easier to use than epinephrine.

### Growth Hormone

Daily injections of porcine growth hormone by Machlin (1972) have been shown to improve daily gain, feed efficiency, and carcass measurements. Chung et al. (1985) used a porcine preparation that was more highly purified than Machlin's and found similar responses in growing pigs, but at a much lower dosage rate. Bacterially synthesized human growth hormone is also active in stimulating growth rate and carcass improvement (Baile et al., 1983). Both the natural and bacterially synthesized hormones must be administered by daily injections, which is a distinct disadvantage for their use.

## IMMUNOLOGY

Immunization of growing boars against androstene steroids—the compounds responsible for boar taint and odor—controls these undesirable characteristics without significantly affecting other characteristics such as weight gain and feed efficiency (Brooks et al., 1986; Williamson et al., 1985). A reduction in androstene steroids might also be attained through selection, since Booth et al. (1986) detected positive correlations between the bulbourethral and submaxillary gland weights and concentrations of 3-α-androstenol and 5-α-androstenone in market weight boars.

Encouraging results with immunology have been obtained in lambs by autoimmunizing the lambs against somatostatin (Spencer and Garssen, 1983). Somatomedin concentration increased (nonsignificant) and growth rate improved compared with control lambs. A similar approach has been reported by Flint and Futter (1986), in which rats immunized against their fat cells were found upon postmortem examination to have about 30 percent less carcass fat than untreated rats.

## TISSUE COMPOSITION

The type of dietary fat fed to the pig will influence the fat composition of the carcass. The percentage of unsaturated fat in back fat samples reflects the type of oil fed (Ellis and Isbell, 1926). Changing carcass fat composition can be accomplished more readily in the pig than in any other large farm animal.

The amount and type of fat found in the lean tissue of the pig longissimus dorsi muscle will respond to differences in diet and management. Restricted feeding reduces the fat content and the level of unsaturation in the muscle, as does feeding barley instead of corn (Greer et al., 1965). And increasing the protein level or reducing the energy concentration of the diet reduces the fat content of the longissimus dorsi lean tissue (Wagner et al., 1963). From these examples, it seems that carcass back fat and the fat content of lean tissue are positively correlated. If this is true, then as producers in the United States strive for leaner animals, they could encounter some of the problems that have surfaced in England. According to a technical report of the Meat and Livestock Commission of the United Kingdom (Phelps, 1985), the marked reduction in back fat that has occurred in

England's pig population has been accompanied by an increase in retailer and consumer complaints that the very lean carcasses produce meat that looks unattractive, lacks succulence and flavor, and has a tendency to be tough.

## REFERENCES

Allee, G. L., B. A. Koch, and R. H. Hines. 1976. Effect of fat level and calorie:protein ratio on performance of finishing pigs. J. Anim. Sci. 42:1349.

Asche, G. L., A. J. Lewis, E. R. Peo, Jr., and J. D. Crenshaw. 1985. The nutritional value of normal high lysine corns for weanling and growing-finishing swine fed at four lysine levels. J. Anim. Sci. 60:1412.

Ashton, G. C., J. Kastelic, D. C. Acker, A. H. Jensen, H. M. Maddock, E. A. Kline, and D. V. Catron. 1955. Different protein levels with and without antibiotics for growing-finishing swine: Effect on carcass leanness. J. Anim. Sci. 14:82.

Baile, C. A., M. A. Della-Fera, and C. L. McLaughlin. 1983. Performance and carcass quality of swine injected daily with bacterially synthesized human growth hormone. Growth 17:225.

Baker, D. H., C. E. Jordan, W. P. Waitt, and D. W. Gouwens. 1967. Effect of a combination of diethylstilbestrol and methyltestosterone, sex and dietary protein level on performance and carcass characteristics of finishing swine. J. Anim. Sci. 26:1059.

Booth, W. D., E. D. Williamson, and R. L. S. Patterson. 1986. 16-Androstene steroids in the submaxillary salivary gland of the boar in relation to measures of boar taint in carcasses. Anim. Prod. 42:145.

Braude, R. 1972. Feeding methods. P. 279 in Pig Production, D. J. A. Cole, ed. London: Butterworth.

Brooks, R. I., A. M. Pearson, M. G. Hogberg, J. J. Pestka, and J. I. Gray. 1986. An immunological approach for prevention of boar odor in pork. J. Anim. Sci. 62:1279.

Cassens, R., F. Giesler, and Q. Kolb. 1972. Proceedings of the Pork Quality Symposium. Madison: Cooperative Extension Service, University of Wisconsin.

Chung, C. S., T. D. Etherton, and J. P. Wiggins. 1985. Stimulation of swine growth by porcine growth hormone. J. Anim. Sci. 60:118.

Cunningham, H. M. 1968. Effect of caffeine on nitrogen retention, carcass composition, fat mobilization and oxidation of $C^{14}$-labeled body fat in pigs. J. Anim. Sci. 27:424.

Cunningham, H. M., and D. W. Friend. 1964. Effect of nicotine on nitrogen retention and fat deposition in pigs. J. Anim. Sci. 23:717.

Cunningham, H. M., D. W. Friend, and J. W. G.

Nicholson. 1963. Effect of epinephrine on nitrogen and fat deposition of pigs. J. Anim. Sci. 22:632.

Davey, R. J., and D. P. Morgan. 1969. Protein effect on growth and carcass composition of swine selected for high and low fatness. J. Anim. Sci. 28:831.

Ellis, N. R., and H. S. Isbell. 1926. Soft pork studies. II. The influence of the character of the ration upon the composition of the body fat of hogs. J. Biol. Chem. 69:219.

Evans, R. 1986. Fall 1985 summary. Iowa Swine Testing Station. Ames, Iowa: Iowa Swine Testing Station.

Flint, D. J., and C. E. Futter. 1986. Immunological manipulation of body fat. P. 123 in Hannah Research 1985. Ayr, Scotland: Hannah Research Institute, University of Glasgow.

Greer, S. A. N., V. W. Hays, V. C. Speer, J. T. McCall, and E. G. Hammond. 1965. Effects of level of corn- and barley-base diets on performance and body composition of swine. J. Anim. Sci. 24:1008.

Jensen, A. H., D. C. Acker, H. M. Maddock, G. C. Ashton, P. G. Homeyer, E. O. Heady, and D. V. Catron. 1955. Different protein levels with and without antibiotics for growing-finishing swine: Effect on growth rate and feed efficiency. J. Anim. Sci. 14:69

Johnson, R. A. 1965. Substitution Rates and Economic Optima in Corn-Soybean Rations for Growing-Finishing Swine. Ph.D. dissertation. Iowa State University, Ames.

Jones, R. W., R. A. Easter, F. K. McKeith, R. H. Dalrymple, H. M. Maddock, and P. J. Bechtel. 1985. Effect of the β-adrenergic agonist cimaterol (CL 263,780) on the growth and carcass characteristics of finishing swine. J. Anim. Sci. 61:905.

Machlin, L. J. 1972. Effect of porcine growth hormone on growth and carcass composition of the pig. J. Anim. Sci. 35:794.

Moser, R. L., R. H. Dalrymple, S. G. Cornelius, J. E. Pettigrew, and C. E. Allen. 1984. Evaluation of a repartitioning agent on the performance and carcass traits of finishing pigs. J. Anim. Sci. 59(Suppl. 1):255.

Phelps, A. 1985. Consumer backlash against U.K.'s drive for leaner pork. Feedstuffs 57(40):S-6.

Plimpton, R. F., Jr., and H. S. Teague. 1972. Influence of sex and hormone treatment on performance and carcass composition of swine. J. Anim. Sci. 35:1166.

Speer, V. C. 1966. Floor feed or self feed? Hog Farm Management 3(7):13.

Spencer, G. S. G., and G. J. Garssen. 1983. A novel approach to growth promotion using auto-immunization against somatostatin. I. Effects on growth and hormone levels in lambs. Livestock Prod. Sci. 10:25.

Stahly, T. S., and G. L. Cromwell. 1979. Effect of environmental temperature and dietary fat supplementation on the performance and carcass characteristics of growing and finishing swine. J. Anim. Sci. 49:1478.

Wagner, G. R., A. J. Clark, V. W. Hays, and V. C. Speer. 1963. Effect of protein-energy relationships on the performance and carcass quality of growing swine. J. Anim. Sci. 22:202.

Williamson, E. D., R. L. C. Patterson, E. R. Buxton, K. G. Mitchell, I. G. Partridge, and N. Walker. 1985. Immunization against 5-α-androstenone in boars. Livestock Prod. Sci. 12:251.

# Processing Options for Improving the Nutritional Value of Animal Products

ROBERT E. RUST

The issue of altering meat products to fit dietary requirements must address these points:

1. Effect on product safety;
2. Effect on economics of manufacture;
3. Effect on storage life;
4. Effect on sensory characteristics such as flavor, texture, and color; and
5. Product identity—for example, a mortadella without dices of fat is no longer a mortadella.

## NITRATES AND NITRITES

Let us examine some of the areas where dietary concerns have been expressed. Nitrates and nitrites are one. About a decade ago we agonized over the potential hazard presented by these processing ingredients. Nitrates largely passed out of the picture once their mechanism of action was understood. Nitrites, in most products, have been voluntarily reduced by processors. The current use level is 156 ppm, except for pumped bacon, where it is 120 ppm.

In most cured meats, sausages, and luncheon meats, the addition of 156 ppm nitrite will generally yield around 30 to 50 ppm residual. It has been my experience that 125 ppm nitrite in cured bacon will produce residuals of less than 15 ppm, and probably more like 10 to 12 ppm. Are these significant from a dietary standpoint? Most likely not, since most reliable estimates indicate that nitrite intake from processed meats equals only 3 to 5 percent of total dietary nitrite intake.

Current U.S. Department of Agriculture (USDA)-Food Safety Inspection Service (FSIS) regulations (318.7) permit nitrite to be used at the levels given in Table 1. It might be wise for the USDA to bring these regulations further into line with current good manufacturing practice.

## SALT

Salt (sodium chloride) is a processing adjunct about which I feel no definite conclusion can be reached that would justify a recommendation to impose limits. To a certain extent, the use of salt is self-limiting, depending on consumer tastes. The general trend toward lower salt levels in food has forced the meat industry to reduce its ingoing levels. Although no general survey

TABLE 1 Levels of Curing Agents for Products Other Than Bacon

| Curing Agent | Dry Cure/ 100 lb of Meat (oz) | Sausage/ 100 lb of Meat (oz) | Curing Pickle/ 100 gal, 10 percent Pump (lb) |
|---|---|---|---|
| Sodium nitrate | 3.5 | 2.75 | 7 |
| Potassium nitrate | 3.5 | 2.75 | 7 |
| Sodium nitrite | 1.0 | 0.25 | 2 |
| Potassium nitrite | 1.0 | 0.25 | 2 |

NOTE: In all cases, residuals shall not exceed 200 ppm calculated as sodium nitrite.

data are available, it has been my experience that sodium levels in cooked sausage have declined by perhaps 20 percent over the past 10 years.

Sodium chloride performs three major functions in a meat product: It helps preserve it, it adds flavor, and it develops the binding properties of the proteins. From a preservation standpoint, the role of salt is still critical in dry cured meats such as hams as well as in dry sausage. Salt also plays a small role in shelf-life extension of cooked sausages. Levels in these products are commonly 2 to 2.75 percent of the meat block* used in formulation.

In Europe, a 2 percent salt addition is customary, but distribution chains are much shorter and shelf-life expectations much less than in the United States. Through good manufacturing practices, the United States can, I believe, achieve adequate shelf-life. However, there are those who would argue that this is the low end of the safety limit. It must be kept in mind that there are certain interactions between salt and nitrite

in the inhibition of *Clostridium botulinum* that are significant from a public health standpoint. Some research indicates an increased danger of toxin formation as salt levels decrease; however, no clear-cut recommendations for minimum salt levels have been proposed to date. Most other pathogens of major public health concern, such as *Staphylococcus* species, are salt-tolerant in the ranges being discussed, so salt reduction probably would have no significant impact on their prevalence (still, the evidence here is less than conclusive).

In terms of flavor, the preference for sodium is an acquired taste that can be modified by total dietary intake. As consumers have reduced their sodium intake, the meat industry has been obligated to follow suit. Proposals to substitute other chlorides (it is the chloride ion that is significant) have encountered flavor problems. Potassium chloride, for instance, could perhaps partially substitute for sodium chloride but the bitter flavor is undesirable. Furthermore, there is still the question of whether added dietary potassium would have any significant impact on health. The effect of reduced sodium on flavor can be somewhat compensated for by other flavorings such as spices and spice extracts. There are no hard-and-fast recommendations that can be made here, since flavorings are a highly variable consideration.

The role of salt in developing the binding properties of proteins is critical. Actually, this is twofold. First, sodium chloride ex-

---

* The notion of meat block is illustrated in the following example. Say that in producing a batch of frankfurters, you start with 100 pounds of meat. All the adjuncts are calculated based on a percentage of this 100 pounds. Thus, if you add 2.5 percent salt, 3.5 percent extender, 0.5 percent sugar, and 10 percent water, you will end up with 116.5 pounds of finished product. The actual salt level in the finished product would therefore be 2.15 percent. (The curing ingredients were deliberately omitted from this example.)

tracts the salt-soluble myofibrillar proteins, which, in turn, encapsulate the fat particles to form a stable "emulsion" or meat batter. Second, it promotes the swelling of these proteins to allow for exposure of more bonding sites for water binding. This is crucial for the production of a stable sausage.

In practical terms, salt levels of much less than 1.5 percent of the meat block are not functional. Even then, optimum technology must be exercised to make this level operational. There are some significant interactions between sodium chloride and the alkaline phosphates that improve the functioning of low sodium chloride. For the most part, however, these alkaline phosphates are mostly the sodium salts; hence, actual sodium reduction is minimal. The alkaline potassium phosphates currently allowed under USDA-FSIS regulations are dipotassium phosphate, monopotassium phosphate, potassium tripolyphosphate, and potassium pyrophosphate. These are not commonly used, though, because of solubility problems, flavor problems, and the fact that they function somewhat less effectively than do their sodium counterparts.

In dry cured products, particularly dry and semi-dry sausage, the salt levels needed for preservation become much more significant. It appears that a level of 3 percent ingoing, which translates to 4.25 to 5 percent salt in the finished product, is optimum. Only recently did the USDA recognize levels less than 3.3 percent ingoing for trichina inactivation. This recognition provides a sliding scale of extended drying times in proportion to ingoing salt levels. However, it would be far better to exercise trichina control through an identification program or raw material control rather than through processing treatment.

In addition to controlling trichina, it is necessary to achieve a sufficiently high brine concentration to inhibit microbial growth, including the more salt-tolerant molds and yeasts. A brine concentration of 12 percent is generally considered necessary for shelf

stability. Percent concentration is calculated as:

$$\frac{\text{Percent salt}}{\text{Percent salt} + \text{Percent water}} \times 100.$$

## FAT

Reduction of caloric intake from fats, particularly the saturated fatty acids, is another major area of concern. This discussion does not focus on modification of animal fat depots by dietary or other means. Nevertheless, such modification must be looked at in light of its effect on the manufacturing characteristics of the meat raw materials, such as flavor, texture, color, and susceptibility to oxidation.

Reduction of fat in a processed meat product is not as simple as it sounds. A notable success in this area is the commercial production of "95 percent fat free" hams. This probably represents the ultimate in fat reduction, since a muscle with all the visible intermuscular fat removed still contains at least 5 percent fat in the form of intramuscular fat and extractable intra- and intercellular lipids.

In cooked sausage, such as a frankfurter, the common accepted fat levels of 25 to 30 percent defy significant reduction without sacrificing textural and other sensory properties. A few commercial attempts at straightforward fat reduction have, in general, resulted in a product with a distinct rubbery texture and reduced consumer demand. If the reduction in textural characteristics is to be overcome, other components will have to be modified. For example, the addition of water will offset the fat reduction by softening the texture of the product. Here, however, we encounter USDA regulations that restrict water levels in a product. Right now, the USDA does not permit substitution of water for fat. These interacting regulations need careful examination. I would suggest regulating product composition based on minimum protein rather than the current fat/water maximums.

Another textural modification involves the substitution of a nonbinding protein—generally originating from a by-product source—for some of the fat. There has been success in substituting 10 percent cooked pork skins for 10 percent pork fat in dry sausage. However, this has run afoul of regulatory restrictions in labeling requirements. The inclusion of mechanically separated meat (MSM) has generally been shown to reduce textural firmness, but, again, its labeling is in fact restrictive to the point that most processors assume that consumers will be driven away from products containing MSM. In its quest for truth in labeling, the USDA may have erected barriers to intelligent dietary modification of meat products. Clearly, the whole area needs examination. Regulatory tradition should not be allowed to interfere with efforts at dietary modification of meat products when such modification is based on sound scientific data.

One promising area in the modification of fat in processed meat products is the substitution of fats and oils of vegetable origin for the animal fat. Through a technique common in Europe, that of preemulsifying the fat with milk proteins such as sodium caseinate or its calcium counterpart, two-thirds of the animal fat has been replaced with preemulsified vegetable oil in a slicing bologna without any practical reduction in sensory properties. Preemulsions are usually made up of eight parts oil, eight parts water, and one part milk protein, which in effect gives a finished emulsion with approximately 48 percent fat.

It is likely that somewhat similar results can be obtained with soy or blood plasma proteins. Once again, though, USDA regulations restrict the inclusion of vegetable fats and oils in meat products. Also, calcium caseinate, despite its widespread use in nonmeat products, is not on the Generally Recognized As Safe list (as is sodium caseinate), and the USDA is reluctant to extend

approval for use until there is greater clarification from the Food and Drug Administration.

Inclusion of stabilized preemulsions that can effectively reduce fat content of the "show fat" appears to be another area worth pursuing. Again, the question of labeling must be considered. A fat/water/protein emulsion diced and incorporated as show fat in a meat product would trigger labeling problems under current regulations. Obviously, labeling requirements are a significant stumbling block. What is needed, above all, is a thorough scientific review of labeling regulations and policies totally divorced from emotion, tradition, and the like.

### LABELING

A few more words should be said on the subject of labeling. I view the policies (or lack thereof) regarding such fanciful labels as Lean and Lite as a regulatory quagmire that is totally out of hand. There needs to be a firm, definitive policy established that would clarify these promotional labels, which currently are being exploited to the confusion of the consumer, despite the USDA's recent attempts to clarify them.

Another labeling issue that comes to mind is the USDA grades for beef and lamb. These still place an unwarranted emphasis on fat. Even though most responsible scientists agree that only about 10 to 15 percent of the palatability differences are explained by the factors considered in USDA grades for beef, this system is still in use. Clearly, it is an emotionally charged issue that has been debated extensively, but can't it be resolved rationally? Personally, I wonder if USDA grades of beef serve any useful purpose, and I challenge this committee to reach a consensus on this system, particularly insofar as it hinders the consumer in making wise decisions on selecting meat and meat products. The application of present USDA grade standards, particularly yield grades, may be the major limitation to processing developments such as immediate postslaughter fat removal.

There appears to be very little that can be done under current regulatory constraints to achieve modification of meat products through the inclusion of various nutrients (that is, vitamins, minerals, and the like). If I read current regulations correctly, the direct inclusion of, say, thiamine to a sausage product would not be approved. At the very least it would trigger nutritional labeling, an activity that is cumbersome and often beyond the capabilities of the small processor, since present USDA policy requires a Partial Quality Control program as a minimum. Even calcium, one of the nutrients whose inclusion appears to be a "plus," is in fact restricted when it appears as a component in mechanically separated meat. Does this make sense, if, indeed, additional calcium is an asset to our diets?

The United States is the only major developed country to restrict the incorporation of blood in meat products. I can find no sound scientific reason for this restriction. Indeed, it makes little sense considering that blood provides an excellent source of such nutrients as iron and protein. Are we, because of purely esthetic considerations, ignoring some potential good sources of nutrients? It would seem so.

## CONCLUSIONS

Our regulatory bodies too often base their decisions on unsupported opinion and esthetic considerations rather than scientific fact. Are regulations in effect hampering positive dietary modification of meat and meat products, especially insofar as processing adjuncts are concerned? This is a question that must be addressed. Following is a list of specific considerations that must be examined, as well as areas important for research.

### Considerations

1. Regulate composition of meat products on the basis of a minimum protein standard, thus allowing interchange of water/fat for textural purposes.

2. Remove esthetic considerations from labeling requirements (that is, flagging of "variety meats," mechanically separated meats, and so on).

3. Change fat labeling to allow separation and recombination of fats in manufactured products.

4. Develop simplified procedures for nutritional labeling to enable small processors to apply nutritional labeling.

5. Set definitive standards for such fanciful labels as Lean and Lite or recommend their elimination.

6. Define the roles of beef and lamb grades. Are they a marketing tool or a label for consumer information?

7. Should consideration be given to control of pathogenic microorganisms such as *Staphylococcus* and *Salmonella* species as part of dietary considerations?

### Areas for Research

1. Salt/nitrite/phosphate interactions and their effect on pathogens;

2. Nutritional contributions of meat byproducts and processing adjuncts after inclusion in a processed meat product; and

3. Modification of current beef and lamb grades to a system similar to that used for pork (quantitative and age).

# Integrated Nutrition, Genetics, and Growth Management Programs for Lean Beef Production

F. M. BYERS, H. R. CROSS, and G. T. SCHELLING

We have evolved into a "lean-conscious society," where *fats* has become a four-letter word and a high priority is placed on getting and staying trim. In no area is this more evident than in our selection of and desire for leaner beef products.

Efficient production of palatable lean beef must be a primary objective of the beef cattle industry if it is to compete in the long term. Current yearly production of the 5 billion pounds of waste and trim fat must be reduced as rapidly as possible. Although beef fat is trimmed extensively at slaughter and by the consumer, which results in a reasonably lean beef product, only the prevention of this excessive fat deposition where it occurs will correct the image of beef as a fat, high-calorie product.

A diversity of beef products are needed, all of which must be separated from the current image of fat cattle and fat beef. Industry must focus on producing and effectively marketing lean beef and work to associate beef with active life-styles and healthful living. Products must be engineered to coincide with consumer needs and to address consumer fears, both perceived and real. Since it is easier to create

new attitudes than to change old ones, the industry must use innovative marketing strategies to reposition beef products with a new identity.

Unique challenges face the beef industry to design and develop new technologies that will allow production of lean beef rather than beef that must be extensively trimmed to make it lean. This will require greater lean tissue deposition throughout the life cycle and extensive redirection of feed energy from fat to protein deposition through all phases of growth. This can only be accomplished if all segments of the industry target on the same goal and integrate available technology to effectively manage growth.

## INDUSTRY PERSPECTIVE

The beef cattle industry has evolved from production of extremely lean beef, based largely on Longhorn-type cattle in extensive grazing systems in the nineteenth century, to production of very fat beef from small-size English breeds in the mid-twentieth century. During the second half of the twentieth century, the trend has shifted back toward leaner beef, with selection of large-framed, later-maturing, large mature size exotic types of cattle. Recent consumer pressure for leaner beef has accelerated this change and encouraged consideration of many new cattle breeds not formerly part of the U.S. beef cattle industry.

The current beef cattle population includes cattle of all types and sizes. They are fed a wide variety of feedstuffs, both grazed and harvested, ranging from poor-quality mature range grasses to high-energy feedlot rations, with most combinations in between. They are managed in systems including wintering, backgrounding, summer grazing, growing, forage finishing, and high-grain feedlot programs. The traditional end product of these diverse cattle-resource combinations is Choice grade beef with 30 to 35 percent carcass fat. Consumer preference for a leaner beef product indicates the need to devise systems to economically produce this kind of beef.

## MECHANISMS TO PRODUCE LEAN BEEF

The traditional method used to increase the production of lean beef is to feed larger mature size cattle. However, an increase in mature size means a larger cow that has greater requirements per unit of weight and greatly increased levels of maintenance energy committed to beef production. For example, Chianina cattle produce large, lean carcasses, but because of their size they require more maintenance feed energy.

Therefore, a more effective approach for producing lean beef is to modify the patterns of growth in cattle to produce more lean beef from all cattle. While this is the eventual target of genetic engineering initiatives, systems using these concepts are not likely to surface any time soon. An understanding of growth and its regulation is required to effectively use growth management strategies to produce leaner beef products. An outline of options and factors involved in

regulation through genetics, nutrition, and growth follows:

*Genetics*
    Establishes upper limit of growth
    Determines base patterns of growth
    Sets priorities for growth of tissues—
        At any rate of growth
        During intervals of growth
    Targets composition at any weight
    Sets physiological maturity at points of growth

*Nutrition: Energy*
    Schedule versus phase of growth
        Growing versus later stages
        Current versus earlier nutritional history
        Deferred versus advanced systems
    Level and source
        Forage versus grain
        Quantity/day versus limits for lean tissue growth
        Rate and composition of growth
        Substrates for tissue growth
    Nutrition and function
        Optimize lean tissue growth
        Feedback on lean tissue priorities
        Storage and retrieval of tissues
        Nutrition and physiological limits

*Growth management: Synchronizing nutrients and needs*
    Endogenous regulation
        Bulls, steers, heifers
        Patterns during growth
    Exogenous regulation
        Repartitioning agents
            Estrogens
            Zeranol
            Growth hormone
            Beta-adrenergic agonists
        Mechanisms of regulation
            Priorities for protein versus fat
            Redirection of nutrients
            Tissue mobilization
            Limits for daily deposition
            Other effects

## Role of Genetics in the Production of Leaner Beef

Mature size and genetics establish the limits (both daily and cumulative), base patterns, priorities, and type of growth predominating through phases of growth. In addition, the genetic directives provide general targets for body and carcass composition and degree of physiological maturity over time and weight intervals through growth. However, other factors really determine the extent to which these theoretical limits will actually be reached, or how patterns and priorities for growth will be followed or translated into and realized as growth.

Some general principles that are usually associated with genetic regulation may be useful as a reference point. In general, cattle of larger mature size have greater limits for daily protein growth and have accumulated more protein than smaller cattle at any point during growth and when mature size is reached (Byers and Rompala, 1980; Byers et al., 1986). Large mature size cattle are typically physiologically younger at any point during growth than smaller mature size cattle. They also place a higher priority on protein growth and deposit a greater fraction of protein at any rate of growth, but especially at lower rates. However, many cattle types violate these notions. For instance, all small-size cattle are not early maturing; Longhorn or Scottish Highlanders, for example, are small and late maturing. Also, limits for daily protein growth do not automatically follow potential cumulative storage. While both Simmental and Limousin accumulate large quantities of protein, rates of protein growth in Limousin may be no greater than in Red or Black Angus, while Simmental have the potential to deposit protein more rapidly. However, both Simmental and Limousin are leaner at most weights through growth than Angus. In Simmental this occurs because of rapid

protein growth, while in Limousin it is primarily a reflection of lower energy intake and lower rates of fat deposition. It becomes immediately evident that rate and composition of growth are directly related and not independent of each other. Available energy translates genetic directives through tissue regulation into patterns of growth.

## Role of Nutrition in Growth

Nutrition is directly linked to rate and composition of growth in several ways (Byers, 1982). Available energy is used to meet the needs for maintenance, protein growth, and fat deposition, primarily in that order. Thus, composition of growth reflects levels of available substrates provided relative to maintenance and limits for protein growth, with additional energy usually deposited as fat. In general, rates of protein deposition increase at decreasing rates and rates of fat deposition increase at increasing rates with rate of growth. Consequently, percentage protein in growth decreases while percentage fat in growth increases with rate of growth. Empty body and carcass composition reflects these patterns of tissue growth, and cattle growing rapidly through higher levels of nutrition are fatter at subsequent points in growth and at slaughter. The magnitude of nutritionally regulated changes in body composition at a given weight reflect animal priorities, rates of growth, and length of time that animals are growing at respective rates. Slower (deferred) growth for extended periods of time invariably results in leaner carcasses at any selected weight. However, most cattle deposit some fat, even at slow rates of growth, and the priorities for protein versus fat deposition at any rate of growth are established through genetic directives that are implemented through physiological mechanisms. Physiological mechanisms exist to allow retrieval of fat to provide energy for protein growth if sufficient stored fat is available from a previous phase of growth. Important components of nutrition include the stage of growth versus nutritional schedule, level and source—that is, forage versus grain—and level relative to growth process priorities.

Nutrition is normally considered relative to phase of growth such as preweaning, stocker, or finishing, and ranges of nutritional levels are implied in each phase. However, the general relationship of rate to composition of growth applies to all phases of growth; only the relative priorities for protein versus fat deposition change with stage of growth. Commonly used beef cattle feeding and management systems include a range of nutritional programs where periods of rapid and deferred growth are included. All periods of deferred growth where protein growth is allowed result in restriction of fat deposition such that the animal is older and has had more time to deposit protein and thus has accumulated more lean tissue. Animals that have been managed in deferred feeding programs will be leaner at any slaughter weight and will be heavier when typical slaughter end points are reached.

Common systems of deferred feeding include growing feeder calves after weaning in winter grazing or backgrounding programs to yearling weight before placement on high-energy feedlot finishing rations that maximize rate of growth. Cattle managed in this system will be more than 150 pounds heavier at slaughter when similar in composition to cattle placed on feedlot rations at weaning (Byers, 1980). It follows that they will be leaner at any slaughter weight than cattle fed to grow rapidly immediately after weaning. While this deferred system allows smaller mature size cattle to produce larger and more acceptable carcasses when slaughter end points are reached, large mature size cattle will yield unacceptably large carcasses weighing in excess of 1,000 pounds. This provides the basis for genotype by nutrition interactions, indicating the utility of deferred feeding programs for smaller

mature size cattle and high-energy feedlot programs for large mature size cattle as soon as feasible after weaning. Some of the greatest real opportunities for growth management exist within cattle types and involve modifying an animal's inherent priorities for growth.

## Integrated Growth Management

The objective of growth management is to regulate growth and synchronize nutrient supplies with nutrient needs to support the desired type of growth. This can be accomplished through both endogenous mechanisms inherent to an animal (that is, castration) or through exogenous mechanisms such as estrogenic repartitioning agents (Byers, 1982; Lemieux et al., 1983b). The mechanisms involved in redirection of growth include modification of (1) priorities for nutrient use for protein versus fat deposition, (2) tissue turnover (Roeder et al., 1984), (3) daily tissue deposition limits, and (4) nutrient supply. Eventually, growth hormone, releasing factors for growth hormone, beta-adrenergic agonists, or immunization strategies to remove negative feedback on growth (that is, somatostatin) may provide additional ways to regulate growth. They may work with or in place of current growth regulation technology. These alternatives are in the early stages of development and probably will not be available any time soon.

In the interim, effective systems of growth regulation must be implemented to allow more lean tissue and less fat deposition in production of carcass beef. Anabolic estrogenic implants are effective repartitioning agents that modify growth by shifting nutrients from fat to protein accretion, resulting in priorities for growth more analogous to those for bulls (Byers et al., 1985a, 1985c; Lemieux et al., 1985a). In addition, they usually enhance rate of growth, serving to further increase lean tissue production (Byers et al., 1985b). Rate and efficiency of lean tissue growth are critical to enhancing lean beef production through conventional cattle feeding and management systems. In addition to more efficient production, anabolic implants provide the opportunity to regulate growth so as to tailor beef production to meet consumer demand for leaner beef products. While implants have been used for several decades, the basis for their growth regulator functions have only recently begun to be understood (Lawrence et al., 1985). This is important for the development of growth regulation systems that allow programmed growth of cattle.

## Rationale for Anabolic Implant Response

Recent research has provided new insights into mechanisms by which growth-promoting implants modify growth in beef cattle. Protein growth is a daily function, and cellular mechanisms establish the maximum rates for daily protein synthesis. Cellular limits for protein growth are not often reached because of physiological factors, such as hormonal and nutritional mechanisms, that set priorities for and limits to protein deposition. Cattle of different types have different priorities for protein deposition at different rates of growth, and larger mature size cattle direct more energy toward protein growth at any rate of growth. Priorities for protein growth are enhanced by anabolic implants, which redirect nutrients from fat to protein in a "daily double play"—increasing lean growth at the expense of fat, especially at rapid rates of gain.

The effectiveness of repartitioning implants increases with rate of growth (Byers, 1982), with maximal redirection of nutrients from fat to protein at the most rapid rates of gain (Lemieux et al., 1983b). The effectiveness of anabolic regulators is predicated on inherent rates of fat deposition providing the opportunity for repartitioning of nutrients from fat to protein accretion. Estradiol-17-beta and zeranol are currently available compounds that occur naturally and

are very effective repartitioning agents, enhancing rates of protein and lean tissue production whenever present at effective levels in cattle depositing fat. In recent studies, implants consistently increased overall rates of carcass and total protein accretion and yield of lean retail product.

Just as we are what we eat, cattle are what they accrete, with carcass beef reflecting cumulative growth from birth to slaughter. Consequently, use of anabolic implants from birth to slaughter provides lifetime growth regulation and provides the maximal redirection of nutrients from fat to protein and lean tissue production. The longer anabolic agents are provided in efficacious doses, the greater is the increase in total beef lean with a simultaneous reduction in fat.

## PRODUCING MARKETABLE LEANER BEEF

The leaner beef product must be acceptable and, hopefully, even desirable in the marketplace. Thus, the impact of strategies to produce leaner beef on product acceptability must be included in an assessment of production options.

### Effects of Breed Type on Acceptability

The following general observations can be made after evaluating 29 separate research studies:

1. Carcasses from English-type cattle ranked first in the U.S. Department of Agriculture (USDA) quality grade and marbling ratings. Continental breeds were intermediate, while Zebu and dairy purebreds ranked last.

2. Flavor and juiciness appeared not to be affected by breed or breed type.

3. Meat from Zebu and their crosses were rated less tender than the English, dairy, or continental breeds or crosses. These low ratings were supported by significantly higher Warner-Bratzler shear force values.

In conclusion, with the exception of the Zebu influence, breed appears to have little practical influence on muscle quality (Cross et al., 1984; McKeith et al., 1985).

### Forage- Versus Grain-Fed Beef

A considerable amount of data has been published on the effect of forage versus grain feeding on carcass traits (Byers, 1980; Lemieux et al., 1983a, 1985b) and muscle quality (Bidner et al., 1986; Crouse et al., 1984). Animals from forage-fed systems produce carcasses that have less marbling, darker lean color, softer lean, coarser-textured lean, and lower USDA quality grades than grain-fed animals. Grain-fed animals averaged two-thirds of a quality grade advantage over forage-fed animals. The quality grade difference was significant in 12 of 29 comparisons. When the difference was not significant, the trend was almost always in favor of the grain-fed animals. Forage-fed beef, because of its darker and softer lean, will not have the retail shelf-life of grain-fed beef. This presents a serious problem from the consumer acceptance standpoint.

Grain-fed animals produced carcasses that were significantly more tender than forage-fed animals in more than 41 percent of the comparisons. Perhaps even more important, 62 percent of the flavor desirability ratings favored grain-fed beef. The flavor-intensity ratings were almost always higher in meat from forage-fed animals. These intensity ratings were likely related to "off" flavors rather than to desirable flavors.

Limited data are available on taste acceptance of forage-fed versus grain-fed beef as evaluated by consumer panels. Generally, the differences were either very small or in favor of the grain-fed beef. Obviously, differences in the literature with regard to quality traits of forage- versus grain-fed beef vary considerably, partly because of the variability in quality of forage, age of the animal, and amount of grain supplemented to the diet.

In summary, forage-fed animals produce carcasses that are borderline in acceptability in terms of color, firmness, and retail shelf-life. Meat from these carcasses is borderline in taste acceptability. To date, the U.S. beef industry has not been willing to risk losing its "taste" image by moving to a total forage production system. Such a system would be impractical for other reasons, too, such as retained ownership because of the time required to reach acceptable market weights and the inability to supply the marketplace on a consistent basis.

### Bulls Versus Steers

Castration of meat-producing animals has long been practiced in the United States. It is intended to produce an animal more acceptable to current management systems and to provide a more desirable carcass for marketing. During the past four decades, a number of research studies have been conducted to assess the performance and meat characteristics of castrates versus noncastrates (Griffin et al., 1985; Seideman et al., 1982). In general, the results have indicated that bulls grow more rapidly, utilize feed more efficiently, and produce leaner carcasses. Increased production efficiency obtained through the use of intact males has often been offset by management problems, particularly with animal behavior. Meat production from young bulls has met with strong resistance from meat packers, in part because of carcass size variability, difficulty of hide removal, and inability to obtain an acceptable USDA quality grade. Retailers have resisted using meat from young bulls because their meat has been labeled as less tender and less desirable in color and texture.

The obvious advantages of using the young bull for meat production are efficiency of growth, leanness, and muscling. The disadvantages are in the area of carcass traits and tenderness. Some of the problems associated with tenderness can be corrected with adequate postmortem handling of the carcass, such as postmortem aging and electrical stimulation. Electrical stimulation can also improve muscle color and retail appearance.

Variability in size and quality has been associated with young bulls. The North Central Regional Research Group (NRC-132) prepared guidelines for the production of young bulls of differing frame sizes to meet certain compositional end points. Under varying market conditions, it is possible that end points for young bulls in each frame size could shift, but it is very unlikely that large-framed bulls should ever be fed to reach the Choice grade. Small- and medium-sized bulls are better suited to reach a particular compositional end point without obtaining excessively heavy market weights.

When properly managed, young bulls provide a good option for efficiently producing lean beef that is acceptable in quality. Considerable effort should be made to develop markets for meat from these animals. This will involve the education of some segments of the meat industry to correct misconceptions about young bulls.

## Impact of Growth Regulators on Beef Quality

Growth regulators and repartitioning agents function by reducing fat deposition. Since a relationship between fatness and marbling exists, a reduction in marbling and resulting quality grade can be expected when fatness is reduced. However, in most instances, acceptability, shear force, palatability, and tenderness are altered to a lesser extent than expected from the reduction in fat. Also, electrical stimulation of carcasses yields taste values equivalent to those for carcasses from nonimplanted cattle without electrical stimulation.

While the need to produce a leaner beef product has become clear, the segmentation of industry and the resulting divergent goals, objectives, and profit centers result in mixed signals at best, and incentives to produce fatter beef often prevail. Incentives for producing leaner beef must be established in all segments of the industry to ensure coordination of growth toward optimal market end points.

Currently, profit incentives favor maximal weaning weight in the cow/calf phase, maximal rate of gain in stocker and growing programs, maximal rates of gain in feedlot phases, and extended feeding in finishing phases to increase dressing percent and quality grade. For any specific animal type or breed, these goals enhance fat deposition while reducing the period of time allowed for protein and lean tissue growth, thereby limiting progress toward producing a leaner beef product (Figure 1).

Faster growth through nutrition invariably increases the percentage of fat produced in each phase of growth. This is true whether the energy comes from milk or creep in cow/calf operations; supplementation, better forage, or higher energy growing diets in stocker systems; or the combination of rapid rates of gain, packer/buyer requests to "feed them another 3 weeks," and feedlot priorities to move more grain in the feedlot phase.

## Shelf-Life in the Feedlot

One of the major problems the industry faces is the short shelf-life of cattle nearing slaughter end points. The concept of shelf-life (Perry et al., 1986) was developed to define the time and/or weight interval over which an animal maintains its current quality or yield grade. For some cattle types, shelf-life in the feedlot may not be appreciably longer than postharvest shelf-life in the retail trade. Extending this interval would provide more flexibility in marketing, and cattle would increase in fatness at a slower rate such that overfeeding would be less deleterious to lean beef production. The use of larger mature size cattle and implants as repartitioning agents provides

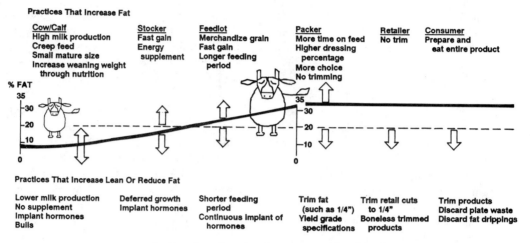

**FIGURE 1** Practices that alter fat content in beef products.

options for increasing the shelf-life of cattle. Shelf-life is shortest for small mature size cattle growing rapidly without growth regulators and longest for large mature size cattle receiving implants and growing at slower rates.

## CONCLUSIONS

Synchronization of nutritional levels with needs for protein growth, continuous delivery of repartitioning agents in all phases of growth from birth to slaughter, and use of intact males where possible will allow industry to reduce fat deposition across the board; produce, rather than trim to produce, lean beef; maintain desirable beef quality, flavor, and taste; and reposition beef's image as a lean product in the market.

To be successful, industry must systematically develop programs to produce the priority lean beef products that integrate breeds, feeds, and growth management regimes to optimize growth and development from conception to consumption.

Diet/health concerns, beef image problems, and animal efficiency in producing quality lean beef all require immediate attention to increasing lean tissue and reducing fat deposition in beef cattle.

Research programs must provide information on consumer preferences, implementation of currently available technology to provide leaner beef, and development of long-term technology to allow more precise regulation of growth through an animal's lifetime. The focus must be on protein production, rather than live weight and fat, and on systems that optimize energetic and economic efficiencies in protein and lean beef production. Rate of gain and feed efficiency criteria will not allow us to make progress toward this goal.

## REFERENCES

Bidner, T. D., A. R. Schupp, A. B. Mohamad, N. C. Rumore, R. E. Montgomery, C. P. Bagley, and K. W. McMillin. 1986. Acceptability of beef from Angus-Hereford or Angus-Hereford Brahman steers finished on all-forage or a high-energy diet. J. Anim. Sci. 62:381.

Byers, F. M. 1980. Systems of beef cattle feeding and management to regulate composition of growth to produce beef carcasses of desired composition. Ohio Agric. Res. Dev. Cent. Res. Circ. 258:1–18.

Byers, F. M. 1982. Nutritional factors affecting growth of muscle and adipose tissue in ruminants. Fed. Proc. 14:2562.

Byers, F. M., and R. E. Rompala. 1980. Level of energy effects on patterns and energetic efficiency of tissue deposition in small or large mature size beef cattle. Pp. 141–146 in Proceedings of the 8th

International Symposium on Energy Metabolism. Cambridge, England: Butterworth.

Byers, F. M., G. T. Schelling, H. R. Cross, and L. W. Greene. 1985a. Anabolic agent modification of protein and fat deposition in steers of two sizes. Proc. W. Sec. ASAS 36:440.

Byers, F. M., G. T. Schelling, H. R. Cross, and L. W. Greene. 1985b. Efficacy of anabolic implants in enhancing protein synthesis and carcass lean tissue in large and small frame steers. J. Anim. Sci. 61(Suppl. 1):93.

Byers, F. M., G. T. Schelling, H. R. Cross, and L. W. Greene. 1985c. Homeorhetic repartitioning to enhance protein growth in steers with anabolic effectors. Fed. Proc. 44:547.

Byers, F. M., G. T. Schelling, H. R. Cross, and L. W. Greene. 1986. Growth regulation in steers with respect to mature size and carcass endpoints. J. Anim. Sci. 63(Suppl. 1):144.

Cross, H. R., J. D. Crouse, and M. D. MacNeil. 1984. Influence of breed, sex, age and electrical stimulation on carcass and palatability traits of three bovine muscles. J. Anim. Sci. 58:1358.

Crouse, J. D., H. R. Cross, and S. C. Seideman. 1984. Effects of a grass or grain diet on the quality of three beef muscles. J. Anim. Sci. 58:619.

Griffin, C. L., D. M. Stiffler, G. C. Smith, and J. W. Savell. 1985. Palatability characteristics of loin steaks from Charolais crossbred bulls and steers. Meat Sci. 15:235.

Lawrence, M. E., R. A. Roeder, G. T. Schelling, F. M. Byers, and L. W. Greene. 1985. Influence of zeranol implants on serum growth hormone levels in growing steers. Fed. Proc. 44:760.

Lemieux, P. G., F. M. Byers, G. T. Schelling, L. M. Schake, and G. C. Smith. 1983a. Anabolic effects on protein and fat deposition in cattle fed forage and grain diets. Fed. Proc. 42:533.

Lemieux, P. G., F. M. Byers, G. T. Schelling, G. C. Smith, L. M. Schake, and T. R. Dutson. 1983b. Anabolic effects on rate of protein and fat deposition and energy retention in cattle fed forage and grain diets. Proc. W. Sec. ASAS 34:240.

Lemieux, P. G., F. M. Byers, G. T. Schelling, and L. W. Greene. 1985a. Redirection in priorities of protein and fat deposition in cattle with anabolic regulators in growing versus finishing phases. J. Anim. Sci. 61(Suppl. 1):267.

Lemieux, P. G., F. M. Byers, G. T. Schelling, G. C. Smith, and T. R. Dutson. 1985b. Carcass merit of steers receiving anabolic implants and fed forage and grain diets. J. Anim. Sci. 61(Suppl. 1):93.

McKeith, F. K., J. W. Savell, G. C. Smith, T. R. Dutson, and Z. L. Carpenter. 1985. Tenderness of major muscles from three breed types of cattle at different times-on-feed. Meat Sci. 13:151.

Perry, R. J., F. M. Byers, G. T. Schelling, D. Hale, H. R. Cross, and L. W. Greene. 1986. A microcomputer model for estimating body composition, yield grade and quality grade of feedlot cattle. J. Anim. Sci. 63(Suppl. 1):144.

Roeder, R. A., S. D. Thorpe, J. M. Gunn, G. T. Schelling, and F. M. Byers. 1984. Influence of anabolic agents on protein synthesis and degradation in muscle cells grown in culture. Fed. Proc. 43:790.

Seideman, S. C., H. R. Cross, R. R. Oltjen, and B. D. Schanbacher. 1982. Utilization of the intact male for red meat production: A review. J. Anim. Sci. 55:826.

# Processing Technologies for Improving the Nutritional Value of Dairy Products

DAVID H. HETTINGA

Milk is a liquid food designed to provide nourishment for rapidly growing young mammals. Bovine milk is an excellent source of nutrients for humans; it contains 3.5 to 3.7 percent fat, 3.5 percent protein, 4.9 percent lactose, and 0.7 percent ash on an "as is" basis. In addition, milk contains nearly all the vitamins required for human nutrition and has a high calcium bioavailability (Kansal and Chaudhary, 1982).

Milk is widely considered nature's most perfect food because of its balanced availability of protein, fat, carbohydrates, vitamins, and minerals, and its high content of essential nutrients such as calcium, essential amino acids, and essential fatty acids. Concentrating these nutrients through processing further enhances the nutritional value of milk and its by-products. For instance, the cheese-making process concentrates the protein and fat, reduces the water, and eliminates the carbohydrate component. The whey derived from cheese making can be further processed through a technique called ultrafiltration to concentrate the alpha-lactalbumin and beta-lactoglobulin, proteins of high nutritional value.

## ULTRAFILTRATION

Ultrafiltration is a high-pressure microfiltration process that selectively segregates components of various molecular weights. For milk processing, membranes with varying pore sizes are used to retain the fat and protein while allowing the lactose, water, and salts to pass through. Ultrafiltration has multiple applications in the dairy industry. Examples include the concentration of whey proteins, the manufacture of cheese base for processing, and the concentration of total milk proteins and fat for the manufacture of all cheese varieties.

The application of heat during milk or product processing can be helpful or harmful. On one hand, heating reduces microbial loads and eliminates pathogens; it also denatures milk proteins to create specific properties, such as the melting of components in cheese processing to create a homogeneous mass. On the other hand, heating destroys, through protein denaturation, valuable components such as immunoglobulins, enzymes such as lactoperoxidase, and vitamin activity.

Multiple processing techniques can be applied to prevent or reduce the destructive effects of heat. For instance, in dealing with a heat-sensitive element for which preservation is necessary, such techniques can be used as freeze-drying (versus spray-drying in a heated atmosphere); freeze concentration, ultrafiltration, or reverse osmosis (versus heated evaporator concentration); or microfiltration or irradiation (versus heat pasteurization or sterilization). Simply reducing heat to reduce bacterial loads can also be effective; of course, the heat level must be high enough to eliminate pathogens but not so high as to affect the desired elements.

## ALTERING THE CARBOHYDRATE IN DAIRY PRODUCTS

Lactose is the primary carbohydrate in milk. A segment of the population is lactose intolerant (that is, these individuals cannot metabolize lactose). Many dairy products (for example, yogurt and sour cream) are manufactured via fermentative processes that eliminate or reduce lactose and can therefore be consumed even by those who cannot tolerate lactose. In these cases, the fermentative process converts the lactose to lactic acid, an element digestible by almost everyone. In addition, yogurt has been shown to contain an inactive form of lactase (the enzyme which breaks down lactose), which is activated in the neutral pH environment of the small intestine (Kolars et al., 1984).

Conventional milk, rich in lactose, can be enzymatically treated with the enzyme lactase to hydrolyze about 80 percent of the lactose. This process, which substantially reduces the intolerance, creates a milk product that is nutritionally unaffected. The product is available under the trade name Lactaid®. Also available are packets of the enzyme lactase, which the consumer can add to conventional milk.

## ALTERING THE FAT IN DAIRY PRODUCTS

Considerable effort has undoubtedly been expended in finding new uses for milk fat. However, because milk fat is the second most expensive edible fat, the economic equation works against its increased use as a food ingredient in its native form. Nevertheless, if the desirable and undesirable characteristics of milk fat, relevant to its utilization, are evaluated, some viable pathways begin to emerge. On the positive side, milk fat is a rich source of essential fatty acids and possesses a uniquely pleasing flavor found in no other fat. It contains a higher proportion of short-chain fatty acids than other fats, which contributes to its ease of digestibility. On the negative side, its high melting range (30 to 41°C) makes butter chilled to below 15°C hard to spread and unsuitable for use in a number of important areas of utilization such as the production of flaky bakery products. Walker (1972) reported that the concentrations of lactose and methyl ketone precursors in fractions with low melting points were slightly higher than those in the anhydrous milk fats. Furthermore, fractions with high melting points contain only 50 to 60 percent of the lactose potential and 60 to 70 percent of the methyl ketone potential of fractions with low melting points.

If the dairy industry is to achieve any success in utilizing its abundant milk fat, technological modifications will have to be undertaken to improve milk fat's utility as a food ingredient of choice. In terms of surplus butter fat, it would be both practical and profitable to extract butter flavor and concentrate it. This product could then be used in pastries, cooking oils, breads, edible creams, and imitation dairy products (Kinsella, 1975).

## ALTERING THE CHOLESTEROL IN DAIRY PRODUCTS

The concentration of cholesterol in bovine milk ranges from 10 to 15 mg/100 ml.

LaCroix et al. (1973) reported that 95 percent of the cholesterol in milk was unesterified; the remainder was esterified to long-chain, usually saturated, fatty acids. According to Jenness (1974), about 75 percent of the cholesterol present in whole milk is dissolved in the milk fat, 10 percent resides in the fat globule membrane, and the rest is present in the skim milk. The effects of commercial processing on the concentrations and distribution of milk cholesterol are poorly defined, but such information is necessary for proper interpretation of data and application of methods for decreasing the cholesterol concentration of milk.

A hypothesis exists that the cholesterol reductase from *Eubacterium* species can be used to convert the cholesterol in fluid milk to products (primarily coprostanol and cholestanol) that are either poorly absorbed or completely unabsorbed in the human intestine and that will therefore be excreted. MacDonald et al. (1983) report that the major end product of cholesterol reduction (coprostanol) by *Eubacterium* species is indeed poorly absorbed by humans. Furthermore, a lesser amount of cholesterol would be available in the intestine for oxidation to compounds that are potentially carcinogenic. Products from the chemical reduction of cholesterol are not carcinogenic. Conversion of cholesterol to chemically reduced and poorly absorbed compounds should therefore decrease the concerns of cholesterol-conscious people about consuming milk and other dairy products.

Supercritical fluid extraction (SFE) is a state-of-the-art unit operation that exploits the dissolving power of supercritical fluids at temperatures and pressures above their critical values. It involves the use of a gas elevated above its critical pressure and temperature as a solvent for selected components of a solid or liquid mixture. Under supercritical conditions, the solvent displays an increase in density, approaching that of a liquid, but retains the diffusivity associated with a gas. These properties allow a super-critical fluid to penetrate the structure of a material to be separated, dissolve soluble components, and carry them out of the extraction vessel. The extract can be easily recovered from the solvent by manipulation of pressure and/or temperature conditions such that they become insoluble and precipitate out of solution. The solvent can be vented off or recirculated through the extraction vessel.

A number of advantages have been cited for SFE compared with conventional extraction techniques currently used in the food industry. These include reduced energy costs, higher yields, better quality products owing to lower operating temperatures, and elimination of explosive or toxic solvents. It is anticipated that the use of supercritical fluid extraction and its range of applications will continue to grow during the coming years.

Supercritical carbon dioxide is receiving increased attention from the food industry as a solvent to replace hydrocarbons and chlorinated hydrocarbons currently used in vegetable oil extraction, decaffeinating coffee, and spice extraction. It has one obvious advantage in food in that it is nontoxic in any concentration. Its low critical temperature (31°C) combined with its pressure-dependent dissolving power make it attractive for separating particularly heat-labile flavor and aroma constituents at near-ambient temperatures.

Supercritical carbon dioxide has been used for the supercritical fluid extraction of oils from soybeans (Friedrich et al., 1982) and corn and cottonseed (List et al., 1984). The oil from these three oilseeds obtained by SFE, compared to hexane-extracted oil, was reported to be much less pigmented, require less refining, and have greater resistance to oxidative rancidity (Friedrich and Pryde, 1984). The last trait was attributed to the lower levels of free fatty acids and free iron and phosphorus (phospholipids) and the higher levels of tocopherols (Friedrich and Pryde, 1984) in the oil after SFE.

This indicates that supercritical carbon dioxide is able to remove a specific lipid fraction while leaving the other fractions intact.

The main structural units of milk are fat globules, casein micelles, globular proteins, and lipoprotein particles (Walstra and Jenness, 1984). Fat globules are the primary source of lipids in milk. Their structure and composition are exceedingly complex. A typical fat globule is probably 2 to 3 $\mu$m in diameter. Its core is composed of triacylglycerols (99 percent), with the remaining 1 percent composed of cholesterol and trace amounts of other lipid components.

To effectively remove the cholesterol from the milk lipid system, the fat globule must be penetrated, since it contains the largest deposit of cholesterol in milk. However, the cholesterol must be removed from the fat globule without destroying any of the globule's ability to function. Therefore, a crucial factor affecting the ability of the supercritical fluid to extract the lipids from the fat globule is the status of the fat globular membrane.

## ALTERING THE TRACE ELEMENTS IN DAIRY PRODUCTS

The addition of trace elements to the diet of a lactating human or other animal can, under certain conditions, increase to a limited extent the concentration of metals in the milk. In lactating humans, iron status seems to have little influence on milk iron concentration, and neither overt iron deficiency nor iron supplementation appreciably alters milk iron (Vuori et al., 1980). A similar observation has been made for cows (Archibald, 1985). In mice, however, iron supplementation of the lactating dams significantly increases milk iron (Carmichael et al., 1977). In humans, addition of copper to the diet causes little change in the milk copper concentration (Vuori et al., 1980).

Unfortified milks and formulas are poor sources of iron. However, the percentage of iron absorbed by infants varies widely with the source. About 50 percent of the iron in breast milk is absorbed compared to 10 to 12 percent for cow's milk or formula (Dallman et al., 1980). Fortification of cow's milk with iron sulfate or iron gluconate increases the total iron assimilated. Prolonged breast-feeding protects against iron deficiency; fortified cow's milk or infant formulas are also effective. The total amount of iron absorbed from fortified cow's milk can be four times that absorbed from breast milk.

Fortification must use chelated forms of the metals to ensure initial transfer to the phosphoserine groups of casein; this ligand-exchange reaction removes the metals from the reactive environment of milk lipids and ensures more effective utilization.

Milk is an important food of high nutritional value, wide distribution, and reasonable price. The opportunity to fortify it with several essential trace element gives us the chance to make it even more nourishing, particularly for infants, children, adolescents, and pregnant women who are at risk of iron and other trace metal deficiencies.

## REFERENCES

Archibald, J. 1985. Trace elements in milk: A review. Dairy Sci. Abstr. 20:712–725, 800–812.

Carmichael, D., J. Hegenauer, M. Lem, L. Ripley, P. Saltman, and L. Hatlen. 1977. Iron supplementation of the lactating mouse and suckling neonates. J. Nutri. 107:1377–1384.

Dallman, P. R., M. A. Siimes, and A. Stekel. 1980. Iron deficiency in infancy and childhood. Nutrition Foundation. Am. J. Clin. Nutr. 33(1):86–118.

Friedrich, J. P., and E. H. Pryde. 1984. Supercritical $CO_2$ extraction of lipid-bearing materials and characterization of the products. J. Am. Oil Chem. Soc. 61:223–228.

Friedrich, J. P., G. R. List, and A. J. Heakin. 1982. Petroleum-free extraction of oil from soybeans with supercritical $CO_2$. J. Am. Oils Soc. 59:288–292.

Jenness, R. 1974. The composition of milk. In Lactation III, Nutrition and Biochemistry of Milk, B. L. Larson and V. R. Smith, eds. New York: Academic Press.

Kansal, V. K., and S. Chaudhary. 1982. Biological availability of calcium, phosphorus and magnesium from dairy products. Milchwissenschaft 37:261–263.

Kinsella, J. E. 1975. Butter flavor. Food Technol. 29(5):82–98.

Kolars, J. C., M. D. Levitt, M. Avugi, and D. A. Savaiana. 1984. Yogurt: An autodigesting source of lactose. N. Engl. J. Med. 310:1.

LaCroix, D. E., W. A. Mattingly, N. P. Wong, and J. A. Alford. 1973. Cholesterol, fat and protein in dairy products. J. Am. Diet. Assoc. 62:275–279.

List, G. R., J. P. Friedrich, and D. D. Christianson. 1984. Properties and processing of corn oils obtained by the extraction with supercritical carbon dioxide. J. Am. Oil Chem. Soc. 61:1849–1851.

MacDonald, I. A., V. D. Bokkenheuser, J. Winter, A. M. McLernon, and E. H. Mosbach. 1983. Degradation of steroids in the human gut. J. Lipid Res. 24:675–700.

Vuori, E., S. M. Makinen, R. Kara, and P. Kuitunen. 1980. Iron supplementation in infancy and childhood. Am. J. Clin. Nutr. 33:227–231.

Walker, N. J. 1972. Distribution of flavour precursors in fractionated milkfat. N.Z. J. Dairy Sci. Technol. 7(4):135–139.

Walstra, P., and R. Jenness. 1984. Pp. 58, 229, and 254 in Dairy Chemistry and Physics. New York: John Wiley & Sons.

# Technological Options for Improving the Nutritional Value of Poultry Products

ROY GYLES

People in the United States are becoming more concerned with the nutritional value of the food they consume. But nutritional improvement per se is ineffective if the product is not consumed by the population at large. For example, there were high expectations for food yeast as a source of protein for developing countries after World War II. The production of large quantities of food yeast was realized and the protein quality was unexcelled. However, tropical workers found no appeal in a light flaky material with no gustatory attributes, and thus the project failed. Therefore, the nutritional status of a product is a function of its nutritional value and the extent of its consumption. To be of nutritional benefit to a population, there are two prerequisites for any food product: The cost must not be prohibitive, and the product must be palatable.

Poultry meat and eggs excel in both respects. Mass production of poultry meat and eggs became established through a combination of individual initiatives by private enterprise and research at land-grant colleges. Hybrid corn research at the University of Connecticut in 1911, the development of coccidiostats, the eradication of

*Salmonella pullorum* and *Mycoplasmas*, the application of genetic selection through population genetics, and the introduction of high-energy feeds have all contributed to the elevation of chicken meat from its former status as a Sunday luncheon luxury meal to its current status as an everyday meal for the general public. Eggs for the breakfasts of people accustomed to hard manual labor were supplied from numerous small flocks owned by independent egg producers. Mass production by large centralized farms came about when research and development provided the technological means for ensuring feed supplies, poultry health, and the improved genetic strains that were required.

Ongoing research, keen competition, and integration of the poultry industry have held down the cost of production of poultry meat and eggs. This has given poultry a competitive edge against other animal products. Relative costs and consumption of animal products have been reported by the U.S. Department of Agriculture (USDA) and show the following trends.* The cost per pound

* U.S. Department of Agriculture, Economic Research Service, Poultry and Egg Situation Report No. 249, and Economics Statistics and Cooperatives Service, Poultry and Egg Situation Report No. 300.

297

of ready-to-cook broilers was 54.8 cents in 1940 and 81.4 cents in 1984. Choice grade beef was 75.4 cents per pound in 1940 and 239.6 cents in 1984. Pork was 54.4 cents in 1940 and 162.0 cents in 1984. Broiler meat rose 49 percent versus 218 percent for beef and 198 percent for pork. In the United States, the per capita consumption of broilers rose from 2.0 pounds in 1940 to 53.0 pounds in 1984. The per capita consumption of turkey meat rose from 2.9 pounds in 1940 to 11.4 pounds in 1984. However, the per capita consumption of eggs dropped from 391 in 1940 to 261 in 1984. This decline may be attributed to several factors, including a greater awareness of the possible link between heart disease and cholesterol.

## BROILERS

Fat, protein, minerals, and water are the basic components of poultry meat. The composition of the fat-free tissue in poultry is relatively constant over a wide range of body weights and ages and is not affected by the degree of fatness (Leenstra, 1984; Lin, 1981). However, the most variable component of dressed ready-to-cook broilers is fat (Lohman, 1973). As the percentage of fat increases, the percentages of protein, minerals, and vitamins decrease. Thus, the fat content of poultry meat affects the variation in its nutritional value more than any other ingredient.

The fat in broiler meat can be categorized as either physiologically necessary fat or extraneous wasteful fat. Cell membranes, which are primarily lipid, control the permeability of cells. In addition, some intracellular and intramuscular fat appears to be necessary for normal growth and reproduction (Brody et al., 1984; Gyles et al., 1982). Extraneous wasteful fat may be found subcutaneously, at the crop; intermuscularly, attached to mesentery and gizzard; and as leaf fat in the abdomen.

The most frequently used measure of fatness in broilers is abdominal fat, which is the combined weight of the leaf fat and the fat attached to the gizzard. Because abdominal fat is highly correlated with total body fat and fat in the various depots, it is used as the main measure of fatness in chickens and tissues (Cahaner et al., 1986; Chambers and Fortin, 1984; LeClercq and Simon, 1982; LeClercq et al., 1980; Whitehead and Griffin, 1984). Abdominal fat is the most variable fat deposit (Becker et al., 1979; Leenstra, 1984). It represents the greatest inefficiency in feed usage and is the largest source of loss when discarded at cooking. Hood (1984) suggests that from an evolutionary standpoint, the purpose of extraneous fat was to provide a reserve of energy when food supplies became low. Today, domestication and mass production of poultry meat ensures a constant food supply. Therefore, excessive deposition of abdominal fat and extraneous fat at other depots is no longer required and represents unnecessary wastage of feed. Ricard et al. (1983) and Becker et al. (1984) point out that large changes in reduction of abdominal fat are possible without affecting the lipids required for optimum growth and reproduction.

Broilers currently contain about 2 to 3 percent of the live body weight as abdominal fat; total body fat ranges between 15 and 20 percent of the live body weight (Griffin et al., 1982). The coefficient of variation for abdominal fat may be as high as 53 percent in broilers (Gyles et al., 1984). The coefficients of variation for protein, minerals, and water in poultry meat are about 3, 8, and 2 percent, respectively (Leenstra, 1984).

During the second half of the 1970s, the broiler industry became aware of a problem with excessive fatness of ready-to-cook broiler carcasses. Consumers complained about throwing away large quantities of leaf fat at cooking and about too much subcutaneous fat and intermuscular fat in cooked broiler meat. Poultry processors complained about losing abdominal fat when the carcasses were cut up to sell by parts, as well as at evisceration. In response to current consumer demand, some processors are now trimming fat from broilers and deboned meat.

The onset of the problem has been developing over several generations of selection. Poultry breeders produced broilers in 1950 that were marketed at 4.0 pounds live body weight at 12 weeks of age using 3.0 pounds of feed per 1-pound gain in weight. Intense genetic selection by poultry breeders for increased body weight at younger ages resulted in broilers being marketed in 1986 at 4.0 pounds live body weight at 6 weeks and 5 days of age using 1.98 pounds of feed per pound of gain. Genetic selection for body weight caused chickens with above-average appetites to be chosen as breeders. As a result, broilers were produced that ate more feed at a given age and became unable to synthesize protein and lean meat fast enough to keep pace with increased intake of food energy. The excess food energy was deposited as lipids, and broilers became fatter.

Age and sex have a distinct influence on the relative amount of fat in young chickens. Older broilers have higher quantities of fat than younger broilers (Edwards et al., 1973; Leenstra, 1984; Lin, 1981). Pfaff and Austic (1976) and March and Hansen (1977) found that fatness in broilers up to 14 weeks of age increased through a proliferation in the number of fat cells. After 14 weeks of age, the numbers of fat cells were fairly constant, but the sizes of the cells increased.

## Management Options

Numerous management options are available that may improve the nutritional status of the dressed broiler carcass. A discussion of these follows.

### Marketing Broilers at Younger Ages

Marketing broilers at younger ages with smaller body size and weight than is currently practiced may be useful for certain marketing requirements to reduce fatness. However, the current thrust in broiler marketing is toward deboned meat for further processed items. (A detailed description of "further processing" is given by Mast and Clouser in this volume.) Processing larger broilers at older ages has an economic advantage for these requirements because older broilers yield more meat.

### Growing Males and Females Separately

Growing the sexes separately for broiler production offers opportunities for reducing carcass fatness. Males may be processed at standard ages or older to provide more deboned meat for further processing, whereas females may be marketed at younger ages before they become undesirably fat. And because females require less protein in their feed than males, formulation of two separate feeds for males and females has potential for economic gain. Furthermore, increased uniformity of carcass size is obtained by processing sexes separately. This increases the efficiency of processing with associated economic gains.

To grow sexes separately requires that the sex of each broiler chicken be determined on the day of birth. Sexing by the vent method is too costly to be feasible for this purpose; therefore, autosexing by genetics is required. Two options are available. Feather sexing based on rate of feathering at day of age is easily accomplished by mating fast-feathering males to slow-feathering females. However, there is a cost for manual evaluation of the feather status in the wing of each day-old broiler to determine sex. Also the producer sometimes experiences difficulties in growth and carcass quality from slow-feathering male broilers. Autosexing by down color is possible and highly attractive because there are no extra expenses for this type of procedure and no production problems. The poultry industry would benefit from the availability of genetic strains that produce autosexing broiler offspring by down color. These strains are available, but because their growth and feed conversion performance are substandard, they are uneconomical at this time.

## Cage Versus Floor Rearing

Almost all broilers in the United States are reared on the floor. However, there are aspects of rearing broilers in cages that are appealing. Cages require less floor space of housing per broiler and negate the laborious task of catching chickens on the floor at marketing. However, Deaton et al. (1974) found that broilers reared in cages had more abdominal fat than those grown on the floor. This suggests that the current industry practice of raising broilers on the floor contributes less to fatness than does cage rearing.

## Texture of Feed

For high-density diets, the texture of the feed has no influence on abdominal fat. However, for low-density diets, more time is taken to consume the feed in mash form as compared with crumbles or pellets. Pesti et al. (1983) found that feeding crumbles increased abdominal fat by 23 percent.

### Genetic and Other Options

The following genetic and other options to reduce fatness in broilers have been considered, and some are currently being used by poultry breeders.

## Family Selection Against Abdominal Fat

Genetic selection against abdominal fat cannot be accomplished by a direct measure of individual performance, because this requires killing the chicken to obtain the weight of abdominal fat. However, family average performance of abdominal fat may be obtained by killing full siblings or half siblings. This procedure requires the de-struction of some outstanding candidate breeders and involves time and expense at the processing plant. Becker et al. (1982) determined that a selection index of carcass weight and abdominal fat weight (0.1108 carcass weight − abdominal fat weight) reduces abdominal fat weight in a population and at the same time allows body weight to increase. Cahaner (1986) reported that divergent selection for abdominal fat based on measurement of abdominal fat among full siblings gave a heritability of 0.77 for reduction of abdominal fat and a realized heritability of 0.73 for separation of the lines. Cahaner further reported that for every gram of reduction in abdominal fat there was a general reduction of 0.8 gram in other body fat. This method of genetic selection is probably being used to some extent by poultry breeders.

## Specific Gravity of Broiler Carcasses

Fortin and Chambers (1981) found that using the specific gravity of the chilled dressed broiler carcass or the individual carcass parts was an unreliable, indirect indicator of fatness, apparently because of entrapment of air in the abdominal cavity and the existence of air sac extensions in the parts.

## Abdominal Fat in Spent (Killed) Parents

The determination of the weight of abdominal fat in spent parents is a destructive procedure, but the chickens are sent to the processing plant at the end of their productive year as normal practice. Therefore, killing the chickens does not incur the loss of a potential breeder. Gyles et al. (1982, 1984) reported that there was a significant ($P < 0.05$) relationship between the abdominal fat in spent females and their broiler offspring when the female parents were fed ad libitum, but not when they were on feed restriction as practiced commercially. Spent females that are switched from restricted to ad libitum feeding for a few weeks before killing for fat determination may show a positive relationship between fatness of parents and offspring at broiler ages. Selection of young candidate breeders based on the abdominal fat content of spent dams is a possible option for reducing abdominal fat but is probably not currently practiced by poultry breeders.

### Selection for Improved Feed Efficiency

Selection for feed efficiency is an effective way to maintain or reduce abdominal fat while improving growth rate and carcass yield. Brody (1935) pointed out that increased weight per age should change the lean/fat ratio in favor of lean tissue deposition. Thomas et al. (1958) found that broilers with higher feed efficiencies tended to have less body fat. Shook et al. (1966) pointed out variations in feed conversion among turkey toms of similar body weights and suggested a way for turkey breeders to use genetic selection to improve feed efficiency of turkeys. Gyles (1968) proposed a new concept in poultry breeding termed "conversion breeding," which was applied to a commercial male parent line for broiler production. Subsequent work by Washburn et al. (1975), Pym and Solvyns (1979), and Chambers et al. (1983) reported that selection for increased feed efficiency reduced the fat content of broiler carcasses. Chambers et al. (1983) found that a correlation of −0.48 between carcass fat and feed efficiency was −0.62 after adjusting for differences in weight gain. Selection for improved feed efficiency of both male and female parent lines of broilers in order to reduce abdominal fat is widely practiced in the poultry industry.

### Selection Against Very-Low-Density Lipoproteins (VLDL) in Sera

Grunder et al. (1984) found that the percentage of abdominal fat and plasma VLDL increased while abdominal fat lipase decreased as broilers advanced in age. The decrease in lipase activity may be associated with an increase in lipogenesis and serve as an indirect measure of fatness.

### The Cloaca Probe

Pym and Thompson (1980) developed a set of calipers to measure indirectly the amount of abdominal fat in live chickens. Chickens were placed on their backs and a probe was inserted into the cloaca. The distance was then measured between the probe and the ventral abdominal skin. The authors reported a significant ($P < 0.05$) correlation of 0.80 between caliper measurement and weight of abdominal fat pad. Other researchers, however, have been unsuccessful in duplicating these results. Mirosh and Becker (1982) reported a correlation of 0.30 between caliper measures at the midline of the abdomen and abdominal fat weight. Gyles et al. (1982) obtained correlations below 0.20. This method is probably not being used by poultry breeders.

### Skin Pinches

Mirosh et al. (1981) removed feathers from the left wing-web of broilers and used calipers to measure the skin thickness at the center of the wing-web. The broilers were subsequently killed and dressed. A pinch (double skin thickness) at the center of the humeral feather tract on the left and right shoulder region of each carcass was measured with calipers. Correlation coefficients between wing-web thickness and abdominal fat weight were 0.14 for males and 0.05 for females. Correlations for humeral tract pinch with abdominal fat weight were 0.12 and 0.17 for males and 0.18 and 0.13 for females. These small associations suggest that both these measures are unsuitable for estimating abdominal fat.

## Lipids of Pectoral Feathers

Becker et al. (1981) found a genetic correlation of 0.90 between percent lipids of pectoral feathers and percent abdominal fat, but this procedure requires further investigation.

## Ultrasonics

Ultrasonic techniques for determining fatness in poultry have been disappointing. Gillis et al. (1973) found that ultrasonics gave unreliable predictions of the percentage of fatness in turkeys. The correlations between two methods of ultrasonic measurement and breast fat and back fat were 0.06 and −0.06, respectively. Miller and Moreng (1963) used a somascope (ultrasonic flow detector) to measure fat thickness on dressed turkey carcasses. Highly significant ($P < 0.01$) correlations of 0.85 and 0.84 were found between somascope readings and fat thickness in the breast feather tract and back feather tract, respectively.

## Selection Against Sartorial Fat

Burgener et al. (1981) suggested that the sartorial (*Musculus sartorius*) fat depot was a useful indirect measure of broiler fatness. They found highly significant ($P < 0.01$) correlations of 0.78 and 0.79 between the total weight of left and right sartorial fat and abdominal fat in 42- and 56-day-old broilers, respectively. They infer that since the sartorial fat is outside the body cavity, it may be readily biopsied. However, the practicality of using this procedure on large flocks is questionable.

## Heritability Estimates of Abdominal Fat

The genetic options are well established and supported by moderate to large estimates of the heritability of abdominal fat based on the sire component of variance and reported by several researchers: Leen-

stra (1984), 0.38; Friars et al. (1983), 0.42; Becker et al. (1984), 0.38; Gyles et al. (1984), 0.72 and 0.23; and Cahaner (1986), 0.77 and 0.73.

## Nutrition Options

Several nutrition options have been reported in the literature that reduce the amount of fat in broilers. However, nutrition options are short term and palliative compared with genetic solutions. Furthermore, the consequences of nutrition options must be carefully evaluated as to whether the reduction in fat is accompanied by some loss in performance that adversely affects net profits. Each option must be evaluated in accordance with the particular goals and circumstances of individual production organizations. The following options may be considered.

## Manipulation of the Energy/Protein Ratio

The energy/protein ratio of the diet has a central role in fat deposition in broilers. Fraps (1943) was among the first to describe this effect. Since then many other investigators have reported on its ramifications (Bartov et al., 1974; Donaldson et al., 1956; Farrell, 1974; Jackson et al., 1982).

Energy levels fed in excess of maintenance requirements result in fat deposition. The energy/protein ratio affects the amount of feed consumed by chickens because the chicken tends to regulate consumption to meet its protein requirements. Decreasing dietary energy while maintaining the same protein level causes a reduction in feed consumption and fat deposition. Maintaining the energy level and increasing the amount of protein has the same effect (Yamashita et al., 1975). Therefore, the amount of fat in broilers can be influenced by changing the energy/protein ratio in accordance with desired product quality and net economic gain. The goal must be to formulate a well-balanced diet to maximize growth rate without increasing fat (Marion and Woodroof, 1966). When the diet is not balanced and chickens are fed insufficient protein, they consume more energy than is required and fat deposition increases. This may occur when there is only a slight protein deficiency (Waldroup et al., 1976).

### Restriction of Feed During Early Life of Broilers

Changing diets during the course of rearing broilers may produce rapid changes in fatness. Khalil et al. (1968) showed that groups of chickens fed low-protein diets for 8 days developed obese (24.1 percent body fat) carcasses. Chickens fed high-protein diets developed lean (1.8 percent body fat) carcasses. When both groups were switched to a balanced diet for 9 days, their carcass fat differences were narrowed (13.6 and 10.3 percent).

The determination that proliferation of fat in broilers is primarily due to an increase in the number of adipose cells has lead to the concept that restriction of feed during the early life of a broiler, followed by normal feeding, may result in reduced fatness. Results reported by March and Hansen (1977) tended to support fat reduction by this feeding regimen, but Griffiths et al. (1977) found that restricting the energy intake of chicks from hatching to 3 weeks of age had no significant ($P < 0.05$) effect on the fat pad size at 8 weeks of age.

### Restriction of Energy in Feed Shortly Before Marketing

Arafa et al. (1983) restricted feeding of broilers for 10 days before marketing and reduced abdominal fat by 79 percent compared with broilers fed ad libitum. The energy intake was 80 percent of the ad libitum intake. The live body weight at marketing and the dressed carcass weight of the restricted groups were slightly less

than those of the chickens fed ad libitum, but the average weights of the cooked broilers were the same for both groups. Commercial organizations that have a high percentage of their business in further processing should examine this option.

Recent work by Cabel et al. (1986) showed that the addition of feather meal from 2 to 6 percent of the diet fed for the 14 days before marketing at 49 days of age significantly ($P < 0.05$) reduced the abdominal fat in the carcasses.

### Formulation of Separate Feeds for Males and Females

Formulation of separate feeds for male and female chickens requires growing the sexes separately. (This was also discussed in the section on genetic options.) Female broilers require less protein in feed than males (Siegel and Wisman, 1962; Wells, 1963). Lowering the protein below 20 percent with an energy/protein ratio of 160 was found to increase the carcass fat in males but had no effect on females until the protein level was reduced below 16 percent with an energy/protein ratio of 200 (Lipstein et al., 1975). Formulation of separate feeds to meet more exactly the nutritional requirements of the sexes and produce less fat and more uniform size of carcasses at the processing plant should increase the overall efficiency of broiler production.

### Protein Quality of Feed

Fisher and Shapiro (1961) observed that a proper balance of amino acids was essential for optimum growth of broilers. Chickens on a diet deficient in some amino acids tended to compensate for the deficiency by overeating, consuming more energy, and depositing more fat. Carew and Hill (1961) found that a slight methionine deficiency did not reduce the growth rate of chickens significantly ($P < 0.05$) but did increase fat deposition. On the other hand, when there was more than the optimum amount of protein in a diet, fatness was reduced. Leveille et al. (1975) observed that addition of excess protein or amino acids to an already balanced diet reduced abdominal fat, probably due to utilization of energy to synthesize uric acid, which is the main end product of nitrogen metabolism in the chicken.

### Feeding Fat as a Form of Energy

Edwards et al. (1973) reported that chickens on a diet supplemented with fats of animal or vegetable sources had slightly more carcass fat than controls. However, the difference was not significant ($P < 0.05$). Fuller and Rendon (1977) confirmed that the addition of fat in place of carbohydrate, without altering the energy/protein ratio, did not affect the amount of carcass fat. Therefore, the form in which energy is supplied in the diet does not seem to influence significantly the degree of fatness.

### Type of Fat in Diet Affects Chemical Composition of Carcass Fat

Marion and Woodroof (1966) pointed out that because carcass fat is deposited in two ways—directly from diet fat and through liver lipogenesis—the dietary constituents significantly influence the chemical composition of the carcass fat. The feeding of unsaturated fatty acids increased unsaturated fatty acids in the carcass, thereby reducing the carcass's shelf life. Edwards et al. (1973) reported that the type of fatty acids in the diet affected the composition of carcass fat. Chickens fed beef tallow had much firmer carcasses than those fed fats of vegetable origin. Beef tallow increased the stearic and oleic acid levels in place of the linolenic acid of vegetable fats.

### TURKEYS

Genetic selection for increased body weight at younger ages has not been as intense for turkeys as for chickens. Rather, selection has been directed primarily toward body conformation to increase yield of breast meat, and also to increase body weight at a standard age. Therefore, while the modern turkey has shown significant gains in body weight and breast meat, excessive fatness has not occurred (Nestor and Bacon, 1985). Bacon et al. (1985) reported that three large-bodied lines were selected from a random-bred control population over 17 generations. The three heavy lines of turkeys, selected in different ways from a common random-bred control, were similar in percentages of protein, ash, dry matter, and fat of dressed carcasses. The abdominal fat as a percent of body weight in the three selected lines was similar at 0.94 to 0.95, as compared with 0.49 for the random-bred control population. Females had larger quantities of leaf fat than males.

Turkey breeders have recently instituted changes in their selection criteria to prevent or delay any development of excessive fatness in turkeys. They are currently testing all the candidate male breeders of their commercial lines for individual feed-converting ability. The young toms are placed in individual floor pens, and their feed-converting abilities over several weeks are determined. Final selection of male breeders is made on more than one trait, but feed-converting ability is strongly emphasized.

### EGGS

The hen's egg is regarded as the near-perfect food. However, egg consumption has declined during the past 40 years, primarily because of changing life-styles (fewer individuals eating "hearty" breakfasts), increased awareness of the importance of food quality to health, and the evidence that cholesterol is linked to cardiovascular disease. Gilbert (1971) describes the yolk of the egg, on which the germinal disc floats, as an orange-yellow viscid fluid of oil-water emulsion with the continuous phase as aqueous protein. Chemically, it contains proteins, lipids, cholesterol, pigments, and a variety of minor organic and inorganic substances. In contrast, the albumin, or egg white, is described as almost pure aqueous protein, consisting of about 40 proteins.

The obvious single nutritional improvement in eggs in terms of human consumption is the reduction of cholesterol. Turk and Barnett (1971) found that the concentration of cholesterol in eggs did not differ significantly ($P < 0.05$) with age of hen, cage versus floor management, strain of commercial hen, or geographic location of feed source. Eggs from meat-type hens contained higher levels of cholesterol than eggs from commercial layers. Turkey, duck, and *Coturnix* quail eggs contained greater concentrations of cholesterol than chicken eggs. These differences are of little concern to the U.S. consumer, however, because chicken eggs from commercial layers are consumed almost exclusively. However, in some Oriental countries, duck eggs are widely consumed.

Differences in egg size that occur along with disproportionate differences between yolk and albumin result in changes in the percentage of yolk and albumin. Marion et al. (1964) found that differences in egg size are highly associated with egg components and that variation in any component is primarily because of covariation with egg size. The percentage yolk of egg tended to increase with a decrease in egg size. Correspondingly, the percentage albumin increased in larger eggs. Therefore, there are genetic and nutritional reasons for improving the nutritional value of eggs.

## Genetic Options

### Cholesterol

Reducing the amount of cholesterol in eggs by genetic selection is the most desirable way to improve their nutritional value.

Cunningham et al. (1974) reported a realized heritability of 0.21 for divergent selection on cholesterol concentration in yolks for one generation of selection. Washburn and Nix (1974) found sufficient genetic variation of cholesterol concentration that resulted in heritability estimates ranging from 0.14 to 0.22. These early reports implied that cholesterol concentration was responsive to selection. Marks and Washburn (1977) practiced divergent selection in one population for four generations and in another for three generations and obtained realized heritability estimates of 0.11 to 0.25 for separation of cholesterol concentration. However, in both populations the divergent separations of cholesterol concentration were due entirely to an increase in cholesterol in the high-cholesterol lines. There were no reductions in cholesterol in the low lines. Interestingly, numbers of eggs produced were reduced in the high-cholesterol lines, and consequently, when the high-cholesterol lines were compared with the low-cholesterol lines for total daily mass output of cholesterol, there were no differences between them. Becker et al. (1977) got similar results in that they were unable to obtain a response to selection for lower cholesterol in the yolk, but they did get a positive response to increased cholesterol. In this divergent selection study, realized heritabilities ranged from 0.04 to 0.13.

The measurements of cholesterol in the above experiments were based on the amount of cholesterol in the total wet yolk. Conceivably, cholesterol measured in milligrams per gram of wet yolk could have been reduced in the low-cholesterol lines without being detected by total cholesterol per wet yolk if yolk size increased. Accordingly, Washburn and Marks (1985) conducted another divergent selection experiment in which cholesterol was measured in milligrams per gram of wet yolk. When total cholesterol was expressed as total amount in yolk or grams of dry matter, the separation between the lines was similar to that when calculated as milligrams of cholesterol per gram of wet yolk. Therefore, it appears that regardless of the mode of expression of cholesterol concentration in eggs, genetic selection thus far has not been successful in significantly ($P < 0.05$) reducing cholesterol in eggs.

There are no breeds or strains of chickens that lay eggs of superior nutritional value with significantly ($P < 0.05$) lower cholesterol than other chickens. In the past an advertisement in the press stated that the blue eggs laid by the Araucana breed were lower in cholesterol than eggs from other breeds. Cunningham (1976) and Somes et al. (1977) refuted this allegation and found that eggs of the Araucana breed were equal to or higher in cholesterol than eggs of other breeds.

### Proteins, Fatty Acids, and Vitamins

There are several reports that ascribe genetic influences to the polymorphic proteins in egg white (for example, see Washburn, 1979). Strain differences for fatty acids in yolks have been shown to be small or negligible (Chen et al., 1965; Sell et al., 1968). Differences between breeds for vitamin A (Arroyave et al., 1957), thiamine (Howes and Hutt, 1956), and riboflavin (Mayfield et al., 1955) have been reported. Considering the excellent nutritional value of eggs (except for high cholesterol), there is no need to use genetic selection to influence the status of these nutrients.

## Nutrition Options

### Cholesterol

Naber (1979) stated that the nutrient composition of the egg had not changed greatly in response to modern industry practices. Naber (1976) pointed out that there appeared to be little variation in cholesterol content of eggs from hens fed the usual commercial diets. Given this ob-servation, it is important to note that deviations from a normal diet may significantly increase or decrease cholesterol. However, these deviations may negatively affect the nutritional value of the egg or the performance of the hen. Weiss et al. (1964) showed that diets containing 30 percent fats or 1 percent cholesterol caused a significant increase in the cholesterol content of eggs. Addition of certain drugs to the hens' diet—namely, triparanol (Burgess et al., 1962), certain azasterols (Singh et al., 1972), and probucol (Naber et al., 1974)—have caused significant reductions of cholesterol in the eggs. Use of these drugs was experimental, and harmful side effects have made them undesirable.

### Vitamins

Hill et al. (1961) found that the vitamin A content of egg yolks increased when levels in the diet were increased. However, the levels of increase in the egg were much less in proportion to those in the feed, because significant amounts were stored in the liver. In the case of vitamin D, there was negligible storage in the liver, and the quantities of the vitamin increased in the egg yolk in proportion to increases in the feed. Denton et al. (1954) pointed out that among the water-soluble vitamins, only the vitamin $B_{12}$ content of the egg may be significantly ($P < 0.05$) enhanced by feeding quantities of the vitamin above the normal dietary requirements.

### Minerals

Wilder et al. (1933) showed that the iodine content of the egg varies according to the quantities in the diet. Latshaw and Osman (1975) were able to significantly ($P < 0.05$) increase the levels of selenium in the egg white by feeding increased levels of either natural sources of the mineral or inorganic selenite.

## BIOTECHNOLOGY

### Meat Production

Work is being done on identifying a single gene in the poultry population that reduces abdominal fat to an acceptably low level and that can then be isolated, cloned, and inserted into the germ plasm of commercial broiler lines. Identification, cloning, and transfer of a single gene from an avian species other than poultry may provide a similar genetic scenario. Identification, cloning, and transfer of a single gene from a species other than avian may provide a third similar genetic situation. In each instance, population geneticists will have to determine whether insertion of a specific gene allows the broiler lines to be significantly ($P < 0.05$) superior in net bioeconomic performance to lines under conventional genetic selection.

### Egg Production

Since genetic selection has so far failed to reduce the cholesterol level of eggs, biotechnology should be investigated as a way to improve the nutritional value of eggs. Identification, cloning, and insertion into the germ plasm of commercial egg layers of a single gene that reduces cholesterol in eggs should be attempted, and the search for this gene should be made within and without the avian species.

### Determination of Sex

Biotechnology may make a significant contribution to the poultry industry by developing a way to determine the sex of fertilized eggs, embryos, or chicks at hatching. Such a procedure would allow broilers to be grown separately by sex, with the advantages mentioned previously for reducing abdominal fat and increasing production efficiency.

## SUMMARY AND RECOMMENDATIONS

Poultry products are widely consumed and contribute greatly to the nutrition of people in the United States. The commercial poultry industry and land-grant colleges must continue their traditional cooperation through research and teaching to maintain the relatively low cost of production and high overall palatability of poultry products. The nutritional value of poultry products can be improved by reducing the amount of fat in broiler carcasses, preventing the occurrence of excessive fatness in turkeys, and producing eggs with a greatly reduced cholesterol content. Several technological options have been discussed for improving the nutritional value of poultry products. The following are recommended for their effectiveness and practicality.

### Broilers

#### Genetic Options

Family selection against abdominal fat and very-low-density lipoproteins in blood sera and selection for improved feed efficiency have been shown to be effective in reducing fatness. A poultry breeding organization should pursue whichever of these or other avenues are considered suitable for the particular breeding program.

#### Nutrition Options

Manipulation of the energy/protein ratio in the diet should be done to suit the marketing needs of each integrated poultry organization and with the knowledge that this ratio is the main option available to nutritionists to reduce fatness in broilers. Restriction of energy in feed shortly before marketing may be effective. In this regard, the recent report (Cabel et al., 1986) on addition of feather meal to the diet for the 14-day period before marketing should be considered.

## Turkeys

Turkey producers should gain from the experience of broiler producers and prevent excessive fatness in turkeys. Breeders are well advised to test and select their candidate male breeders on the basis of individual feed-converting ability.

## Eggs

Researchers in biotechnology should be encouraged to cooperate with population geneticists in reducing the cholesterol in eggs.

## REFERENCES

Arafa, A. S., M. A. Boone, D. M. Janky, M. R. Wilson, R. D. Miles, and R. H. Harms. 1983. Energy restriction as a means of reducing fat pads in broilers. Poultry Sci. 62:314–320.

Arroyave, G. N., S. Schrimshaw, and O. B. Tandon. 1957. The nutrient content of the eggs of five breeds of hens. Poultry Sci. 36:469–473.

Bacon, W. L., K. E. Nester, and P. A. Renner. 1985. The influence of genetic increases in body weight and shank width on the abdominal fat pad and carcass composition of turkeys. Poultry Sci. 64(Suppl. 1):60.

Bartov, I., S. Bornstein, and B. Lipstein. 1974. Effect of calorie to protein ratio on the degree of fatness in broilers fed on practical diets. Br. Poultry Sci. 15:107–117.

Becker, W. A., J. V. Spencer, J. A. Verstrate, and L. W. Mirosh. 1977. Genetic analysis of chicken egg yolk cholesterol. Poultry Sci. 56:895–901.

Becker, W. A., J. V. Spencer, L. W. Mirosh, and J. A. Verstrate. 1979. Prediction of fat and fat free live weight in broiler chickens using back-skin fat, abdominal fat and live weight. Poultry Sci. 58:835–842.

Becker, W. A., J. V. Spencer, L. W. Mirosh, and J. A. Verstrate. 1981. Genetic correlation between pectoral feather tract lipids and abdominal fat in female broilers. Poultry Sci. 60:1621–1622 (Abstr.).

Becker, W. A., J. V. Spencer, L. W. Mirosh, and J. A. Verstrate. 1982. Selection of broilers for large carcass weight and low abdominal fat. Poultry Sci. 61:1415 (Abstr.).

Becker, W. A., J. V. Spencer, L. W. Mirosh, and J. A. Verstrate. 1984. Genetic variation of abdominal fat, body weight and carcass weight in a female broiler line. Poultry Sci. 63:607–611.

Brody, S. 1935. Nutrition. Annu. Rev. Biochem. 4:383–412.

Brody, T. B., P. B. Siegel, and J. A. Cherry. 1984. Age, body weight, and body composition requirements for the onset of sexual maturity of dwarf and normal chickens. Br. Poultry Sci. 25:245–252.

Burgener, J. A., J. A. Cherry, and P. B. Siegel. 1981. The association between sartorial fat and fat deposition in meat-type chickens. Poultry Sci. 60:54–62.

Burgess, T. L., C. L. Burgess, and J. D. Wilson. 1962. Effect of MER-29 on egg production in the chicken. Proc. Soc. Exp. Biol. Med. 109:218–221.

Cabel, M. C., T. L. Goodwin, and P. W. Waldroup. 1986. Reduction in abdominal fat content of broilers by addition of feather meal during the finisher period. Poultry Sci. 65(Suppl. 1):157.

Cahaner, A. 1986. Direct and correlated responses to divergent selection on abdominal fat. Pp. 71–88 in Proceedings of the 35th Annual National Breeders Roundtable, St. Louis, Mo., May 1–2, 1986. Decatur, Ga.: Poultry Breeders of America and Southeastern Poultry and Egg Association.

Cahaner, A., Z. Nitsan, and I. Nir. 1986. Weight and fat content of adipose and non-adipose tissues in broilers selected for or against abdominal adipose tissue. Poultry Sci. 65:215–222.

Carew, L. B., and F. W. Hill. 1961. Effect of methionine deficiency on the utilization of energy by chicks. J. Nutr. 74:185.

Chambers, J. R., and A. Fortin. 1984. Live body and carcass measurements as predictors of chemical composition of carcasses of male broiler chickens. Poultry Sci. 63:2187–2196.

Chambers, J. R., A. Fortin, and A. A. Grunder. 1983. Relationships between carcass fatness and feed efficiency and its component traits in broiler chickens. Poultry Sci. 62:2201–2207.

Chen, P. H., R. H. Common, N. Nikolaiczuk, and H. F. MacRae. 1965. Some effects of added dietary fat on the lipid composition of hen's egg yolk. J. Food Sci. 30:838–845.

Cunningham, D. L., W. F. Krueger, R. C. Fanguy, and J. W. Bradley. 1974. Preliminary results of bidirectional selection for yolk cholesterol level in laying hens. Poultry Sci. 53:384–391.

Cunningham, F. E. 1976. Composition of Araucana eggs. Poultry Sci. 55:2024.

Deaton, T. W., L. F. Kubena, T. C. Chen, and F. N. Reece. 1974. Factors influencing the quantity of abdominal fat in broilers. 2. Cage versus floor rearing. Poultry Sci. 53:574–576.

Denton, C. A., W. L. Kellogg, J. R. Sizemore, and R. J. Lillie. 1954. Effect of injection and feeding vitamin $B_{12}$ to hens on content of the vitamin in the egg and blood. J. Nutr. 54:571–577.

Donaldson, W. E., G. F. Combs, and G. L. Romoser. 1956. Studies on energy levels in poultry rations. 1. The effect of calorie protein ratio of the ration on growth nutrient utilization and body composition of chicks. Poultry Sci. 35:1100.

Edwards, H. M., Jr., F. Denman, A. Abou-Ashour, and D. Nugara. 1973. Carcass composition studies. 1. Influences of age, sex, and type of dietary fat supplementation on total carcass and fatty acid composition. Poultry Sci. 52:934–948.

Farrell, D. J. 1974. Effects of dietary energy concentrations on utilization of energy by broiler chickens and on body composition determined by carcass analysis and predicted using tritium. Br. Poultry Sci. 15:25–41.

Fisher, H., and R. Shapiro. 1961. Amino acid balance. Rations low in tryptophan, methionine and lysine and the efficiency of utilization of nitrogen in unbalanced rations. J. Nutr. 75:395.

Fortin, A., and J. R. Chambers. 1981. Specific gravity of the carcass and of its parts as predictors of carcass composition in broiler chickens. Poultry Sci. 60:2454–2462.

Fraps, G. S. 1943. Relation of protein, fat and energy of the ration to the composition of chickens. Poultry Sci. 22:421.

Friars, G. W., C. Y. Lin, D. L. Patterson, and L. N. Irwin. 1983. Genetic and phenotypic parameters of fat deposition and associated traits in broilers. Poultry Sci. 62:1425 (Abstr.).

Fuller, H. L., and M. Rendon. 1977. Energetic efficiency of different dietary fats for growth of young chickens. Poultry Sci. 56:549.

Gilbert, A. B. 1971. Poultry. P. 423 in Physiology and Biochemistry of the Domestic Fowl, D. J. Bell and B. M. Freeman, eds. New York: Academic Press.

Gillis, W. A., H. L. Orr, and W. R. Osborne. 1973. Ultrasonic estimation of carcass yield in turkey broilers. Poultry Sci. 52:1439–1445.

Griffin, H. D., C. C. Whitehead, and L. A. Broadbent. 1982. The relationship between plasma triglyceride concentrations and body fat content in male and female broilers—a basis for selection? Br. Poultry Sci. 23:15–23.

Griffiths, L., S. Leeson, and J. D. Summers. 1977. Fat deposition in broilers: Effect of dietary energy to protein balance and early life caloric restriction on productive performance and abdominal fat pad size. Poultry Sci. 56:638.

Grunder, A. A., J. R. Chambers, and A. Fortin. 1984. Abdominal fat lipase, plasma very low density lipoproteins and fatness of meat-type chickens during growth. Poultry Sci. 63(Suppl. 1):107 (Abstr.).

Gyles, N. R. 1968. Conversion breeding shoots for feed efficiency, then growth. Turkey World 43:12–14.

Gyles, N. R., A. Maeza, and T. L. Goodwin. 1982. Regression of abdominal fat in broilers on abdominal fat in spent parents. Poultry Sci. 61:1809–1814.

Gyles, N. R., A. Maeza, and T. L. Goodwin. 1984. Regression of abdominal fat in broilers on abdominal fat in spent parents on severe feed restriction. Poultry Sci. 63:1689–1694.

Hill, F. W., M. L. Scott, L. C. Norris, and G. F. Heuser. 1961. Reinvestigation of the vitamin A requirements of laying and breeding hens and their progeny. Poultry Sci. 40:1244–1254.

Hood, R. L. 1984. Cellular and biochemical aspects of fat deposition in the broiler chicken. World Poultry Sci. 40:160–169.

Howes, C. E., and F. B. Hutt. 1956. Genetic variation in efficiency of thiamine utilization by the domestic fowl. Poultry Sci. 35:1223–1229.

Jackson, S., J. D. Summers, and S. Leeson. 1982. Effect of dietary protein and energy on broiler carcass composition and efficiency of nutrient utilization. Poultry Sci. 61:2224–2231.

Khalil, A. A., O. P. Thomas, and G. F. Combs. 1968. Influence of body composition, methionine deficiency or toxicity and ambient temperature on feed intake in the chick. J. Nutr. 96:337.

Latshaw, T. D., and M. Osman. 1975. Distribution of selenium in egg white and yolk after feeding natural and synthetic selenium compounds. Poultry Sci. 54:1244–1252.

LeClercq, B., J. C. Blum, and J. P. Boyer. 1980. Selecting broilers for low or high abdominal fat: Initial observations. Br. Poultry Sci. 21:107–113.

LeClercq, B., and J. Simon. 1982. Selecting broilers for low or high abdominal fat: Observations on the hens during the breeding period. Ann. Zootechnol. 31:161–170.

Leenstra, F. R. 1984. Influence of diet and genotype on carcass quality in poultry and their consequences for selection. Pp. 3–16 in Recent Advances in Animal Nutrition, W. Haresign and D. J. A. Cole, eds. London: Butterworth.

Leveille, G. A., D. R. Romsos, Y. Y. Yeh, and E. K. O'Hea. 1975. Lipid biosynthesis in the chick. A consideration of site of synthesis, influence of diet and possible regulatory mechanisms. Poultry Sci. 54:1075.

Lin, C. Y. 1981. Relationship between increased body weight and fat deposition in broilers. World Poultry Sci. 37:106–110.

Lipstein, B., S. Bornstein, and I. Bartov. 1975. The replacement of some of the soya bean meal by the first limiting amino-acids in practical broiler diets. Br. Poultry Sci. 16:627.

Lohman, T. G. 1973. Biological variation in body composition. J. Anim. Sci. 32:647–653.

March, B. E., and G. Hansen. 1977. Lipid accumulation and cell multiplication in adipose bodies in White Leghorn and broiler-type chickens. Poultry Sci. 56:886–894.

Marion, J. E., and J. G. Woodroof. 1966. Composition and stability of broiler carcasses as affected by dietary protein and fat. Poultry Sci. 45:241.

Marion, W. W., A. W. Nordskog, H. S. Tolman, and R. H. Forsythe. 1964. Egg composition as influenced by breeding, egg size, age and season. Poultry Sci. 43:255–264.

Marks, H. L., and K. W. Washburn. 1977. Divergent selection for yolk cholesterol in laying hens. Br. Poultry Sci. 18:179–188.

Mayfield, H. L., R. R. Roehm, and A. F. Beeckler. 1955. Riboflavin and thiamine content of eggs from New Hampshire and White Leghorn hens fed diets containing condensed fish or dried whale solubles. Poultry Sci. 34:1106–1111.

Miller, B. F., and R. E. Moreng. 1963. Studies on turkey body composition. 2. Measuring carcass fat of turkeys by ultrasonic detection. Poultry Sci. 42:268–273.

Mirosh, L. W., and W. A. Becker. 1982. Components which form the thickness of the abdomen region in broiler chickens. Poultry Sci. 61:1515.

Mirosh, L. W., W. A. Becker, J. V. Spencer, and J. A. Verstrate. 1981. Prediction of abdominal fat in broiler chickens using wing web and humeral feather tract measurements. Poultry Sci. 60:509–512.

Naber, E. C. 1976. The cholesterol problem, the egg and lipid metabolism in the laying hen. Poultry Sci. 55:14–30.

Naber, E. C. 1979. The effect of nutrition on the composition of eggs. Poultry Sci. 58:518–528.

Naber, E. C., J. F. Elliot, and T. L. Smith. 1974. Effect of Probucol on reproductive performance and liver lipid metabolism in the laying hen. Poultry Sci. 53:1960.

Nestor, K. E., and W. L. Bacon. 1985. Turkey fat problem? Canada Poultryman 72(10):54.

Pesti, G. M., T. S. Whiting, and L. S. Jensen. 1983. The effect of crumbling on the relationship between dietary density and chick growth, feed efficiency and abdominal fat pad weights. Poultry Sci. 62:490–494.

Pfaff, F. E., and R. E. Austic. 1976. Influence of diet on development of the abdominal fat pad in the pullet. J. Nutr. 106:443–450.

Pym, R. A. E., and A. J. Solvyns. 1979. Selection for food conversion in broilers. Body composition of birds selected for increased body weight gain, food consumption and food conversion ratio. Br. Poultry Sci. 20:87–97.

Pym, R. A. E., and J. M. Thompson. 1980. A simple caliper technique for the estimation of abdominal fat in live broiler chickens. Br. Poultry Sci. 21:281.

Ricard, F. H., B. LeClercq, and C. Touraille. 1983. Selecting broilers for low or high abdominal fat: Distribution of carcass fat and quality of meat. Br. Poultry Sci. 24:511–516.

Sell, J. L., S. H. Choo, and P. A. Kondra. 1968. Fatty acid composition of egg yolk and adipose tissue as influenced by dietary fat and strain of hen. Poultry Sci. 47:1296–1302.

Shook, J. G., J. E. Valentine, L. D. Andrews, and N.

R. Gyles. 1966. How turkey breeders may select for feed conversion. Ark. Agric. Exp. Stn. Bull. 710.

Siegel, P. B., and E. L. Wisman. 1962. Protein and energy requirements of chicks selected for high and low body weight. Poultry Sci. 41:1225.

Singh, R. A., J. F. Weiss, and E. C. Naber. 1972. Effect of azasterols on sterol metabolism in the laying hen. Poultry Sci. 51:449–457.

Somes, R. G., Jr., P. V. Francis, and J. J. Tlustohowicz. 1977. Protein and cholesterol content of Araucana chicken eggs. Poultry Sci. 56:1636–1640.

Thomas, C. H., E. W. Glazener, and W. L. Blow. 1958. The relationship between feed conversion and ether extract of broilers. Poultry Sci. 37:1177–1179.

Turk, D. E., and B. D. Barnett. 1971. Cholesterol content of market eggs. Poultry Sci. 50:1303–1306.

Waldroup, P. W., R. J. Mitchell, J. R. Payne, and Z. B. Johnson. 1976. Characterization of the response of broiler chickens to diets varying in nutrient density content. Poultry Sci. 55:130.

Washburn, K. W. 1979. Genetic variation in the chemical composition of the egg. Poultry Sci. 58:529–535.

Washburn, K. W., and H. L. Marks. 1985. Changes in egg composition of lines selected for divergence in yolk cholesterol concentration. Poultry Sci. 64:205–211.

Washburn, K. W., and D. F. Nix. 1974. Genetic basis of yolk cholesterol content. Poultry Sci. 53:109–115.

Washburn, K. W., R. A. Guill, and H. M. Edwards, Jr. 1975. Influence of genetic differences in feed efficiency on carcass composition of young chickens. J. Nutr. 105:1311–1317.

Weiss, J. F., E. C. Naber, and R. M. Johnson. 1964. Effect of dietary fat and other factors on egg yolk cholesterol. 1. The "cholesterol" content of egg yolk as influenced by dietary unsaturated fat and the method of determination. Arch. Biochem. Biophys. 105:521–526.

Wells, R. G. 1963. The relationship between dietary energy level, food consumption and growth in broiler chicken. Br. Poultry Sci. 4:161.

Whitehead, C. C., and H. D. Griffin. 1984. Development of divergent fat lines of lean and fat broilers using plasma very low density lipoprotein concentration as selection criterion: The first three generations. Br. Poultry Sci. 25:573–582.

Wilder, O. H. M., R. M. Bethke, and P. R. Record. 1933. The iodine content of hen's eggs as affected by the ration. J. Nutr. 6:407–412.

Yamashita, C., Y. Ishimoto, T. Yamada, H. S. Medada, and S. Ebisawa. 1975. Studies on the meat quality of broilers. 1. Effect of dietary protein and energy levels on abdominal fat content and meat taste. Jpn. Poultry Sci. 12:78.

# Processing Options for Improving the Nutritional Value of Poultry Meat and Egg Products

M. G. MAST and C. S. CLOUSER

American consumers are becoming more aware of the nutritional value of the foods they eat. This knowledge, together with the current emphasis on being physically fit and trim, has led to an increase in the emphasis on "diet" foods and labels such as Light, Lean, low-fat, reduced-fat, and reduced calories.

Poultry and egg products are natural candidates to meet this emerging demand because of their high nutrient content and relatively low caloric value. They are a good source of high-quality, easily digested proteins; egg proteins have traditionally been a standard by which other proteins are evaluated.

In spite of these attributes, there are still nagging issues—some real, some exaggerated, some imagined—facing the poultry industry. For eggs, cholesterol continues to be a concern; the steady decline in shell egg consumption undoubtedly reflects this. For poultry meat, the current focus is on reducing the fat content of the final product. This emphasis on fat comes partly from the consumer and, more recently, from the industry itself, as individual companies compete to capture the market that desires the "leaner" product.

This paper reviews the impact of processing steps on the nutritional value of poultry products and explores some processing options for improving nutritional value.

## THE INFLUENCE OF PRIMARY PROCESSING OF POULTRY MEAT ON NUTRITIONAL VALUE

Processing and its effects on the nutritional value of poultry have become more of a concern during the past few years (Demby and Cunningham, 1980; Mast and Clouser, 1985; Post, 1984). Processing can be divided into primary processing (stunning, scalding, plucking, chilling, postmortem aging, and cold storage) and further processing (heating, storage, freeze-drying, irradiation, and creation of restructured or ready-to-eat products).

Primary processing, with the possible exception of wet chilling, does very little to alter the nutritional value of poultry. Stunning has no effect. Although semiscalding (50–54°C) and subscalding (57–58°C) can cause loss of the pigmented epidermal layer (Demby and Cunningham, 1980), Harris and von Loesecke (1960) reported no evidence of significant nutritional losses at these temperatures. Scholtyssek et al. (1970) found that semiscalding produced less drip, a lower pH, and better tenderness than subscalding.

In the United States, most poultry chilling is accomplished by immersing the carcasses in ice water for 30 to 60 minutes. An alternative method is air chilling; carcasses are not immersed but instead are chilled by refrigerated air. Air chilling is used by the European Economic Community for broilers that are sold fresh (that is, nonfrozen) to consumers.

Several authors have indicated that immersion chilling may affect the water-soluble nutrients in poultry meat. Hurley et al. (1958) reported increases in calcium, sodium, phosphorus, potassium, chlorine, and nitrogen in chill water during immersion chilling; they recorded losses of solids from the poultry (4.8 mg/gram of meat) after 24 hours of immersion in water. Pippen and Klose (1955) also indicated losses of sodium and phosphorus to the chill water from broiler carcasses; they reported that about 4 g of dry solids/kg of meat leached out of the tissue during wet chilling. If chicken is 70 percent water, this would mean that 4 grams/300 grams of solids, or 1.3 percent, leached into chill water during 18 hours of immersion. Harris and von Loesecke (1960) also stated that wet chilling may leach as much as 1 percent of the total solids.

Ang and Hamm (1983) compared the nutrients of breast meat from broilers that were immersion chilled or hot-deboned (no chilling). Hot-deboned birds had significantly less moisture (0.9 percent), more ash (12 percent), more phosphorus (5.2 percent), more potassium (5.8 percent), and less sodium (10 percent) than water-chilled broilers. The authors suggested that the higher sodium content in the water-chilled meat may be attributed to absorption from the skin during the 24-hour chilling period in crushed ice.

Wet chilling also causes water uptake,

leading to a dilution effect on other components and yielding an increase in drip loss and a further leaching of solids (Froning et al., 1960; Pippen and Klose, 1955). Hale and Stadelman (1973) determined that initial weight gains from wet chilling were negated upon cooking and that net losses of 20 grams after cooking (as compared with air-chilled birds) were recorded.

Therefore, it does appear that water chilling may lead to a slight loss in some water-soluble nutrients, primarily minerals. However, no significant losses occur for proteins or lipids.

Although kosher processing of poultry is accomplished in a similar manner to the conventional processing discussed above, three practices differentiate the two processing methods. In kosher processing, no hot-water scalding is permitted, additional mechanical pickers are required, and eviscerated carcasses are liberally salted inside and out and held for 1 hour to draw out residual blood (Powers and Mast, 1980). This salting process significantly increased the ash and sodium content of the meat and skin. Mast and MacNeil (1983) reported that the sodium content of raw breast meat was 291 mg/100 grams for kosher processing and 66 mg/100 grams for conventional processing; corresponding values for thigh meat were 243 versus 64 mg/100 grams and for skin, 357 versus 55 mg/100 grams. Dukes and Janky (1985) also reported an increase in sodium chloride of broiler breast meat that had been subjected to chilling solutions containing varying amounts of sodium chloride. In deference to consumers who wish to restrict sodium intake, labeling of the sodium content of kosher processed poultry is desirable.

After chilling, the next primary processing step is postmortem aging. Khan and Lentz (1965) found that time of aging may make a difference in the nutritional content of poultry meat. Three periods of time were defined in their experiments: prerigor, or within 15 minutes of slaughter; rigor, or 4 hours postslaughter; and postrigor, 24 hours or more postslaughter. Freezing during rigor caused the most drip loss during thawing, the lowest protein solubility, and the greatest cooking loss. Larger losses of nitrogen constituents and ribose also occurred in birds frozen during rigor. Khan and van den Berg (1964) reported maximum extractability of nitrogen from broiler meat after 24 hours (postrigor).

Hay et al. (1973) also reported lipid changes in postmortem chicken muscle with an increase in free fatty acids and decreases in phosphatidyl choline and phosphatidyl ethanolamine. Long-chain polyunsaturated fatty acids were produced in aged muscle, but not in unaged muscle.

## THE EFFECT OF STORAGE ON PRIMARY PROCESSED POULTRY

Storage time and storage conditions can affect the vitamin, mineral, and fat content of foods. Losses depend on the type of processing preceding storage, the length of storage time, and the temperature at which the food is held.

### Chilling

Fresh poultry, if chilled and stored under ideal conditions, can have a shelf-life of 2 to 3 weeks. Ang et al. (1982) used four treatments (control, iced whole, iced breast, deep-chilled breast) to determine nutritional losses in fresh poultry. Thiamine and riboflavin losses were negligible over the entire 14 days of the study. Magnesium, potassium, and phosphorus decreased significantly ($P < 0.01$) in the iced breast treatment, while significant losses of potassium and magnesium were reported in the iced whole treatment. Only potassium decreased significantly in the deep-chilled breast treatment. Calcium levels in all treatments significantly increased; the authors hypothesized a leaching of calcium from the bone over time. Proximate analysis indicated no

statistically significant differences, although moisture content was higher in the two iced treatments.

Conclusions indicate that deep chilling is the best method tested for retaining mineral content of the meat. Vitamin and protein retention were the same for all methods.

### Freezing

Vitamin retention is excellent in frozen foods if proper temperature ($-20°C$) is maintained (Somers et al., 1974). The Institute of Food Technologists Expert Panel and Committee on Public Information (1974) stated that storage temperatures of $-18°C$ or below result in excellent retention of the vitamin content of frozen foods. Nutrient levels can actually be higher in frozen foods than in fresh, depending on how old the fresh product is and how soon the frozen product was processed. The rate of freezing can also influence drip losses resulting in losses of B vitamins during thawing and subsequent cooking (Bender, 1978). Studies conducted by Kahn and Livingstone (1970) and Singh and Essary (1971) report B vitamin losses of 10 percent because of drip loss.

In most cases, the freezing process itself was shown to have little effect on nutritional values. Details on methods of freezing were not given in most cases, and differences in values may have arisen from differences in standing time and rate of freezing. Losses during frozen storage do occur, particularly with thiamine. Freezing does not affect the nutritional value of protein. Bowers and Fryer (1972) showed that no significant loss of riboflavin or thiamine occurs in a cooked product after 5 weeks of storage at $-17.5°C$. Singh and Essary (1971) used four different methods of thawing birds stored for 10 months (running cold water 21–22°C, running warm water 44–46°C, room temperature, and refrigerated 3–5°C). All birds were in sealed plastic bags. Niacin, thiamine, and riboflavin were measured before freezing and after thawing. The only significant loss ($P < 0.05$) occurred in niacin from the birds thawed at room temperature. The authors stated that "the lower value of niacin observed in birds thawed at room temperature was apparently due to some reason not understood."

West et al. (1959) found that after 2 and 4 months of frozen storage ($-29°C$), precooked, frozen chicken breasts had the same thiamine content as those frozen raw, thawed, and then cooked. Samples frozen for 2 months were found to have thiamine values of 0.18 to 0.19 µg/100 grams, while 4-month samples with similar moisture content had levels of thiamine ranging from 0.13 to 0.14 µg/100 grams. Although statistical differences were not mentioned, a decreasing trend in thiamine retention can be seen.

Thiamine was well retained (96 percent) in a freshly prepared chicken à la king frozen at $-10°C$ (Kahn and Livingstone, 1970). Morgan et al. (1949) found that riboflavin and niacin were fairly stable in three groups of chickens for up to 8 months. Thiamine was significantly lower after 4 months in one of the groups but appeared to be stable in the others. Cook et al. (1948) found similar results, reporting no significant losses in thiamine, riboflavin, or niacin after 3 to 9 months of storage at $-23°C$.

In a study conducted by Lee and Dawson (1973), precooked and raw chickens that were subsequently frozen were tested for retention of linoleic acid. The raw chicken had linoleic acid levels of 20 percent of the total lipid, which increased to 34 percent upon cooking (fried). Slow losses occurred over the storage period. Linoleic acid levels in the raw and frozen chicken dropped to 20 percent after 3 months and 16 percent after 6 months.

## INFLUENCE OF FURTHER PROCESSING OF POULTRY MEATS ON NUTRITIONAL VALUE

The term "further processed" is used in the poultry industry in a similar manner as the term "processed meats" is used in the red meat industry. U.S. Department of Agriculture (USDA) economists compile data for further processing under the category of "beyond cut-up." Examples of methods used in preparing further-processed poultry products are size reduction, deboning, restructuring, emulsifying, batter/breading, heating, and freezing. Many of the products are "ready to eat" at the time they leave the processing plant, in contrast to the "ready to cook" status of non-further-processed whole birds. Further processing reduces the preparation efforts of the consumer, hence, the term "convenience foods," which is frequently used for such products.

Critics of further processing have implied that the additional steps involved in preparing these products reduce their nutritional value. A review of some of the individual processes and their impact on nutritional value of poultry meat follows.

### Heat Processing

Heat is by far the most destructive of all processing methods. Most affected of the amino acids are lysine and threonine. Of the B vitamins, thiamine is the most heat labile, and large losses can occur depending on the amount of time heated and the degree of heat.

#### Oven

Mulley et al. (1975) demonstrated the time/temperature relationship of thiamine destruction. Hall and Lin (1981) found significant differences in thiamine content of broiler breast muscle and thigh muscle roasted to an internal temperature of 82°C at both 204°C (46 minutes) and 121°C (131 minutes). Retention of thiamine was significantly higher ($P < 0.01$) for the higher temperature, shorter cooking time. A significantly higher percent of thiamine ($P < 0.01$) was also retained in breast meat versus dark meat; the authors felt this was due to a lower end temperature of the breast meat (82°C) compared to the thigh meat. Since the breast muscle is thicker and larger, it would heat more slowly. The latter part of this study concurred with one conducted by Cook et al. (1948), which showed a twofold increase in thiamine loss in turkey leg meat (62 to 87 percent) compared to turkey breast meat (38 to 43 percent). An end point temperature was not reported. These meat samples were cooked for 2 to 3 hours at 168°C. Again, breast and thigh were cooked together.

Percent losses of riboflavin and niacin are always less than percent losses of thiamine; riboflavin is stable up to 130°C and niacin is also stable at even higher temperatures. Niacin is also stable to air and light at all pH levels, while riboflavin can be destroyed under alkaline conditions (Bender, 1978).

No significant loss of riboflavin in chicken after 45 minutes of roasting was reported by Hodson (1941). Similarly, Rowe et al. (1963) found no decrease of riboflavin in chicken cooked 15 minutes in a pressure saucepan. Losses of only 20 to 30 percent in turkey and chicken muscle were reported by Cook et al. (1948) and Morgan et al. (1949) for both riboflavin and niacin. It should be noted that cooking times for the studies by Hodson (1941) and Cook et al. (1948) were very different. Additionally, two different methods were used (fluorometric and microbiological, respectively) to determine losses.

The effects of heating on protein appear to be minimal. The following studies all used acid hydrolysis to calculate amounts of amino acids present. Sheldon et al. (1980) found no significant differences in the protein efficiency ratios of rats fed rations containing turkey meat roasted to end points of 74, 79, 85, or 91°C; however, the rats fed the ration containing the turkey with the highest end point temperature gained the least amount of weight. Millares and Fellers (1949) showed small losses of all amino acids except tryptophan, leading to the conclusion that "destruction of amino acids is probably not a principal factor in the alteration of the nutritive values of proteins as a result of heating." Finally, Thomas and Calloway (1961) found no loss in essential or semiessential amino acids subjected to heat processing. However, they did find losses in availability of many of the amino acids upon pepsin digestion of the treated samples, indicating that acid hydrolysis does indeed camouflage the biological availability of the amino acids. Studies by Warner et al. (1962), Myers and Harris (1975), and Chang and Watts (1952) indicate that no significant losses of fatty acids occur in poultry or meat products.

## Frying

Both Cheldelin et al. (1943) and Hodson (1941) found no significant losses in riboflavin upon frying. Cheldelin et al. (1943) also reported no significant loss of thiamine. In both studies, chicken parts were fried for 15 minutes in an open pan. Warner et al. (1962) found no change in the biological value of the fats in skillet-fried chicken. Nakai and Chen (1984) point out that although total amounts of fat in chicken meat do not change after frying, there is an alteration of fatty acid composition. Using four different coatings for treatments (battered, battered and breaded, breaded, and no coating), chicken parts were deep fat fried and evaluated for changes in fatty acid content. Decreases in palmitic ($C_{16:0}$), palmitoleic ($C_{16:1}$), and linoleic ($C_{18:2}$) acids and an increase in oleic acid indicated that the shortening was being absorbed into the meat. These changes were not as great in chicken that was battered and flour dusted or battered and breaded as in chicken that was just breaded or noncoated, suggesting that batter and breading may help "seal" the meat. Chang and Watts (1952) also verified that there was some increase in unsaturated fats because of the vegetable oil.

## Broiling

Hodson (1941) found no significant losses in riboflavin after chicken thighs were broiled for 20 minutes.

## Boiling

Boiling probably affects the B vitamin content more than any other treatment. Some of the thiamine, riboflavin, and niacin leaches into the water during boiling. The amount of each vitamin lost depends on the cooking time and the surface area involved. An extreme example was presented by Bender (1978) in the manufacture of meat extract. The meat was cut up into small pieces and boiled for 15 minutes; 80 percent of the water-soluble vitamins and muscle extractives were lost.

Proteins, on the other hand, are denatured by boiling, but this does not affect nutritional value (Bender, 1978).

## Canning

Thomas and Calloway (1961) reported a loss in thiamine due to canning, but the amount and significance of the loss were not reported. Riboflavin and niacin did not decrease, and total amino acid levels were unaffected. However, in vitro pepsin digestion revealed that less than 50 percent of the available lysine, cystine, methionine, and tryptophan found in the raw state remained available after canning. Similar results were indicated in a study by Millares and Fellers (1949), but losses in thiamine were reported as significant, with the instability of thiamine at high temperatures with pH values close to neutrality given as a possible explanation. Microbiological assays indicate riboflavin retention as 100 percent or better (complex molecules released riboflavin upon heating) and no significant losses of niacin. Amino acid content was changed only slightly, with a 50 to 80 percent decrease in tryptophan.

Ascorbic acid and thiamine, both present in only minimal quantities in poultry meat, are susceptible to loss during prolonged storage of conventionally canned foods. Hellendoorn et al. (1969) found most vitamins stable to processing and storage at 22°C in canned whole meals. Immediately after processing, a 50 percent loss was observed for thiamine and vitamin C. After 1.5 years, all the vitamin C was destroyed and losses of thiamine were 75 percent. Niacin loss was 10 percent owing to processing and an additional 10 percent because of storage. Riboflavin was not affected.

## Curing and Smoking

Significant losses in thiamine and niacin of cured, smoked, and cured canned chicken versus canned chicken were observed by Millares and Fellers (1949). Greenwood et al. (1943) noted significant (12 to 69 percent) thiamine losses in the presence of 0.02 to 0.10 percent sodium nitrite in thiamine solutions. Higher pH (6.1 versus 5.6) and length of heating increased the losses. But when Greenwood et al. (1943) investigated the possibility of loss in the presence of sodium nitrite in pork, they found no significant loss when the pork was heated in the presence or absence of meat-curing ingredients or in meat cured 10 days and held 1 hour at 98°C.

## Microwave Cooking

Microwave cooking can alleviate two major destructive components of conventional heating: external heat and time of heating. Goldblith et al. (1968) reported no loss of thiamine by microwaves when held at 0°C for 45 minutes or at 33°C for 30 minutes. However, continuous loss over time was observed when thiamine in solution was held at 102.8°C for 50 minutes. The loss was roughly equivalent to losses occurring at the same temperature in a conventional oven. Goldblith et al. (1968) used thiamine in solution for this experiment, which is more easily destroyed than thiamine found in muscle tissue. McMullen and Cassilly (1976), however, demonstrated no difference in thiamine or riboflavin losses between microwaved or conventionally heated chicken.

Similar results were obtained by Hall and Lin (1981), who looked at two different wattages of microwaves versus two different cooking temperatures in a conventional oven. No significant differences in the retention of thiamine in pectoralis muscles cooked at 400°F (204°C) in an 800-watt microwave or a 1,600-watt microwave were found. However, a significantly higher loss of thiamine was found in birds cooked at 250°F (121°C) for more than 2 hours.

This study points out the obvious problem of the time/temperature relationship. The temperature of the oven and, consequently, the time of cooking significantly affect outcome.

Wing and Alexander (1972) reported a 91 percent retention of vitamin $B_6$ in chicken cooked by microwave and only an 83 percent retention for conventional cooking. The microwaved chicken was cooked for 1.5 minutes, while the conventionally heated chicken was heated to an internal temperature of 88°C (45 minutes, no oven temperature given). Retention of vitamin $B_6$ found in the drippings was then added to the retention in the meat, resulting in a total loss of 7.5 percent in the microwaved chicken and 11.6 percent in the conventionally cooked chicken. Bender (1978) points out that findings by Miller et al. (1973) indicate that the coefficient of variation of analysis of $B_6$ is 9 percent; therefore, a real difference between the values reported by Wing and Alexander (1972) may not exist.

No studies on the effects of microwaves on poultry protein were identified in the literature. Causey et al. (1950) reported no statistical differences in lysine retention between beef patties cooked in a microwave (90 percent retention) and those cooked in a conventional oven. Campbell et al. (1958) found losses of five essential amino acids to be about 15 percent in both microwaved and conventionally cooked beef.

Myers and Harris (1975) studied the effects of microwave cooking on fatty acids and concluded that there were no significant differences between fatty acids of conventionally cooked chicken and microwaved chicken. Additionally, no differences were found between raw or cooked chicken.

Microwave cooking apparently causes no more nutrient loss than does conventional cooking. Any benefit would come from decreased drip loss and shorter cooking time, but only when compared with prolonged conventional cooking. Riboflavin and niacin losses were minimal in both cases. Amino acid and fatty acid losses were also found to be insignificant.

### Irradiation

Irradiation is still considered a food additive by the U.S. Food and Drug Administration. Most researchers, however, treat it as a food process, and it is considered as such in this review.

Irradiation of poultry is not approved in the United States. Although the World Health Organization has unlimited clearances on irradiation levels of 2 to 7 kGy, only The Netherlands and South Africa have set clearances (up to 3 kGy) for use on poultry. The USSR has approved test batches (radurization only) up to 6 kGy, and Canada is test marketing poultry irradiated up to levels of 7 kGy (Goresline, 1983).

Irradiation of food is considered a "cold" process because of only slight temperature rises. This minimizes nutritional losses (Thomas and Josephson, 1970). Two forms of radiation processing, radurization and radicidation, are used on chilled poultry in a few countries to prolong shelf life. Radurization, pasteurization designed to kill or inactivate food spoilage organisms, and radicidation, pasteurization designed to kill or inactivate all disease-causing organisms, are accomplished at processing levels below 10 kGy. Foods are then stored refrigerated. Both processes show minimal, if any, losses in protein, fat, and vitamin levels. However, these processes only pasteurize, and shelf-life can be extended by 2 weeks at most (Froning, 1978).

A third form of irradiation processing, radappertization, incorporates heating. Radappertization is sterilization by irradiation. Precooked foods in vacuum-sealed containers are exposed to ionizing radiation while frozen ($-20$ to $-40°C$) at absorbed doses high enough to achieve commercial sterility (25 to 70 kGy). Care must be taken that absorbed radiation does not exceed 70 kGy, or palatability may be affected. Packaging is critical as exposure to light, oxygen, moisture, and microorganisms could quickly deteriorate food quality. Precooking must achieve an internal temperature of at least 70 to 80°C to inactivate enzymes that would cause food degradation upon storage. After irradiation, the product is thawed and stored at room temperature. Because of the processing in sealed containers and storage at room temperature, radappertization has been equated to thermal canning.

In early studies, radappertization done at room or chilled temperatures resulted in the formation of off flavors and odors. A study by Brasch and Huber (1948) indicated that irradiation at low temperatures ($-20$ to $-40°C$) could reduce or eliminate these problems. Holding the food at these temperatures in an oxygen-free environment during the irradiation process also helps to retain nutrients.

Radiation, at levels envisioned for food processing, has minimal effects on the nutritional value of protein, although other physical properties can be affected. Irradiation in meat causes intermolecular cross-linking reactions of proteins, leading to decreases in molecular weight, solution weight, tensile strength, and solubility. Irradiation also causes a decrease in water-holding capacity, while drip loss increases (Josephson and Peterson, 1983). Similarities exist between the effects of freeze-drying and irradiation in that solubility and water-holding capacity are diminished (Diehl, 1983).

In a study by Ley et al. (1969), rats fed diets of radappertized (up to 70 kGy) meat and bone meal showed no significant differences from rats fed nonirradiated diets in total digestibility, biological value, and net protein utilization or in amino acid composition. Levels of cystine, methionine, and tryptophan were measured, since these are considered the most sensitive to ionizing radiation.

DeGroot et al. (1972), in comparing irradiated versus nonirradiated chicken, found that lysine availability and protein efficiency ratios in both groups were unaffected by irradiation (6 kGy) after 6 days of refrigeration followed by conventional cooking. The authors concluded that irradiation did not affect the nutritional value of the protein fraction.

Sheffner et al. (1957) found no changes in content or enzymatic availability of amino acids in ground turkey meat at irradiation levels of 19.4 kGy and concluded that irradiation was superior to canning. The observations of Calloway et al. (1957), which indicated that neither irradiation nor cooking altered the biological value of turkey protein, concurred with those of Sheffner et al. (1957).

Thiamine is the most radiation-sensitive B vitamin. As absorbed radiation levels are decreased, thiamine levels in aqueous solution increase (Groninger and Tappel, 1957). Thomas and Josephson (1970) also commented on studies showing increased vitamin retention as temperatures decreased, which indicated that vitamins are affected by the heat and not the irradiation process.

Riboflavin and niacin were found to be stable to all forms of radiation processing in several studies, with maximum loss levels of 20 percent (Alexander et al., 1956; DeGroot et al., 1972; Proctor et al., 1956).

Radappertization causes oxidation, degradation, and decarboxylation of the lipid fraction (Thomas and Josephson, 1970). Unsaturated fats are the most affected. Antioxidant factors form in the nonlipid constituents of irradiated meat that protect the lipid fraction. The antioxidant factors work best in ground products where lipid and nonlipid components are in intimate contact with one another. In whole-meat products, where fat and lean are separated, autooxidation of the lipid fraction occurs rapidly in the presence of oxygen. Chemical changes are minimized by packaging (to exclude light and oxygen) and freezing irradiation (Josephson and Peterson, 1983). Digestibility of fats seems unaffected.

Conclusions of most of the authors cited here are that losses of nutrients do occur in irradiated foods but that they are comparable to those observed in other processing methods and therefore are considered acceptable.

### Dehydration and Freeze-Drying

Freeze-drying and low-temperature dehydration produce few changes in the nutritional value of poultry since heat is not used. In a study by Thomas and Calloway (1961), five different processes (dehydrated, raw state; cooked, dehydrated; enzyme inactivated, then irradiated; precooked, irradiated; and conventionally canned) were tested for their nutrient retention. Thiamine retention was most favored by freeze-drying raw poultry and least favored by irradiation. Riboflavin levels increased in the canning process, but changes were not statistically different in any other process. Niacin was well preserved in all processes, with no one method better than any other. Pyridoxine was completely stable after freeze-drying, as was pantothenic acid. A 20 percent loss in dienoic fatty acids occurred during freeze-drying. Although total levels of essential and semiessential amino acids remained unchanged for both the raw and cooked

dehydrated chicken, pepsin digestibility of the cooked dehydrated chicken was significantly lower.

Digestibility of the freeze-dried chicken was good by both pepsin and humans. The overall conclusions were that freeze-drying least affected the nutrient content of poultry as compared with all other methods studied, with excellent vitamin stability during subsequent storage. This was confirmed by a later study done by Rowe et al. (1963) that demonstrated that freeze-drying was not destructive to thiamine, niacin, or riboflavin in chicken muscle, although losses of thiamine occurred if the meat was cooked before freeze-drying or after freeze-drying and rehydrating.

### Size Reduction—Mechanically Deboned Meat

Mott et al. (1982) showed differences between levels of protein, fat, water, ash, iron, and fluoride in mechanically deboned meat from whole birds, frames with skin, and frames without skin. Whole birds had lower protein, higher fat, lower water, and lower iron contents than did bird frames with or without skin. Fluoride content was higher in the frames without skin, as was ash (indicative of higher bone content). The kilocalories per 100 grams were significantly higher in the whole, deboned birds. Protein efficiency ratios were not significantly different.

In vitro digestibility of homogenates of mechanically or hand-deboned chicken (using hydrogen chloride, pepsin, and pancreatin) showed a 79 to 93 percent retention, with no differences between raw versus cooked or hand versus mechanically deboned meat (Schoenhauser et al., 1980).

Marriot et al. (1982) showed that chicken hot dogs provided 104 mg of calcium in a 100-gram serving. This was attributed to limited amounts of pulverized bone and larger amounts of bone marrow. Higher values (than beef or pork hot dogs) for cobalt, iron, magnesium, and phosphorus were also attributed to the use of mechanically deboned poultry in the hot dog formulation.

## THE EFFECTS OF PROCESSING, STORAGE, AND FURTHER PROCESSING ON THE NUTRITIONAL VALUE OF EGGS

Shell eggs lose very few nutrients when stored properly. Everson and Souders (1957), in a comprehensive literature review on egg composition, cited several studies showing no significant losses of protein, fat, or minerals in shell eggs. Changes in solids were attributed to the transfer of water from the white to yolk or evaporation through the shell. Riboflavin, thiamine, and vitamin A decreased slightly during cold-storage times of 3 to 4 months.

The quality of eggs stored at room temperature deteriorates at a much faster rate than does the nutritional value. Imai (1981) demonstrated that although coating the eggs slowed the rate of deterioration at room temperature in a 4-week storage study, egg quality was much higher in both coated and noncoated eggs stored for up to 4 months at 3°C.

Cooking of eggs (frying, scrambling, poaching, and hard boiling) results in very few compositional changes. The most notable decreases are in thiamine and riboflavin (17 percent and up to 11 percent, respectively). Protein, iron, calcium, and fats remain stable, although frying may increase saturated or unsaturated fats, depending on the type of butter or shortening used. Vitamin A increases in fried products if butter is used.

Spray-drying is the most common form of drying. The drying process itself results in no nutritional loss. Sugar is removed from dried egg products to prolong shelf-life. Everson and Souders (1957) reported that vitamin A, niacin, riboflavin, and thiamine were stable at storage temperatures below 15°C but that higher storage temperatures

resulted in losses of these nutrients. Packaging of eggs stored at room temperature in sealed tins increased vitamin A retention. Vitamin D was not significantly affected by drying or subsequent storage. Protein, fats, and minerals were also not affected. Cotterill (1981) reported that dried whole egg and yolk products should be stored at 10°C or less. Egg white is stable at room temperature for several years.

## PROCESSING OPTIONS FOR INCREASING NUTRITIONAL VALUE

### Collection and Utilization of Blood

According to Satterlee (1981), animal blood is not used in human foods in the United States because the consumer has an unfavorable image of blood as a food. Disadvantages of blood protein as a food ingredient are the strong taste and odor of dried plasma and hemoglobin and the red color of hemoglobin, which may be disagreeable to consumers (Calvi et al., 1984a). The off flavor, which is probably due to lipid breakdown, can be minimized with newer, low-temperature drying methods (Stevenson and Lloyd, 1979).

Blood from larger animals is routinely collected, decolorized when desired, and used in foods such as blood sausage in other countries. In the United States, blood is currently used in nonfood products such as fertilizers and as a feed additive. However, like soy and milk proteins, blood protein could be used to enrich food (Calvi et al., 1984a).

In a recent issue of *Meat Industry* (Anonymous, 1986a), the editors, commenting on a rumor that USDA is close to approving limited use of blood in U.S.-produced meat products, stated that "blood may turn out to be yet another of those things that's considered a delicacy in other parts of the world but doesn't excite the American appetite."

Animal blood is a potential source of high-quality protein. Beef blood, for example, contains 18 percent protein and is rich in lysine, valine, tryptophan, phenylalanine, and leucine. However, blood proteins are very low in isoleucine, which can result in an amino acid imbalance (Olson, 1970). The plasma component of blood contains about 70 percent protein and the cellular fraction (red and white cells) about 94 percent protein (Stevenson and Lloyd, 1979). Young et al. (1973) demonstrated that the protein efficiency ratio of a diet containing dried bovine plasma could be increased from −1.05 to 2.88 by adding 1.2 percent DL-isoleucine to the diet. The composition of dried poultry blood is 80 percent protein, 8 percent moisture, 1 percent fat, and 11 percent fiber or ash (Mountney, 1976).

Broiler chickens contain about 7.5 percent of their body weight in blood, 45 percent of which is collectible during slaughter operations (Kotula and Helbacka, 1966). In 1985, more than 23 billion pounds of poultry were inspected in the United States (U.S. Department of Agriculture, 1986). Therefore, some 800 million pounds of blood could have been collected.

Efficient processes for hygienic blood collection from large animals using hollow knives and sodium citrate (to prevent coagulation) have been reported by Stevenson and Lloyd (1979) and Wismer-Pedersen (1979). Systems for collecting blood have also been constructed and commercially tested in poultry-processing plants (Childs et al., 1976). These systems were effective and reliable in handling the blood and also reduced the pollution entering the plant effluent. However, they were not designed for collecting blood for use in human food.

Although a sanitary system for blood collection may be technologically possible, the economic aspects of protein recovery from blood remain a problem. Satterlee (1981) stated that the "problem is the cost of recovering protein from dilute solutions and resulting energy needed to dry the whole solution, to concentrate and preserve the protein." New energy-efficient recovery processes are required to make such recovery feasible.

## Increased Use of Giblets

Poultry giblets—heart, gizzard, and liver—are not fully used in the United States. In some processing plants, especially those slaughtering birds for use in further processing, it has become economically infeasible to harvest, clean, and package giblets.

These three foods are high in protein, iron, and niacin. In addition, liver is high in vitamins A and C.

The undesirable texture of gizzard and heart tissue has been a factor in the underuse of these foods. In addition, the functional properties of the proteins in these tissues are not as acceptable as those in the skeletal muscle of poultry. A number of studies have demonstrated that protein modification can improve the functional properties of various tissues: beef (DuBois et al., 1972); fish (Spinelli et al., 1972); beef heart (Smith and Brekke, 1984); and mechanically deboned fowl (Smith and Brekke, 1985a,b). According to Franzen (1977), modification refers to the intentional alteration of the physiochemical properties of proteins by chemical, enzymatic, or physical agents to improve functional properties.

According to Brekke and Eisele (1981), acylation reactions, involving the direct addition of chemical groups to functional groups of amino acid side chains via substitution, have the most potential for chemically modifying food proteins. The anhydrides of acetic and succinic acids are usually the acylating agents, since they are easy to use, safe, and inexpensive and produce acylated derivatives that are functionally important. When a protein is reacted with acetic anhydride, the acylation reaction is termed acetylation; when succinic anhydride is used, the reaction is referred to as succinylation.

Succinylation affects the physical character of proteins by increasing the net negative charge, changing conformation, and increasing the propensity of proteins to dissociate into subunits, breaking up protein aggregates, and increasing protein solubility (Franzen, 1977).

For acylated proteins to be incorporated into foods, they will need to be safe, digestible, and probably approved by the Food and Drug Administration and USDA as food ingredients since the protein has been modified. Groninger and Miller (1979) indicated that the influence of acylation on protein utilization and nutritional quality depends on the type of protein, the amount of protein modification, and the acylating agent used. Similar techniques may also be useful in improving the functional properties of poultry giblets, thereby making these products, with good nutritional properties, more usable by the poultry further-processing industry.

### Hot-Deboning and Hot-Stripping

Hot-deboning is the removal of meat from the eviscerated carcass before the onset of rigor mortis. Hot-stripping is a modification of hot-deboning in that the muscle is removed from a noneviscerated bird.

As much as 1 percent of the total solids in poultry meat may be lost during water chilling of the carcass. These losses, although minor, do occur with water-soluble components such as vitamins and minerals. Air chilling or hot deboning alleviates this loss, since the carcass is not in contact with water for a prolonged period.

Of probably greater importance than this 1 percent loss in solids content, however, is the potential economic advantage of hot-deboning or hot-stripping. The economic savings that could be expected with these techniques include energy savings through a decrease in cooling costs, decreased water consumption, lowered equipment expenditures, reduced labor and time, and improved yields.

For hot-stripping to be used, changes in USDA inspection regulations are necessary, since muscle tissue is removed from carcasses prior to the inspection of the viscera.

### Removal of the Abdominal Fat Pad

Consumers do not like to buy chicken containing the abdominal fat pad. Most remove it themselves before preparing the chicken. Several large poultry companies are currently removing this fat at the processing plant in an effort to sell a product that is lower in total fat than their competitor's chicken. The average abdominal fat pad weighs about 40 grams, which constitutes 2.5 percent of the total weight of the carcass and 10 percent of the total body fat (F. E. Pfaff, personal communication, 1986). These values are based on whole carcass composition determinations and not on specific cuts of boneless meat.

### Reduction in Sodium Content of Further-Processed Products

In recent years, considerable attention has been focused on sodium and its potential impact on public health. Although the value of low-sodium diets is questioned by some scientists (Kolata, 1982), there is sufficient concern within the scientific community (Putnam and Reidy, 1981) and by many consumers to warrant production of food products containing less sodium.

Poultry meat itself is not high in sodium content; cooked breast meat contains 63 mg of sodium/100 grams of meat, and cooked thigh meat contains 75 mg/100 grams. However, during the further processing of poultry meat into products, the sodium content may increase dramatically as sodium chloride and various sodium phosphates are added to the product.

Sodium chloride is generally used in further-processed products such as frankfurters at levels of 1.5 to 2.5 percent. Salt influences the flavor, may affect the shelf-life, and affects the functional properties of the my-ofibrillar proteins.

One option for lowering sodium content is to use substitutes for all or part of the sodium chloride, such as calcium chloride, magnesium chloride, and potassium chloride (Hand et al., 1982; Maurer, 1983). Hand et al. (1982) reported that replacing 100 percent of the sodium chloride with magnesium chloride or potassium chloride was detrimental to the flavor of the frankfurters prepared from mechanically deboned turkey. The authors suggested that 35 percent of the sodium chloride could be successfully replaced with potassium chloride; magnesium chloride caused off flavors, even at the 35 percent level.

Smith and Brekke (1985b) varied the sodium chloride content of frankfurters prepared from enzyme-modified, mechanically deboned fowl. They found that 0.5 percent salt was the least amount that could be added and still produce a satisfactory frankfurter from which the casing could be easily removed. Brekke and Eisele (1981) had earlier reported that enzymatic modification also has potential as a partial substitute for salt in processed meat products. The low-salt (0.5 percent) frankfurters were rated as having less chicken frankfurter flavor than products prepared with 2 percent salt. The authors stated that if low-salt frankfurters are to gain consumer acceptance, appropriate spice formulations will need to be developed to compensate for the salty flavor.

Barbut et al. (1986) reported that turkey frankfurters with 1.5 percent salt combined with phosphate were as acceptable as "reference" frankfurters, which contained 2.5 percent salt.

The sodium chloride in poultry frankfurters could be reduced to at least 1.5 percent (590 mg of sodium/100 grams of meat) without detracting from the flavor and to as low as 0.5 percent (197 mg of sodium/ 100 grams of meat) if additional spices can be found to improve the flavor.

## Reduction of Fat Content in Poultry Frankfurters

Chicken and/or turkey frankfurters traditionally contain 18 to 22 percent fat, compared to pork and/or beef franks, which usually contain 25 to 30 percent fat. Some producers of poultry franks have lowered the fat content of their product to 13 to 16 percent by using mechanically deboned meat from portions of the poultry such as the front quarter, breast cage, or skinless necks, which contain less fat than backs or legs. According to a study in *Consumer Reports* (Anonymous, 1986b), poultry frankfurters ranged in caloric content from 180 to 300 kcal/100 grams of meat; the mean was 243 kcal/100 grams.

From a sensory standpoint, fat is an important component in increasing the palatability in a food such as frankfurters. If the fat content is too low, the resulting product tends to be rubbery and tough. Therefore, although consumers may think they want a much leaner frankfurter, such a product may not be acceptable to them.

## Reduction in Fat Content of Fried Poultry Products

Batter/breaded, deep-fried poultry products have been a mainstay of the further-processed and fast-food industry for many years. The current emphasis is toward boneless products, such as nuggets and patties. According to Przybyla (1985), the single fastest growing area within the processed chicken category is frozen, boneless, breaded chicken, partly because of increased sales of chicken-based finger foods in fast-food outlets. Retail sales of such items increased 71 percent from 1982 to 1984. There is also more interest in producing a product that is lower in fat and therefore lower in calories.

Baker et al. (1986) recently evaluated four cooking methods for battered and breaded broiler parts: FF (full frying in 177°C oil),

FSF (fry, steam, fry: brief fry, followed by longer steam cook plus additional short fry), WC (water cook: thoroughly cooked in hot water followed by 45 seconds of frying), and FOC (fry, oven cook: fried for 2.5 minutes followed by thorough heating in a 218°C oven). The three most commonly used methods for commercial preparation of retail frozen, fully cooked and browned, battered and breaded chicken are WC, FF, and FOC, respectively. Baker et al. (1986) found that the fat content was slightly higher in breasts cooked by FF and FSF compared with breasts cooked by WC and FOC, but the differences were not significant; for thighs, there was very little difference in fat content due to cooking treatments. Generally, there were no differences in the flavor or acceptability of parts heated by any of the four methods; yields were highest for pieces cooked by FSF, followed by FOC.

Stadelman (1985) illustrated that breaded chicken products can be produced with reduced caloric content by using hot air cooking instead of deep-fat frying, which resulted in a 23 to 31 percent decrease in fat content of parts and a 13 to 15 percent decrease in calories, and by removing the skin before breading and hot air cooking, which resulted in a 42 to 65 percent decrease in calories (see Table 1).

According to Stadelman (1985), when breaded, fried chicken contains 20 percent fat, as it frequently does with open kettle frying, 60 percent of the calories come from the fat. By removing the skin and cooking in hot air, a chicken breast or drumstick can be prepared with only 27 percent of the calories coming from the fat.

Cooking systems such as the one mentioned above and/or broiling will become more commonplace in the future as the demand for poultry products with less fat and fewer calories increases.

### Increased Utilization of Proteins Recovered from Bone Residue of Mechanically Deboned Poultry

Bones from slaughtered animals, especially larger animals such as beef and swine, are usually used for animal feed, gelatin, and glue. However, they could be used as ingredients in certain processed products; they are high in protein and provide a dietary source of minerals such as calcium. Bone products are used as food ingredients in some European countries. Some countries consider bone-derived protein added to a meat product to be meat; others consider it to be a nonmeat ingredient. In the United States, bone-derived protein is not currently permitted in food products (Calvi et al., 1984b).

TABLE 1   Analyses of Chicken Parts

| Source | Breast | | Thigh | | Drumstick | |
|---|---|---|---|---|---|---|
| | Percent Fat | Kcal/100 g | Percent Fat | Kcal/100 g | Percent Fat | Kcal/100 g |
| USDA[a] | 13.2 | 260 | 16.2 | 275 | 15.8 | 268 |
| Lab fried[b] | 15.7 | 275 | 16.9 | 279 | 14.0 | 244 |
| Lab modified[c] | 10.8 | 233 | 13.0 | 243 | 9.9 | 209 |
| Lab ultimate[d] | 5.7 | 186 | 9.8 | 218 | 4.9 | 166 |

[a]Data from U.S. Department of Agriculture. 1979. Composition of Foods—Poultry Products. Agricultural Handbook No. 8-5. Washington, D.C.: U.S. Department of Agriculture.
[b]Pressure deep fat fried, commercial equipment.
[c]Pieces with skin; hot air, no frying.
[d]Pieces without skin; hot air, no frying.

SOURCE: W. J. Stadelman. 1985. This chicken product breaks "grease barrier." Broiler Ind. 48:46.

Recent estimates indicate that 300 million pounds of mechanically deboned poultry are produced annually in the United States. This represents yields of about 60 to 70 percent mechanically deboned poultry depending on the type of machine used. On the basis of these estimates, 150 million pounds of bone residue (BR) are produced annually, most of which is used in fertilizer, pet food, or animal feeds. Bone residue is the material remaining when mechanically deboned poultry is prepared. Bone residue has characteristics that make it a valuable potential source of human food. It contains 20 percent protein, which represents an additional 30 million pounds of protein available annually for human use, assuming all protein could be extracted.

Bone residue contains approximately 18.9 percent protein, 7.7 percent fat, 11.7 percent ash, and 60.0 percent moisture (Mast and Opiacha, 1987; Opiacha et al., 1986). The two methods that have been developed to extract protein from BR are use of sodium chloride solutions (Kijowski and Niewiarowicz, 1985; Young, 1976) and use of mild alkali solutions (Jelen et al., 1982; Opiacha et al., 1986).

Freeze-dried protein isolates from BR using sodium chloride, prepared by Young (1976), contained 60 to 65 percent lipid, 5 to 10 percent ash, and 4 to 6 percent moisture. The freeze-dried protein extract obtained by Opiacha et al. (1986), using alkali, contained 45 percent protein, 47 percent fat, and 14 percent ash. Yields of dried extract represented 7 percent of the original BR.

Limited information is available on the nutritional quality of protein from BR. Lawrence and Jelen (1982) state that severe alkali treatments of protein may cause racemization or destruction of certain amino acids; in addition, unusual new amino acids may be produced, such as lysinoalanine, lanthionine, and ornithinoalanine. These authors concluded that the alkali extraction methods, as usually conducted with BR,

should not produce material such as lysinoalanine that could pose health hazards for consumers.

Protein extracts from BR have relatively good functional properties (water-holding capacity, emulsifying capacity, solubility) and could serve as ingredients in other poultry proteins. The poultry industry should be encouraged to explore the economic feasibility of using this protein source, which is currently underutilized or discarded.

### Reduction of Cholesterol Content of Liquid Egg

Much research has focused on reducing the cholesterol content of chicken eggs by altering the diet or through genetic selection. These approaches have met with varying degrees of success. Another alternative is to modify the egg yolk after the egg is laid. Since this disrupts the shell, albumin, and yolk, only processed eggs (currently about 15 percent of all eggs consumed) are available for this procedure.

Approaches used to date include dilution of whole liquid egg with egg white, thereby reducing the cholesterol content of the final product; removal of portions of the yolk lipids and cholesterol with various "solvents," thereby producing a product lower in cholesterol; and complete removal of the yolk and formulation of a substitute "yolk" from vegetable oils and other ingredients, thereby producing a product that is cholesterol-free.

Numerous U.S. patents have been obtained to accomplish the above goals. A few are discussed below.

*Melnick (1971), U.S. Patent 3,563,765:* Egg yolk solids were treated with nonpolar solvents (for example, hexane) at ≤160°F (71°C) to extract 50 to 90 percent of the fat and 70 to 98 percent of the cholesterol. The author indicated that *n*-hexane caused "little, if any, damage to the functional properties of the remaining protein."

*Melnick et al. (1971), U.S. Patent 3,594,183:* A specific objective of this patent was to provide an egg yolk product high in polyunsaturates, low in saturates, and low in cholesterol. Egg yolk solids, from which most of the fat and cholesterol have been extracted with *n*-hexane, were mixed with vegetable oil, salt, emulsifiers, and coloring compounds. After emulsifying, pasteurizing, and drying, "refatted egg yolk solids" were obtained. These can be used as a replacement for conventional egg yolk solids.

*Seeley (1974), U.S. Patent 3,843,811:* A frozen egg product was prepared that contained 0 to 1.1 percent fat, 8 to 18 percent protein, and <0.05 percent cholesterol. The product contained ≥92 percent egg white and ≤8 percent egg yolk. Other ingredients added were 2 to 2.6 percent potato flour, 0.1 to 0.2 percent carboxymethyl cellulose, 1.4 to 1.8 percent nonfat milk solids, and citric acid.

*Glasser and Matos (1976), U.S. Patent 3,941,892:* This patent differed from others in that a frozen "sunny-side up" egg product was developed; the mold used to form the shape was also used as the package. The "yolk" portion was synthesized with 20 to 45 percent dried egg white, 5 to 35 percent oil (with a polyunsaturated/saturated [P/S] fatty acid ratio > 0.6), dry milk protein, vegetable gum, colors, flavorings, and emulsifiers.

*Seeley et al. (1976) and Seeley and Seeley (1980), U.S. Patents 3,987,212 and 4,200,663, respectively:* A frozen egg product that contains no cholesterol or egg fats was produced that was suitable for making scrambled eggs, omelets, and so on. The product was prepared by blending egg whites and small amounts of nonfat milk solids, vegetable gums, and flavor enhancers.

*Fioriti et al. (1978), U.S. Patent 4,103,040:* The goal of these authors was to produce wet egg yolks and egg products that were low in cholesterol and had a P/S ratio > 1, while maintaining the functional properties of natural eggs. Wet egg yolks were prepared using a high-energy, higher shear mixer for a short time. During mixing, cholesterol was extracted from the yolk by the oil. At the same time, the P/S ratio increased. The wet yolk was then separated (centrifuged) from the oil. Egg yolk products were produced in which > 70 percent of the cholesterol was removed and the P/S ratio was > 1.3.

*Boldt (1981), U.S. Patent 4,296,134:* A 99 percent cholesterol-free egg blend was prepared that was low in fat (1.25 percent) and calories (80 kcal/100 grams). The blend contained 60 to 96 percent liquid egg white, 0 to 18 percent water, 2 to 10.5 percent protein replacement (nonfat dried milk solids, powdered egg albumin, and soy protein), stabilizers, flavoring, and coloring.

*Tan et al. (1982), U.S. Patent 4,360,537:* These authors developed a "lipoprotein emulsion system composed of protein, edible oil, and other selected food ingredients" that could be used to replace egg yolk. Their primary objective was to improve the composition and processes for preparing a product with good functional properties.

The nutritional quality of one egg substitute has been compared to whole eggs by several investigators. Navidi and Kummerow (1974) reported that raw egg substitute caused severe nutritional deficiencies in weanling rats and that all animals died within 4 weeks of weaning. Francis (1975) reported 100 percent mortality of chicks within 12 days when fed egg substitute as their only food. Since eggs are not usually the only food in a diet, Ryan and Kienholz (1979) prepared diets for chicks in which egg substitute or whole eggs constituted only 40 percent of the diet. These authors concluded that when cooked and fed in a palatable form, egg substitute is a satisfactory source of protein to support chick growth. Chicks fed whole-egg diets weighed 787 grams after 28 days, whereas chicks fed egg substitute averaged 687 grams (about 13 percent less).

Baker and Darfler (1977) and Baker and Bruce (1986) prepared egg blends by varying the yolk to white ratio from 1:1 to 1:10. Liquid egg with a 1:3 ratio of yolk to white produced scrambled eggs and omelets comparable to those made with whole eggs but contained only 50 percent as much cholesterol and 30 percent fewer calories. In the 1977 study, the authors found that egg blends containing as little as one-fourth the normal amount of egg yolk, with protein and lipid raised to the content of normal egg by the addition of dried albumin and corn oil, made egg products that were as acceptable as those made with whole eggs.

The patents and research studies reviewed have focused on cholesterol elimination or reduction in egg yolk products. Larsen and Froning (1981) suggested that fractionating egg yolk into its lipid, protein, and aqueous components may also lead to entities with new properties that could then be used in food systems. After trying several solvent systems, they reported that either hexane-isopropyl alcohol or hexane-ethyl alcohol was the most efficient for separating the egg oil fraction. If a protein isolate is desired, ethyl alcohol or isopropyl alcohol is the appropriate solvent; the use of hexane altered the integrity of the protein so that it was no longer an effective emulsifier.

Tokarska and Clandinin (1985) described a method for the preparation of egg yolk oil that did not cause decomposition of unstable polyunsaturated fatty acids. They obtained optimal extraction of lipid from egg yolk with ethanol/hexane/water. They reduced the cholesterol content of the egg yolk oil by 80 percent by washing with 90 percent ethanol; the cholesterol content of the product was 7 mg/gram of oil.

Solvent extraction procedures do not selectively remove cholesterol and can impair the functional properties of certain components. An alternative to solvent extraction is supercritical fluid extraction (SFE); the lipid components need not be extracted and functional properties are not destroyed.

A supercritical fluid is produced when the temperature of a gas is raised above the critical point and is then subjected to high pressure. As pressure is applied to a gas above critical temperature, the density of the gas will increase and may approach that of a liquid, while the viscosity of the gas is virtually unchanged. This combination of high density and low viscosity allows it to be an excellent extracting agent. The supercritical fluid has the ability to readily diffuse in and out of the food, thereby increasing extraction efficiency. By varying the density of the fluid through pressure changes, the solubility of the fluid can be adjusted to preferentially extract certain components. For egg products, the goal is to selectively extract cholesterol without removing the polar lipids responsible for functional and sensory properties of the resulting product (G. W. Froning, personal communication, 1986).

The food industry is currently using SFE to decaffeinate coffee; other applications may be extraction of spices; removal of oil from snack foods; extraction of oil from cottonseed, corn, and soybeans; and extraction of flavors from foods. To date, no one has used SFE with eggs or egg products; however, scientists at the University of Nebraska have initiated research to extract egg yolk with supercritical carbon dioxide at various pressures and temperatures to obtain extraction of cholesterol. SFE is further discussed by Hettinga in this volume.

## Incorporation of Eggs To Increase Nutritional Value of Foods

The consumption of shell eggs is rapidly declining in the United States. One approach to curbing an overall (that is, shell plus processed) decline in egg consumption is to increase efforts for developing new products made entirely or partly from yolk, albumin, or whole eggs.

## SUMMARY

From a nutritional point of view, poultry and egg products are good because they contain high-quality protein and provide many other essential nutrients. Even with their excellent nutritional quality, however, these products are not the "perfect" food— nor should they be. No one food can be expected to provide all the nutrients we require; a balanced diet of many different foods is essential for well-being.

Nutrient loss during primary or further processing of poultry is minimal. Aspects of processing that may further enhance the nutritional value of poultry are increasing the utilization of blood, giblets, and bone residue protein; hot-deboning; removal of the abdominal fat pad in ready-to-cook carcasses; and reduction of fat and sodium content in further-processed products.

The primary negative aspect of egg nutrition is the high amount of cholesterol in the yolk. Numerous methods have been proposed to reduce or remove cholesterol from processed egg products. The industry needs to look at these approaches as it develops much-needed, new, egg-based products.

## REFERENCES

Alexander, H. D., E. J. Day, H. E. Sauberlich, and W. D. Salmon. 1956. Radiation effects on water soluble vitamins in raw beef. Fed. Am. Soc. Exp. Biol. Fed. Proc. 15:921.

Ang, C. Y. W., and D. Hamm. 1983. Comparison of commercial processing methods vs. hot deboning of fresh broilers on nutrient content of breast meat. J. Food Sci. 48:1543, 1544, 1565.

Ang, C. Y. W., D. Hamm, and G. K. Searcy. 1982. Changes in nutrient content during chill-holding of ice-packed and deep-chilled broilers. J. Food Sci. 47:1763.

Anonymous. 1986a. Inside stuff. Meat Ind. 32(7):118.

Anonymous. 1986b. Hot dogs. Consumer Reports June, 364.

Baker, R. C., and C. Bruce. 1986. Development of a low cholesterol and low calorie egg blend. Poultry Sci. 65(Suppl. 1):8.

Baker, R. C., and J. M. Darfler. 1977. Functional and organoleptic evaluation of low cholesterol egg blends. Poultry Sci. 56:181.

Baker, R. C., D. Scott-Kline, J. Jutchison, A. Goodman, and J. Charvat. 1986. A pilot plant study of the effect of four cooking methods on acceptability and yields of prebrowned battered and breaded broiler parts. Poultry Sci. 65:1322.

Barbut, S., A. J. Maurer, and R. C. Lindsay. 1986. Effects of reduced sodium chloride and added phosphates on sensory and physical properties of turkey frankfurters. Poultry Sci. 65(Suppl. 1):10.

Bender, A. E. 1978. Food Processing and Nutrition. New York: Academic Press.

Boldt, W. A. 1981 (October 20). Liquid egg blend. U.S. Patent 4,296,134.

Bowers, J. A., and B. A. Fryer. 1972. Thiamine and riboflavin in cooked and frozen, reheated turkey. J. Am. Diet. Assoc. 60:399.

Brasch, A., and W. Huber. 1948. Reduction of undesirable by-effects in products treated by radiation. Science 108:536.

Brekke, C. J., and T. A. Eisele. 1981. The role of modified proteins in the processing of muscle foods. Food Technol. 35(5):231.

Calloway, D. H., E. R. Cole, and H. Spector. 1957. Nutritive value of irradiated turkey. J. Am. Diet. Assoc. 33:1027.

Calvi, B., G. Kasaoka, A. Jarboe, and G. Kuester. 1984a. Animal blood protein as a food ingredient. Memorandum of Screening and Surveillance 3(1):5. Washington, D.C.: U.S. Department of Agriculture.

Calvi, B., G. Kasaoka, A. Jarboe, G. Kuester, and C. Spenser. 1984b. Edible bone protein. Memorandum of Screening and Surveillance 3(3):25. Washington, D.C.: U.S. Department of Agriculture.

Campbell, C. L., T. Y. Lin, and B. E. Proctor. 1958. Microwave vs. conventional chicken. J. Am. Diet. Assoc. 34:365.

Causey, K., M. E. Hausrath, P. E. Ramstad, and I. Fenton. 1950. Effect of thawing and cooking methods on the palatability and nutritive value of frozen ground meat. 2. Beef Food Res. 15:249.

Chang, I. C., and B. M. Watts. 1952. The fatty acid content of meat and poultry before and after cooking. J. Am. Oil Chem. Soc. 29:334.

Cheldelin, V. H., A. M. Woods, and R. J. Williams. 1943. Losses of B vitamins due to cooking of foods. J. Nutr. 26:477.

Childs, R. E., W. K. Whitehead, and E. J. Lloyd. 1976. Automated Blood and Lung Collecting and Handling Systems for Poultry Processing Plants. Marketing Research Report No. 1062. Washington, D.C.: U.S. Department of Agriculture.

Cook, B. B., A. F. Morgan, and M. B. Smith. 1948. Thiamine, riboflavin, and niacin content of turkey tissues as affected by storage and cooking. Food Res. 14:449.

Cotterill, O. J. 1981. A Scientist Speaks about Egg Products. American Egg Board Report No. 1460. Park Ridge, Ill.: American Egg Board.

DeGroot, A. P., L. P. van der Mijll Dekker, P. Slump, H. J. Vos, and J. J. L. Willems. 1972. Composition and Nutritive Value of Radiation-Pasteurized Chicken. Report No. R3787. Zeist, Netherlands: Central Institute for Nutrition and Food Research.

Demby, J. H., and F. E. Cunningham. 1980. Factors affecting composition of chicken meat. A literature review. World Poultry Sci. 36:25.

Diehl, J. F. 1983. Radiolytic effects in food. Ch. 10 in Preservation of Food by Ionizing Radiation, Vol. II, E. S. Josephson and M. S. Peterson, eds. Boca Raton, Fla.: CRC Press.

DuBois, M. W., A. F. Anglemier, M. W. Montgomery, and W. D. Davidson. 1972. Effect of proteolysis on the emulsification characteristics of bovine skeletal muscle. J. Food Sci. 37:27.

Dukes, M. G., and D. M. Janky. 1985. Physical characteristics and sensory evaluation of cooked Pectoralis superficialis from broiler carcasses chilled in water or brine solutions under commercial time and temperature conditions. Poultry Sci. 64:664.

Everson, G. J., and H. J. Souders. 1957. Composition and nutritive importance of eggs. J. Am. Diet. Assoc. 33:1244.

Fioriti, J. A., H. D. Stahl, R. J. Sims, and C. H. Spotholz. 1978 (July 25). Low cholesterol egg product and process. U.S. Patent 4,103,040.

Francis, D. W. 1975. Students learn by experience. Poultry Sci. 54(5):1763.

Franzen, K. L. 1977. Chemically modified food proteins—A research review. P. 101 in Proceedings of the 37th Annual Meeting of the International Food Technologists, Dallas, Tex., June 5–8, 1977. Abstract 89.

Froning, G. W. 1978. Final report of the panel on irradiation of poultry and poultry products. In Food Irradiation in the United States. Interdepartmental Committee on Radiation Preservation. U.S. Army, Natick Research Laboratory.

Froning, G. W., M. Swanson, and H. Benson. 1960. Moisture levels in frozen poultry as related to thawing losses, cooking losses, and palatability. Poultry Sci. 37:328.

Glasser, G. M., and H. Matos. 1976. Low cholesterol egg product and process. U.S. Patent 3,941,892.

Goldblith, S. A., S. R. Tannenbaum, and D. I. C. Wang. 1968. Thermal and 2450 MHz microwave energy effect of the destruction of thiamine. Food Technol. 22:1266.

Goresline, H. E. 1983. Historical aspects of the radiation preservation of food. P. 8 in Preservation of Food by Ionizing Radiation, Vol. I, E. S. Josephson and M. S. Peterson, eds. Boca Raton, Fla.: CRC Press.

Greenwood, D. A., B. W. Beadle, and H. R. Kraybill. 1943. Stability of thiamine to heat. II. Effect of meat curing ingredients in aqueous solution and in meat. J. Biol. Chem. 149:349.

Groninger, H., and A. L. Tappel. 1957. The destruction of thiamine in meats and in aqueous solution by gamma radiation. Food Res. 22:519.

Groninger, H. S., and R. Miller. 1979. Some chemical and nutritional properties of acylated fish protein. J. Agric. Food Chem. 27:949.

Hale, K., and W. Stadelman. 1973. Effects of electrolyte treatments and dry-chilling on yields and tenderness of broilers. Poultry Sci. 52:244.

Hall, K. N., and C. S. Lin. 1981. Effect of cooking rates in electric or microwave oven on cooking losses and retention of thiamine in broilers. J. Food. Sci. 46:1292.

Hand, L. W., R. N. Terrell, and G. C. Smith. 1982. Effects of chloride salts on physical, chemical and sensory properties of frankfurters. J. Food Sci. 47:1800.

Harris, R. S., and H. von Loesecke. 1960. Nutritional Evaluation of Food Processing. Westport, Conn.: AVI Publishing Co.

Hay, J. D., R. W. Currie, and I. H. Wolfe. 1973. Effect of postmortem aging on chicken muscle lipids. J. Food Sci. 38:696.

Hellendoorn, E. W., A. P. deGroot, and P. Slump. 1969. Effect of sterilization and three years storage on the nutritive value of canned prepared meals. Voeding 30:44.

Hodson, A. Z. 1941. Effect of cooking on riboflavin content of chicken meat. Food Res. 6:175.

Hurley, W. C., O. J. Kahlenberg, E. M. Funk, L. G. Maharg, and N. L. Webb. 1958. Factors affecting poultry flavour. 1. Inorganic constituents. Poultry Sci. 37:1436.

Imai, C. 1981. Effects of coating eggs on storage stability. Poultry Sci. 60:2053.

Institute of Food Technologists Expert Panel and Committee on Public Information. 1974. The effects of food processing on nutritional values. Food Technol. 28:77.

Jelen, P., R. A. Lawrence, and M. Cerrone. 1982. Evaluation of alkali extracted chicken protein for use in luncheon meats. Can. Inst. Food Sci. Technol. J. 15:289.

Josephson, E. S., and M. S. Peterson. 1983. Radappertization of meat, poultry, finfish, shellfish and special diets. Ch. 8 in Preservation of Food by Ionizing Radiation, Vol. III, E. S. Josephson and M. S. Peterson, eds. Boca Raton, Fla.: CRC Press.

Kahn, L. N., and G. E. Livingstone. 1970. Effects of heating methods on thiamine retention in fresh or frozen prepared foods. J. Food Sci. 35:3459.

Khan, A. W., and C. P. Lentz. 1965. Influence of prerigor, rigor, and postrigor freezing on drip losses and protein changes in chicken meat. J. Food Sci. 30:787.

Khan, A. W., and L. van den Berg. 1964. Some protein changes during post-mortem tenderization in poultry meat. J. Food Sci. 28:425.

Kijowski, J., and A. Niewiarowicz. 1985. A method of protein extraction from chicken bone residue and the chemical and electrophoretic characteristics of the extract. J. Food Technol. 20:43.

Kolata, G. 1982. Value of low-sodium diets questioned. Science 216:38.

Kotula, A. W., and N. V. Helbacka. 1966. Blood volume of live chickens and influence of slaughter technique on blood loss. Poultry Sci. 45:684.

Larsen, J. E., and G. W. Froning. 1981. Extraction and processing of various components from egg yolk. Poultry Sci. 60:160.

Lawrence, R. A., and P. Jelen. 1982. Formation of lysino-alanine in alkaline extracts of chicken protein. J. Food Prot. 45:923.

Lee, W. T., and L. E. Dawson. 1973. Chicken lipid changes during cooking in fresh and reused cooking oil. J. Food Sci. 38:1232.

Ley, F. J., J. Bleby, M. E. Coates, and J. S. Patterson. 1969. Sterilization of laboratory animal diets using gamma radiation. Lab. Anim. 3:221.

Marriot, N. G., A. Lopez, and H. L. Williams. 1982. Essential elements in unprocessed and processed frankfurters. J. Food Prot. 45(8):707.

Mast, M. G., and C. S. Clouser. 1985. The effect of further processing on the nutritive value of poultry products. P. 219 in Proceedings from 7th European Symposium on Poultry Meat Quality, T. Ambrosen, ed. Vejle, Denmark, May 6–10, 1985.

Mast, M. G., and J. H. MacNeil. 1983. Effect of kosher vs. conventional processing on yield, quality, and acceptability of broiler chickens. J. Food Sci. 48:1013.

Mast, M. G., and J. O. Opiacha. 1987. Extraction of protein from bone residue now feasible. Poultry 3(5):17, 18.

Maurer, A. J. 1983. Can sodium be reduced in poultry products? Turkey World (July-August):34.

McMullen, E. A., and J. P. Cassilly. 1976. Thiamine and riboflavin retention in meats cooked uncovered and in oven film. Home Econ. Res. J. 5(1):34.

Melnick, D. 1971 (February 16). Low cholesterol dried egg yolk and process. U.S. Patent 3,563,765.

Melnick, D., M. I. Wegner, and D. R. Davis. 1971 (July 20). Egg food product and process for the preparation thereof. U.S. Patent 3,594,183.

Millares, R., and C. R. Fellers. 1949. Vitamin and amino acid content of processed chicken meat. Food Res. 14:131.

Miller, C. F., D. G. Guadagni, and S. Kon. 1973. Vitamin retention in bean products; cooked, canned, and instant bean powders. J. Food Sci. 38:493.

Morgan, A. F., L. E. Kidder, M. Hunner, B. D. Sharokh, and R. M. Chesbro. 1949. Thiamine, riboflavin, and niacin content of chicken tissues as affected by cooking and frozen storage. Food Res. 14:439.

Mott, E. L., J. H. MacNeil, M. G. Mast, and R. M. Leach. 1982. Protein efficiency ratio and amounts of selected nutrients in mechanically deboned spent layer meat. J. Food Sci. 47(2):655.

Mountney, G. J. 1976. P. 285 in Poultry Products Technology, 2nd ed. Westport, Conn.: AVI Publishing Co.

Mulley, E. A., C. R. Stumbo, and W. M. Hunting. 1975. Thiamine: A chemical index of the sterilization efficacy of thermal processing. J. Food Sci. 40:993.

Myers, S. J., and N. D. Harris. 1975. Effect of electronic cooking on fatty acids in meat. J. Am. Diet. Assoc. 67:232.

Nakai, Y., and T. C. Chen. 1984. Effects of coating preparation methods on yields and compositions of deep-fat fried chicken parts. Poultry Sci. 65:307.

Navidi, M. K., and F. A. Kummerow. 1974. Nutritional value of Egg Beaters compared with farm fresh eggs. Pediatrics 53(4):565.

Olson, F. C. 1970. Nutritional aspects of offal proteins. P. 23 in Proceedings of the Meat Industry Research Conference. Chicago, Ill.: American Meat Institute Foundation.

Opiacha, J. O., J. Kijowski, and M. G. Mast. 1986. Functional properties of protein extracted from mechanically deboned poultry bone residue. P. 104 in the 46th Annual Institute of Food Technologists Meeting Abstracts, J. B. Klif, ed. Chicago, Ill.: Institute of Food Technologists.

Pippen, E. L., and A. A. Klose. 1955. Effects of ice water chilling on flavor of chicken. Poultry Sci. 34:1139.

Post, R. C. 1984. Variables in broiler production and processing in the U.S.A. which influence yields and nutrient composition of carcasses sold at the retail level. World Poultry Sci. 41:240.

Powers, J. M., and M. G. Mast. 1980. Quality differences in simulated kosher and conventionally processed chicken. J. Food Sci. 45:760.

Proctor, B. E., J. T. R. Nickerson, C. Campbell, and J. J. Licciardello. 1956. Annual Report on Contract No. DA-19-129-QM-521. Chicago, Ill.: Quartermaster Food and Container Institute for the Armed Forces.

Przybyla, A. 1985. Prepared chicken items offer versatility, low cost. Prepared Foods 154(8):159.

Putnam, J. J., and K. Reidy. 1981. Sodium: Why the concern? Natl. Food Rev. NFR-15:27.

Rowe, D. M., G. J. Mountney, and I. Prudent. 1963. Effect of freeze drying on the thiamine, riboflavin, and niacin content of chicken muscle. Food Technol. 17:1449.

Ryan, J. R., and E. W. Kienholz. 1979. Comparison of whole egg to Egg Beaters as a source of dietary protein. Nutr. Rep. Int. 19(3):363.

Satterlee, L. D. 1981. Proteins for use in foods. Food Technol. 35(6):53.

Schoenhauser, E., R. Schoenhauser, and A. Blumenthal. 1980. Digestibility of the proteins of different types of poultry meat. Nutr. Abstr. Rev. 41(11):7669.

Scholtyssek, S., P. Heimbach, and H. Berner. 1970. Investigation into new methods of chilling poultry. IV. Investigation of carcass quality. Fleishwirtschaft 50:77.

Seeley, R. D. 1974 (October 22). Low fat egg product. U.S. Patent 3,843,811.

Seeley, R. D., and R. B. Seeley. 1980 (April 29). Cholesterol-free egg product having improved cooking tolerance. U.S. Patent 4,200,663.

Seeley, R. D., H. J. Hartmann, and D. R. Sodoti. 1976 (October 19). Cholesterol free egg product. U.S. Patent 3,987,212.

Sheffner, A. L., R. Adachi, and H. Spector. 1957. The effect of radiation processing upon the in vitro digestibility and nutritional quality of proteins. Food Res. 22:455.

Sheldon, B. W., E. O. Essary, K. P. Bovard, and R. W. Young. 1980. Effect of endpoint cooking temperature upon the nutritive value and composition of turkey meat. Poultry Sci. 59:2725.

Singh, S. P., and E. O. Essary. 1971. Vitamin content of broiler meat as affected by age, sex, thawing and cooking. Poultry Sci. 50:1150.

Smith, D. M., and C. J. Brekke. 1984. Functional Properties of enzymatically modified beef heart protein. J. Food Sci. 37:604.

Smith, D. M., and C. J. Brekke. 1985a. Enzymatic modification of the structure and functional properties of mechanically deboned fowl proteins. J. Agric. Food Chem. 33:631.

Smith, D. M., and C. J. Brekke. 1985b. Characteristics of low-salt frankfurters produced with enzyme-modified mechanically deboned fowl. J. Food Sci. 50:308.

Somers, I. I., R. P. Farrow, and J. M. Reed. 1974. Influence of storage and distribution upon vitamin-mineral content and biological availability in processed foods. Ch. 6 in Nutrients in Processed Foods: Vitamins, Minerals. Acton, Mass.: American Medical Association Publishing Sciences Group.

Spinelli, J., B. Koury, and R. Miller. 1972. Approaches to the utilization of fish for the preparation of protein isolates. Enzymatic modifications of myofibrillar fish proteins. J. Food Sci. 37:604.

Stadelman, W. J. 1985. This chicken product breaks "grease barrier." Broiler Ind. 48:46.

Stevenson, T. R., and G. T. Lloyd. 1979. Better uses for abattoir blood. Agric. Gaz. N.S. Wales 90:42.

Tan, C. T., G. P. Howard, and E. W. Turner. 1982 (November 23). Lipoprotein emulsions for food use and methods for improving the same. U.S. Patent 4,360,537.

Thomas, M. H., and D. H. Calloway. 1961. Nutritional value of dehydrated foods. J. Am. Diet. Assoc. 39:105.

Thomas, M. H., and E. S. Josephson. 1970. Radiation preservation of foods and its effects on nutrients. Sci. Teacher 37:53.

Tokarska, B., and M. T. Clandinin. 1985. Extraction of egg yolk oil of reduced cholesterol content. Can. Inst. Food Sci. Technol. J. 18:256.

U.S. Department of Agriculture. 1986. Poultry Slaughter. Crop Reporting Board, SRS. February. Washington, D.C.: Agricultural Statistics Board.

Warner, W. D., P. N. Abell, P. E. Mone, C. E. Poling, and E. E. Rice. 1962. Nutritional value of fats in cooked meats. J. Am. Diet. Assoc. 40:422.

West, L. C., M. C. Titus, and F. O. VanDuyne. 1959. Effect of freezer storage and variations in preparation on bacterial count, palatability, and thiamine content of ham loaf, Italian rice, and chicken. Food Technol. 13:323.

Wing, R. W., and J. C. Alexander. 1972. Effect of microwave heating on vitamin B retention in chicken. J. Am. Diet. Assoc. 61:661.

Wismer-Pederson, J. 1979. Utilization of animal blood in meat products. Food Technol. 33:76.

Young, C. R., R. W. Lewis, W. A. Landmann, and C. W. Dill. 1973. Nutritive value of globin and plasma fractions from bovine blood. Nutr. Rep. Int. 8:211.

Young, L. L. 1976. Composition and properties of animal protein isolate prepared from bone residue. J. Food Sci. 41:606.

# Possible Impacts of Changes in USDA Grade Standards and Labeling/Identification Procedures

G. C. SMITH

U.S. Department of Agriculture (USDA) grades for carcasses of red meat animals are based on criteria presumed to be related to palatability (flavor, juiciness, and tenderness) of the meat when cooked and on estimations of relative cutability (yield of trimmed cuts from the carcass). Nomenclature for the grading systems is not identical for beef, pork, and lamb; but, in general, words (for example, Prime, Choice) are used to characterize palatability and numbers (for example, 1, 4) are used to indicate cutability.

Relative palatability assessments for beef and lamb are assigned by USDA graders using a hierarchical arrangement of word descriptors wherein the USDA quality grade names—Prime, Choice, Good/Select, and Standard for beef; Prime, Choice, Good, and Utility for lamb—indicate the relative level of palatability or the relative probability that a specific piece of meat will be flavorful, juicy, and tender. A leg roast from a U.S. Prime grade lamb should be more flavorful, juicy, and tender than a leg roast from a U.S. Choice grade lamb; the probability of obtaining a steak that is bland, dry, and tough should be greater if it is from a U.S. Good/Select grade beef carcass

than if the steak is from a U.S. Prime grade beef carcass. Pork quality is not equated hierarchically. Rather, a bipartite system is used in which quality is judged to be either "acceptable" (in which case the carcass is assigned the grade prefix "U.S." and a number—1 through 4—depending on its relative cutability) or "unacceptable" (in which case the carcass is assigned the grade designation U.S. Utility, regardless of its relative cutability, and thus there is no numerical suffix).

The USDA meat grading service for red meat animals was instituted as a means for setting and reporting prices of commodities in the wholesale meat trade. It eventually evolved to facilitate trading in live animals and merchandising of retail cuts. Meat grading was made compulsory under the Office of Price Administration during World War II and then again, under the Office of Price Stabilization during the Korean conflict, but not between those periods or since. In 1946, the program was authorized by the Agricultural Marketing Act and was made voluntary; packers who wished to use the grading service had to pay for it. The grades, assigned by USDA graders acting in the role of a third party, identify the quality/ cutability of meat for wholesalers and retailers who purchase it without previously viewing it. In 1984, 65.1 percent of steer and heifer beef (53.3 percent of total beef) in the U.S. federally inspected slaughter was officially graded and stamped; of that, 3 percent was Prime, 93 percent was Choice, and 4 percent was Good, while 3 percent was yield grade 1, 42 percent was yield grade 2, 49 percent was yield grade 3, and 5 percent was yield grade 4. Of the 12 billion pounds of red meat (beef, lamb, calf, and veal) that was officially graded and stamped in 1984, more than 90 percent was beef.

Assurance of wholesomeness and freedom from disease attributed to red meat by USDA inspection does not relate to its grade, but USDA grades are assigned only if a carcass has passed inspection. USDA policy is that beef, pork, and lamb can be graded only as carcasses to ensure that grading decisions are accurate and consistent; thus, grading is done only at the slaughter site. Once the meat has been cut up and packaged for sale, its equivalent carcass grade cannot be determined.

Cutability ("yield") grades are in numerical order: USDA yield grade 1 signifies the highest comparative cutability (yield of closely trimmed wholesale or retail cuts as a percentage of carcass weight); yield grade 4 for pork carcasses or 5 for lamb and beef carcasses denotes the lowest relative cutability. For pork and beef carcasses, the USDA quality and yield grades are said to be "coupled"; that is, neither grade can be assigned without the other. The grading systems are "uncoupled" for lamb carcasses; a lamb carcass can be assigned a quality grade, a yield grade, or both quality and yield grades. In practice, lamb carcasses are seldom yield graded because the industry does not use yield grades in the determination of trading price.

Trading of cattle and sheep and beef, lamb, and mutton carcasses and wholesale cuts relies heavily on USDA quality/yield grading. For example, price quotations for cattle coming from the feedlot to a slaughter plant are usually set by specifying a price per hundred-weight for animals that are described using a four-part (live weight, sex class, quality grade, yield grade) system (for example, 1,125 pounds, steers, Choice, yield grade 3). Because descriptions of market animals depend heavily on subjective evaluations of live weight, quality grade, and yield grade, market reporters often use ranges in weight, the sex class, an estimated percentage expected to grade U.S. Choice, and a generalization about yield grades (for example, 1,075 to 1,200 pounds, steers, 65 percent Choice, mostly yield grade 2's with a few yield grade 4's). Swine and lambs are similarly described for market reporting purposes; in fact, grades are much more useful for describing live pigs and lambs than for facilitating trading of their carcasses.

When it is to the advantage of the seller, the USDA quality grade is used to merchandise the commodity. Certain restaurants, steakhouses, supermarkets, and the like advertise and identify beef or lamb that is U.S. Prime or U.S. Choice, but terminology related to USDA quality grade is never specified for pork. USDA quality grade names are imprinted, using purple ink, on the surface of beef carcasses and lamb carcasses, but essentially are never imprinted on pork carcasses.

To imprint the USDA grade name, a round metal wheel (known as a grade roll) with a series of identical official USDA shields on its outer surface is continuously coated with purple ink and used to mark the carcass at strategic locations. The wheel is rolled down the length of the carcass and across it so that the USDA stamp appears on almost every solid-muscle retail cut that can be obtained from that carcass. (A beef ribeye roll is a solid-muscle retail cut but would not show the grade roll without special care.) Beef and lamb carcasses that are not officially graded are described in meat trade vernacular as "No-Roll" carcasses. Pork carcasses are almost never graded for quality or yield and are not often sold as intact carcasses to wholesalers and retailers because so many of the cuts—for example, the belly, jowl, picnic shoulder, ham, and clear plate—are usually cured and smoked before retail sale and because the two major wholesale cuts (Boston butt and loin) that are sold fresh (unprocessed) have heavy layers of subcutaneous fat and skin that are removed before preparation of retail cuts.

Essentially all beef and lamb carcasses are presented to USDA officials for grading; but only those that qualify for merchantable grades—Prime and Choice quality grades and, for beef, 1, 2, and 3 yield grades—are normally identified with official grade stamps. Over the years, quality grade names of Good/Select, Standard, and Utility have come to signify inferior quality; and yield grade designations of 4 and 5 result in punitive price discounts, so packers seldom if ever allow such words or numbers to be affixed to carcasses. Most packers have a category of carcasses that they call No-Roll and they attempt to merchandise the conglomerate as one kind of carcass. Depending on company policy, carcasses from young intact males (bullocks or lambs) and carcasses from females of advanced age ("heiferettes" or young cows and yearling ewes, for example) may also be included in the product mix of No-Rolls; as a result, the palatability and cutability of No-Roll beef and lamb may be quite variable within and between lots and over time.

USDA quality grades for beef carcasses are based on evaluations of (1) the estimated physiological age of the animal at the time of slaughter, called "maturity" and assessed by looking at the color and texture of the exposed ribeye muscle (longissimus dorsi muscle exposed by cutting between the 12th and 13th ribs of the carcass), and by evaluating the amount of ossification of cartilage

in the skeletal system and (2) the estimated amount and distribution of intramuscular fat (called "marbling") in the exposed ribeye muscle. The more youthful the carcass and the more heavily marbled the ribeye muscle, the higher the USDA quality grade for beef.

USDA quality grades for lamb carcasses are based on evaluations of (1) the estimated physiological age of the animal at the time of slaughter, called "maturity" and assessed by looking at the color of muscles on the interior surfaces of the body cavity and by evaluating color and shape of rib bones and ossification of the cannon bones; (2) the amount and distribution of streaks of fat across the surface of the primary flank muscle (in the abdominal cavity of the carcass), which is an indirect estimate of the amount of marbling expected in the ribeye muscle; and (3) the conformation of the carcass, evaluated as the width, bulge, and plumpness of muscles and thus of the muscle/bone ratio of the carcass. The more youthful the carcass, the more extensive the streakings of fat in the flank, and the higher the muscle/bone ratio, the higher the USDA quality grade for lamb.

Quality is assessed for pork carcasses based on evaluations of (1) acceptability of the belly for bacon production, determined by its thickness and firmness; (2) color of the muscles on the interior surfaces of the body cavity; (3) firmness of the fat and lean throughout the carcass; and (4) the amount and distribution of streaks of fat across the surfaces of the primary flank, secondary flank, and intercostal muscles. If the belly is firm and thick, the muscles grayish pink or darker, the fat and lean at least slightly firm, and the fat streaking present in at least Slight amounts, the carcass is considered "acceptable" in quality and is then yield graded. The crux of the quality grading systems for carcasses of red meat animals is intramuscular fat content (the higher the fat content in the muscles, the higher the quality grade), because marbling improves the chance that the meat will be flavorful, juicy, and tender when cooked.

USDA yield grades for beef carcasses are based on evaluations of (1) carcass weight; (2) surface area of the ribeye muscle at the juncture of the 12th and 13th ribs; (3) thickness of external fat at the specified point over the ribeye exposed in the cross-sectional surface exposed between the 12th and 13th ribs; and (4) the estimated percentage weight as kidney, pelvic, and heart fat. At a given carcass weight, the larger the ribeye, the less the external fat thickness; and the lower the percentage of kidney/pelvic/heart fat, then the lower the yield grade number (thus, the higher the cutability).

USDA yield grades for lamb carcasses are based on evaluations of (1) bulge and plumpness of muscles in the leg, (2) thickness of external fat at the specified point opposite the ribeye muscle between the 12th and 13th ribs, and (3) the estimated percentage of carcass weight as kidney and pelvic fat. The more muscular the leg, the less the external fat thickness; and the lower the percentage of kidney and pelvic fat, the lower the yield grade number (thus, the higher the cutability; in other words, the greater the amount of the carcass that can be sold as trimmed, boneless cuts).

Cutability in pork carcasses is determined by assessments of (1) length or weight of the carcass, (2) thickness of external fat at the specified point on the midline of the carcass, and (3) bulge and plumpness of muscles in the carcass. At a given carcass weight or length, the less the external fat thickness and the more muscular the carcass, the lower the yield grade number (thus, the higher the cutability; in other words, the greater the amount of the carcass that can be sold as partially trimmed, bone-in, ham/loin/shoulder). The crux of the yield grading systems for carcasses of red meat animals is the muscle/fat ratio—the higher the fat content of the carcass (as external, seam, and body cavity depots), the higher the yield grade number (thus, the lower the cutability). Yield grade predicts the amount of the carcass that will be salable as wholesale (pork) or retail (beef and lamb) cuts and is intended for use by the packer, wholesaler, and retailer but never by the consumer (since by the time the consumer sees the piece of meat, its excess fat has been removed).

Although the USDA quality and yield grade systems may appear to be paradoxical—one (quality grade) encourages fatness, the other (yield grade) penalizes fatness—it must be understood that fat is deposited in an animal's body in a number of specific anatomical locations called fat depots and that the depots are filled with fat in an ordered sequence. The fat depots are (1) the mesenteric region—around the stomach and intestines; (2) those adhering to the thoracic/abdominal/pelvic cavities—around the heart as a sac, around the kidney as a capsule, and lining the pelvic cavity; (3) the subcutaneous region—under the skin of the live animal and over the external surfaces of the skinned carcass; (4) the intermuscular seam areas—between two muscles and between a muscle and bone/cartilage; and (5) the intramuscular sites—within muscles. Accumulation of fat in depots (1), (2), (3), and (4) listed above is of little or no consequence in assessing prospective flavor, juiciness, or tenderness of the muscles from that carcass; deposition of fat as marbling, in fat depot (5) above, is positively related to palatability of cooked beef, pork, and lamb. Unfortunately, in most red meat animals, deposition of fat in depots 1 through 4 occurs earlier in the animal's life than deposition of fat as marbling, so that generally by the time the animal has deposited enough intramuscular fat to qualify for the highest USDA quality grades, it has deposited too much fat in the body cavity, between the muscles, and over the exterior of the skinned carcass to have desirable composition (proportions of muscle and fat). Also, as animals are fed high-concentrate diets for progressively longer periods of time to increase chances that they will have enough marbling to grade Choice or Prime (for lamb or beef, but not for pork), their yield grade suffers because of a greater probability that the trimmable fats are present in excessive quantities.

The USDA quality grading system per se can be a deterrent to increasing leanness of beef cattle and their carcasses because in certain market situations it encourages overfattening. Such is not the case for lambs, because they can attain the Choice grade without ever having been fed grain, or for swine, because the pork grading system is not hierarchical and it is not used by the trade to determine prices. For beef, Choice carcasses are worth 1 to 3 cents more per pound ($6 to $24 per carcass) than Good/Select carcasses most of the time, but—at times—can be worth substantially more than Good/Select carcasses, with premiums for Choice sometimes reaching 7 to 11 cents per pound ($42 to $88 per carcass). Such differences, though they occur infrequently, provide incentive to overfeed cattle.

For some breeds or crossbreeds of cattle and for some lines/strains within breeds and crossbreeds, increasing the time-on-feed will result in increased deposition of marbling, but there are cattle that do not have the inherent ability to deposit intramuscular fat and that will not achieve the level of marbling needed to qualify for the Choice grade regardless of length of feeding period. In these cases, it is futile to extend time-on-feed in the hope of increasing value by improving the USDA quality grade. Rather, the cattle simply get fatter in depots that detract from leanness, lower the yield grade number, and make the end product less acceptable to consumers.

However, lengthening time-on-feed almost always increases the "dressing percentage" (the ratio of carcass weight to live weight, expressed in percentage points) for cattle, swine, and lambs, regardless of their genetic capability to respond to feeding by depositing more intramuscular or superficial streaks of fat. The extent to which meat packers encourage producers to lengthen time-on-feed in order to (1) increase the number of animals achieving a certain USDA quality grade versus (2) increase dressing percentage and thereby decrease the cost per pound of the carcass differs depending on the genetics of the livestock involved and cannot be precisely assessed because quality grade and dressed yield are highly related to each other.

When buyers for meat packers purchase cattle, sheep, and swine on a live-animal basis, they do so by deciding on a price per pound alive that will minimize the cost per pound of the carcass and that is still high enough to beat out other buyers. Price determination starts with estimations of carcass value plus drop (edible and inedible offal) value minus cost to slaughter/fabricate; that sum is divided by estimated carcass weight to obtain carcass value per pound. The price a buyer will then pay per pound for a live animal is determined by multiplying carcass value per pound times the dressing percentage; as the dressing percentage increases, the price paid increases. Knowing that the dressing percentage increases as the fatness of the animal increases, the buyer will push for greater fatness (by encouraging that the animals be fed longer) up to, and sometimes beyond, the point at which a yield grade line (between 3 and 4, for example) will be crossed at a punitive discount. For example, suppose a buyer evaluates a pen of lambs that he estimates will have a dressing percentage of 50. If he bids 75 cents per pound for the live animals and they dress 50 percent, the carcasses will have cost him—hanging on the rail—$1.50 per pound. If he believes the lambs could be fed an additional 3 weeks without becoming yield grade 4's and—because they are much fatter—dress 54 percent, he will encourage the producer to feed them longer, because although he will still pay 75 cents per pound alive, he can rail the carcasses at a cost of $1.39 per pound. Unfortunately, though, the composition of the carcasses of lambs fed for the additional 3 weeks will have suffered greatly. The same scenario applies for beef; additional time-on-feed to increase dressing percentage and decrease carcass cost has been abetted by the fact that, until very recently, primal cuts of beef moved freely in the trade with as much as 1 inch of external fat covering.

If dressing percentage (and carcass cost) could somehow be removed from the pricing logic currently used for the purchasing of red meat animals, the incentive to feed the animal longer would be greatly lessened. In fact, the practice of fattening the animal to increase dressing percentage has worked only because wholesalers and retailers tolerated the additional fat knowing they could pass it along to their customers, the end product consumer. As that changes—and it is doing so rapidly with the advent of quarter-inch fat trim at retail and adoption of three-eighths to one-half inch fat trim at the packer level—the impetus to minimize carcass cost by encouraging overfattening to improve dressing percentage will decline. Indeed, the dressing percentage/carcass cost pricing logic used routinely in the trading of live red meat animals is a deterrent to improving leanness, as are the USDA quality grading standards. So long as feeders demand to sell cattle on a live weight basis—rather than on the basis of carcass grade and weight—dressed yield/carcass cost is an imperative component of the pricing system.

There remains incentive to increase the fatness of red meat animals if it is true that as fatness increases, the flavor, juiciness, and tenderness of cooked meat improves. There is, however, enough genetic variability among swine, sheep, and cattle to make it possible to select animals that will deposit marbling in the muscles to a degree sufficient to qualify them for the U.S. Choice

or even Prime grades without having deposited excessive quantities of subcutaneous, intermuscular, or kidney/pelvic/heart fat. Also, U.S. consumers are attuned to the presence of certain quantities of fat intermingled with lean such that "acceptable" or superior palatability in beef, pork, and lamb depends on deposition of marbling in specific amounts. This is especially the case for customers in hotel, restaurant, and food service establishments who, because they pay high prices for a meal, expect consistently high palatability in the meat they are served. Therefore, meat purveyors sell Prime or Choice beef and lamb to restaurateurs and food-service-unit operators who serve affluent clientele. Because such products are in limited supply yet in substantive demand, their prices are higher than those of beef and lamb of lower quality grades. Price incentives encourage packers and feeders to strive to produce beef of the highest grades. For most animals, the likelihood that they will grade Prime or Choice is improved with increased feeding time. That being the case, cattle producers will—especially if grain prices are low—feed their cattle longer than is economically optimal from growth, efficiency, and carcass composition standpoints, striving for the minimum intramuscular fatness required to achieve the U.S. Choice grade. The Choice grade is achieved in beef when a chemical fat level of about 4.3 percent is attained in the longissimus dorsi, or "ribeye," muscle. That fatness level is very low and well within caloric constraints for a healthful diet. However, by the time—chronologically or in time-on-feed—that the 4.3 percent intramuscular fat level is attained, the entire carcass will be composed of 25 to 40 percent fat (subcutaneous, intermuscular, intramuscular, and kidney/pelvic/heart). Because deposition of fat in subcutaneous, intermuscular, and kidney/pelvic/heart regions usually precedes deposition of fat as marbling, feeding cattle to achieve some set point in marbling deposition will far too often result in production of carcasses that are excessively fat.

A possible way to reduce the overall fatness of lamb and beef carcasses is to lower the marbling requirement for each USDA quality grade. If, for example, the minimum marbling requirement for the U.S. Choice grade in beef were reduced from 4.3 percent (described as a Small amount of marbling in official USDA quality grade standards) to 3.0 percent (a Slight amount), time-on-feed could be reduced by about 30 days and percentage of fat in the carcass by about 10 percentage points. However, this solution ignores the fact that beef of 3.0 to 4.3 percent intramuscular fatness is currently available (as USDA Good/Select grade beef) yet has found only limited consumer demand.

The National Cattlemen's Association (NCA) concluded in January 1986 that (1) consumers want lean beef regardless of USDA quality grade, (2) changing the USDA beef quality grading standards is not a prerequisite for producing leaner beef, (3) the retail consumer market is segmented between those who emphasize taste and those who emphasize leanness, (4) combining the Choice and Good/Select grades into one grade would reduce the industry's ability to market beef effectively to either market segment, and (5) any attempt to change the USDA beef quality grading standards will be interpreted by consumers as negative. In 1981, NCA asked USDA to allow part of the Good/Select grade of beef to be designated Choice (because such beef was leaner but still tasty); USDA rejected the idea partly because of opposition by some retailers, consumers, and cattle producers but largely because of opposition by restaurateurs and purveyors as well as consumer groups who contended that the proposal was a ploy to sell lean meat at higher prices.

Nevertheless, for more than 10 years consumer advocates have been calling for a change in the USDA beef quality grading standards so that the system will not discriminate against leaner beef. Additional consumer efforts have called for a complete overhaul of USDA grades to reflect nutritional content of meat rather than the subjective characteristics of taste. In 1974, the National Consumers League recommended that the USDA beef quality grading system be modified so that one additional grade designation be added between Choice and Good/Select in order to "encourage the production and marketing of leaner beef which uses less grain, costs less to produce, and at the same time would allow prices to reflect this producer-cost reduction." Six years later, the Community Nutrition Institute stated that "the marketplace is ready and eager to accept a leaner, cheaper beef that must be promoted without imposing subjective opinions of eating pleasure" and that "the discrimination against lean beef inherent in the nomenclature of the present system could be eliminated by developing a new grade name [they suggested 'USDA Choice Lean,' 'USDA Choice Light,' or 'USDA Lean Choice'] to replace USDA Good." In February 1986, the Public Voice for Food and Health Policy suggested that USDA could either create a new grade (e.g., "Choice Lean," "Leaner Choice") that is lower in fat than Choice but that is clearly palatable and that could perhaps replace Choice, or restructure the entire quality grading system to reflect nutritional content of the meat.

In the 1985 National Consumer Retail Beef Study, beef of two quality levels was offered to participants (U.S. Choice as Choice and U.S. Good as Select). Overall acceptability of the two kinds of beef was the same, but for different reasons. Consumers who preferred Choice beef did so because of its advantages in palatability, while those who preferred Select beef did so because of its advantages in leanness. Choice beef was recognized as being somewhat fatter and Select beef as somewhat less desirable in palatability; yet consumers preferring each type of beef were willing to make the trade-off to achieve the attribute most important to them. (A more thorough discussion of the National Consumer Retail Beef Study is given by Savell and Cross in this volume.)

Results of the National Consumer Retail Beef Study were sufficiently encouraging to prompt the Public Voice for Food and Health Policy to petition USDA to "change the name of the 'Good' federal beef grade to reflect that it is leaner than 'Prime' or 'Choice' and to stop discrimination against lean beef." Public Voice asked that the word "Select" replace the word "Good" as a grade name for beef carcasses having a Slight amount of marbling and thus containing 3.0 to 4.3 percent fat in the longissimus dorsi muscle. The USDA ruled in late September 1987 to implement the name change from Good to Select, effective November 23, 1987.

The National Academy of Sciences (NAS) Committee on Technological Options for Nutritional Improvements in the Food Supply with Emphasis on Animal Products concluded that such change in grade nomenclature—though purely semantic—would be in the best interest of all concerned. At present, essentially no beef is officially identified as U.S. Good; as a result, those who might wish to buy such beef cannot find it so identified. Packers sell the equivalent of U.S. Good beef as a part of the No-Roll category, for which there is no minimum quality indicator (marbling or maturity) level. As a result, no true test of the acceptability of Good grade beef to consumers can be achieved because the beef is in a mixture of the commodity (No-Rolls) that is highly variable in palatability.

In May 1986, the American Meat Institute supported the Public Voice objective of changing the nomenclature of the Good grade to give leaner beef a more positive image. The NAS committee also considered recommending changes in the U.S. standards for beef grading that would parallel those made in 1972 by Canada. The Canadians premised their changes in beef grading on the following conclusions: (1) Although fatness helps to ensure tenderness and flavor, beef does not have to be fat to be flavorful and tender; (2) it is wasteful and inefficient to produce overfat cattle only to have their carcasses trimmed to retail standards; (3) a potent force encouraging excess fatness is the obvious desire of packer buyers to purchase cattle as cheaply as possible on the rail by increasing dressing percentages so as to lower carcass cost; and (4) changes in cattle through breeding would be a long and difficult process and rapid changes in carcass characteristics through changes in cattle feeding are unlikely, so by far the most important change that could be made—a change that would result in an immediate and dramatic response—would be to "harvest" the cattle as they reach the point of optimum finish. Before 1972, the Canadian beef carcass grading system was similar to that currently used in the United States; in 1972, the Canadians adopted a system based on dual grading. This system consists of five quality/maturity designations (A, B, C, D, E) and four subgrades (1, 2, 3, 4) based on single fat thickness measurements taken opposite the ribeye muscle between the 11th and 12th ribs. Since implementation of those grade standards, the percentage of beef carcasses grading A-1 has increased from about 32 percent in 1972 to about 52 percent in 1986. The primary difference between quality grading in Canada versus that in the United States is the essential disregard of marbling as a grade-determining factor in the Canadian system.

The NAS committee received testimony from Canadian officials acknowledging that they have a perceived and possibly real problem with unsatisfactory tenderness, juiciness, and flavor of their beef and that this inadequacy in eating satisfaction may well be the result of ignoring marbling in determining quality grade. Much of the beef sold to the food service trade in Canada is Prime or Choice beef produced in the United States. Therefore, the NAS committee could not support any change that would eliminate marbling as a grade-determining factor and thereby eliminate the ability of the industry to differentiate beef of the present Prime, Choice, Good/Select, and Standard grades. Because some consumers want and are willing to pay for a product having the characteristics of and identified as Prime or Choice, it is best to continue such identification protocol. As long as products are identified as such, consumers can find them and select or reject them—thereby exercising their right to an option in the marketplace.

A goal, then, of the NAS committee was to ensure that American consumers have the opportunity to exercise personal informed choice in the selection of foods to include in their diet and that such choices are identifiable and available. A review of the research at the Texas Agricultural Experiment Station (reported in more detail by Savell and Cross in this volume) indicates that a minimum level of 3 percent chemical fat in the ribs and loins of cattle, swine, and sheep is necessary to ensure acceptable palatability in beef, pork, and lamb. They contend that, in terms of nutritional merit, the maximum level of intramuscular fat that should be in the rib and loin cuts is 7.0 percent. A "window of acceptability" (3.0 to 7.0 percent intramuscular fat) is thus created that considers diet/health/nutrition as well as flavor/juiciness/tenderness factors. Within that window are two other thresholds of chemical fatness associated with progressive increases in palatability—at approximately 5 percent chemical fat (midpoint of the Small amount of marbling) and at approximately 7 percent chemical fat (at the lower end of the Moderate amount of marbling).

These hierarchical rankings in palatability associated with increasing levels of intramuscular fatness would allow segmentation of the beef, pork, and lamb supplies into expected palatability groupings that would facilitate targeting and servicing the wants and needs of a segmented consumer market

with varying tastes. Identification of beef with 3.0 to 4.3 percent intramuscular fatness with a new grade designation—Select—will make it possible for those who seek beef of that kind to find it and might encourage grocers/restaurateurs to stock it. Because this change will create "identifiable consumer choices" and give customers the option to buy leaner beef in the marketplace, the committee encourages merchants to promote the sale of Select beef as an alternative or adjunct to beef of the Choice grade. If beef of that fatness level is acceptable to consumers, its production will be encouraged by price, encouraging a supply commensurate with the demand expressed at that price.

The committee evaluated the trend toward promotion of red meat products labeled "Natural" and "Light" (with the variant "Lite"). The exact implications of such claims are in the purview of the USDA Standards and Labeling Division, Food Safety and Inspection Service (FSIS). While the term "Natural" is being promoted by some elements of the industry as representing meat from animals that have not been exposed to drugs, growth promotants, hormones, antibiotics, pesticides, or feed additives and—by others—as representing meat from animals that are reared in open spaces (as opposed to feedlots) and fed forages/roughages (rather than grains), such connotation is not codified in state or federal regulations. USDA FSIS Policy Memo 055 states that the term "Natural" may be used on the label of meat and poultry products providing that (1) the product does not contain any artificial flavoring, coloring ingredient, chemical preservatives, or any other artificial or synthetic ingredient and (2) the product and its ingredients are not more than minimally processed ("minimal processing" may include smoking, roasting, freezing, drying, fermenting, and grinding). This being the case, all fresh red meat could be labeled "Natural."

The committee considers present use of

the term "Natural" by certain producers/processors to connote that meat from animals produced by use of health and growth/efficiency aids is somehow unnatural and thus unhealthy to be misleading and inappropriate. Because it is not in the best interest of the consumer to create unwarranted fear about the safety/healthfulness of the food supply, the committee recommends that use of the term "Natural," in the manner that some promoters now use it, not be allowed.

By the same token, the terms "Light" and "Lean" are being used inappropriately by some elements of private enterprise to imply superiority in leanness when such is not the case. USDA FSIS Policy Memos 070A and 070B state that the terms "Lean" and "Low Fat" can be used only on meat and poultry products containing less than 10 percent fat and that the terms "Light," "Leaner," and "Lower Fat" can be used only on products that contain at least 25 percent less fat than the majority of such products in the marketplace. Before issuance of these policy memoranda, fat claims such as "Light," "Lean," and "Extra Lean" could be used interchangeably on meat and poultry products containing 25 percent less fat than a comparable product and on products containing no more than 10 percent fat. The committee is concerned about the use of descriptive adjectives like "Light," when verification of relative fatness/leanness is made at the carcass level (comparing carcass traits of two kinds of beef, pork, or lamb), because retail cuts from fat or lean carcasses can be either fat or lean (and not different from each other) after fabrication and trimming at the retail level. The committee strongly urges USDA not to allow certification as "Light" or "Lean" on the basis of carcass data and to restrict use of such terminology to products as they would be presented to consumers at the retail level. Fresh red meats or poultry, if they are to be labeled as "Light" or "Lean" at the retail level, must in fact be low in fat

or the industry will suffer further loss of consumer confidence. The USDA should consider developing a program to certify fatness of wholesale and retail cuts and should offer a "Certi-Light" or "Certi-Trim" specification that industry could use as a third-party verification that fatness does not exceed some critical set point (for example, no more than 10 percent chemical fat). Such USDA certification, although it might be perceived as government intervention, would make possible industry standardization of the term "Light" and would make feasible equal opportunity for market entry by firms of small, medium, or large size. Unless USDA controls the use of terms like "Natural" and "Light," these terms will soon lose credibility and the red meat industry will lose the opportunity to capitalize on well-documented desires of certain segments of the consumer market to purchase lower calorie or residue-safe meat products.

The committee also supports action to uncouple the yield grading/quality grading of beef carcasses. At present, carcasses that are categorized as No-Roll because they have too little marbling to grade Choice are not identified for cutability (specifically, they are not yield graded). Those carcasses that are categorized as No-Roll because they have too much fat to qualify for the 3 or better yield grade are not identified for expected palatability (specifically, they are not quality graded). This disrupts the communicative function of the grading system and is thus a deterrent to increasing leanness of cattle. Furthermore, carcasses that are trimmed before presentation for grading cannot be accurately yield graded and so are ineligible for quality grading. Some packers would remove, at the time of slaughter, most or all of the subcutaneous or kidney/pelvic/heart fats from beef carcasses that were too fat if USDA would allow such carcasses to be quality graded.

There is presently no disincentive in the U.S. marketing system to prevent the feeding of grain—when it is cheap—to the point that it causes overfattening of red meat animals. Until such disincentive is in place—and a governmental policy change may be necessary to effect such a change—the industry will continue to produce animals with too much fat. The quickest available means to make beef, pork, and lamb leaner and to discourage overfeeding and excessive fattening would be to allow packers to remove, during the slaughter/dressing process, all external fat in excess of that amount (for example, one-fourth inch) that can remain on retail cuts.

In late 1986, the American Meat Institute (AMI) decided that trimming of retail cuts to leave only one-fourth inch of external fat, as initiated by some retailers in 1986, is a systematic and real improvement and that the place to accomplish such fat removal is in the packing plant—on the slaughter floor. In November 1986, AMI and NCA members reviewed hot-fat trimming at the Monfort of Colorado plant in Greeley and received results of a Texas A&M University study evaluating that process. AMI suggested that use of hot-fat trimming would (1) remove dressing percentage as a price-determining factor in purchases of live cattle, (2) discourage overfeeding and overfattening of cattle, (3) allow for removal of excess fat at a point where its value (as edible tallow) is highest, and (4) make possible payment of the highest prices for the leanest cattle. If excess external fat is removed on the slaughter floor and cattlemen are paid only for that amount of fat left on the carcass when the carcass is weighed, there will be excellent incentive to not overfatten cattle.

The committee considered AMI's suggestions and, as a result, favors uncoupling the yield and quality grades to allow for hot-fat trimming of beef carcasses and encourages USDA to implement such changes in grading protocol.

The yield grades are useful to certain segments of the beef industry (producers, packers, wholesalers, purveyors, retailers) but do nothing to assist the consumer in making purchasing decisions that would benefit from knowledge of relative fatness/caloric content of meat cuts. The committee considered numerous options for providing relative fatness information to consumers and decided that at least three alternatives existed for accomplishing that end. The information could be provided by mandating nutrition labeling for retail cuts, but there is little evidence that such information would actually be useful or used. Because consumers make purchasing decisions very quickly, a system of identification by fatness level that would carry through the marketing sequence and appear at the retail level in alphanumerical form might be helpful. For example, in the code A-2-3, A could indicate maturity of the animal at slaughter, 2 the amount of marbling (or perhaps marbling plus subcutaneous and intermuscular fat), and 3 the yield grade of the carcass. Identification as A-1-1 would therefore signify a young animal with a "Moderate" amount of marbling and very high cutability. Because not every piece of meat from an A-1-1 carcass would actually be an A-1-1 retail cut, the last number could be dropped and individual cuts from an A-1 could be labeled, at the retail meat counter, as A-1, A-2, A-3, or A-4, depending on their marbling level and subcutaneous plus intermuscular fat content. More severe trimming of retail cuts would improve the numerical grade, moving it, for example, from A-4 to A-1 if trimming was severe enough.

A second means for identifying relative fatness/caloric content of retail cuts might involve the use of a color system (red, white, blue) or a medal system (gold, silver, bronze) affixed to retail packages. Such a system would be based on the identification of three levels of fatness of retail cuts that would determine the size of serving that could be consumed on a daily basis while conforming to a healthy diet. Compliance could be voluntary or mandatory depending on local, state, or federal ordinances or laws. The advantage of a color-coding or medal system is that it would be very easy to interpret and consumers could make selections very quickly. As opposed to a system of identification based solely on a criterion like "calories from fat," which would essentially preclude any consumption of certain animal products (for example, butter), a system of identification based on serving size or frequency would allow any and all animal products to be consumed in some amount and at some interval of time as part of a balanced diet. There is a dangerous tendency on the part of some health professionals to identify certain animal products as "too high" in calories, "too high" in saturated fatty acids, or "too high" in cholesterol and thus to advise consumers never to eat them. The errors in such advice are that not all health professionals agree that all people will benefit from dietary modification, not all research indicates that these chemical entities are involved in a causal relationship to heart disease or cancer, and consumption of an undesirable entity per se probably does not endanger health—rather, it is the amount and frequency of consumption that is critical. Therefore, if a meat product carried a silver sticker and consumers had been told the meaning of that sticker, they would know, instantly, that they could purchase that cut and consume, say, 6 ounces of it up to three times per week without exceeding a target level of certain dietary substances. Such a procedure would ensure that consumers have "identifiable choices" and "options in the marketplace" that would assist them in selecting foods.

A third approach is that of the Nutritional Effects Foundation (NEF), which was established to encourage the production, processing, marketing, and consumption of lean meat by ensuring the availability of low-fat meat products to replace high-fat meat in the diet. Two levels of composition—NEF1 and NEF2—would be identified, and seals of approval would be placed on all cuts meeting a predesignated standard. Products accepted for labeling could be eaten in moderate amounts as parts of diets recommended by the National Institutes of Health, the Consensus Development Conference Statement—Lowering Blood Cholesterol to Prevent Heart Disease, the U.S. Department of Agriculture/Department of Health and Human Services Dietary Guidelines for Americans, the American Heart Association, and the American Cancer Society.

It is currently recommended that to reduce the dietary risks associated with coronary heart disease, cancer, and other chronic diseases, no more than 30 percent of the total daily caloric intake for the general population and no more than 20 percent for the high-risk population should come from dietary fat. To provide a wide range of reasonable portion sizes for use in both the 20 and 30 percent calories-from-fat diets, two categories of meat are accepted for labeling: NEF1 products contain no more than 3.5 percent fat (uncooked) and NEF2 products contain no more than 6 percent fat (uncooked). In most cases, these meat products, if eaten in a reasonable quantity on any single day, will provide less than 30 percent of the recommended intake of total fat and less than 25 percent of the recommended intake of saturated fatty acids. In addition, products in both of these categories could contain the minimum level of intramuscular fat (approximately 3 percent) necessary to ensure palatability.

Any retail identification system based on total fatness or total caloric content of animal products and means for monitoring compliance should be based on both palatability and nutritional merit with the goal of identifying different kinds of retail cuts of beef, pork, or lamb in a simplified manner. Identification according to palatability/nutritional merit by USDA, for example, would make possible "identifiable consumer choices" and minimize selection time.

In summary, the changes in USDA grade standards or labeling/ identification procedures most likely to improve nutritional attributes, increase consumer options in the marketplace, and enhance consumer acceptability of beef, pork, and lamb are (1) changes in grade nomenclature that would identify a lean yet palatable product with a new name, (2) changes in grade-application regulations that would allow hot-fat trimming at slaughter without eliminating the possibility of quality grade identification, (3) control of use of the terms "Light" and "Natural" to prevent confusion in the marketplace, and (4) identification of red meat at the retail level according to fatness level or nutritional merit to signal to consumers that specified quantities of a product could be consumed and still allow for compliance with current dietary guidelines and health recommendations.

# The Role of Fat in the Palatability of Beef, Pork, and Lamb

J. W. SAVELL and H. R. CROSS

Within the past two decades, fat in the diet has come under scrutiny with respect to its role in coronary heart disease and other health-related problems. Recent recommendations have centered on eating moderate amounts of lean red meat, but there is a problem with consumer acceptance when fat is absent from meat. Meat that is tough or dry or that does not taste good probably will not be eaten, even by people on restricted diets. Thus, some fat is necessary to ensure that meat is enjoyed when eaten, but the level should be low enough so that meat can be included in a restricted diet.

In this paper we describe the role of fat in improving the tenderness, juiciness, and flavor of beef, pork, and lamb and recommend the minimum level of fat necessary to ensure consumer acceptability.

## FAT'S INFLUENCE ON TENDERNESS, JUICINESS, AND FLAVOR

The most comprehensive review of fat and palatability to date is that of Smith and Carpenter (1974), who summarized how fat affects tenderness, juiciness, and flavor in meat. Following is a brief description of these mechanisms.

### Tenderness

Of the three factors influencing the tenderness of meat—actomyosin effect, background effect, and bulk density or lubrication effect—only lubrication effect deals with fat. It is associated with the amount and distribution of intramuscular fat, or marbling. Marbling probably influences meat tenderness based on the individual or collective effects of the following mechanisms (Smith and Carpenter, 1974):

*Bite theory.* This theory suggests that within a given bite-size portion of cooked meat, the occurrence of marbling decreases the mass per unit volume, lowering the bulk density by replacing protein with lipid. Because fat is much less resistant to shear force than is coagulated protein, the decrease in bulk density is accompanied by an increase in real or apparent tenderness.

*Strain theory.* As marbling is deposited in the perivascular cells inside the walls of the perimysium or endomysium, the connective tissue walls on either side of the deposit are thinned, thereby decreasing their effective width, thickness, and strength.

*Lubrication theory.* Intramuscular fats, present in and around the muscle fibers, lubricate the fibers and fibrils and so make for a more tender and juicier product that potentiates the sensation of tenderness. Thus, tenderness is closely associated with juiciness.

*Insurance theory.* The presence of higher levels of marbling allows the use of high-temperature, dry-heat methods of cooking and/or a greater degree of doneness without adversely affecting the palatability of the meat. Marbling thus provides some insurance that meat that is cooked too long, too rapidly, or incorrectly will still be palatable.

### Relationship Between Fat and Tenderness

Based on their review of the data, Smith and Carpenter (1974) found that fatness had a moderate relationship to tenderness in pork and a low to moderate relationship to tenderness in beef and lamb.

### Juiciness

Juiciness is made up of the combined effects of initial fluid release and the sustained juiciness resulting from the stimulating effect of fat on salivary flow (Weir, 1960). These two factors can be described as follows (Bratzler, 1971): (1) initial fluid release—the impression of wetness perceived during the first chews, produced by the rapid release of meat fluids, and (2) sustained juiciness—the sensation of juiciness perceived during continued chewing, created by the release of serum and due, in part, to the stimulating effect of fat on salivary flow. According to Pearson (1966), the initial fluid release is affected by degree of doneness and method of cooking, while sustained juiciness is related to intramuscular fat content.

Fat may affect juiciness by enhancing the water-holding capacity of meat, by lubricating the muscle fibers during cooking, by increasing the tenderness of meat and thus the apparent sensation of juiciness, or by stimulating salivary flow during mastication (Smith and Carpenter, 1974).

### Relationship Between Fat and Juiciness

According to Smith and Carpenter (1974), fatness has a moderate relationship to juiciness in lamb, a moderate to high relationship to juiciness in pork, and a low to moderate relationship to juiciness in beef.

### Flavor

Hornstein (1971) believes that fat may affect flavor in two ways: (1) Fatty acids, on oxidation, can produce carbonyl compounds that are potent flavor contributors, and (2) fat may act as a storage depot for odoriferous compounds that are released on heating. Volatile compounds released from fat or produced from triglyceride or phospholipid fractions may be responsible for the species-specific flavors of beef, pork, and lamb. Smith and Carpenter (1974) stated that although the basic meaty flavor is nonlipid in origin, some quantity of fat is undoubtedly necessary to make beef taste rich, full, and "beefy." Smith et al. (1983) stated that U.S. Department of Agriculture (USDA) beef quality grades are related to flavor of beef because grade indirectly assesses the extent to which flavor and aroma compounds are likely to be present in the meat.

### Relationship Between Fat and Flavor

Fatness has a low relationship to flavor in lamb and a low to moderate relationship to flavor in pork and beef (Smith and Carpenter, 1974).

## SPECIFIC RESEARCH ON PORK, LAMB, AND BEEF PALATABILITY

This section covers pertinent information on species-specific research that helps to determine how much fat is necessary for acceptable palatability. The work that is reported is from the Texas Agricultural Experiment Station and represents a portion of the palatability/grade/ consumer acceptance research conducted on pork, lamb, and beef by the Meats and Muscle Biology Section during the past three decades.

### Pork Palatability Research

The study by Davis et al. (1975) with 403 pork loins showed that when three categories of loins were created based on marbling level ("typical-Modest" or higher, "typical-Slight" to "Modest-minus," and "Slight-minus" or lower), scores for juiciness and overall satisfaction were significantly lower in the "Slight-minus" or lower category. Juiciness, tenderness, and overall satisfaction ratings were significantly higher for chops from loins that were from the "typical-Modest" or higher category. Davis et al. (1978), using the same sample of pork loins used by Davis et al. in 1975, designed a system for segmentation of fresh pork loins into quality groups of "Superior," "Acceptable," or "Inferior." Using the sirloin end as the scoring surface, loins that were light in color, that were soft, and that had low marbling scores were rated as "Inferior," while those with intermediate color, firmness, and intermediate to high levels of marbling were rated as "Superior." With respect to the level of marbling necessary in pork longissimus dorsi muscle to ensure acceptable palatability, Davis (1974) recommended between 3.5 and 4.5 percent intramuscular fat.

### Lamb Palatability Research

In a study of lamb rib chops, Carpenter and King (1965) evaluated the influence of cooking method, marbling, color, and core position (for Warner-Bratzler shear determinations) on tenderness. Chemical fat was determined on the rib chops and was stratified by marbling score of the longissimus

dorsi muscle as follows: Practically Devoid = 2.05, Traces = 2.49, Slight = 3.15, Small = 3.54, Modest = 4.10, Moderate = 4.79, Slightly Abundant = 4.39, Moderately Abundant = 5.17, and Abundant = 6.67. Tenderness (as measured by the Warner-Bratzler shear machine) was most affected by cooking method and core position. Highly significant correlations were found between tenderness and the fat content of the longissimus dorsi muscle, but the coefficients were of low magnitude.

Lamb carcass quality was extensively evaluated by Smith et al. (1970a,b) and Smith and Carpenter (1970). Smith et al. (1970a), in evaluating the palatability of leg roasts, found that individual or combined USDA scores for carcass quality—feathering, flank streaking, firmness, and maturity—were associated with less than 15 percent of the variation in overall satisfaction ratings. Segmentation into USDA quality grades indicated that roasts from Prime carcasses possessed the highest percentage of desirable ratings and the lowest percentage of undesirable ratings for juiciness, tenderness, and overall satisfaction compared with the other grades evaluated. Small and inconsistent differences appeared between roasts from carcasses in the Choice and Good/Select grades, but leg roasts from Utility carcasses were decidedly inferior in palatability to those from the higher USDA grades.

Smith et al. (1970b), in the companion study on palatability of rib, loin, and sirloin chops, found that segmentation into USDA quality grades indicated that chops from Prime carcasses were superior to those of the other grades in percentage of desirable ratings for juiciness, tenderness, and overall satisfaction. As grade decreased from Prime through Good/Select, there were corresponding decreases in the proportion of chops considered desirable in juiciness, tenderness, and overall satisfaction. With the exception of scores for tenderness, differences between chops from Good/Select versus Utility carcasses were small.

When Smith and Carpenter (1970) collected chemical data from a sample of carcasses used in the studies by Smith et al. (1970a,b), they found that differences in intramuscular fat were associated with significant changes in juiciness, tenderness, and overall satisfaction ratings for all the cuts studied. Based on the conclusions of three studies, increased fatness was generally associated with increased palatability, but fatness appeared to have a greater impact on the cuts from the rack and loin than on the cuts from the leg.

Jeremiah et al. (1971) evaluated the impact of chronological age and marbling on the palatability of individual muscles from leg steaks of lamb. Marbling appeared to be of little consequence in determining the tenderness of the rectus femoris, vastus lateralis, biceps femoris, semitendinosus, or semimembranosus muscles of the leg, but chronological age was highly related to the tenderness of these muscles. The authors concluded that increased marbling was of little importance for increasing the tenderness of leg muscles, but that increased marbling was associated with higher juiciness scores for the rectus femoris, vastus lateralis, and semitendinosus muscles.

Smith et al. (1976) evaluated the influence of fatness—subcutaneous and marbling—on the palatability of lamb. They found that lamb carcasses that have increased quantities of fat chill more slowly, maintain muscle temperatures conducive to autolytic enzyme degradation for greater periods of time postmortem, sustain less shortening of sarcomeres, have muscles with lower ultimate pH values, have less perceptible or softer connective tissue, and are more tender than lamb carcasses that have limited quantities of subcutaneous or intramuscular fat. The authors theorized that deposition of increased quantities of subcutaneous or intramuscular fat (particularly in carcasses with limited quantities of subcutaneous fat) increases tenderness by changing postmortem chilling rate. Thus, an increased quan-

tity of fat decreases the rate of temperature decline, enhances the activity of autolytic enzymes in muscle, lessens the extent of myofibrillar shortening, and thereby increases the ultimate tenderness of cooked meat from a fatter carcass.

## Beef Palatability Research

### Physical, Chemical, and Histological Studies

Davis et al. (1979) investigated variations in tenderness among beef steaks from carcasses of the same USDA quality grade to better understand why some steaks are less palatable than others even when the USDA quality grade is the same. For Choice, A maturity beef loins, the most tender steaks had more intramuscular fat, less intramuscular moisture, higher water-holding capacity, and a lower fragmentation index. Intramuscular fat percentages for steaks from the four tenderness groups of Choice, A maturity beef loins were as follows: very tender = 7.6 percent, moderately tender = 6.1 percent, slightly tender = 5.6 percent, and slightly tough = 4.4 percent. For Choice, B maturity beef loins, very tender steaks had 7.2 percent fat while slightly tough steaks had 5.6 percent fat. Although in the other grade/maturity groups, other physical, chemical, and histological factors were more important than fatness, high tenderness scores were most often associated with intramuscular fat percentages of 6 to 8.

### Time-on-Feed and Beef Palatability

The length of time that cattle are fed high-concentrate feeds is associated with increased palatability, irrespective of quality grades. Tatum et al. (1980) reported that rib steaks from high Choice and average Choice carcasses were juicier, more flavorful, and overall more palatable than steaks from low Good/Select and high Standard carcasses; however, steaks from low Choice, high Good/Select, and average Good/Select carcasses did not differ in palatability. Increased time-on-feed was associated with increased carcass maturity, increased fat deposition, decreased yield grade, and increased percentage of carcasses grading Choice. Increased feeding time from 100 to 160 days had a beneficial effect on flavor desirability but did not significantly affect juiciness, tenderness, or overall palatability. Tatum et al. (1980) suggested that a knowledge of feeding history may be a useful adjunct to—or substitute for—USDA quality grade for predicting beef palatability.

Dolezal et al. (1982a), in a study of feeding groups of steers and heifers for periods ranging from 30 to 230 days, found that extending feeding time beyond 90 to 100 days did little to ensure additional palatability. Within time-on-feed strata from 100 through 230 days, few differences in palatability were found between rib steaks from carcasses of different USDA quality grades. Dolezal et al. (1982a) recommended that the minimum marbling requirement for the Choice grade could be lowered with no appreciable loss in palatability if it was stipulated that cattle had been fed a high-concentrate diet for at least 90 days.

### Subcutaneous Fat Thickness and Marbling

Several studies have been conducted that explored the combined role of subcutaneous fat and marbling in the palatability of beef. Tatum et al. (1982) found that compared with marbling, fat thickness was ineffective as a predictor of cooked beef palatability and, therefore, would appear to be an unsuitable substitute for marbling. However, marbling, used in combination with a minimum subcutaneous fat thickness constraint of 7.6 mm for carcasses with a Slight amount of marbling, facilitated more equitable stratification of carcasses according to their expected palatability than did marbling alone. Dolezal et al. (1982b) found that assigning

carcasses to three expected palatability groups based on fat thickness was at least equivalent to, and perhaps slightly more precise than, the use of USDA quality grades for grouping the carcasses according to expected palatability. There were progressive increases in palatability of cooked beef as fat thickness of carcasses increased from less than 2.5 to 7.6 mm, but quantities greater than 7.6 mm did not further improve palatability.

In studies involving young bulls, Riley et al. (1983a,b) found that the combination of subcutaneous fat and marbling was an important factor in the determination of beef palatability. Subcutaneous fat thickness was found to be more important than "masculinity" in ensuring that beef from young bulls would be acceptably tender (Riley et al., 1983a). Riley et al. (1983b) recommended that the USDA grade standards for beef could be revised to allow those carcasses with Slight marbling and at least 7.6 mm of fat thickness to grade Choice, irrespective of sex. When steaks from Standard bulls and steers and steaks from Good/Select bulls and steers that had less than 7.6 mm of fat thickness were compared with steaks from Choice steers or steaks from Good/Select bulls with at least 7.6 mm of fat thickness, they were found to be significantly less palatable (Riley et al., 1983b).

### USDA Beef Quality Study

In the mid-1970s, the Texas Agricultural Experiment Station conducted a comprehensive study for the U.S. Department of Agriculture on USDA beef quality grades and palatability. This study involved 1,005 carcasses ranging in maturity from A to E and in marbling from Moderately Abundant to Practically Devoid. In their report on the effect of maturity groups on palatability, Smith et al. (1982) found that in comparison to carcasses of B, C, or E maturity, carcasses of A maturity produced broiled steaks that had higher palatability ratings in 62 to 86 percent of comparisons, were decidedly less variable in sensory traits, were more likely to be assigned high (≥6.00) and less likely to be assigned low (≤2.99) sensory panel ratings, and were more likely to have low (≤3.63 kg) shear force values. They found that position within the A or A + B maturity groups explained ≤4 percent (loin steaks) and 10 to 18 percent (round steaks) of the observed variation in overall palatability ratings and/or shear force values.

In the report on the relationship between marbling and palatability, Smith et al. (1984) found that as marbling increased from Practically Devoid to Moderately Abundant, loin steaks were more palatable about two-thirds of the time, round steaks were more palatable about one-eighth of the time, and loin steaks were more likely to be assigned high (≥6.00) panel ratings and to have low (≤3.63) shear force values. However, increases in marbling from Slight to Moderately Abundant (A + B maturity) had little or no effect on percentage incidence of loin or round steaks with panel ratings ≤2.99 or ≥4.00, or with shear force values ≥6.35 kg or ≤4.99 kg. Differences in marbling explained about 33 percent (loin) and 7 percent (top round) of the variation in overall palatability ratings in A, B, C, and A + B maturity carcasses.

Smith et al.'s (1987) report on the influence of USDA quality grades on beef palatability indicated that Prime carcasses produced loin and round steaks that were more palatable than the steaks from Choice through Canner carcasses in 85.7 percent of comparisons and more palatable than the steaks from Choice through Standard carcasses in 69.0 percent of comparisons. Comparable percentages were 71.4 percent (for Choice through Canner), 42.9 percent (for Choice through Standard), 74.3 percent (for Good/Select through Canner), and 35.7 percent (for Good/Select compared to Standard). Among Prime through Standard carcasses, grade predicted flavor, tenderness, and overall palatability of loin steaks with 30 to 38 percent accuracy, but could only explain

about 8 percent of the variation in sensory panel ratings or shear force values of round steaks.

### National Consumer Retail Beef Study

The National Consumer Retail Beef Study was an industry-wide program supported by government, producer, feeder, packer, and retailer segments of the industry (Cross et al., 1986). The program was led by the Texas Agricultural Experiment Station of the Texas A&M University System with coordination of the Beef Industry Council of the National Live Stock & Meat Board and the National Cattlemen's Association. The beef industry identified two challenges to achieving a market-driven orientation: What are the demands of specific segments of consumers, and what kinds of beef will satisfy them?

The relationship between quality grade and taste appeal was first addressed by Savell et al. (1987). The study (called Phase I) was carried out in Philadelphia, Kansas City, and San Francisco. Steaks from carcasses that varied in marbling were evaluated by 540 households. For the first time, a nationwide study was conducted to see (1) if consumers, rather than trained sensory panelists, could detect differences in palatability of steaks that differed in marbling and (2) if there were regional consumer preferences for steaks according to level of marbling. Results showed that consumers could detect palatability differences due to marbling and that there were indeed regional differences with respect to the way consumers rated steaks that differed in marbling. Consumers in all three cities rated steaks with high marbling the same. Consumers in San Francisco and Kansas City gave consistently high ratings that were only slightly reduced as marbling decreased from Slightly Abundant to Traces. But ratings given by Philadelphia consumers were sharply reduced as marbling decreased. Thus, it appeared that different consumer market segments might need to be identified to more effectively reflect consumer tastes in each city.

Because the information gathered in Phase I addressed only one issue in the selection of beef—taste—specific demands for the other major selection criteria—price and leanness—remained unanswered. Therefore, it became necessary to conduct further research (Phase II) to determine (1) what amount of taste, if any, would be sacrificed by the consumer to obtain the leanness advantages of lower grading beef and (2) what degree of external fat trim would consumers seek and be willing to pay for.

Phase II of the National Consumer Retail Beef Study (Cross et al., 1986; Savell et al., in press) was conducted in San Francisco and Philadelphia (the two cities in Phase I with the greatest difference between consumer ratings of steaks from the various marbling levels). With respect to the marbling or quality grade findings from Phase II, retail cuts from Choice and Good/Select carcasses were rated equally high for consumer acceptance, but for different reasons. Choice retail cuts were rated high in taste, but when objections were voiced, they concerned fatness. Good/Select retail cuts were rated high in leanness, but when objections were voiced, they concerned taste or texture. A major recommendation from this study was to merchandise the two grades of beef based on their strengths—Choice should be marketed for its taste appeal and Good/Select for its leanness.

## MINIMUM FAT IN MEAT NEEDED FOR ACCEPTABLE PALATABILITY

Before a recommendation can be made with respect to the level of fatness needed for acceptable palatability, it is important to know how much chemical fat is present in steaks from the various marbling levels. Savell et al. (1986) reported the amount of chemical fat in the uncooked longissimus dorsi muscle of 518 beef carcasses that

ranged in marbling from Moderately Abundant to Practically Devoid (Figure 1). Mean values for chemical fat ranged from 10.42 percent in Moderately Abundant to 1.77 percent in Practically Devoid. The authors generated a regression equation to calculate the amount of chemical fat in a raw loin steak for known marbling level:

$$\text{Percentage ether-extractable fat} = (\text{Marbling score} \times 0.0217) - 0.8043.$$

For this equation ($r^2 = 0.78$), marbling score is converted to a numerical code where Moderately Abundant = 800–899, Slightly Abundant = 700–799, Moderate = 600–699, Modest = 500–599, Small = 400–499, Slight = 300–399, Traces = 200–299, and Practically Devoid = 100–199. Using the equation, the amounts of fat in Traces, Slight, Small, Modest, and Moderate are 1.74, 3.00, 4.28, 5.55, and 6.82 percent, respectively. These levels of fat are low compared with the 10 to 50 percent levels in processed meat products.

The key question asked of us was, what level of fatness is necessary for acceptable palatability? After reviewing the research we have conducted over the years under many different circumstances and with many different objectives, we conclude that the minimum fat percentage required for acceptable palatability of broiling cuts (rib, loin, sirloin, and so on) is 3 percent on an uncooked basis (associated with the minimum Slight degree of marbling). As in all biological relationships, there is no magic point where at one concentration or level something is acceptable and at the next increment it is not, but our findings are based on the overwhelming evidence of many observations where steaks with less than 3 percent animal fat (or the marbling levels associated with less than 3 percent fat—Practically Devoid and Traces) are tougher, drier, and less flavorful, whether evaluated by trained panelists or by consumers. Note that this is only a minimum

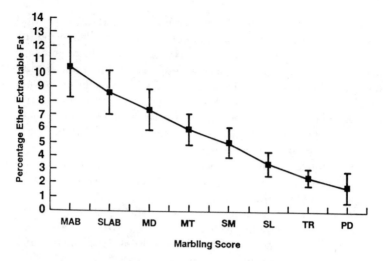

**FIGURE 1** Marbling score and ether extractable fat. NOTE: MAB is moderately abundant; SLAB, slightly abundant; MD, moderate; MT, modest; SM, small; SL, slight; TR, traces; and PD, practically devoid.

fat percentage for "acceptable" palatability; it is our belief that there are two other levels or plateaus of chemical fat associated with increasing palatability: approximately 5 percent (midpoint of the Small amount of marbling) and approximately 7 percent (the lower end of the Moderate amount of marbling). These hierarchical rankings in palatability as associated with increasing fatness allow the beef supply to be sorted into expected palatability groups that can best serve a segmented consumer market with widely varying tastes.

The following discussion will help to further defend our choice of 3 percent or Slight marbling as the minimum level of fat needed for acceptable palatability. Tatum et al. (1982) found that marbling had a low, but positive, relationship to all the palatability traits of beef, but that more than 90 percent of the steaks with Slight or higher degrees of marbling were desirable in tenderness, flavor, and overall palatability. In unpublished data generated by the USDA Beef Quality Study, the relationship between actual chemical fat levels and overall palatability shows a distinct downturn in ratings once fat is below 3 percent. The relationship

between overall desirability ratings and marbling level for the three cities used in Phase I of the National Consumer Retail Beef Study supports our contention that once marbling drops below minimum Slight, consumers are likely to find the meat less palatable. Finally, in Phase II of the National Consumer Retail Beef Study (Cross et al., 1986; Savell et al., in press), although consumers could detect differences in taste between steaks and roasts from Choice and Good/Select, they still rated those from Good/Select (Slight amount of marbling) very high in overall acceptance primarily because of the leanness and absence of waste of the cuts.

Our recommendation of a minimum 3 percent fat is only for those cuts from the rib and loin. Palatability evaluations of cuts from the chuck and round fail to show strong relationships between fatness and palatability. Griffin et al. (1985) found that consumers could detect differences in palatability between steaks from the rib and loin of higher grading steer carcasses when compared with steaks from lower grading bull carcasses, but that they could not detect differences in palatability between roasts from the chuck and round from the two groups. Smith et al. (1984, 1987) reported that neither marbling nor quality grade was closely associated with the sensory panel ratings or shear force values of steaks from the round. Overall palatability of the strip loin does reach a point—at minimum Slight—that the ratings start to diminish quite drastically, but the overall palatability ratings for the top round are fairly level from Slightly Abundant to Practically Devoid marbling. Therefore, it is our opinion that in young cattle, there is no minimum level of marbling or chemical fat necessary to ensure acceptable palatability for cuts from the round or chuck, primarily because of the way they are cooked (moist-heat roasting, braising, pan frying, and so on) and because of lower consumer expectation for these cuts compared with higher priced steaks from the rib and loin.

Although the data for minimum chemical fatness are not as well documented for pork and lamb as they are for beef, because most studies have focused their attention on the relationship between general fatness of carcasses and palatability, we still recommend a minimum level of 3 percent chemical fat for those cuts from the loin of pork and from the loin and rack of lamb. Most of the studies mentioned earlier in the sections on pork and lamb found that there were certain levels of fatness where undesirable chops were encountered. Chemical fat is less important for palatability in the cuts from the shoulder and leg of pork or lamb because in pork they are further processed and in lamb they are most often roasted, which probably minimizes the influence of fat on palatability. For lamb leg roasts, we recommend a minimum of 2 percent chemical fat to ensure acceptable palatability.

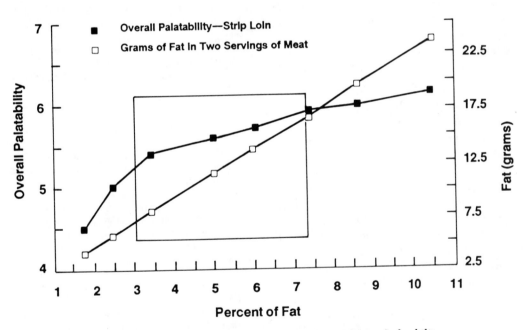

**FIGURE 2** Window of acceptability for fat content of meat (palatability versus grams of fat, two servings). The window is based on a fat content range of 3 percent to 7.3 percent. This is equivalent to meat cuts that grade in the lower range of Good/Select (3 to 4.27 percent fat content) to those that grade in the high range of Choice (4.28 to 8.0 percent fat content).

## MAXIMUM FAT ALLOWABLE IN MEAT FOR ACCEPTABLE NUTRITIONAL MERIT

The point at which fat stops being an asset (in terms of taste) and starts becoming a liability (in terms of health) must also be considered. We conclude that the maximum amount of fat that should be present in cuts of meat to ensure nutritional merit is 7.3 percent (uncooked basis). We arrived at this figure based on the following assumptions:

- An intake of 2,000 kcal/day;
- No more than 30 percent of calories from fat, based on the American Heart Association's Dietary Guidelines;
- Of the calories from fat, no more than 25 percent from fat in beef, pork, and lamb;
- No more than 600 kcal from fat and no more than 150 kcal from fat from red meat;
- A maximum of 16.6 grams of fat from red meat per day;
- Two servings per day from the meat group, based on good nutrition practice; and 4 ounces, uncooked, per serving;
- 16.6 grams of fat divided by 226.8 grams (number of grams in 8 ounces) = 7.3 percent chemical fat in uncooked portion.

Based on these calculations and our recommendations of 3 percent minimum fat, Figure 2 was developed, which shows the "window of acceptability" of fat in meat products. This target is amply wide, since it allows most cuts from carcasses that grade low Good/Select to the middle of high Choice to qualify. In addition, smaller or fewer servings of red meat per day would accommodate a slightly higher fat level without exceeding the American Heart Association's Dietary Guidelines. This "window" will cause some controversy from those who are proponents of fat for taste reasons (minimum level set too low) and those who are opponents of fat for health reasons (maximum level set too high), but

we feel that these levels are very realistic goals from both production and consumption points of view.

## REFERENCES

Bratzler, L. J. 1971. Palatability factors and evaluation. Pp. 328–348 in The Science of Meat and Meat Products, 2nd ed., J. F. Price and B. S. Schweigert, eds. San Francisco: W. H. Freeman.

Carpenter, Z. L., and G. T. King. 1965. Tenderness of lamb rib chops. Food Technol. 19(11):102.

Cross, H. R., J. W. Savell, and J. J. Francis. 1986. National Consumer Retail Beef Study. Pp. 112–116 in Proceedings of the 39th Reciprocal Meat Conference. Chicago, Ill.: National Live Stock & Meat Board.

Davis, G. W. 1974. Quality Characteristics, Compositional Analysis and Palatability Attributes of Selected Muscles from Pork Loins and Hams. Master's thesis. Texas A&M University, College Station.

Davis, G. W., G. C. Smith, Z. L. Carpenter, and H. R. Cross. 1975. Relationships of quality indicators to palatability attributes of pork loins. J. Anim. Sci. 41:1305.

Davis, G. W., G. C. Smith, Z. L. Carpenter, and R. J. Freund. 1978. Segmentation of fresh pork loins into quality groups. J. Anim. Sci. 46:1618.

Davis, G. W., G. C. Smith, Z. L. Carpenter, T. R. Dutson, and H. R. Cross. 1979. Tenderness variations among beef steaks from carcasses of the same USDA quality grade. J. Anim. Sci. 49:103.

Dolezal, H. G., G. C. Smith, J. W. Savell, and Z. L. Carpenter. 1982a. Effect of time-on-feed on the palatability of rib steaks from steers and heifers. J. Food Sci. 47:368.

Dolezal, H. G., G. C. Smith, J. W. Savell, and Z. L. Carpenter. 1982b. Comparison of subcutaneous fat thickness, marbling and quality grade for predicting palatability of beef. J. Food Sci. 47:397.

Griffin, C. L., D. M. Stiffler, G. C. Smith, and J. W. Savell. 1985. Consumer acceptance of steaks and roasts from Charolais crossbred bulls and steers. J. Food Sci. 50:165.

Hornstein, I. 1971. Chemistry of meat flavor. Pp. 348–363 in The Science of Meat and Meat Products, 2nd ed., J. F. Price and B. S. Schweigert, eds. San Francisco: W. H. Freeman.

Jeremiah, L. E., G. C. Smith, and Z. L. Carpenter. 1971. Palatability of individual muscle from ovine leg steaks as related to chronological age and marbling. J. Food Sci. 35:45.

Pearson, A. M. 1966. Desirability of beef—its characteristics and their measurement. J. Anim. Sci. 25:843.

Riley, R. R., J. W. Savell, C. E. Murphey, G. C. Smith, D. M. Stiffler, and H. R. Cross. 1983a. Effects of electrical stimulation, subcutaneous fat thickness and masculinity traits on palatability of beef from young bull carcasses. J. Anim. Sci. 56:584.

Riley, R. R., J. W. Savell, C. E. Murphey, G. C. Smith, D. M. Stiffler, and H. R. Cross. 1983b. Palatability of beef from steer and young bull carcasses as influenced by electrical stimulation, subcutaneous fat thickness and marbling. J. Anim. Sci. 56:592.

Savell, J. W., H. R. Cross, and G. C. Smith. 1986. Percentage ether extractable fat and moisture content of beef longissimus muscle as related to USDA marbling score. J. Food Sci. 51:838.

Savell, J. W., R. E. Branson, H. R. Cross, D. M. Stiffler, J. W. Wise, D. B. Griffin, and G. C. Smith. 1987. National Consumer Retail Beef Study: Palatability evaluations of beef loin steaks that differed in marbling. J. Food Sci. 52:517.

Savell, J. W., H. R. Cross, J. J. Francis, J. W. Wise, D. S. Hale, and G. C. Smith. In press. National Consumer Retail Beef Study: Interaction of leanness, price and palatability on consumer acceptance of steaks and roasts of different grades and trimness levels. J. Food Sci.

Smith, G. C., and Z. L. Carpenter. 1970. Lamb carcass quality. III. Chemical, physical and histological measurements. J. Anim. Sci. 31:697.

Smith, G. C., and Z. L. Carpenter. 1974. Eating quality of animal products and their fat content. Proceedings of the Symposium on Changing the Fat Content and Composition of Animal Products. Washington, D.C.: National Academy of Sciences.

Smith, G. C., Z. L. Carpenter, G. T. King, and K. E. Hoke. 1970a. Lamb carcass quality. I. Palatability of leg roasts. J. Anim. Sci. 30:496.

Smith, G. C., Z. L. Carpenter, G. T. King, and K. E. Hoke. 1970b. Lamb carcass quality. II. Palatability of rib, loin and sirloin chops. J. Anim. Sci. 31:310.

Smith, G. C., T. R. Dutson, R. L. Hostetler, and Z. L. Carpenter. 1976. Fatness, rate of chilling and tenderness of lamb. J. Food Sci. 41:748.

Smith, G. C., H. R. Cross, Z. L. Carpenter, C. E. Murphey, J. W. Savell, H. C. Abraham, and G. W. Davis. 1982. Relationship of USDA maturity groups to palatability of cooked beef. J. Food Sci. 47:1000.

Smith, G. C., J. W. Savell, H. R. Cross, and Z. L. Carpenter. 1983. The relationship of USDA quality grade to beef flavor. Food Technol. 37(5):233.

Smith, G. C., Z. L. Carpenter, H. R. Cross, C. E. Murphey, H. C. Abraham, J. W. Savell, G. W. Davis, B. W. Berry, and F. C. Parrish, Jr. 1984. Relationship of USDA marbling groups to palatability of cooked beef. J. Food Qual. 7:289.

Smith, G. C., J. W. Savell, H. R. Cross, Z. L. Carpenter, C. E. Murphey, G. W. Davis, H. C. Abraham, F. C. Parrish, Jr., and B. W. Berry. 1987. Relationship of USDA quality grades to palatability of cooked beef. J. Food Qual. 10:269.

Tatum, J. D., G. C. Smith, B. W. Berry, C. E. Murphey, F. L. Williams, and Z. L. Carpenter. 1980. Carcass characteristics, time on feed and cooked beef palatability attributes. J. Anim. Sci. 50:833.

Tatum, J. D., G. C. Smith, and Z. L. Carpenter. 1982. Interrelationships between marbling, subcutaneous fat thickness and cooked beef palatability. J. Anim. Sci. 54:777.

Weir, C. E. 1960. Palatability characteristics of meat. Pp. 212–221 in The Science of Meat and Products. American Meat Institute Foundation. San Francisco: W. H. Freeman.

# Index